STEP-UP
TO
SURGERY

SECOND EDITION

STEP-UP

TO

SURGERY

SECOND EDITION

STANLEY ZASLAU, MD, MBA, FACS

Professor, Chief, Urology Residency Program Director
Associate Chair, Education and Research
Department of Surgery
West Virginia University
Morgantown, West Virginia

RICHARD A. VAUGHAN, MD, FACS

Professor
Department of Surgery
West Virginia University
Morgantown, West Virginia

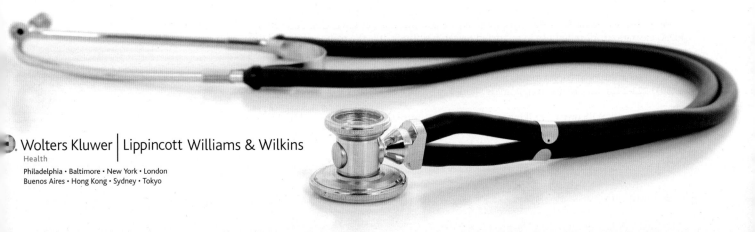

Wolters Kluwer | Lippincott Williams & Wilkins
Health

Philadelphia · Baltimore · New York · London
Buenos Aires · Hong Kong · Sydney · Tokyo

Publisher: Michael Tully
Acquisitions Editor: Tari Broderick
Product Development Editor: Jenn Verbiar
Marketing Manager: Joy Fisher-Williams
Designer: Holly Reid McLaughlin
Production Manager: Joan Sinclair
Compositor: Absolute Service, Inc.

2nd Edition

351 West Camden Street   Two Commerce Square
Baltimore, MD 21201   2001 Market Street
                                Philadelphia, PA 19103

Printed in China

First Edition, 2009

9 8 7 6 5 4 3 2 1

Library of Congress Cataloging-in-Publication Data

Step-up to surgery / [edited by] Stanley Zaslau, Richard A. Vaughan. — Second edition.
    p. ; cm.
  Includes bibliographical references and index.
  ISBN 978-1-4511-8763-2 (alk. paper)
  I. Zaslau, Stanley, editor of compilation. II. Vaughan, Richard A., editor of compilation.
  [DNLM: 1. Surgical Procedures, Operative—Outlines. 2. Surgical Procedures, Operative—Problems and Exercises. WO 18.2]
  RD37.2
  617.0076—dc23

                        2013048668

To purchase additional copies of this book, call our customer service department at **(800) 638-3030** or fax orders to **(301) 223-2320**. International customers should call **(301) 223-2300**.

Visit Lippincott Williams & Wilkins on the Internet: http://www.lww.com. Lippincott Williams & Wilkins customer service representatives are available from 8:30 am to 6:00 pm, EST.

Dedication

To our students, whose interest in surgery fuels our energy and enthusiasm to further our own knowledge of this great specialty.

Editors

STANLEY ZASLAU, MD, MBA, FACS
Professor, Chief, Urology Residency Program Director
Associate Chair, Education and Research
Department of Surgery
West Virginia University
Morgantown, West Virginia

RICHARD A. VAUGHAN, MD, FACS
Professor
Department of Surgery
West Virginia University
Morgantown, West Virginia

ASSOCIATE EDITOR

CYNTHIA F. GRAVES, MD
Assistant Professor
Program Director, General Surgery Residency Program
Department of Surgery
West Virginia University
Morgantown, West Virginia

Chapter Editors

FARRELL ADKINS, MD
Resident
Department of Surgery
West Virginia University
Morgantown, West Virginia

ROBERT ANDRES, MD
Resident
Department of Surgery
West Virginia University
Morgantown, West Virginia

AMANDA BAILEY, MD
Resident
Department of Surgery
West Virginia University
Morgantown, West Virginia

ZACHARY BAKER, MD
Resident
Department of Surgery
West Virginia University
Morgantown, West Virginia

JAMES BARDES, MD
Resident
Department of Surgery
West Virginia University
Morgantown, West Virginia

PATRICK BONASSO, MD
Resident
Department of Surgery
West Virginia University
Morgantown, West Virginia

MICHELLE BRAMER, MD
Assistant Professor
Department of Orthopedic Surgery
West Virginia University
Morgantown, West Virginia

STEPHANIE BURKHARDT, PA-C
Physician Assistant
Department of Orthopedic Surgery
West Virginia University
Morgantown, West Virginia

JORDAN CAIN, MD
Resident
Department of Otolaryngology
West Virginia University
Morgantown, West Virginia

RIAZ CASSIM, MD
Assistant Professor
Department of Surgery
West Virginia University
Morgantown, West Virginia

RICHARD CASUCCIO, MD
Associate Professor
Division of Plastic Surgery, Department of Surgery
West Virginia University
Morgantown, West Virginia

JORGE CON, MD
Assistant Professor
Department of Surgery
West Virginia University
Morgantown, West Virginia

MOUNGAR COOPER, MD
Resident
Department of Surgery
West Virginia University
Morgantown, West Virginia

KEVIN DAY, MD
Attending Surgeon
Samaritan Plastic Surgery
Corvallis, Oregon

BRENNER DIXON, MD
Resident
Department of Surgery
West Virginia University
Morgantown, West Virginia

ROBERT FERGUSON, MD
Resident
Department of Surgery
West Virginia University
Morgantown, West Virginia

JARED FEYKO, DO
Resident
Department of Surgery
West Virginia University
Morgantown, West Virginia

DAVID MICHAEL FOURQUREAN, MD
Resident
Department of Surgery
West Virginia University
Morgantown, West Virginia

BRUCE FREEMAN, MD (POSTHUMOUS)
Associate Professor
Department of Surgery
West Virginia University
Morgantown, West Virginia

CYNTHIA F. GRAVES, MD
Assistant Professor
Program Director, General Surgery Residency Program
Department of Surgery
West Virginia University
Morgantown, West Virginia

SYED HASHMI, MD
Assistant Professor
Department of Surgery
University of Massachusetts
Worcester, Massachusetts

HANNAH HAZARD, MD
Chief, Division of Surgical Oncology
Associate Chair, Oncology
Assistant Professor
Department of Surgery
West Virginia University
Morgantown, West Virginia

CHAD HUBSHER, MD
Resident
Division of Urology, Department of Surgery
West Virginia University
Morgantown, West Virginia

GLEN JACOB, MD
Assistant Professor
Department of Surgery
West Virginia University
Morgantown, West Virginia

LISA JACOB, MD
Assistant Professor
Department of Surgery
West Virginia University
Morgantown, West Virginia

ANTONY JOSEPH, MD
Attending Surgeon
Williamson Memorial Hospital
Williamson, West Virginia

FAWAD J. KHAN, MD
Assistant Professor
Department of Surgery
West Virginia University
Morgantown, West Virginia

UZER KHAN, MD
Resident
Department of Surgery
West Virginia University
Morgantown, West Virginia

JENNIFER KNIGHT, MD
Assistant Professor
Department of Surgery
West Virginia University
Morgantown, West Virginia

TARUN KUMAR, MD
Attending Surgeon, Pediatrics
Mercy Medical Center
Des Moines, Iowa

JAMES LONGHI, DO
Attending Surgeon
Bassett Healthcare Network
Cooperstown, New York

MATTHEW LOOS, MD
Vice President of Medical Affairs
Associate Chair, Safety and Quality
Associate Professor
Department of Surgery
West Virginia University
Morgantown, West Virginia

BRANDON MARR, MD
Assistant Professor
Department of Surgery
West Virginia University
Morgantown, West Virginia

JASON McCHESNEY, MD
Assistant Professor
Department of Otolaryngology
West Virginia University
Morgantown, West Virginia

DAVID W. McFADDEN, MD
Professor and Chairman
Department of Surgery
University of Connecticut Health Center
Farmington, Connecticut

STEPHEN McNATT, MD
Assistant Professor
Division of Bariatric Surgery
Wake Forest Baptist Medical Center
Winston-Salem, North Carolina

CHAD MORLEY, MD
Resident
Division of Urology, Department of Surgery
West Virginia University
Morgantown, West Virginia

MUHAMMAD NAZIM, MD
Assistant Professor
Department of Surgery
Texas Tech University
Amarillo, Texas

OLUSOLA ODUNTAN, MD
Assistant Professor
Department of Surgery
West Virginia University
Morgantown, West Virginia

AMANDA PALMER, MD
Resident
Department of Surgery
West Virginia University
Morgantown, West Virginia

JESSICA PARTIN, MD
Assistant Professor
Department of Surgery
West Virginia University
Morgantown, West Virginia

LAKSHMIKUMAR PILLAI, MD
Associate Professor and Chief
Division of Vascular and Endovascular Surgery
Department of Surgery
West Virginia University
Morgantown, West Virginia

SHELLEY REYNOLDS HILL, MD
Resident
Department of Surgery
West Virginia University
Morgantown, West Virginia

IRFAN A. RIZVI, MD
Attending Surgeon
St. James Mercy Hospital
Hornell, New York

ROBERT RODDENBERRY, MD
Resident
Department of Surgery
West Virginia University
Morgantown, West Virginia

CHARLES ROSEN, MD
Professor and Chairman
Department of Neurosurgery
West Virginia University
Morgantown, West Virginia

DANIEL ROSSI, DO
Attending Surgeon
Department of Surgery
Geisinger Medical Center
Danville, Pennsylvania

DAVEN J. SAVLA, MD
Resident
Department of Surgery
West Virginia University
Morgantown, West Virginia

GREGORY SCHAEFER, DO
Assistant Professor, Co-Director, Surgery Medical
    Student Education
Department of Surgery
West Virginia University
Morgantown, West Virginia

SANTOSH SHENOY, MD
Attending Surgeon
Louis A. Johnson VA Medical Center
Clarksburg, West Virginia

SMARIKA SHRESTHA, MD
Resident
Department of Surgery
West Virginia University
Morgantown, West Virginia

MAGESH SUNDARAM, MD
Chief, Surgical Oncology
Associate Director
Carle Cancer Center
Urbana, Illinois

JOHN TIDWELL, MD
Resident
Department of Orthopedic Surgery
West Virginia University
Morgantown, West Virginia

JASON TURNER, MD
Resident
Department of Surgery
West Virginia University
Morgantown, West Virginia

KEVIN J. TVETER, MD
Assistant Professor
WVU Heart Institute, Department of Surgery
West Virginia University
Morgantown, West Virginia

RICHARD A. VAUGHAN, MD, FACS
Professor
Department of Surgery
West Virginia University
Morgantown, West Virginia

MARY CAROLYN C. VINSON, MD
Resident
Department of Surgery
West Virginia University
Morgantown, West Virginia

GLENN WARDEN, MD
Professor
Department of Surgery
West Virginia University
Morgantown, West Virginia

ALISON WILSON, MD
Vice-Chairman
Chief, Division of Trauma
Associate Professor
Department of Surgery
West Virginia University
Morgantown, West Virginia

STANLEY ZASLAU, MD, MBA, FACS
Professor, Chief, Urology Residency Program Director
Associate Chair, Education and Research
Department of Surgery
West Virginia University
Morgantown, West Virginia

PAMELA ZIMMERMAN, MD
Assistant Professor, Co-Director, Surgery Medical
    Student Education
Department of Surgery
West Virginia University
Morgantown, West Virginia

Reviewers

SAMUEL BARKER
Medical Student
Texas Tech University Health Sciences Center
School of Medicine
Lubbock, Texas

JENNIFER BENTLEY
Medical Student
University of Arkansas for Medical Sciences
Little Rock, Arkansas

SHANNON BOGAN
Medical Student
Meharry Medical College
Nashville, Tennessee

TYFANNY CHEN
Medical Student
Vanderbilt University School of Medicine
Nashville, Tennessee

COURTNEY HENTZ
Medical Student
University of Cincinnati
College of Medicine
Cincinnati, Ohio

CHRISTOPHER HOM
Medical Student
Meharry Medical College
Nashville, Tennessee

SETTY MEGANA
Medical Student
University of Minnesota Medical School
Minneapolis, Minnesota

AMBER VAN DEN RAADT
Medical Student
A.T. Still University
Mesa, Arizona

AGATHE STREIFF
Medical Student
The University of Texas Medical School at Houston
Houston, Texas

RYAN WILLINGHAM
Medical Student
Texas Tech University Health Sciences Center
School of Medicine
Lubbock, Texas

Preface

Step-Up to Surgery evolved from our desire to provide medical students with a concise, easy-to-read, up-to-date overview of the key concepts of general surgery, applicable to students taking the third-year clerkship rotation. We wanted our book to be different from others currently available in the following ways:

1. Provide a core overview of not only general surgery topics but also key concepts in the surgical subspecialties.
2. Provide numerous "quick hits" to illustrate important points for licensure examinations.
3. Provide authentic, case-based questions to further illustrate concepts and allow students to apply them to typical patient presentations.
4. Provide many pictures, figures, and tables to further illustrate key concepts and allow for easy recall when students are questioned on rounds, in the operating room, and on written examinations.
5. Provide students with a full-length comprehensive simulated shelf-examination to serve as a study aid for end of rotation examinations.

To this end, we have recruited the authors from our department of surgery faculty and residents. These dedicated teachers are our front-line educators for our students and have provided didactic education to them.

Because of their location in rural West Virginia and three campuses throughout the state, it is our hope that *Step-Up to Surgery* will allow a standardization of general surgical clerkship education at all sites. We are hopeful that our readers will share the same enthusiasm for surgical education as we do.

Stanley Zaslau
Richard A. Vaughan

Acknowledgments

To Stacey Sebring and Susan Rhyner for their support and guidance throughout this process. To our families who have allowed us to spend more times on our laptops than with them.

Contents

CHAPTER 12. Skin and Soft Tissue

CHAPTER 13. Vascular Surgery

CHAPTER 14. Pediatric Surgery

CHAPTER 15. Orthopedic Surgery

CHAPTER 16. Neurosurgery

CHAPTER 17. Urology

CHAPTER 18. Otolaryngology

CHAPTER 19. Cardiothoracic Surgery

CHAPTER 20. Transplantation

Surgical Physiology

1

Gregory Schaefer and Jared Feyko

FLUIDS AND ELECTROLYTES

The diversity and complexity of fluid and electrolyte disorders managed by surgeons mirrors that of our patients in general. The general surgeon must be well acquainted with the fluids available in their facility's formulary, indications, and appropriate use. The importance of understanding electrolyte disorders in regard to etiology and treatment cannot be understated. A concise and organized approach is essential to resolve these disorders quickly.

I. **Body Water and Distribution**
   A. Total body water (TBW) varies from 45% to 70% of body weight depending upon age and gender. This value is also influenced by disease processes and administration of intravenous (IV) solutions. Although TBW is described in a compartmentalized fashion, the astute clinician is attuned to the regular shifting of fluids between compartments in response to treatments and pathologies.
   B. TBW is distributed in the following ways:
      1. Extracellular compartment (40% TBW)
         a. Intravascular/plasma space (25% extracellular water)
         b. Extravascular/interstitial space (75% extracellular water)
      2. Intracellular compartment (60% TBW)
   C. Extracellular water electrolyte composition is primarily that of sodium, chloride, and bicarbonate. The intracellular water electrolyte composition is primarily that of potassium, organic phosphate, and sulfate.
   D. Intravascular water also has many proteins (mostly albumin), which account for plasma colloid oncotic pressure.
   E. The kidneys maintain volume and composition of body fluid by two mechanisms: regulation of water excretion via antidiuretic hormone (ADH) and reabsorption of sodium.
      1. By regulating sodium and water metabolism, the kidneys maintain volume and body fluid composition in a very narrow range.
      2. Osmolality throughout all compartments remains similar even if the solutes are different. Regulation is primarily by the kidneys: If water intake decreases, the kidneys can concentrate the urine to a solute concentration four times that of the plasma, thus maintaining body osmolality.

II. **Volume Disorders**
   A. Starling fluid flux equation
      1. Movement of fluids and proteins between the intravascular and interstitial spaces is governed by the Starling fluid flux equation:

   $$Q = K_f (P_{mv} - P_t) - \sigma(p_{mv} - p_t)$$

   where σ is the osmotic reflection coefficient, p_{mv} is the capillary colloid osmotic pressure, p_t is the tissue interstitial colloid osmotic pressure, K_f is the filtration coefficient, P_{mv} is the capillary hydrostatic pressure, and P_t is the tissue interstitial hydrostatic pressure.

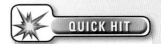

QUICK HIT

In a 70-kg adult, the intravascular volume is $70 \times 0.4 \times 0.25 = 7$ L.

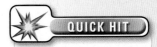

QUICK HIT

Urinalysis is a valuable tool because changes in the urine reflect changes in body water composition.

2. Net fluid flux in normal patients favors movement of fluid from the intravascular to the interstitial space.
3. It should be understood that water and sodium movements across barriers are intimately related. A change in the concentration of one will elicit movement of the other molecule to maintain concentrations.
4. *Example:* During hemorrhage, the initial P_{mv} drops, favoring the influx of fluid from the interstitial to the intravascular space. In cardiac failure, P_{mv} increases, and fluid flux into the interstitial space can result in pulmonary edema.

B. Volume overload (hypervolemia)
1. Syndrome of inappropriate antidiuretic hormone secretion (SIADH): This syndrome can occur after head injury, some cancers, and burns. The patient is hyponatremic and hypervolemic (the extracellular fluid volume is increased). The patient also has highly concentrated urine and high urine sodium concentrations. Lethargy and coma can ensue. Treatment includes free-water intake restriction, replacing lost sodium with IV saline infusion, and a loop diuretic such as furosemide (Lasix).
2. Hypervolemia can be associated with hyponatremia. Conditions frequently associated are congestive heart failure, cirrhosis, and nephrosis.
3. Iatrogenic conditions. In the majority of hospitalized surgical patients, volume overload is iatrogenic (caused by management of the health care team). Attention to the volume of administered fluids is required and can be anticipated by the increase in patient weight.
4. Daily patient weights, both at home and during hospitalization, can be an accurate method to trend volume status and may be more accurate than "measured" intake output (I/O).

C. Volume depletion
1. Central diabetes insipidus (CDI) occurs in head trauma patients due to damage in the hypothalamic nuclei or hypophyseal stalk. Large-volume urine output is noted and in combination with low specific gravity. Urine sodium and osmolarity levels are low while serum values are elevated. A dilute urine is produced that can result in severe hypovolemia if not identified and corrected in a timely fashion.
   a. Treatment is supportive, with replacement of free water as guided by the following estimate:

   $$(\text{Body weight}) \times (\% \text{ water}) = \text{normal TBW}$$

   $$(140 / \text{current serum sodium}) \times \text{TBW} = \text{current body water}$$

   $$\text{TBW} - \text{current body water} = \text{water deficit}$$

   b. *Example:* In a 70-kg man with a serum sodium of 156 mEq/L:

   $$(70) \times (0.6) = 42 \text{ L normal TBW}$$

   $$(140 / 156) \times (42 \text{ L}) = 37.7 \text{ L current TBW}$$

   $$42 \text{ L} - 37.7 \text{ L} = 4.3 \text{ L water deficit}$$

   c. Free water correction should be done with a mind to following the serum sodium and rate of correction. Typically, correction should not exceed 0.5 to 1 mmol/L/hr.
2. Gastrointestinal (GI) fluid losses
   a. Table 1-1 lists the typical electrolyte compositions and volumes of different GI fluids. Often, this can aid in fluid and electrolyte replacement strategy.
   b. *Example:* In a patient on a proton-pump inhibitor or H_2 blocker therapy (i.e., low acid stomach fluid) and who has emesis, the typical replacement fluid would be 0.45% normal saline with 20 mEq KCl ($Na^+ = 72$, $Cl^- = 92$, $K^+ = 20$), and to maintain isotonicity, the commercially available fluid adds 5% dextrose. Therefore, D5½ NS with 20 mEq KCl is the typical crystalloid fluid replacement for protracted emesis.
   c. Choosing fluids and amounts: In response to hypotension and hypovolemia, angiotensin I is released and converted to angiotensin II

TABLE 1-1 Electrolyte Composition and Volumes of Gastrointestinal Fluids

	Na$^+$(mEq/L)	K$^+$(mEq/L)	Cl$^-$(mEq/L)	HCO$_3^-$(mEq/L)	Volume (mL/24 hr)
Stomach, high acid	20	10	120	0	1,000–9,000
Stomach, low acid	80	15	90	15	1,000–2,500
Pancreas	140	5	75	80	500–1,000
Bile	148	5	100	35	300–1,000
Proximal small bowel	110	5	105	30	1,000–3,000
Distal small bowel	80	8	45	30	1,000–3,000
Colon/diarrhea	120	25	90	45	500–17,000

by angiotensin-converting enzyme. This causes vasoconstriction. Angiotensin II also stimulates the release of aldosterone from the adrenal gland. Aldosterone affects the kidney by reabsorbing more sodium and thereby "holding onto" more water. A byproduct is renal potassium wasting, or excretion of potassium in the urine.

(1) In most surgical patients, a balanced isotonic salt crystalloid solution is used for IV fluid replacement and management. The body loses water in the urine, stool, and via insensible (evaporative) losses. Open wounds dramatically increase the latter. It is estimated that during open abdominal surgery, up to 1 L insensible losses occur per hour.

(2) Use of large volume crystalloid resuscitation in acutely bleeding patients has come into question recently. Approximately 3 L of crystalloid are used to replace every liter of blood loss. Crystalloid has no oxygen-carrying capacity, can contribute to worsening acidosis, and, in large volumes, may contribute to acute respiratory distress syndrome (ARDS) and anasarca. Crystalloids readily leave the intravascular space within 20 minutes after a 1-L infusion of crystalloid, and only 200 mL remain intravascularly! Among patients with systemic inflammatory response syndrome (SIRS), the amount of fluid shift may be even greater. The clinical scenario, mechanism of injury, and local resources must guide the volume and type of fluid resuscitation. Further, the mechanism of injury should guide and may influence treatment strategies.

(3) In the healthy adult, fluid maintenance requirements approximate 30 mL/kg body weight/24 hours. Maintenance fluid after resuscitation is also estimated using the 4-2-1 formula:

$$\left[\begin{array}{l} \text{4 mL/kg for the first 10 kg body weight} \\ \text{2 mL/kg for the second 10 kg body weight} \\ \text{1 mL/kg for all additional weight} \end{array} \right.$$

(4) Daily fluid requirements are also influenced by losses from the GI and respiratory tracts, which should be included when prescribing IV fluids.

(5) The postoperative, or physiologically stressed, patient is glucose intolerant as a result of high circulating glucagon levels and relative insulin resistance. Diabetics tend to be particularly hyperglycemic at these times, and the high serum glucose can function as an osmotic agent to promote inappropriate diuresis. During the first 48 to 72 hours post-surgery and after trauma, it is unlikely that exogenous glucose will provide an energy substrate. Commonly, lactated Ringers or normal saline solutions are appropriate choices for surgical patients until specific restrictions are necessary.

TABLE 1-2 Electrolyte Abnormality Clinical Manifestations

Electrolyte Abnormality	Clinical Manifestation
Hypernatremia	Thirst, restlessness, irritability, ataxia, altered mental status
Hyponatremia	Headache, delirium, nausea, malaise, lethargy, confusion; if more severe, acute seizures and coma
Hypokalemia	If severe: <3.0 fatigue, weakness, cramps, constipation, ileus Flat T-waves, ST depression, appearance of U waves
Hyperkalemia	If severe: weakness, flaccid paralysis Peaked T-waves, prolonged PR and QRS interval
Hypercalcemia	If severe: >12 and acute: weakness, confusion, vomiting, anorexia, abdominal pain, polyuria Short QT interval · Chronic: nephrolithiasis, pathologic fractures
Hypocalcemia	Confusion, seizures, carpopedal spasm, perioral paraesthesias, tetany, Trousseau sign, Chvostek sign; QT prolongation with severe deficits
Hypermagnesemia	Occur when >4. Hyporeflexia; weakness; lethargy; paralysis; ileus; respiratory failure; prolonged PR, QRS, and QT intervals
Hypomagnesemia	Occur with levels <1.2; lethargy, confusion, tetany, seizures. Prolonged PR and QT interval, wide QRS and presence of U waves, Torsades de pointes
Hyperphosphatemia	Signs and symptoms attributable to hypocalcemia
Hypophosphatemia	If severe: <1 weakness, impaired diaphragmatic function, ileus, confusion, stupor

III. Electrolyte Abnormalities (see Table 1-2)

A. Hypernatremia: Commonly, hypernatremia is seen in free water deficit. This condition may occur as a result of diabetes insipidus (DI) or a significant renal condition. Please refer to the section on volume deficit.

B. Hyponatremia: This condition, which may occur as a result of isotonic fluid loss, can be seen in SIADH (discussed previously), in adrenal insufficiency, or in hyperglycemia, where the osmotic effects of glucose lead to inappropriate fluid loss from the kidney. In usual circumstances, a balanced salt solution can be used to replace sodium deficits.

C. Hyperkalemia

1. This serious condition mandates prompt attention. It can result from any catabolic state, such as crush injuries in trauma, burns, prolonged illness, hemolysis, renal failure, and adrenal insufficiency (addisonian crisis). Depolarizing paralytics such as succinylcholine (commonly used for rapid-sequence induction anesthesia) can cause massive muscle potassium release and acute hyperkalemia. In acute scenarios, most clinical manifestations are absent. However, an abnormal electrocardiogram (EKG) demonstrating progressive peaked T-waves and widening of the QRS complex can ultimately lead to cardiac arrest. Hyperkalemia also occurs in acidosis (see later in the chapter).

2. Treatment is based on rapidity of rise of serum potassium and the underlying cause. Some treatments simply displace the potassium intracellularly whereas others facilitate excretion from the body. If not treating the underlying problem or excreting an excess of potassium, displaced potassium may return and result in recurrent hyperkalemia.

   a. Serum potassium is actively transported intracellularly with insulin. Therefore, initial treatment is administration of IV glucose (1 ampule of $D_{50\%}$) and IV regular insulin (10 U).

   b. Correcting a metabolic acidosis with sodium bicarbonate can lower serum potassium levels.

    c. Calcium gluconate is another option—calcium antagonizes the tissue effects of hyperkalemia to stabilize cardiac membrane potentials. Calcium administration should be considered in any hyperkalemic patient manifesting arrhythmia. The infusion of calcium does not by itself lower serum potassium levels.

    d. Inhaled beta-agonist bronchodilators (i.e., albuterol)

    e. If hyperkalemia is due to adrenal insufficiency, hydrocortisone can be administered. Hyperkalemia due to renal failure may require hemodialysis or peritoneal dialysis.

    f. A slower treatment is Kayexalate (sodium polystyrene sulfonate, a cation exchange resin), which can be given orally or by enema and binds potassium in the GI tract in exchange for sodium.

    g. Refractory hyperkalemia or cases manifesting with arrhythmia should prompt consideration of hemodialysis to remove excess potassium.

D. Hypokalemia

  1. Obligatory potassium losses occur in both the urine (30 to 60 mEq/day) and stool (30 to 90 mEq/day). Increased potassium loss can result from emesis, diarrhea, diuretic use, DI, and metabolic alkalosis.

  2. Increased urinary excretion of potassium occurs when the serum potassium level rises above 4 mEq/L. Aldosterone release is increased as a result of hyperkalemia, promoting excretion of potassium in the distal tubule of the kidney. In patients with emesis, the loss of hydrogen ion in the emesis results in potassium retention in the kidney (to maintain electrical neutrality) at the expense of hydrogen ion excretion. The emesis causes a hypochloremic, hypokalemic metabolic alkalosis, worsened paradoxically over time by the kidney, leading to a paradoxical aciduria. This is commonly seen in children with pyloric stenosis.

  3. Another cause of hypokalemia is potassium loss, primarily from the kidney. This is called renal wasting of potassium. Greater than 30 mEq/L of urinary potassium when the serum potassium is <3.5 mEq/L defines renal potassium wasting. The three causes of renal potassium wasting are diuretic therapy, effects of aldosterone, and alkalosis.

  4. When assessing for hypokalemia, the acid-base status of the patient must be ascertained first. If the patient is alkalemic, the hypokalemia may simply be an ion exchange issue; the more alkalemic the intravascular space is, the more hydrogen ion is shifted intravascularly and potassium shifted extravascularly. Figure 1-1 suggests a replacement strategy for potassium when alkalosis exists. Often, correcting the underlying alkalosis resolves the hypokalemia and should be considered first. This is depicted in Table 1-3.

FIGURE 1-1 Relationship of serum potassium to total body potassium stores at different blood pH levels.

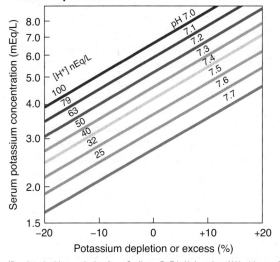

(Reprinted with permission from Scribner B, Ed. *University of Washington Teaching Syllabus for the Course on Fluid and Electrolyte Balance.* University of Washington; 2008.)

TABLE 1-3	Prediction of Serum Potassium Concentrations in Acid-Base Abnormalities Assuming no Potassium Wasting
If Serum pH Is:	**Predicted Serum K+ (mEq/L)**
7.10	5.9
7.20	5.1
7.30	4.7
7.40 (normal)	4.1
7.50	3.8
7.60	3.1
7.70	2.6

5. Treatment most often consists of potassium replacement once the acid-base status of the patient has been ascertained. IV potassium (usually potassium chloride) generally is given at rates of 20 mEq/hr via a central line and 10 mEq/hr peripherally. Preferred routes for patient comfort are via a central line or orally. If the cause of hypokalemia is diuretic therapy, consider alternatives to that therapy. If hypokalemia is persistent despite adequate replacement, check for and correct coexistent hypomagnesemia.

E. Hypercalcemia: This condition occurs with hyperparathyroidism, cancer, hyperthyroidism, adrenal insufficiency, and prolonged immobilization. Serum calcium levels of 12 g/dL and greater are a medical emergency and should be managed with IV saline. Loop diuretics, steroids, and calcitonin are additional treatments.

F. Hypocalcemia: This is a more common calcium abnormality in surgical patients and may result from hypoparathyroidism, pancreatitis, severe trauma and crush injuries, necrotizing fasciitis, and severe renal failure. Patients undergoing total thyroidectomies or multiple parathyroidectomies should be followed clinically and with labs for hypocalcemia. Clinically, patients develop hyperactive deep tendon reflexes, abdominal cramps, carpopedal spasm, Chvostek sign (tetany of the facial nerve), or Trousseau sign (tetany of the arm when blood pressure cuff inflated), all of which can be extremely painful. Treatment initially involves treating a metabolic alkalosis if it exists then replacing calcium with calcium chloride or gluconate. Hypocalcemia may also be seen chronically among malnourished patients. Correction based on serum albumin or investigation of an ionized calcium level will determine true extent of hypocalcemia.

G. Hypermagnesemia: This condition is rare in surgical patients but can occur with renal disease. Iatrogenic hypermagnesemia can occur in these patients with excessive magnesium intake through antacid and laxative therapy, those being treated for spontaneous subarachnoid hemorrhage with vasospasm, or women with preeclampsia. Patients with hypermagnesemia are lethargic and weak. EKG abnormalities are similar to those in hyperkalemia. Progressive hypermagnesemia results in the loss of deep tendon reflexes, somnolence, coma, and death. Treatment consists of withholding additional magnesium, IV normal saline, calcium infusions (similar to hyperkalemia, calcium antagonizes the neuromuscular effects of hypermagnesemia), and possible dialysis if the patient has severe renal failure.

H. Hypomagnesemia
1. This abnormality occurs as a result of poor dietary intake, malabsorption in the GI tract, excessive GI loss (e.g., diarrhea), enteric fistulas, chronic alcohol use and abuse, acute pancreatitis, severe burns, prolonged use of total

parenteral nutrition (TPN) with insufficient magnesium, hyperaldosteronism, and hypercalcemia. Symptoms are similar to those of hypocalcemia (hyperactive deep tendon reflexes, Chvostek sign, tremors, delirium, and seizures).

    2. Treatment consists of replacing magnesium. Oral replacement is best. IV magnesium in the form of magnesium sulfate is often used, especially in more severe deficiencies. While replacing magnesium, the EKG should be monitored, and in renal failure, any magnesium must be given with great caution.

I. Hypophosphatemia: This condition occurs in hyperparathyroidism and malnourished patients (e.g., alcoholics). Neuromuscular effects (fatigue, weakness, convulsions, and even death) predominate when serum phosphorus levels fall below 1 mg/dL. Replacement is accomplished either orally or parenterally (potassium or sodium phosphate).

J. Hyperphosphatemia: This disorder occurs in severe crush injury, muscle breakdown, and in severe renal failure. Elevated serum phosphorus decreases intravascular calcium. Phosphate-binding antacids (such as aluminum hydroxide) can be used, as well as diuretics to promote urinary excretion of phosphorus. In severe renal failure, hemodialysis may be necessary.

IV. Acid-Base Disorders

A. General principles

    1. Hydrogen ions are generated in the body at a rate of about 70 mEq/kg/day. Carbon dioxide is formed from aerobic metabolism. The Henderson–Hasselbalch equation depicts the relationship of bicarbonate to carbonic acid and pH:

$$pH = pK + \frac{\log([HCO_3^-])}{(0.03p \times CO_2)}$$

A simpler form of this same equation is:

$$[H^+] = \frac{(24 \times pCO_2)}{[HCO_3^-]}$$

and it must be remembered that:

$$H_2O + CO_2^- = H_2CO_3 = HCO_3^- + H^+$$

    2. The serum pH is a reflection of the amount of carbon dioxide that is produced, the efficiency of elimination in the lung (ventilation), and the buffering capability (in the serum, and either elimination or retention of bicarbonate by the kidney) according to the previous equations. Hydrogen ion can also be excreted by the kidney in the form of ammonium ion.

    3. The myriad chemical reactions occurring in humans do so within a narrow range of optimal pH. Acid-base disorders can result in ineffective coagulation and vasopressor/inotrope function among critically ill patients.

B. Respiratory disorders

    1. Acidosis: Patients who inadequately eliminate CO_2 develop respiratory acidosis. As a result, hydrogen ion accumulates as the previous equation is forced to the "right." Treatment acutely is to improve ventilation and elimination of CO_2. Patients with a metabolic alkalosis (high HCO_3^-) drive the equation to the right, resulting in a compensatory respiratory acidosis. Clinically, this may be found among somnolent head injury patients or those suffering from excessive ingestion of intoxicants that have compromised the airway or suppressed the respiratory drive. This may also be a finding in patients suffering from early respiratory failure because they have become fatigued from work of breathing and have an inadequate minute volume.

    2. Alkalosis: Patients may hyperventilate for many reasons, including anxiety, hypoxia, sepsis, and a mechanically induced small tidal volume. Elimination of excessive CO_2 results in the equation being driven to the "left," causing an alkalosis. Patients who have a metabolic acidosis (high H^+) also drive the equation to the left, prompting hyperventilation and a compensatory respiratory alkalosis.

C. Metabolic disorders
   1. Acidosis: Excessive production of hydrogen ion or increased excretion of bicarbonate results in a metabolic acidosis. The decrease in bicarbonate is exchanged for an increase in serum chloride, maintaining a normal anion gap (AG). The AG is simply measured by:

   $$[HCO_3 + Cl^-] - Na < 8–12 \text{ mEq/L}$$

   If the AG is greater than 8 to 12 mEq/L, an unmeasured anion (such as lactate or ketoacid) is present.
      a. Distinguishing anion gap acidosis (AGA) from non-anion gap acidosis (NAGA) is critical in determining the etiology of a metabolic acidosis. This will direct subsequent treatment. In NAGA, bicarbonate depletion is primarily the cause related to diarrhea, emesis, fistulas, or renal tubular acidosis. AGA has many etiologies and common among them are iatrogenesis, diabetic ketoacidosis, poisonings, and hypoperfusion.
      b. In the presence of AGA among septic or trauma patients, hypovolemia and hypoperfusion are the most likely and sinister etiologies. Correlating base deficit, serum lactate, and clinical markers of perfusion are important to confirm the hypothesis and identify other potential etiologies.
      c. *Example:* In AGA, the presence of lactate may signify inadequate perfusion and anaerobic metabolism, generating lactate. In this case, treatment is directed at restoring perfusion.
      d. *Example:* A severely head-injured patient receiving normal saline and hypertonic saline may develop a hyperchloremic metabolic acidosis with a normal AG.
   2. Alkalosis: The kidneys play a significant role in acid-base homeostasis. Active hydrogen ion secretion occurs in response to acidosis, and bicarbonate combines with hydrogen ion to form carbonic acid and CO_2, thereby facilitating reabsorption of bicarbonate.
D. Mixed disorders: In the acute phase of injury or surgery, many acid-base disorders are purely respiratory or metabolic. However, patients with premorbidities and medical conditions, as well as those who are beyond the acute phase of their disease, often manifest mixed acid-base disorders. Despite efforts to compensate, mixed acid-base disorders will not achieve a pH of 7.40. Respiratory compensation is able to begin with minutes to hours, whereas metabolic compensation occurs over a period of hours to days.
   1. *Example:* A patient who suffers an injury and is in shock develops lactic (metabolic) acidosis (AGA). The patient hyperventilates to remove CO_2 and develops a compensatory respiratory alkalosis. However, it is uncommon for the compensation to ever exceed the primary process. Therefore, despite the patient's best efforts, he or she remains acidotic with a primary metabolic acidosis and compensatory respiratory alkalosis until the shock and poor perfusion are corrected with resuscitation.
   2. *Example:* A patient suffers ARDS, and this results in the inability of the lungs to ventilate adequately. Therefore, the $PaCO_2$ rises, resulting in a respiratory acidosis. Over time (more than 24 hours), the kidneys respond and excrete hydrogen ion and chloride in order to retain bicarbonate. This results in a compensatory metabolic alkalosis. However, until the lung condition improves, the compensation is partial, and the patient remains slightly acidotic.
   3. *Example:* A patient who has diarrhea and chronic obstructive pulmonary disease may have a high respiratory rate and therefore a respiratory alkalosis. However, the diarrhea causes loss of fluid and bicarbonate and results in a metabolic acidosis.
   4. *Example:* A patient with vomiting may present with a metabolic alkalosis. The patient may also be breathing rapidly due to abdominal pain and may also have a respiratory alkalosis.

TABLE 1-4 Determining the Primary Disturbance

Condition	pH	CO_2	HCO_3
Respiratory acidosis	↓	↑	N
Respiratory alkalosis	↑	↓	N
Metabolic acidosis	↓	N	↓
Metabolic alkalosis	↑	N	↑

N = no change

E. Arterial blood gas (ABG) and interpretation
1. CO-oximeter analyzer separately can measure oxyhemoglobin, methemoglobin, and carboxyhemoglobin. A normal ABG is: PaO_2 = 100 mm Hg, $PaCO_2$ = 40 mm Hg, pH = 7.40, bicarbonate = 24 mEq/L, base excess/deficit = 0, and HbO_2 = 100%.
2. ABG analyzers must compensate for extremes of body temperature, a problem for hypo- or hyperthermic patients.
3. In an uncompensated metabolic condition, the $PaCO_2$ remains normal, but the pH is low (in a metabolic acidosis) or high (in a metabolic alkalosis). The calculated base deficit or excess, respectively, reflects the degree of metabolic derangement. It is important to remember that base deficit and excess are a reflection of the metabolic acidosis or alkalosis, respectively, and not a reflection of respiratory acid-base conditions.
4. In mixed acid-base disorders, the base deficit/excess as seen on an ABG helps sort out the primary disorder. With metabolic acidosis, the AG further helps sort out the abnormality and direct treatment.
5. Use Table 1-4 to aid in determining the primary underlying disturbance. Once the primary disturbance is identified, if a metabolic acidosis, the AG (as described previously) can be determined to narrow down potential etiologies. Further, the expected compensation component can also be calculated to identify if there is a mixed disorder.
   a. Metabolic acidosis: PCO_2 is expected to decrease 1.2 mm Hg for every 1 mEq decrease in HCO_3 (below 24).
   b. Metabolic alkalosis: PCO_2 is expected to increase 0.7 mm Hg for every 1 mEq rise in HCO_3 (above 24).
   c. Acute respiratory acidosis/alkalosis: pH is expected to change by 0.08 for every 10 mm Hg change in $PaCO_2$.

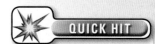

QUICK HIT

In pure respiratory disorders, a rise in $PaCO_2$ by 10 lowers the pH by 0.08. Therefore, in respiratory acidosis, a $PaCO_2$ = 50 results in a pH = 7.32. In respiratory alkalosis, a $PaCO_2$ = 30 results in a pH = 7.48. In both cases, the calculated bicarbonate is still 24 and the base excess/deficit is still 0.

V. Fluid Therapy
A. Crystalloids: The solute concentrations of four typical crystalloids are presented in Table 1-5. Becoming familiar with the composition of typical IV fluids may appear trivial, but understanding their composition can be critical for understanding in which clinical situations certain fluids should be avoided.

TABLE 1-5 Solute Concentrations of Standard Crystalloid Solution

Crystalloid	Na^+(mEq/L)	Cl^+(mEq/L)	K^+(mEq/L)	HCO_3^- (mEq/L)	Ca^+(mEq/L)	Glucose
Normal saline (0.9%)	154	154				
Lactated Ringers	130	109	4	28	2.7	
D5½ NS	77	77				50
D5½ NS + 20 KCl	77	97	20			50

Further, it is helping in knowing when to attribute physiologic derangements to iatrogenic causes secondary to IV fluid administration.

1. Normal saline is ubiquitously used for dehydration and hypovolemia. It is compatible with blood product transfusion and most medications. It is classified as an isotonic fluid; however, the concentration of NaCl is higher than found in humans. Recent literature has raised concerns about the deleterious effects of solutions with supraphysiologic chloride concentrations. It is typically the first-line fluid used in trauma resuscitations, head injuries, acute neurologic conditions where hyponatremia should be avoided, and treatment of mild hyponatremia.

2. Lactated Ringers is a more isotonic fluid, also commonly used for resuscitation. It provides less sodium and chloride than normal saline and offers a small amount of other solutes, including bicarbonate, calcium, and potassium. In severely underperfused patients, the increase in circulating lactate may exacerbate an acidosis. Lactated Ringers is not compatible with blood product transfusions and with some medications, specifically calcium. Despite these considerations, lactated Ringers is widely used and has equal efficacy in most circumstances to normal saline. The L-lactate is converted to bicarbonate in the perfusing liver, thereby helping to resolve acidosis. Advantages include more physiologic levels of sodium and chloride; however, the presence of potassium should prompt reflection before use in those with hyperkalemia or renal dysfunction.

3. D5½ NS
   a. This mildly hypotonic fluid provides a small amount of dextrose along with hypotonic salt. Adding 20 mEq/L of KCl results in an almost isotonic solution whose solute concentrations approach that of stomach fluid. The small amount of dextrose helps decrease the hypotonicity and may help with minimizing ketoacidosis. The dextrose provides caloric content to IV fluids and stimulates insulin release, thereby preventing protein catabolism in patients who otherwise are not receiving nutrition. Additionally, the typically used D5½ NS with 20 mEq is also appropriate for maintenance fluid because it approximates normal sodium (1 to 2 mEq/kg/day) and potassium (0.5 to 1.0 mEq/kg/day) requirements when given in typical maintenance volumes.
   b. *Example:* Initially, in the resuscitative management of the adult patient with emesis, an isotonic solution should be used. Once stabilized, maintenance with D5½ NS with 20 KCl is often used as the replacement fluid.

4. Hypertonic saline: These solutions, ranging from 2% to 23.4%, have been used to treat patients with head injury, hypovolemic shock, spontaneous subarachnoid hemorrhage, or refractory hyponatremia. Benefits include volume expansion, reduction of cerebral edema via osmotic effects, and scavenging of oxygen free radicals. Extreme caution should be used when prescribing concentrated salt solutions. Frequent monitoring of clinical conditions and serum lab values are appropriate to prevent iatrogenesis.

B. Colloids
1. Colloids are large-molecular-weight particles that generally remain intravascular longer than crystalloids and result in an increased oncotic gradient with the extravascular space.
2. Plasmanate is a dilute colloid consisting of 5% albumin in saline. It is occasionally used in anesthesia but is not common in other settings.
3. Albumin solutions are typically available in a 5% or 25% concentration. It may be used as a volume expander and to facilitate concomitant dieresis by transiently pulling fluid into the intravascular space. Caution should be used among immunocompromised patients.

C. Synthetic colloids
1. The hetastarch (Hespan) synthetic colloids have the greatest application in surgery and trauma. They are excellent volume expanders; the volume infused remains intravascularly longer than crystalloids. In addition, there are few side effects. However, large quantities of hetastarch can interfere with coagulation, and therefore, its use must be limited in the trauma patient.

2. Dextran 40 and 70: These two synthetic colloids were once popular as both volume expanders and as hemorheologic modifiers (making the blood less viscous and promoting perfusion). They are still used in some vascular situations.

3. Gelatin synthetic colloids are available in Europe and Asia but not in the United States.

D. Blood products: U.S. blood banks provide an array of blood products, and transfusion is based on clinical need. Although viral and other infections are well-known transmissible complications of blood product transfusions, they occur rarely (1 in 200,000 units for hepatitis B and 1 in 1.6 million units for hepatitis C or HIV). Transfusion reactions are significantly more common (1 in 200 units), can be morbid, and on rare occasion, anaphylaxis can be life threatening. Judicious transfusion with a clear clinical indication is always warranted.

1. Whole blood is not approved in the United States by the American Red Cross. In the United States, blood component therapy is the standard. Interestingly, the U.S. military has used whole blood transfusions overseas in combat with excellent results.

2. Each unit of packed red blood cells (PRBCs) is a volume of approximately 550 mL and weighs 400 g. Generally speaking, one unit of transfused blood equates to a patient hemoglobin rise of 1 g/dL, but it depends on the donor's initial hemoglobin.

3. Platelets are pooled from multiple donors and generally are provided in a six-pack. Because the platelets are pooled from multiple donors, their transfusion must be for clinically appropriate reasons only.

4. Fresh frozen plasma (FFP) is rich in fibrinogen, coagulation factors, and protein. When there is a need for a colloid, as well as to reverse a coagulopathy, FFP is transfused. Often, the amount is determined by the clinical appearance of bleeding and the prothrombin time (PT).

5. Cryoprecipitate is pooled from multiple donors, and similarly to platelets, its administration must be guided by a true need. Cryoprecipitate is especially rich in fibrinogen.

6. Recombinant factor VIIa (rFVIIa) is a U.S. Food and Drug Administration (FDA)-approved agent for hemophilia. However, its use has recently gained popularity in bleeding patients. Some data exist regarding its utility in cardiac surgery. There are no conclusive studies in trauma and in surgery, but rFVIIa appears promising as an adjunct in the bleeding patient, especially one who is already acidotic from hypoperfusion. It is sometimes administered at a dose of 90 μg/kg body weight. rFVIIa currently is quite expensive. Military case series have reported a benefit to use of rFVIIa that has not always been replicated in civilian series.

E. Blood substitutes have been investigated for 40 years. At the moment, there is no FDA-approved blood substitute.

F. In rare cases, acutely bleeding trauma patients may demonstrate a pattern of fibrinolysis that is apparent on a thromboelastogram (TEG) tracing. Consideration should be given to administering tranexamic acid (an antifibrinolytic) based on the results of a recent multinational, randomized, placebo-controlled trial.

HEMOSTASIS/COAGULATION

I. **General Principles.** Hemostasis is a complex interaction of multiple components in the body. Usually, it occurs in an ordered way as the body's response to injury, but can also occur in a dysfunctional manner, leading to significant morbidity.

A. Vasoconstriction is the initial response to injury. It occurs as a reflex to most stimuli.

B. Platelet aggregation results from the release of platelet factors and fibrin. This leads to formation of a platelet plug that acts as a physical barrier to further bleeding.

C. Coagulation is an interaction of factors that leads to the formation of a fibrin and platelet plug. It is a series of enzymatic reactions that can be slowed with hypothermia or a deficiency of factors.

D. Fibrinolysis is the final step in the coagulation cascade. Its main effect is to prevent the thrombosis from going unchecked. It also helps break down the clot once bleeding has been controlled and leads to improved blood flow in the vessel.

II. Testing the Surgical Patient for Hemostatic Risk Factors

A. For minor surgical procedures, all that is needed is a thorough history and physical. It is especially important to ask about excessive bruising after minor injuries or significant bleeding after small cuts or abrasions. Medications are also an important factor.

B. If the history and physical are unrevealing but the patient is to undergo a major surgical procedure (one that involves a large part of the body), or the operation is to involve a part of the body where even a small amount of excessive bleeding would have disastrous complications (i.e., involving the eye or brain), then additional tests need to be ordered. In most circumstances, checking a PT, prothromboplastin time (PTT), and platelets suffices. However, if these are normal but the history or physical suggest some bleeding abnormalities, then tests such as bleeding time can be ordered.

C. Other tests that are useful include a hematocrit and a platelet count (although this gives no information on the function of the platelets).

III. Tests of Hemostasis and Coagulation

A. PT measures mostly the extrinsic factors that lead to clotting. Extrinsic refers to the interaction between platelets, and specifically factors outside the blood vessel, leading to initiation of the clotting cascade. It is also used as a surrogate to reflect the function of the liver.

B. PTT refers to the function of the intrinsic pathway.

C. Bleeding time is not useful as an initial screening test because it is labor intensive and the results can be subjective. It is useful, though, when the bleeding disorder is caused by factors that are not measured by the PT or PTT, such as platelet dysfunction.

D. Thromboelastography (TEG) is a study that provides real-time information to the clinician regarding coagulation factor levels (indirectly), function, and degree of any platelet dysfunction.

IV. Congenital Defects

A. Hemophilia A, or classic hemophilia, is caused by an abnormality in factor VIII. It occurs as a sex-linked recessive trait that occurs almost exclusively in males. Although history may lead to the diagnosis, levels of factor VIII confirm it. Patients also have an elevated PTT with a normal PT. Treatment is with factor VIII or cryoprecipitate.

B. Hemophilia B, or Christmas disease, is caused by a factor IX abnormality. It is also sex-linked and recessive, and so occurs exclusively in males. The disease has a similar presentation to classic hemophilia. Treatment is with factor IX concentrate.

C. Von Willebrand disease is secondary to abnormalities with von Willebrand factor (vWF). Normally, vWF helps in platelet adhesion to collagen and cross-linking platelets in clot aggregation. It is commonly inherited in an autosomal dominant pattern with variable penetrance. Affected people usually have episodes of mucocutaneous bleeding. Bleeding time is commonly prolonged, although the PTT can also be prolonged. Treatment is with cryoprecipitate.

V. Acquired Defects

A. Platelet defects can occur secondary to drugs, uremia, or thrombocytopenia (which may be related to massive blood transfusion or platelet destruction). As more antiplatelet agents are introduced to manage cardiovascular conditions, the frequency with which surgeons encounter these will increase.

B. Fibrinogen deficiency usually occurs with disseminated intravascular coagulation (DIC). DIC can be brought on by multiple causes, including retained placenta, sepsis, or amniotic fluid embolism. Treatment is to remove the underlying cause, if possible.

VI. Hepatic and Renal Disease

A. Liver disease, especially if severe, can lead to depletion in coagulation factors by a decrease in production. All factors, except for factor VIII and vWF, which are produced by the endothelium, are produced by the liver. This can lead to a severe coagulopathy that is difficult to correct.

B. Renal failure leads to a uremic state. This occurs typically when the patient has not undergone dialysis and the blood urea nitrogen has increased significantly. The uremia interferes with the aggregation of platelets and leads to a diffuse bleeding diathesis. The best way to correct this is through dialysis. If that is not immediately available, then IV 1-deamino-8-D-arginine vasopressin or conjugated estrogens have been shown to work.

VII. Anticoagulation

A. Heparin is a naturally occurring heterogeneous mixture of glycosaminoglycans with differing molecular weights. It accelerates the effect of antithrombin III, leading to a systemically anticoagulated state. It is given intravenously or subcutaneously. The heparin antithrombin III complex inactivates several factors in the anticoagulant cascade, especially thrombin and factor X. The level of anticoagulation achieved can be measured by checking the PTT.

B. Low-molecular-weight heparin (LMWH), which is made by fractionating heparin into its lower-weight molecules, acts primarily by inhibiting factor Xa. It is administered subcutaneously. The lower-weight molecule is incapable of inactivating thrombin or antithrombin. Because of this, LMWH does not prolong PTT. Oral forms of factor Xa are now available. Caution should be used among patients with renal failure. Dose adjustments may be appropriate in morbid obesity. Anti-factor Xa levels may be followed but do not correlate with effective anticoagulation.

C. Warfarin leads a deficiency of vitamin K (an important cofactor in certain coagulation factor synthesis), resulting in a decrease in production by the liver of factors II, VII, IX, and X; protein C; and S. The drug is given orally, with a half-life of about 1.5 days, and so it takes a few days to take effect and to reverse. The level of anticoagulation can be measured by checking the PT (the international normalized ratio [INR] is an indirect measure of the PT).

D. Heparin-induced thrombocytopenia (HIT) occurs in two forms:

1. HIT type I, which occurs frequently. It usually occurs with a drop in platelet count of more than 100,000. It occurs by a nonimmune-mediated phenomenon. There is no risk of thrombosis, and discontinuation of heparin is not necessary.

2. HIT type II, which occurs far less frequently (in 2% to 10% of all exposed patients). It should be suspected when the platelet count drops by more than 50% from baseline or to a total less than 100,000. The diagnosis can be confirmed by checking for antibodies to HIT antibody. The cause is an immune-mediated reaction against heparin-platelet factor antibodies. This results in aggregation of platelets, leading to thrombocytopenia and possibly arterial and venous thrombosis. Because up to 30% of patients with HIT type II develop thrombosis even after discontinuation of heparin, anticoagulation with a nonheparinoid product is essential.

VIII. Management of Bleeding.

Local control of bleeding is especially important during, and sometimes after, surgical procedures. The most frequent cause of surgical bleeding is inadequate hemostasis in the wound. Less likely causes include coagulopathies.

A. Direct pressure is a very effective way to control and slow most bleeding. Ligature of vessels also controls most surgical bleeding. Tourniquet use has been reborn via use of new technologies in recent wars. Application for uncontrollable arterial bleeding in extremity wounds has been life-saving.

B. Electrocautery leads to hemostasis by the denaturation of proteins, resulting in coagulation over a large surface area, secondary to the diffusion of the electrical current.

C. Chemical agents can act as procoagulants and vasoconstrictors (epinephrine).

D. Topical hemostatics have been developed to address bleeding that is difficult to control due to accessibility (e.g., axillary or groin wounds).

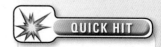

QUICK HIT

Low platelets can also be an indicator that significant liver disease exists.

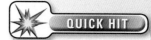

QUICK HIT

The half-life of heparin is just over 1 hour.

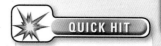

QUICK HIT

The efficacy of LMWH can be measured by checking anti-Xa levels.

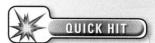

QUICK HIT

Because proteins C and S lead to systemic anticoagulation, their deficiency can lead to a prothrombotic state and may cause a phenomenon known as warfarin-induced skin necrosis if the patient is given warfarin compounds. For this reason, heparinization should always be performed prior to administering warfarin.

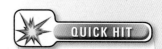

QUICK HIT

HIT is also possible with LMWH (at a lower incidence than with regular heparin).

Surgical Physiology

IX. Replacement Therapy

A. Typing and crossmatching is performed to establish serologic compatibility—to establish A, B, O, and the Rh status of the patient. This may take upward of an hour or so to do. If no knowledge about the patient's blood type is available but PRBCs are urgently needed, then type O Rh-negative blood can be given to women and type O Rh-positive can be given to men. If time permits, a type-and-screen can be done, and type-specific blood can be infused. Crossmatch can be accomplished with even a blood-soaked piece of clothing or gauze at many trauma centers and may obviate the need for collecting a tube specimen in critically ill patients. Further, in the event that blood draws are limited due to severity of illness, crossmatch should be a high priority over other labs.

B. Component therapy has replaced fresh whole blood transfusion due largely to practical consideration related to storage. In the actively bleeding patient, hemorrhage control and restoration of blood volume and clotting factors should occur simultaneously.

C. Platelet concentrates are given for a significant deficiency in either platelet function or quantity. Each unit raises the count by about 10,000/μL.

D. Volume expanders are isotonic or hypertonic crystalloid products, such as lactated Ringers, 0.9% normal saline, or 3% normal saline. Artificial colloids such as hetastarch or natural ones such as albumin are also useful for volume expansion.

E. Concentrates of factors such as FFP or concentrates of specific factors such as factor VIII are useful for replacement of deficiencies or dysfunction.

X. Indications for Replacements of Blood and Its Substitutes

A. Volume replacement is best performed based on amount of blood loss. Initially, isotonic crystalloid solutions are best. As significant amounts of blood are lost, replacement should be completed using a combination of PRBCs and crystalloid solutions. If massive bleeding is occurring and large amounts of transfusions are needed, then FFP is also needed, secondary to the dilutional effect of crystalloid solutions and the PRBCs.

B. Oxygen-carrying capacity can be impaired if severe anemia exists. This is especially significant if an area of ischemia exists in the body. However, in most other circumstances, hemoglobin as low as 5 g/dL may be tolerated well. In most instances clinically, patients are transfused to maintain a target hemoglobin of 7 g/dL, and for those with evidence of active cardiac ischemia, data support a target hemoglobin of >10 g/dL.

C. Patients diagnosed with active coronary disease or acute coronary syndrome may benefit from maintaining a hemoglobin of 10 g/dL during the acute phase.

D. Massive transfusion refers to the transfusion of more than 10 units of PRBCs, or the entire blood volume over a 24-hour period. To prevent complications from massive transfusion, a clinician should be dedicated to managing the process. Ideally, all products will be warmed during administration to prevent hypothermia. Military and civilian literature have demonstrated a benefit to transfusing in a ratio of 1:1:1 for red blood cells, plasma, and platelets, respectively. Consideration should also be given to replacing cryoprecipitate (for factor VIII) and calcium due to depletion that can occur with large-volume transfusions. Serial blood work including TEG and monitoring clinical signs of bleeding are helpful to direct ongoing transfusion.

XI. Complications of Transfusions

A. Febrile and allergic reactions

1. Acute hemolytic transfusion reactions occur because the wrong blood type is given, usually because of clerical error. Typical symptoms include anxiety, chest pain, chills, flank pain, and headaches. The treatment is to stop the transfusion, alert the blood bank, and ensure adequate hydration and diuresis.

2. Nonhemolytic transfusion reactions are secondary to antibodies against donor white blood cells. Patients might become anxious, pruritic, and dyspneic, and they may also develop fevers, flushing, and mild hypotension. Treatment includes ruling out a hemolytic transfusion and stopping the transfusion, followed by supportive therapy.

B. Transmission of bacteria and viruses: Screening for viruses is performed on all donated units, which has led to a significant decrease in infection risk.
   1. The estimated risk of infection with hepatitis B is one case in 60,000 units transfused, whereas the estimated risk of infection with hepatitis C is one case per 100,000 units transfused.
   2. The estimated risk of HIV is about one case in 450,000 units transfused.
   3. Bacterial infections are not common secondary to blood being stored at 4°C. Transfusion-acquired sepsis carries a high mortality rate, usually secondary to the size of the inoculum and impaired immunocompetence of the host.
C. Morbidity and mortality: Emerging data show increased morbidity and even mortality with each unit of blood transfused. Each unit of foreign blood transfused leads to an immunologic suppressed state, which in turn leads to a higher risk of infection. Cell-mediated immunity can be impaired. Also, blood products tend to be given by the blood bank with a "last in, first out" strategy in mind, so some of their functionality may be lost due to time in storage.

SURGICAL NUTRITION

I. **Nutritional Assessment**
   A. History: weight loss, chronic illnesses (malignancy), dietary habits, social habits (predisposing to malnutrition), and medications (that influence food intake)
   B. Physical examination: loss of muscle or adipose tissue; temporal wasting; organ dysfunction; and changes in skin, hair, or neuromuscular function
   C. Anthropometric data: weight change, triceps skin fold thickness, and midarm circumference
   D. Biochemical data: albumin, prealbumin, transferrin, total lymphocyte count, and creatinine excretion. Albumin has a half-life of 20 days and therefore reflects an indicator of long-term nutritional status and is a very important indicator of preoperative morbidity and mortality. Prealbumin has a half-life of 2 to 3 days and therefore reflects more acute changes in nutritional status.

II. **Estimation of Nutritional Requirements**
   A. Energy requirements
      1. Energy is needed for metabolic processes, core temperature maintenance, and tissue repair.
      2. Energy requirements can be estimated by indirect calorimetry and urinary nitrogen excretion.
      3. Basal energy expenditure may be estimated by the Harris-Benedict equation.
      4. Fat contains 9 kcal/g, protein 4 kcal/g, carbohydrates 4 kcal/g, and dextrose 3.4 kcal/g.
   B. Basic caloric need is 25 kcal/kg/day. Most postsurgical patients have an energy requirement of 30 kcal/kg/day. If the degree of surgical stress increases secondary to trauma or sepsis, this requirement goes up to 20% to 40%.
   C. Protein requirements
      1. Proteins are required for wound healing, and the minimum for a nonstressed person is 1g/kg/day.
      2. A nonprotein calorie:nitrogen ratio of 150:1 is needed to prevent the utilization of protein as a source of energy.
      3. In stress, more protein is required, so that a ratio of 90:1 to 120:1 is beneficial.

III. **Nutritional Requirements in Specific Conditions**
   A. Renal failure
      1. Renal failure results in an impaired ability to clear the byproducts of protein metabolism.
      2. These patients are given nutrients in a restricted volume with great care not to overfeed proteins.
      3. Administration of essential amino acids and high biologic value protein, such as egg albumin, results in less frequent need for dialysis.

B. Hepatic failure
1. Liver damage and portosystemic shunting results in a derangement in the level of amino acids in the blood, resulting in an increase in the aromatic to branched-chain amino acids.
2. The aromatic amino acids are precursors of false neurotransmitters that contribute to hepatic encephalopathy.
3. Patients with hepatic failure are therefore given diets enriched in branched-chain amino acids and deficient in aromatic amino acids.

C. Respiratory failure
1. Carbohydrate metabolism produces more CO_2 (respiratory quotient [RQ] = 1) as compared to fat (RQ = 0.7) or protein (RQ = 0.8).
2. Production of higher amounts of CO_2 results in more need for ventilatory support.
3. It is therefore important to prevent overfeeding patients. The amount of carbohydrate intake can be reduced, and that of fat may be increased. However, this must be done cautiously because high-fat diets may exacerbate lung injury.

D. Cardiac failure
1. Fluid overload may exacerbate cardiac failure.
2. Concentrated solutions are therefore given to these patients to limit the amount of fluid administered.

IV. Enteral Nutrition

A. General principles
1. Nutrition via the enteral route is preferred over the parenteral route, hence the commonly used phrase in surgery patients, "if the gut works, use it."
2. Feeding the GI tract functions to preserve the "gut mucosal barrier." This barrier prevents the translocation of bacteria and bacterial toxins across the gut into the host portal venous circulation.
3. Maintenance of the gut mucosal barrier requires (a) normal perfusion, (b) an intact epithelium, and (c) normal mucosal immune mechanisms.
4. Luminal contact of food prevents intestinal mucosal atrophy and stimulates intestinal production of immunoglobulin A (IgA).
5. Surgical patients who are adequately nourished and have not suffered a major complication can tolerate 10 days of partial starvation before any significant protein catabolism occurs. Therefore, most patients can be maintained on a 5% dextrose solution before return of feeding after surgery with no detrimental outcome.
6. Initiation of enteral feeding should occur immediately after adequate resuscitation.

B. Enteral formulas
1. Wide arrays of formulas are commercially available. The choice of an enteral formula is influenced by the degree of organ dysfunction and nutrient needs.
2. Patients who have not been fed for a prolonged period of time are less likely to tolerate complex solutions.
3. Patients with malnutrition benefit from provision of dipeptides, tripeptides, and medium-chain triglycerides because these substances are more easily absorbed.
4. Major categories of enteral formulas are:
   a. Low-residue isotonic formulas
      (1) These first-line formulas for stable patients with an intact GI tract contain no fiber bulk and so leave minimal residue.
      (2) They provide a caloric density of 1 kcal/mL and a nonprotein calorie:nitrogen ratio of 150:1.
   b. Isotonic formulas with fiber
      (1) The formulas contain fiber, which delays intestinal transit time and reduces the incidence of diarrhea.
      (2) The fiber stimulates pancreatic lipase activity and is degraded by gut bacteria into short-chain fatty acids.

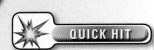

QUICK HIT

Certain nutrients are especially important for the GI tract. Glutamine is the most important fuel for enterocytes. Short-chain fatty acids are the primary energy source for colonocytes.

c. Immune-enhancing formulas
  (1) The formulas contain special nutrients such as glutamine, arginine, branched-chain amino acids, omega-3 fatty acids, nucleotides, and beta carotene.
  (2) The addition of amino acids generally doubles the amount of protein.
d. Calorie-dense formulas
  (1) The formulas provide 1.5 to 2 kcal/mL and are therefore used in fluid-restricted patients.
  (2) They have a higher osmolarity than standard formulas and are therefore used for intragastric feedings.
e. High-protein formulas
  (1) The formulas are used in critically ill patients with high protein requirements.
  (2) They provide nonprotein calorie:nitrogen ratios of 80:1 to 120:1.
f. Elemental formulas
  (1) The formulas contain predigested nutrients and are thus easy to absorb.
  (2) They are deficient in fat, vitamins, and trace elements that limit their long-term use. Instead, they are used in patients with malnutrition, gut impairment, and pancreatitis.
g. Renal failure formulas
  (1) These formulas contain protein exclusively in the form of essential amino acids and have a high nonprotein calorie:nitrogen ratio.
  (2) They require lower fluid volumes and contain lower concentrations of potassium, magnesium, and phosphorus.
h. Pulmonary failure formulas
  (1) These formulas have a reduced content of carbohydrate and a corresponding increased content of fat up to 50% of the total calories.
  (2) This aims to reduce the amount of CO_2 produced to decrease the burden of ventilation.
i. Hepatic failure formulas: These formulas have an increased quantity of branched-chain amino acids and reduced aromatic amino acids.

C. Access for enteral nutrition
1. Nasoenteric tubes (nasogastric and nasoduodenal tubes)
  a. Intragastric feeding permits bolus feeding due to the reservoir capacity of the stomach.
  b. Feeding the stomach results in stimulation of the biliary-pancreatic axis, which is trophic for the small bowel.
  c. Gastric secretions also have a dilutional effect on the osmolarity of the feedings, decreasing the incidence of diarrhea.
  d. Nasogastric feeding should be administered to patients with intact mental status and protective laryngeal reflexes to minimize the risk of aspiration.
  e. Nasoduodenal feedings decrease the risk of aspiration pneumonia by 25%.
  f. Placement of tubes past the pylorus is technically difficult. However, fluoroscopic-guided placement has a high success rate.
2. Percutaneous endoscopic gastrostomy (PEG)
  a. This technique is used for long-term enteral nutrition access.
  b. Catheters are placed in the stomach percutaneously using endoscopic guidance.
  c. Relative contraindications to PEG include ascites, coagulopathy, gastric varices, gastric neoplasm, and lack of suitable abdominal site.
3. Percutaneous endoscopic gastrostomy-jejunostomy (PEG-J) and direct percutaneous endoscopic jejunostomy (DPEJ)
  a. These techniques are used for patients who cannot tolerate gastric feedings or are at risk of aspiration.
  b. PEG-J is performed by passing a tube past the pylorus into the jejunum using an existing PEG tube. This is done endoscopically or fluoroscopically. PEG-J has a more than 50% malfunction rate due to retrograde tube migration, clogging, and kinking.

    c. DPEJ is performed using the same techniques as PEG but requires the enteroscope to reach the jejunum.

4. Surgical gastrostomy and jejunostomy

D. Complications of enteral nutrition

1. Abdominal distension and cramps: This is managed by temporarily discontinuing feeds and resuming at a lower infusion rate.

2. Pneumatosis intestinalis and small bowel necrosis

    a. This occurs as a result of bowel distension and consequent reduction in bowel wall perfusion.

    b. Factors implicated include hyperosmolarity of tube feeds, bacterial overgrowth, fermentation, and metabolic breakdown products.

    c. Initiation of enteric tube feedings in critically ill patients should be delayed until they have been adequately resuscitated so that an already hypoperfused bowel is not stressed further.

    d. Tube feeds can also be diluted, or solutions with low osmolarity can be used so that less digestion is needed by the GI tract.

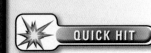

QUICK HIT

DPEJ has a lower rate of malfunction than PEG-J but is technically much more challenging.

V. Parenteral Nutrition

A. General principles: Parenteral nutrition consists of infusion of a hyperosmolar solution containing carbohydrates, proteins, fats, and other important nutrients.

B. Indications

1. Prolonged ileus (less than 7 to 10 days) after a major operation

2. Hypermetabolic patients in whom enteral nutrition is not possible or adequate (e.g., critically ill patients, cancer patients)

3. Short bowel syndrome

4. High-output enterocutaneous fistulas (output >500 mL/day)

5. Malabsorption (e.g., pancreatic insufficiency, celiac disease, inflammatory bowel disease)

6. Functional GI disorders (e.g., esophageal dyskinesia, anorexia nervosa)

C. Routes of parenteral nutrition

1. TPN (also called central parenteral nutrition)

    a. These solutions are hyperosmolar and must therefore be delivered into a high-flow system (i.e., a central vein) to prevent venous sclerosis.

    b. A standard TPN solution contains 15% to 25% dextrose, 10% amino acid, lipids and electrolytes, minerals, and vitamins.

    c. Lipids are primarily in the form of long-chain triglycerides, which provide essential fatty acids (linoleic acid). However, the high content of these polyunsaturated fatty acids has harmful effects on pulmonary and immune function.

2. Peripheral parenteral nutrition (PPN)

    a. These solutions can be administered via peripheral veins because they have low osmolarity, secondary to reduced levels of dextrose (5% to 10%) and protein (3%).

    b. Some nutrients cannot be administered due to inability to concentrate them into small volumes.

    c. Typically, PPN is used for nutritional support for short periods (less than 2 weeks) when central venous access is not available or feasible.

D. Complications of TPN

1. TPN is associated with more complications, compared with enteral feeding, due to intestinal bacterial overgrowth and increased gut permeability, leading to bacterial translocation. However, parenteral feeding still has fewer infectious complications compared with no feeding at all.

2. Complications of TPN can be divided into mechanical, metabolic, and infectious.

    a. Mechanical: central line insertion–related complications

    b. Metabolic

        (1) Hyperglycemia: Glucose should be monitored closely and maintained in a normal range to minimize associated complications.

        (2) Hypoglycemia: due to sudden cessation of TPN. Treated by administering dextrose.

(3) Carbon dioxide retention: due to excess glucose administration. Treated by decreasing glucose calories and replacing with fat.

(4) Azotemia: due to excess amino acid administration. Treated by decreasing amino acids and increasing glucose calories.

(5) Hypertriglyceridemia: due to rapid fat infusion. Treated by decreasing rate of fat infusion.

(6) Liver enzyme elevation: Mild elevation of transaminases, alkaline phosphatase, and bilirubin may occur. However, this is transient, and if liver enzymes do not plateau or return to normal over 7 to 14 days, another cause of the enzyme elevation should be investigated. Excess glucose is stored in the form of fat and results in hepatic steatosis. Long-term TPN administration results in cholestasis and formation of gallstones.

(7) Mineral, vitamin, and essential fatty acid deficiencies

c. Infectious: Sepsis can occur due to line infection or contamination of the solution. TPN should be used cautiously among immunocompromised patients.

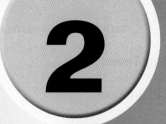

2

Acute Abdomen

Brandon Marr, Amanda Bailey,
Syed Hashmi, and Muhammad Nazim

SEVERE ABDOMINAL PAIN

I. Definition

A. Acute abdomen is defined as severe, persistent abdominal pain, usually of sudden onset, that is likely to require surgical intervention to treat its cause. Although the severity of the pain is a guide to its seriousness, it is critical to decide which patients need surgery because not all of them require an operation to treat their pain.

B. It is one of the most common reasons for presentation to emergency departments and physician offices.

II. Embryology of the Gastrointestinal Tract

A. The organs of the gastrointestinal (GI) tract are externally lined by a layer of mesodermally derived cells called the visceral peritoneum.

B. This is continuous with the inner layer of the abdominal wall called the parietal peritoneum.

C. The GI tract is divided by blood supply into three areas:

1. Foregut: consists of the oropharynx down to the proximal duodenum and includes the pancreas, liver, biliary tract, and spleen. Its blood supply is the celiac axis. It elicits pain in the periumbilical area.

2. Midgut: consists of the distal duodenum down to the proximal two-thirds of the transverse colon. Its blood supply is the superior mesenteric artery. It elicits pain in the periumbilical area.

3. Hindgut: consists of the colon and rectum. It is supplied by the inferior mesenteric artery. It elicits pain in the suprapubic area.

III. Physiology of Abdominal Pain

A. Visceral pain: due to stimuli affecting the visceral peritoneum (overlying the organs of the GI tract)

1. It is mediated by the autonomic nervous system and appreciated at the level of the thalamus.

2. It is stimulated by pulling, stretching, distention, or spasm. It is not stimulated by touch or heat.

3. Chemical stimuli, including substance P, serotonin, prostaglandins, and hydrogen ions, can also cause pain by stimulating the visceral chemoreceptors.

4. Pain is often a dull ache and is poorly localized. It is frequently described in the midline because of the bilateral innervation of the viscera. Because it is not affected by movement, patients are often restless.

B. Parietal pain: pain appreciated in the parietal peritoneum covering the abdominal cavity, which is innervated by peripheral nervous system

1. These stimuli are transmitted by the central nervous system and are interpreted at a specific cortical level.

2. It is induced by touch, pressure, heat, and inflammation.

3. Localized by great accuracy, it is often described as sharp or cutting. Pain is affected by movement, so patients tend to lie still.

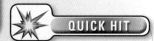

Pain in the foregut is usually felt in the epigastrium.

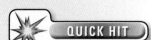

Pain located in the midgut is felt in the periumbilical region.

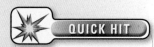

Hindgut pain is usually felt in the suprapubic area.

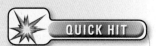

The vagus nerves do not transmit pain from the gut.

C. Referred pain: pain felt at a site distant from the diseased organ but sharing a common development

1. Splenic disease is felt at the tip of the left shoulder because splenic pathology irritates the diaphragm, which is supplied by the phrenic nerve. The phrenic nerve itself comes from the trunks of the fourth cervical nerve, and pain in its distribution is felt in the skin distribution of the fourth cervical nerve.
2. Right subscapular pain is the referred site of pain due to biliary colic or perforated ulcer.
3. Back pain often occurs with patients with pancreatitis or ruptured aortic aneurysms.

D. Combined pain: Visceral and parietal pain can often be combined when there is an alteration of the relationship and proximity of the two types of peritoneum.

1. Contact between an organ with inflamed visceral peritoneum and its pain-sensitive parietal peritoneum results in the perception of pain over the site of the parietal peritoneum.
2. Rebound tenderness is appreciated when an examiner presses down on the patient and then let go to see if this movement elicits pain. By doing this, the examiner alters the relationship between the two peritoneal surfaces and attempts to elicit contact between the parietal peritoneum and the visceral peritoneum.

IV. Etiology and Pathology of Abdominal Pain

A. Etiology: Sources of abdominal pain are listed in Table 2-1. The most common causes of acute abdominal pain requiring hospital admission include:

1. Acute appendicitis. Ex: 19-year-old woman with right lower quadrant (RLQ) pain × 3 days, nausea/vomiting (N/V), decreased appetite, increased white blood cell count (WBC), fever. + McBurney point. Tx: laparoscopic appendectomy and antibiotics.
2. Acute cholecystitis. Ex: 35-year-old obese woman with sharp right upper quadrant (RUQ) pain that radiates to her back for 4 days. + fever, + N/V, pain worse with food. Exam shows RUQ tenderness, + Murphy sign. Leukocytosis, elevated alkaline phosphate (ALP) and liver enzymes. Ultrasound with pericholecystic fluid and gallstones. Tx: antibiotics and laparoscopic cholecystectomy.
3. Small bowel obstruction. Ex: 30-year-old man with diffuse crampy abdominal pain × 5 days, N/V, unable to tolerate oral intake, no bowel movement (BM) or flatus for 5 days. History of ex-lap for trauma. Exam shows abdominal distention, hyperactive bowel sounds, tympany to percussion. Tx: nasogastric (NG) tube and nothing by mouth (NPO) for medical management, OR for complete obstruction.
4. Pain from genitourinary organs. Ex: 18-year-old female escort with abdominal pain, vaginal discharge, fever. Lower abdominal tenderness, cervical tenderness on pelvic exam. Leukocytosis.
5. Acute pancreatitis. Ex: 56-year-old man with stabbing epigastric pain radiation to back for 1 day + fever + N/V, no appetite + binge drinking. Exams shows epigastric tenderness. Leukocytosis, elevated lipase and amylase, hyponatremia. Tx: NPO, intravenous (IV) fluids, total parenteral nutrition (TPN).

TABLE 2-1   Sources of Abdominal Pain

Abdominal
- Abdominal wall
- Intraperitoneal organs
- Retroperitoneal organs and tissues
- Pelvic organs

Extra-abdominal
- Intrathoracic organs
- Systemic dysfunction
- Functional abdominal pain

Reprinted with permission from Sterns EE. *Clinical Thinking in Surgery*. Norwalk, CT: Appleton & Lange; 1988.

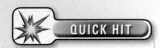

B. Pathology
    1. Peritonitis is intra-abdominal inflammation.
        a. Inflammation of the peritoneal cavity causes increased secretion of fluid containing protein and leukocytes into the peritoneal cavity.
        b. Ongoing inflammation leads to increased secretion and resultant hypotension.
        c. If peritoneal defenses are adequate, an exudate is formed that causes adherence between bowel loops or omentum to wall off the area of inflammation, causing an intra-abdominal abscess, which causes localized findings on examination. If these defenses are overwhelmed, there is diffuse peritonitis, which usually requires surgery.
        d. Intra-abdominal pain can have extra-abdominal pathology. Ex: pneumonia.
    2. Types of peritonitis
        a. Primary or spontaneous peritonitis is inflammation of the peritoneum from a source outside the abdomen. For instance, cirrhotic patients can develop spontaneous bacterial peritonitis.
        b. Secondary peritonitis is inflammation of the peritoneum from an intra-abdominal pathology, such as perforation of the appendix causing appendicitis.
        c. Tertiary peritonitis is the persistent and ongoing infection that results after inadequate treatment for secondary peritonitis.

V. Diagnosis of Abdominal Pain

A. A systemic approach is critical in diagnosing abdominal pain, starting with a thorough history, physical examination, laboratory testing, and then radiologic testing as needed.
B. History (Table 2-2)
    1. With regard to the pain, it is critical to document:
        a. Location: assists in defining the anatomic area that may be involved in the disease (Table 2-3)
        b. Nature of the pain: dull pain more likely to be visceral, whereas sharp pain more likely to be parietal pain
        c. Mode of onset and duration: Sudden sharp, severe pain with hypotension suggests a surgical emergency such as perforated ulcer or a rupture of an abdominal aortic aneurysm. Progressive pain over a few hours to days is more consistent with a process, such as appendicitis or bowel obstruction.
        d. Quality and intensity
        e. Exacerbating or relieving factors, such as relation to meals (e.g., exacerbation of RUQ pain by fatty foods is suggestive of cholelithiasis)

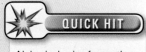

TABLE 2-2   Key Historical Features in Acute Abdominal Pain
Age
Time and mode of onset of pain
Duration of symptoms
Character of pain
Location of pain and site(s) of radiation
Associated symptoms and their relation to pain
Nausea or anorexia
Vomiting
Diarrhea or constipation
Menstrual history

Reprinted with permission from Mulholland MW, Lillemoe KD, Doherty GM, Maier RW, Upchurch GR Jr, eds. *Greenfield's Surgery: Scientific Principles and Practice.* 4th ed. Baltimore, MD: Lippincott Williams & Wilkins; 2006:1210.

TABLE 2-3 Most Common Causes of Pain by Quadrants

Right Upper Quadrant Pain	Left Upper Quadrant Pain
Biliary tract disease	Splenic disease
Liver disease	Perforated gastric ulcer
Pulmonary disease	Pulmonary disease
Renal disease	Myocardial infarction

Right Lower Quadrant Pain	Left Lower Quadrant Pain
Appendicitis	Colonic disease
Renal disease	Renal disease
Pelvic inflammatory disease	Pelvic inflammatory disease
Ovarian torsion	Ovarian torsion

    f. Radiation: Flank pain going to the groin is suggestive of renal calculus disease, whereas RLQ pain going to the back is more suggestive of appendicitis.

    g. Associated factors: anorexia, nausea, vomiting, or change in bowel habits in relation to the pain

      (1) Most patients with abdominal pain of surgical causes lose their appetite.

      (2) In surgical patients, vomiting usually follows the development of abdominal pain, unlike patients with medical conditions such as gastroenteritis. It is important to characterize the vomitus.

        (a) Bilious vomiting suggests an obstruction distal to ampulla of Vater.

        (b) Feculent or foul-smelling vomiting suggests a long-standing small bowel obstruction.

      (3) Change in bowel habits can also give clues to the etiology of abdominal pain. Progressive constipation suggests an obstruction.

  2. Other important historical factors are:

    a. In women: thorough menstrual history

    b. Timing of the last meal: This affects anesthetic management.

    c. Past medical history and surgical history

    d. Review of current medications is also essential.

      (1) If patients are taking steroids, the immunosuppressive effects can modify the inflammatory reaction such that these patients may have minimal findings on examination. They require steroid supplementation if an operation is planned to prevent adrenal insufficiency.

      (2) Anticoagulants may cause bleeding.

    e. Family history (e.g., patients with familial Mediterranean fever or acute porphyria may have recurrent attacks of abdominal pain)

    f. Social history, including substance abuse. Cocaine can cause visceral ischemia.

C. Physical examination

  1. Vital signs

    a. Elevated temperatures are rare in most surgical patients. They are more common in patients with urinary tract infection or gynecologic pathology.

    b. Tachycardia or hypotension suggests significant volume deficits and an aggressive disease process.

  2. Observe and inspect the patient.

    a. Start by observing the patient's position in bed: Patients with renal colic are restless, whereas patients with perforation and peritonitis tend to lie still because movement irritates the parietal peritoneum.

    b. Inspect the abdomen for distention, scars, hernias, or masses.

    c. Auscultate the abdomen, which allows for the detection of bowel sounds, but also to listen for abdominal bruits.

   d. Palpate the abdomen.

     (1) Should be gentle and start away from the area of pain

     (2) Should include all four quadrants and search for hernias (see Table 2-3)

     (3) Assess for presence of guarding (when patient resists movement by tensing abdominal muscles) and rebound tenderness. Percussion of the abdomen is also a useful adjunct because it is a more gentle way to elicit rebound tenderness.

   e. Perform a rectal examination to assess for blood, masses, and tenderness.

   f. Perform a gynecologic examination to assess for tenderness in the adnexa, cervical discharge, and ovarian enlargement.

   g. Elderly, alcoholic, or immunosuppressed patients may have minimal findings on physical examination despite having serious illness.

   h. Special signs

     (1) Murphy sign: Right subcostal pain upon palpation with an inspiratory arrest is elicited by having patient take a deep breath and is suggestive of acute cholecystitis.

     (2) Rovsing sign: Palpation of the left lower quadrant causes pain in the RLQ and is suggestive of acute appendicitis.

     (3) Iliopsoas sign: pain of passively extending the hip, suggestive of acute appendicitis

     (4) Obturator sign: pain on internal or external rotation of the flexed hip, suggestive of acute appendicitis

D. Laboratory tests

  1. Assist in diagnosis but rarely provide it

  2. Include the following:

   a. Complete blood count, which allows assessment of inflammation and anemia

   b. Serum electrolytes can be altered in patients who have been vomiting or who are dehydrated.

   c. Serum amylase lipase levels in patients suspected of having pancreatitis, where the serum lipase is more sensitive. These can also be elevated in conditions other than pancreatitis, such as small bowel infarction.

   d. Liver function tests, which include bilirubin, alkaline phosphatase, and serum transaminases in patients with RUQ pain

   e. Human chorionic gonadotropin in all women of childbearing age

   f. Urinalysis in all patients to check for blood or urinary tract infection

   g. Electrocardiogram (EKG) in patients with heart disease because myocardial infarction can be confused with abdominal pain

E. Radiologic studies

  1. An important adjunct to clinical diagnosis

  2. X-rays are useful as a screening tool, and three X-rays are usually taken.

   a. Chest X-ray to look for free air suggestive of visceral perforation or pneumonia causing abdominal pain

   b. Abdominal X-ray (erect and supine views) to look for:

     (1) Free air, which suggests perforation of a viscus (Fig. 2-1)

     (2) Air–fluid levels suggestive of bowel obstruction

     (3) Abnormal calcification: 90% of renal calculi, and 10% of gallstone calculi have enough calcium to be detected by X-rays. If it is not possible to take upright films, lateral decubitus films can be done to look for free air.

  3. Ultrasound

   a. Allows low-cost evaluation of patient with abdominal pain

   b. Best used to detect liver, gallbladder, or gynecologic pathology

   c. Is both operator and patient dependent (difficult to obtain good windows in the obese)

  4. Computed tomography (CT) scans

   a. Allows anatomical evaluation of the patient with abdominal pain

   b. Usually done with oral and IV contrast (CT scans for renal calculi are done without contrast)

FIGURE 2-1 Example of free air under the diaphragm.

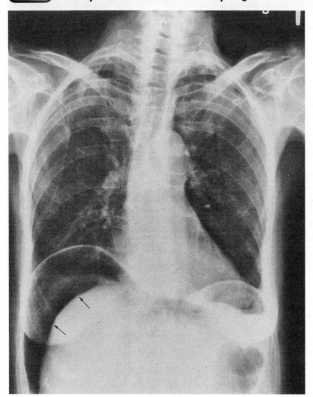

(Reprinted with permission from Blackbourne LH. *Surgical Recall*. 4th ed. Baltimore, MD: Lippincott Williams & Wilkins; 2006:185.)

    c. CT improves diagnostic accuracy but may not need to be performed in all patients.

    d. IV contrast may be contraindicated if there is history of anaphylaxis or renal disease.

  5. Other tests, such as hydroxy-iminodiacetic acid (HIDA) scans, are performed more selectively depending on clinical circumstances (Tables 2-4 to 2-6).

VI. Management

  A. It is critical to decide whether a patient needs an operation and when he or she needs it.

  B. Patients who will probably need an operation include:

    1. Patients with peritoneal signs such as tenderness, guarding, or rebound

    2. Patients with sepsis or worsening abdominal pain

    3. Patients with free air

    4. Patients with hemodynamic instability

  C. If signs are equivocal, patients can be admitted and observed for progression of pain.

TABLE 2-4 Conditions Characterized by Diffuse Abdominal Pain

Peritonitis
Mesenteric ischemia
Diabetic ketoacidosis
Uremia

TABLE 2-5 Most Common Causes of Midline Abdominal Pain
Epigastric
Peptic ulcer Pancreatitis Myocardial ischemia Cholecystitis
Periumbilical
Early appendicitis Intestinal obstruction Pancreatitis Ruptured abdominal aortic aneurysm
Infraumbilical
Appendicitis Diverticulitis Ovarian torsion Cystitis

D. Preparation for an operation involves:
1. Fluid hydration
2. Making sure that the patient is nil per os (NPO), or nothing by mouth
3. Analgesia
4. Antibiotics, depending on circumstances
5. Consent

TABLE 2-6 Warning Signs in Patients with Abdominal Pain
History
Severe, sudden, sharp continuous pain Elderly Immunosuppressed
Physical Examination
Changes in vital signs, especially tachycardia or hypotension Hypoxia Altered mentation Peritoneal signs, especially a rigid abdomen Abdominal pain out of proportion to physical findings
Laboratory Testing
Anemia Leukocytosis Renal failure Acidosis Elevated liver enzymes
Radiology
Free air (pneumoperitoneum) Bowel obstruction with air–fluid levels Air in the portal venous system

Adapted with permission from Flasar MH, Goldberg E. Acute abdominal pain. *Med Clin North Am.* 2006;90:481–503.

E. Choice of an operation is up to the operating surgeon.
   1. Laparotomy involves open exploration of the abdominal contents.
   2. Laparoscopy involves using a laparoscope to evaluate intra-abdominal contents in a less invasive fashion.

VII. Special Patient Populations

A. Pregnant women
   1. Acute abdominal pain can also occur during pregnancy.
   2. Cholecystitis and gallstone pancreatitis can also complicate pregnancy.
      a. Gallstone pancreatitis has significant increased morbidity to fetus.
      b. Laparoscopic cholecystectomy can be performed in any trimester.
   3. Appendicitis complicates 1 in 1,500 pregnancies.
      a. This condition is difficult to diagnose because the enlarging uterus may push the appendix laterally into the flank or RUQ.
      b. Ultrasound can aid in diagnosis, and it also prevents radiation exposure.
      c. Laparoscopic appendectomy can be performed in any trimester.
B. Geriatric patients
   1. One-third of all geriatric patients with acute abdominal pain require surgical intervention.
   2. These patients have more medical conditions.
   3. There is a higher rate of misdiagnosis due to subtle or confusing presentations.
   4. Objective findings may or may not be present.
   5. Medication can alter response to pain or alter the examination, such as beta-blockers blunting the tachycardia of the stress response.
   6. It is essential to perform a thorough examination and obtain an EKG to evaluate for myocardial ischemia.
   7. The threshold for intervention should be low.
C. Immunosuppressed individuals
   1. Patient populations who may have varying degrees of immunosuppression include:
      a. Elderly
      b. Those who are malnourished
      c. Those with diabetes
      d. Those with renal failure
      e. Those with a current malignancy, especially if they are on chemotherapy
      f. Those who are on immunosuppressive medications such as steroids, chemotherapy agents, and antirejection medicines for transplants
      g. Those with HIV and CD4 counts less than 200/mL
   2. Symptoms are vague, and the threshold for intervention needs to be high.
   3. Causes are likely to be either unusual fungal infections or unusual tumors.
   4. Common diseases are GI non-Hodgkin lymphoma, acute appendicitis, cytomegalovirus colitis, and mycobacterium intracellular colitis.
D. Patients with medical conditions
   1. Some conditions may complicate evaluation of abdominal pain and should be considered in the differential diagnosis.
   2. Urinary tract infection may mimic appendicitis, which is why it is critical to do a urinalysis on all patients.
   3. Patients with pneumonia may complain of right or left upper quadrant pain.
   4. History and physical examination assist in diagnosing these conditions.
E. Abdominal pain in women
   1. Relation to menstrual cycle: Evaluate for ectopic pregnancy.
   2. Vaginal discharge and sexual activity: Evaluate for pelvic inflammatory disease (PID).
   3. Evaluate for tubo-ovarian abscess (TOA).
   4. Evaluate for ovarian torsion.

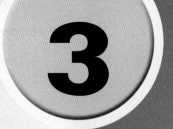

3 Trauma and Burns

Alison Wilson, Daniel Rossi, Jorge Con, and James Bardes

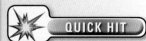

Airway and breathing are the most important priorities in the trauma patient. Facial fractures and injuries can severely compromise and complicate the airway.

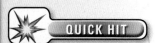

Signs and symptoms of airway compromise include stridor, hoarseness, subcutaneous emphysema, obvious fractures, noisy breathing, and displacement of the trachea.

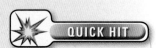

Definition of shock: end organ dysfunction due to inadequate oxygenation and perfusion.

I. General Principles

A. Primary survey: Life-threatening conditions are quickly identified and managed (see Clinical Pearl 3-1).

1. Airway: Is patient talking? Is air being moved?
   a. Airway protection is needed in patients with the following conditions:
      (1) Decreased level of consciousness (Glasgow Coma Scale [GCS] ≤8)
      (2) Severe maxillofacial fractures
      (3) Risk of aspiration such as bleeding or vomiting
      (4) Risk of obstruction such as stridor, neck hematoma, or laryngeal or tracheal injury
   b. Management
      (1) Airway maintenance techniques include chin lift, jaw thrust, oropharyngeal airway, and nasopharyngeal airway.
      (2) Definitive airway: endotracheal/nasotracheal intubation, cricothyroidotomy, tracheostomy
2. Breathing and ventilation
   a. Ensure adequate gas exchange: lungs, chest wall, diaphragm
   b. Management
      (1) Chest tube for pneumothorax
      (2) Bag valve mask/mechanical ventilation
3. Circulation and bleeding: pulse exam. Check blood pressure.
   a. Hemorrhagic shock (Table 3-1)
   b. Nonhemorrhagic shock
      (1) Cardiogenic shock: myocardial dysfunction from blunt cardiac injury, myocardial infarction
      (2) Obstructive shock: obstruction to normal flow, causing inadequate perfusion
         (a) Cardiac tamponade
         (b) Tension pneumothorax
         (c) Pulmonary embolism
      (3) Neurogenic shock: loss of sympathetic tone, causing hypotension without tachycardia
      (4) Septic shock: very unlikely in setting of acute trauma (see Clinical Pearl 3-2)

CLINICAL PEARL 3-1

Primary Survey

- A = Airway maintenance with cervical spine immobilization
- B = Breathing and ventilation
- C = Circulation with hemorrhage control
- D = Disability: neurologic status
- E = Exposure/environment control: undress patient; then prevent hypothermia

---

TABLE 3-1 Categories of Hypovolemic Shock

	Class I	Class II	Class III	Class IV
Blood loss (mL)	Up to 750	750–1,500	1,500–2,000	>2,000
Blood loss (% blood volume)	Up to 15%	15%–30%	30%–40%	>40%
Pulse rate	<100 bpm	>100 bpm	>120 bpm	>140 bpm
Blood pressure	Normal	Normal	Decreased	Decreased
Urine output (mL/hr)	>30	20–30	5–15	None
Mental status	Normal	Anxious	Confused	Lethargic

B. Secondary survey
1. Done only after primary survey is completed and life-threatening conditions have been addressed
2. Complete history and head-to-toe physical exam
3. History includes AMPLE: allergies, medications, past illness, last meal, and events

II. Head and Neck
A. Traumatic brain injury
1. Anatomy and physiology (see Clinical Pearl 3-3)
   a. The scalp is very vascular and can be a source of significant blood loss.
   b. Cerebral perfusion pressure (CPP) is the mean arterial pressure (MAP) minus the intracranial pressure (ICP).
   c. The carotid and vertebral arteries enter at the base of the skull, and an injury to these vessels could further lead to ischemic/embolic injury to the brain.
   d. The third cranial nerve runs along the edge of the tentorium and is compressed with temporal herniation, causing pupillary dilatation.
2. Assessment
   a. The GCS is used to quickly assess for severity (Fig. 3-1).
   b. Types of head injury
      (1) Skull fracture requires significant force and increases the risk of an underlying brain injury.
      (2) Physical signs associated with basal skull fractures are periorbital ecchymosis (raccoon eyes), retroauricular ecchymosis (Battle sign), and rhinorrhea (cerebrospinal fluid [CSF] leakage from the nose).
      (3) Intracranial lesions can be focal or diffuse, although both commonly occur together.
         (a) Diffuse injuries include hypoxia or ischemia.
            i. Computed tomography (CT) scan of the brain may appear normal or diffusely swollen.
            ii. Diffuse axonal injury includes punctuate hemorrhages throughout both hemispheres, primarily at the gray–white matter junction.
         (b) Focal injuries
            i. Epidural hematomas are usually located in temporal regions outside the dura and are biconvex in shape. Usually, they are a result of a tear in the middle meningeal artery.

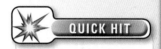

QUICK HIT

The primary focus in caring for patients with severe brain injury is to prevent secondary injury. Secondary injury is caused by hypoxia and hypotension.

Trauma and Burns

CLINICAL PEARL 3-2

Hypovolemic Shock from Bleeding

- Most common cause of shock in trauma patient
- Management consists of bleeding control and replenishing intravascular volume.
- Patients in shock will need adequate IV access for resuscitation with blood products and crystalloids.
- Definitive control of bleeding often requires an operation.

CLINICAL PEARL 3-3

Monro-Kellie Doctrine

- The skull is a confined space that contains the brain, CSF, and blood.
- Intracranial hemorrhage or brain swelling occupy additional volume inside the skull.
- Initially, venous blood and CSF can be compressed out, allowing for a small degree of pressure buffering.
- Once ICP rises, it can result in decreased blood flow to the brain and ultimately in herniation.

    ii. Subdural hematomas are a result of a tearing of the small sur-face vessels of the cortex. They are crescent shaped and can cover the entire surface of the hemisphere.

    (4) Contusions and intracerebral hematomas can evolve with time and therefore are best detected by follow-up CT scan at 12 to 24 hours.

3. Management of traumatic brain injuries
   a. Management of traumatic brain injuries consists of minimizing secondary insults to the injured brain such as hypoxia and hypoperfusion.
   b. Mild injuries to the brain (GCS 13 to 15) are often characterized by disorientation and/or a brief loss of consciousness in a patient who is now talking and appropriate.
      (1) Management of these patients usually consists of a brief period of observation to ensure that the exam does not worsen. Alcohol and other substances can often confound this picture.
      (2) The term "concussion" is often used when there are mild neurologic findings, such as loss of consciousness or nausea, in the setting where the CT scan is normal. By consensus, it is broadly defined as a complex pathophysiologic process affecting the brain, induced by traumatic bio-mechanical forces.
   c. More severe injuries require an evaluation with a CT scan and a neurosurgery consultation.
      (1) Early endotracheal intubation should be performed in patients with severe injuries (GCS ≤8) to protect the airway and ensure adequate oxygenation and ventilation.
      (2) Hypotension causes a secondary insult to the brain and increases the mortality, so causes for hypotension such as bleeding must be addressed quickly.

FIGURE 3-1   Glasgow Coma Scale.

Eye Opening	
Spontaneous	4
To speech	3
To pain	2
None	1
Verbal Response	
Oriented	5
Confused	4
Inappropriate words	3
Moans	2
None	1
Motor Response	
Follows commands	6
Localizes pain	5
Withdrawals	4
Decorticate (Flexion)	3
Decerebrate (Extension)	2
None	1

Note: Glasgow Coma Scale score = E + V + M; minimum score is 3, maximum is 15.

(3) A mass effect causing a midline shift of 5 mm or greater seen on the CT often indicates the need for emergency craniotomy and decompression.

(4) ICP monitoring may be indicated in patients with a GCS ≤8.

(5) Increased ICPs require therapy. These may include mannitol, hypertonic saline, diuretics, sedation, barbiturates, or CSF drainage via ventriculostomy or surgical decompression.

B. Facial trauma

1. Neurologic, airway, and ocular examinations are important.
2. Mandible and midface fractures can compromise the airway.
3. Orbital wall and sinus fractures may cause muscle entrapment or nerve injury.
4. Parotid duct injuries can occur with lateral facial lacerations.

C. Neck

1. Zones of the neck
   a. Zone I: thoracic outlet, cricoid cartilage down to the clavicle
   b. Zone II: cricoid cartilage up to the angle of the mandible
   c. Zone III: angle of the mandible to the base of the skull
2. Diagnosis and evaluation
   a. Ensure adequate airway and breathing while maintaining cervical immobilization.
   b. Nowadays, the CT scan is usually the choice for the initial evaluation of hemodynamically stable patients with zone I or III injuries. Traditional tests were arteriography, endoscopy of the airway and esophagus, and barium swallow.
   c. Penetrating injuries to zone II that violate the platysma often require an operative exploration.

D. Spine and spinal cord injuries

1. Anatomy
   a. Spinal column consists of 7 cervical, 12 thoracic, and 5 lumbar vertebrae.
   b. There are three ligaments that stabilize the spine. The anterior and posterior longitudinal ligaments flank the body of the spine. The ligamentum flavum travels along the laminae of adjacent vertebrae.
   c. Cervical spine is most prone to injury.
   d. The presence of one fracture increases the risk of having other fractures along the spine. Imaging of the entire spine is mandatory to look for them (see Clinical Pearl 3-4).
2. Examination: The examination consists of a sensory examination, including pain, temperature, proprioception, vibration, and light touch, as well as the motor examination throughout all dermatomes and myotomes (Table 3-2).
3. Classification of spinal cord injury
   a. Level: defined at the most caudal segment of the spinal cord with normal sensory and motor function on both sides of the body
   b. Severity
      (1) Injuries are defined as incomplete paraplegia, complete paraplegia, incomplete quadriplegia, and complete quadriplegia.
      (2) Signs of incomplete injury include the following:
         (a) Sacral sparing: perianal sensation or voluntary anal sphincter contraction
         (b) Voluntary movement or sensation distal to the injury

> **QUICK HIT**
>
> All patients with a radiographic abnormality, neurologic deficit, or decreased level of consciousness should be considered to have an unstable spine and should be completely immobilized.

Trauma and Burns

CLINICAL PEARL 3-4

Imaging of the Spine

- The CT scan has a high sensitivity for fractures of the spine.
- Plain films of the cervical spine will miss up to two out of three fractures in adults.
- Flexion and extension plain films of the spine may be useful in determining ligamentous instability.
- MRI is used to evaluate for ligamentous injuries and for spinal cord injuries.

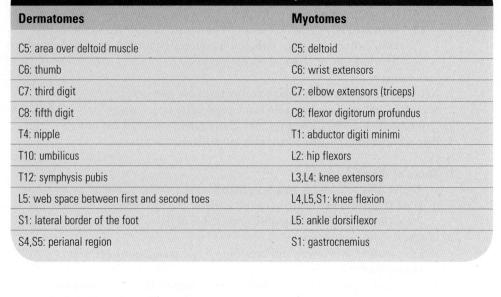

Dermatomes	Myotomes
C5: area over deltoid muscle	C5: deltoid
C6: thumb	C6: wrist extensors
C7: third digit	C7: elbow extensors (triceps)
C8: fifth digit	C8: flexor digitorum profundus
T4: nipple	T1: abductor digiti minimi
T10: umbilicus	L2: hip flexors
T12: symphysis pubis	L3,L4: knee extensors
L5: web space between first and second toes	L4,L5,S1: knee flexion
S1: lateral border of the foot	L5: ankle dorsiflexor
S4,S5: perianal region	S1: gastrocnemius

TABLE 3-2 Nerve Root Association with Myotomes and Dermatomes

4. Spinal cord syndromes
   a. Central cord syndrome shows greater motor loss in upper versus lower extremities with various sensory losses and is often seen with hyperextension injury in a patient with preexisting cervical canal stenosis.
   b. Anterior cord syndrome includes paraplegia with loss of pain and temperature but preserved position, vibration, and deep pressure. Usually due to infarction of anterior spinal artery.
   c. Brown–Sequard syndrome is caused by hemisection of the cord, resulting in ipsilateral motor loss and proprioception with contralateral loss of pain and temperature.
5. Other specific injuries
   a. Atlanto-occipital dislocation is usually fatal due to brain stem injury. Survivors tend to be quadriplegic and ventilator dependent.
   b. C1 fracture/Jefferson fracture is a burst fracture of the ring often not associated with spinal cord injury.
   c. C2 fracture is a hangman's fracture involving posterior elements of C2.
   d. Spinal cord injury without radiographic abnormality (SCIWORA) can present more commonly in the pediatric population given the greater flexibility of their ligaments and joint capsules.
   e. Chance fractures are transverse fractures through the lumbar vertebral body.
      (1) Often associated with lap belt
      (2) High association with retroperitoneal and bowel injuries
6. Management
   a. Maintain in-line stabilization in all trauma patients until spine injury is ruled out, either clinically or with radiographic images.
   b. Unstable spine fractures consist in stabilization either with a brace or with surgery to avoid damage to the spinal cord.
   c. Treatment of spinal cord injury consists of stabilizing the spine to avoid additional mechanical injury while minimizing secondary insults such as hypoxia and hypoperfusion.
   d. In the past, methylprednisolone given within 8 hours of injury was standard. Now, no longer standard, it is used in select circumstances of high spinal cord injuries.

III. Thoracic Trauma
A. Chest wall trauma and pulmonary contusion
   1. Sternal, multiple rib, and scapular fractures often result from a large force and can be indicative of underlying cardiac or pulmonary contusions.

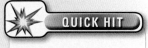

QUICK HIT

Complete imaging of the spine is mandatory in all patients with a spine fracture.

2. Pain from rib fractures can impair oxygenation and ventilation, and management consists in providing adequate analgesia and pulmonary care.
   a. Mild rib fractures may be managed with oral analgesics, whereas more severe ones may require an intravenous route or even an epidural.
3. Flail chest occurs when more than two ribs are fractured in two or more places.
   a. Paradoxical movement of the chest when breathing
   b. Primary problem is severe pulmonary contusion
4. Pulmonary contusion can impair gas exchange and cause respiratory failure.
   a. Managed with supportive care and avoiding fluid overload
   b. Sometimes requires mechanical ventilation

B. Hemothorax
   1. Can be from blunt or penetrating trauma
      a. Intercostal arterial injury can result from a blunt force to the ribs.
      b. Massive hemothorax suggests possibility of injury to great vessels, hilum, or heart.
   2. Treatment
      a. Chest tube in fifth intercostal space
      b. Chest tube output is an indication for emergency operative intervention.
         (1) Greater than 1,500 mL immediately when chest tube placed
         (2) Evidence of ongoing bleeding
         (3) Greater than 200 mL/hr over 4 hours

C. Pneumothorax
   1. Simple pneumothorax
      a. Diagnosed on chest X-ray (CXR); sometimes see a deep sulcus sign
      b. Can convert to tension pneumothorax if untreated
      c. Treatment: chest tube placed in fifth intercostal space
   2. Open pneumothorax is a sucking chest wound.
      a. Large defect in chest wall causing equilibration between intrathoracic and atmospheric pressure
      b. Cover defect and tape on three sides to allow for air to escape on fourth side.
      c. Place chest tube.

D. Tracheobronchial tree injuries are injuries to trachea or bronchus.
   1. Blunt trauma injury usually occurs within 1 inch of the carina.
   2. Signs and symptoms: hemoptysis; tension pneumothorax; pneumothorax with massive air leak; CXR with completely collapsed, nonventilated lung
   3. Diagnosis is made with bronchoscopy.
   4. Treatment is to intubate mainstem bronchus of opposite lung.
      a. Place chest tube on affected side.
      b. Immediate surgical intervention

E. Cardiac tamponade
   1. Pericardium fills with blood, preventing cardiac filling and constricting the heart, causing hemodynamic collapse. Penetrating trauma is a more common cause.
   2. Signs
      a. Beck triad: elevated central venous pressure, decreased blood pressure, and muffled heart tones
      b. Kussmaul sign: rise in venous pressure with inspiration when breathing spontaneously
   3. Transthoracic ultrasound has high sensitivity.
   4. Treatment
      a. Fluid bolus to help venous return and cardiac output
      b. Temporizing maneuver is with pericardiocentesis.
      c. Operative repair is with thoracotomy or median sternotomy, depending on injury.

F. Blunt cardiac injury
   1. Etiology: can result from myocardial muscle contusion, valve disruption, and chamber rupture

2. Signs and symptoms
   a. Most common presentation is arrhythmias.
   b. Pump failure, leading to low cardiac output, respiratory distress
3. Diagnosis
   a. Twelve-lead electrocardiogram: If any new abnormalities, patient should be monitored for 24 hours.
   b. Common dysrhythmias include premature ventricular contractions and right bundle branch block, and may progress to ventricular tachycardia.
   c. Patient may show ischemic changes.
   d. An echocardiogram may show wall dysfunction.
4. Treatment is supportive. Inotropes, diuretics, antiarrhythmics, and a balloon pump may be needed.

G. Traumatic aortic injury
   1. This is a common cause of sudden death after deceleration blunt injury. There is a transection of the aorta at the ligamentum arteriosum (distal to the left subclavian artery).
   2. Diagnosis and management
      a. CXR: wide mediastinum (Fig. 3-2)
      b. Arteriography or helical contrast-enhanced CT
      c. Some require endovascular or open repair.

H. Esophageal injuries
   1. Signs and symptoms
      a. An early sign or symptom is a left pneumothorax without a rib fracture, particulate matter in chest tube, or mediastinal air.
      b. May present late as septic shock
   2. Diagnosis (both of these are required to complete the workup)
      a. Esophagoscopy
      b. Gastrografin swallow
   3. Treatment
      a. Broad-spectrum antibiotics
      b. Early treatment includes primary repair and drainage.
      c. Late treatment includes wide pleural drainage and cervical esophagostomy.

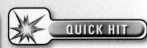

QUICK HIT

Signs of possible traumatic aortic injury on CXR: wide mediastinum, obliteration of aortic knob, deviation of trachea to the right, obliteration of aortopulmonary window, depression of left mainstem bronchus, deviation of esophagus to right, wide paratracheal stripe, and pleural cap.

FIGURE 3-2 Plain CXR demonstrating signs of traumatic aortic injury. Note the wide mediastinum, esophageal deviation, and blurring of the aortic knob.

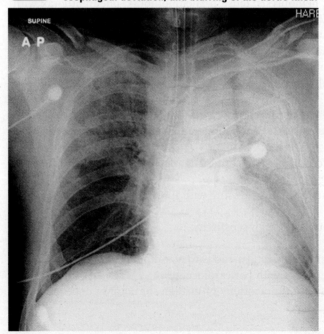

(Reprinted with permission from Mulholland MW, Lillemoe KD, Doherty GM, Maier RV, Upchurch GR, eds. *Greenfield's Surgery: Scientific Principles and Practice.* 4th ed. Philadelphia, PA: Lippincott Williams & Wilkins; 2006.)

TABLE 3-3 Modalities to Evaluate for Abdominal Trauma	FAST	DPL	CT
Sensitivity for solid organ injury	42%–97%	90%–95%	100%
Specificity for solid organ injury	48%–98%	96%–100%	97%
Evaluation of the retroperitoneum	(−)	(−)	(+ +)
Suitable for nonresponders/transient responders	(+ +)	(+)	(−)

Becker A, Ling G, McKenney MG, et al. Is the FAST exam reliable in severely injured patients? *Injury.* 2010;41(5): 479–483.

Miller MT, Pasquale MD, Bromberg W, et al. Not so FAST. *J Trauma.* 2003;54(1):52–60.

Nagy KK, Roberts RR, Joseph KT, et al. Experience with over 2500 diagnostic peritoneal lavages. *Injury.* 2000;31:479–482.

Wing WV, Federle MP, Morris JA, et al. The clinical impact of CT for blunt abdominal trauma. *AJR.* 1985;145(6):1191–1194.

IV. Abdomen/Pelvis

A. Evaluation (Table 3-3)

1. Blunt force injury

a. Hemodynamically stable indicates CT abdomen/pelvis, serial abdominal exams, and focused abdominal sonography in trauma (FAST) (Fig. 3-3).

b. Hemodynamically unstable indicates laparotomy, FAST, and diagnostic peritoneal lavage (DPL).

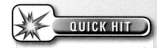

QUICK HIT

Criteria for positive DPL: gross = >10 mL blood, particulate matter; microscopic = >100,000 RBC/hpf, >500 WBC/hpf, bacteria.

Trauma and Burns

FIGURE 3-3 Positive FAST exam. Note that blood appears as a dark stripe around the liver.

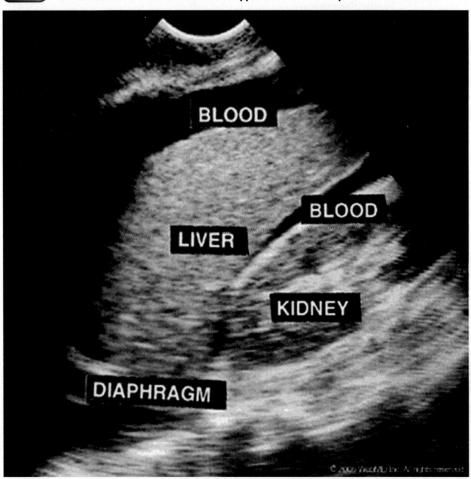

(*ACS Surgery: Principles and Practice,* Chapter 701: Initial Management of Life-Threatening Trauma.)

Trauma and Burns

2. Penetrating injury
   a. Hemodynamically stable
      (1) Stab wound includes local wound exploration, serial abdominal examinations, and laparotomy.
      (2) Gunshot wound usually requires a laparotomy.
   b. Hemodynamically unstable indicates laparotomy.
B. Solid organ injuries
   1. Signs and symptoms
      a. Abdominal pain, referred pain to shoulder from diaphragm irritation, and hypotension
      b. Most commonly injured organs in blunt trauma
   2. Diagnosis
      a. Acute abdomen
      b. FAST, DPL
      c. CT abdomen/pelvis
         (1) May show subcapsular hematoma, laceration, hemoperitoneum, or arterial blush—indicative of ongoing bleeding
         (2) Graded according to severity
   3. Liver injuries
      a. Hemorrhage can come from the liver parenchyma, arterial system, portal system, and the caval system.
         (1) Most lower-grade injuries are managed nonoperatively in the intensive care unit (ICU): bed rest, serial hematocrits, transfusions, and possible angiography and embolization.
         (2) A liver injury that requires an operation to stop it from hemorrhaging is usually a challenge.
         (3) With the Pringle maneuver, a clamp is placed on the porta hepatis, thus controlling the arterial and portal inflow.
         (4) The most common technique to stop the liver from bleeding is packing the abdomen.
   4. Spleen injuries
      a. Stable patients can be observed with bed rest, serial examinations, and hematocrit.
      b. Angiography and embolization may be an adjunct to nonoperative management.
      c. Unstable patients usually require a splenectomy or splenorrhaphy.
      d. Complications (see Clinical Pearl 3-5)
         (1) Postsplenectomy sepsis, which is rare (2% occurrence)
         (2) Injury to tail of the pancreas during splenectomy
         (3) Delayed rupture, which can occur 10 to 14 days after injury
C. Diaphragm injuries
   1. Usually on left—liver protects right side
   2. Penetrating injuries include small holes that may enlarge and herniate over time.
   3. Diagnosis: often missed on various imaging modalities
      a. CXR, which may show elevated hemidiaphragm, air–fluid level above the diaphragm; nasogastric (NG) tube in chest; displacement of mediastinum to right (Fig. 3-4)
      b. May require laparoscopy to diagnose

QUICK HIT

For both liver and spleen trauma, the presence of an arterial blush on CT is seen with ongoing bleeding. It is associated with higher risk of failure of nonoperative management but may also respond to selective embolization.

CLINICAL PEARL 3-5

Vaccines after Splenectomy

- Should cover encapsulated organisms
- *Neisseria meningitidis*
- *Streptococcus pneumoniae*
- *Haemophilus influenzae*

FIGURE 3-4 CXR demonstrating evidence of a traumatic diaphragmatic hernia. Note the cardiac deviation to the right and the elevated air–fluid level in the chest.

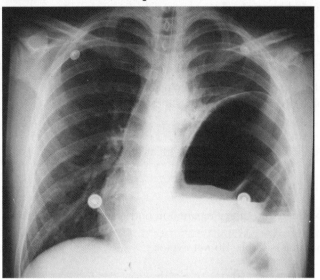

(Reprinted with permission from Mulholland MW, Lillemoe KD, Doherty GM, Maier RV, Upchurch GR, eds. *Greenfield's Surgery: Scientific Principles and Practice.* 4th ed. Philadelphia, PA: Lippincott Williams & Wilkins; 2006.)

4. Treatment
   a. Acute injuries are repaired via a laparotomy because there is a high incidence of associated injuries.
   b. Chronic injuries can be approached through the chest.
D. Pancreas injuries
   1. Signs and symptoms include severe abdominal pain, peritonitis, nausea, vomiting, and elevated pancreatic isoenzymes.
   2. Usually diagnosed with a CT
   3. Management varies from bowel rest and observation to operative resection.
E. Bowel injuries
   1. Duodenum
      a. Differs from jejunum and ileum because of its shared vascular supply with the head of the pancreas, the presence of the ampulla of Vater in the second portion, and its location in the retroperitoneum
      b. Diagnosis
         (1) Clinically may present as peritonitis from a bowel perforation or a proximal bowel obstruction from a hematoma in the retroperitoneum
         (2) May be found in the usual radiographic modalities with oral contrast, but DPL may be negative because of retroperitoneal location of duodenum
      c. Treatment
         (1) Intramural hematoma can be managed nonoperatively with an NG tube and total parenteral nutrition (TPN).
         (2) Perforation can be managed with a primary repair or with diversion and wide drainage.
   2. Small bowel (jejunum and ileum)
      a. Most common organ injured in penetrating injuries
      b. Associated clinical findings: seatbelt sign, chance fracture
      c. Perforation may present in a delayed fashion when primary injury devascularizes a portion of the small bowel.
      d. Treatment
         (1) Primary repair in transverse fashion if less than 50% of wall is involved
         (2) Resection and anastomosis
            (a) Loss of more than 50% circumference or multiple injuries in a segment
            (b) Devascularized segment

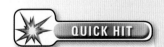

QUICK HIT

A bucket handle injury results from blunt trauma causing a shearing and tearing of the mesentery and vessels, usually occurring at the ileocolic junction and resulting in ischemia.

Trauma and Burns

3. Colon
   a. Primary repair versus resection and primary anastomosis
   b. If hemodynamically stable, minimal contamination, and normal temperature, then repair or resect and anastomosis is needed.
   c. If hemodynamically unstable, significant other injuries, hypothermic, then a diverting colostomy is needed.
4. Rectum
   a. For intraperitoneal, a repair and diverting colostomy is indicated.
   b. For extraperitoneal, a diverting colostomy is indicated.
F. Retroperitoneum
   1. Zones (Fig. 3-5)
      a. Zone 1: central and medial aspects; contains great vessels
      b. Zone 2: flanks
      c. Zone 3: pelvis
   2. Treatment
      a. Zone 1: must be explored and injury repaired in both penetrating and blunt trauma
      b. Zone 2: If the hematoma is stable, do not explore.
      c. Zone 3
         (1) With blunt trauma, do not explore the hematoma.
         (2) With penetrating trauma, explore and repair.
G. Kidney
   1. Often with flank pain and micro- or macroscopic hematuria
   2. Diagnosis is made with a CT in hemodynamically stable patients.
   3. Treatment varies from observation to angiography to operative repair and nephrectomy.

FIGURE 3-5 Zones of the retroperitoneum.

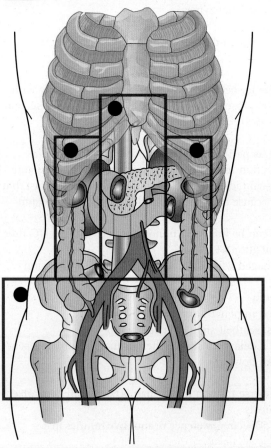

(*ACS Surgery, Operative Exposure of Abdominal Injuries and Closure of the Abdomen.* BC Decker INC; 2006.)

CLINICAL PEARL 3-6

Potential Sources of Hemorrhagic Shock

- Hypotension from hemorrhage requires acute loss of 1,500–2,000 mL of blood.
- In a trauma patient, internal hemorrhage into the chest, abdomen, and pelvis can cause hemorrhagic shock.
- Although femur fractures can be a significant source of blood loss, the thigh compartments are less likely to hold this volume.
- External hemorrhage is the remaining possible location for blood loss leading to hypotension.

H. Ureteral injuries
  1. Rare in blunt trauma but more likely with stab or gunshot wounds
  2. Diagnosis is with intravenous pyelogram.
  3. Treatment
     a. Surgical: primary repair over stent versus reconstruction
I. Urethral injuries
  1. Commonly in the setting of anterior pelvic fractures
  2. Suspect with blood at the meatus or when unable to pass Foley catheter
  3. High-riding prostate on digital rectal examination
  4. Diagnosis is with a retrograde urethrogram.
  5. Treatment is with early realignment over Foley catheter.
J. Bladder injuries
  1. Types of injuries include intraperitoneal, extraperitoneal, and combined. They are often associated with pelvic fractures.
  2. Unlikely in the absence of gross hematuria
  3. Diagnosis is with cystography or CT cystogram.
  4. Treatment
     a. In an intraperitoneal rupture, the treatment is operative with a two-layer repair.
     b. In an extraperitoneal rupture, the treatment is conservative; Foley catheter for 10 to 14 days with follow-up cystography.
K. Pelvic fractures
  1. Anterior fractures
     a. May cause injury to urethra, bladder, prostate, and vagina
     b. If isolated, usually hemodynamically stable
  2. Posterior fractures
     a. May cause severe injury to pelvis arteries, veins, and nerves
     b. Potential source of massive bleeding leading to hemorrhagic shock
  3. Treatment (see Clinical Pearl 3-6)
     a. Stabilize the patient with a sheet, pelvic binder, or external fixator.
     b. Angiography with embolization. Selective if identified or hypogastric artery.

V. Extremity Injuries

A. Assessment
  1. Pay special attention to neurologic and vascular examination.
  2. X-rays of extremity, which include the joint above and below the injury
  3. Mangled extremity severity score
     a. Tool to assess viability for limb salvage
     b. The score is based on bone/soft tissue loss, shock, ischemia, and age.
  4. Vascular injury (see Clinical Pearl 3-7)
     a. Decreased pulses or signs of mild ischemia
        (1) Realign and splint extremity.
        (2) Ankle brachial index (ABI)
           (a) Compare systolic blood pressure (SBP) of dorsalis pedis/posterior tibialis pressures to SBP of brachial artery.
           (b) Low probability of vascular injury = 0.9 or greater
        (3) The arteriogram is the gold standard but is invasive.
        (4) CT angiography

CLINICAL PEARL 3-7

Hard and Soft Signs of Vascular Injury

- Hard signs: expanding hematoma, pulsatile bleeding, bruit, absent pulse (or other signs of obvious arterial occlusion)
  - Operative exploration and repair
- Soft signs: diminished pulse, nonexpanding hematoma, nonpulsatile bleeding, injury in proximity of vessel, history of arterial bleeding at the scene
  - Consider angiography, computed tomography angiography (CTA)

B. Open fractures/joints
   1. Any laceration that communicates with a fracture
   2. Treatment must occur within 6 hours to minimize risk of infection.
      a. Grades I and II: first-generation cephalosporin
      b. Grade III: first-generation cephalosporin and aminoglycoside
C. Compartment syndrome
   1. Risk factors
      a. Tibial and forearm fracture
      b. Fractures in tight dressings, casts
      c. Severe crush injury to muscle
      d. Localized, prolonged external pressure to an extremity
      e. Reperfusion after ischemia
      f. Burns
   2. Signs and symptoms
      a. Pain on passive motion
      b. Paresthesias and lack of pulse are late signs, and damage is irreversible.
   3. Diagnosis
      a. Clinical examination
      b. Compartment pressures can be measured and should be less than 30 mm Hg.
   4. Treatment is with fasciotomy.

VI. Burns
   A. Anatomy
      1. Skin layers
         a. Epidermis
            (1) Acts as a barrier to environment, protecting from infection, toxins, ultraviolet light, and fluid evaporation
            (2) Epidermal layers from superficial to deep: stratum corneum → stratum lucidum → stratum granulosum → stratum spinosum → stratum basale (germinativum)
         b. Dermis
            (1) Consists of the papillary dermis and reticular dermis
            (2) Majority of the dermis consists of the reticular dermis.
   B. Burn types
      1. Thermal
      2. Chemical
         a. Initial treatment involves copious irrigation: 20 L of water for 30 minutes.
         b. Alkali burns
            (1) Occur from cement, lime, potassium/sodium hydroxide, and bleach
            (2) Deeper burns, more damaging than acid burns
         c. Acid burns
            (1) Seen often with formic and hydrofluoric acid
            (2) Do not penetrate as deeply as alkaline
            (3) Hydrofluoric acid results in calcium chelation, which leads to insoluble salt formation, which leads to hypocalcemia and dysrhythmia. The treatment with calcium gluconate is used to treat the dysrhythmia, not the burn.
         d. Hydrocarbon in organic solvents create injury by causing cell membrane dissolution and skin necrosis.

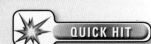

QUICK HIT

Stratum corneum is the most important epidermal layer, consisting of keratin cells.

3. Electrical
   a. High-voltage burns due to greater than 1,000 watts (W) require a full trauma evaluation.
      (1) Check for rhabdomyolysis and follow serial creatinine kinases (CKs).
      (2) Complete an ophthalmologic examination to exclude cataract formation.
      (3) Monitor median nerve function (lies within carpal tunnel).
      (4) Treatment may require escharotomy or fasciotomy.
      (5) Extent of injury is actually greater than the visible areas of tissue necrosis.
   b. Low-voltage burns due to less than 1,000 W
      (1) Systemic sequelae are rare and are not transmitted to deeper tissues.
      (2) Typically, the result of a child chewing on an electric cord and causing burns to the corner of the mouth
   c. Lightning is another source of electrical burn injury.
4. Inhalation
   a. Upper airway thermal injury
      (1) Due to heat or chemical toxins, upper airway injury occurs more often than lower airway injury because heat is absorbed by the oropharynx.
      (2) Diagnosis is confirmed by direct laryngoscopy.
      (3) Symptoms manifest within first 6 hours of injury. The most sensitive sign is lip edema.
      (4) Therapy includes the use of humidified oxygen, pulmonary toileting, and bronchodilators. Endotracheal intubation is indicated if posterior pharyngeal swelling, mucosal sloughing, or carbonaceous sputum are present.
   b. Lower airway burn injury
      (1) Results from the combustion products in smoke. Thermal injury directly to the lungs is rare.
      (2) Mucosal damage, large increase in blood flow, and loss of ciliary clearance leads to parenchymal inflammation, pulmonary edema, pneumonia, and acute respiratory distress syndrome (ARDS).
      (3) Diagnosis: PaO2:FiO2 ratio <200 and bronchoscopy
C. Burn classification (see Clinical Pearl 3-8)
   1. Superficial (first-degree) burn
      a. Burn injury is confined to the epidermis.
      b. Burns are painful, erythematous, and blanch to the touch. However, the epidermal barrier is intact.
      c. Examples of first-degree injuries include minor scalds or sunburn.
      d. Treatment involves the use of salves or nonsteroidal anti-inflammatory drugs
   2. Partial-thickness (second-degree) burns
      a. Involve the dermis to varying degrees
      b. Superficial partial-thickness burns
         (1) Burns present as erythematous, painful, blanching, or blisters, and no scarring occurs.
         (2) Scalding and flash flame injuries are examples of superficial partial-thickness burns.
         (3) Reepithelialization occurs spontaneously in 7 to 14 days.

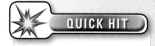

QUICK HIT

No scarring occurs in first-degree burns.

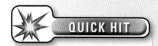

QUICK HIT

Scarring occurs with deep partial-thickness burns.

CLINICAL PEARL 3-8

Burn Classification

- Superficial (first degree)—injury localized to epidermis
- Superficial partial thickness (second degree)—injury to the epidermis and superficial dermis
- Deep partial thickness—injury though the epidermis and into the deep dermis
- Full thickness (third degree)—full-thickness injury through the epidermis and dermis, into subcutaneous fat
- Fourth degree—injury through the skin and subcutaneous fat into underlying muscle or bone

    c. Deep partial-thickness burns
      (1) Burn injury extending into the reticular dermis
      (2) Appearance of burn is described as pale, mottled, nonblanching, or painful.
      (3) Healing occurs in 2 to 4 weeks by reepithelialization from hair follicles and sweat glands.
      (4) Healing begins at the central epidermal appendages and extends peripherally.
  3. Full-thickness (third-degree) burns
    a. Injury extends into the subcutaneous fat.
    b. Burns appear as a painless, hard, leathery eschar, and color varies between black, white, or cherry.
    c. No epidermal or dermal appendages remain, and thus healing occurs by reepithelialization from wound edge peripherally, extending centrally.
    d. Treatment for third-degree burns consists of burn or eschar excision and skin grafting.
D. Area of burn injury
  1. Zone of coagulation: necrotic area where tissue will not recover
  2. Zone of stasis: surrounds the zone of coagulation. The tissue can become necrotic or recover. There is decreased tissue perfusion
  3. Zone of hyperemia: Healing process begins from this viable tissue.
E. Burn size
  1. Rule of nines (Fig. 3-6): First-degree burns are not included in burn calculations.
    a. Modified in children
      (1) Each arm equals 9% total body surface area (TBSA).
      (2) Each leg equals 14% TBSA.
      (3) The anterior and posterior trunk each equal 18% TBSA.
      (4) Head equals 18% TBSA.

FIGURE 3-6 Rule of nines diagram for estimating burn size for both pediatric and adult use.

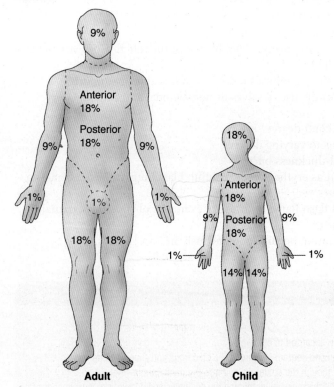

(Reprinted with permission from Mulholland MW, Lillemoe KD, Doherty GM, Maier RV, Upchurch GR, eds. *Greenfield's Surgery: Scientific Principles and Practice.* 4th ed. Philadelphia, PA: Lippincott Williams & Wilkins; 2006.)

TABLE 3-4   Resuscitation Formulas

Formula	Crystalloid Volume	Colloid Volume	Free Water
Parkland	4 mL/kg per % TBSA burn	None	None
Galveston (pediatric)	5,000 mL/m² TBSA burned + 1,500 mL/m² TBSA	None	None
Brooke	1.5 mL/kg per % TBSA burned	0.5 mL/kg per % TBSA burned	2.0 L

TBSA, total body surface area.

F. Resuscitation
   1. Resuscitation formulas (Table 3-4)
      a. Parkland formula: reportedly underestimates needs
         (1) Half of the total volume is given in the first 8 hours.
         (2) The remaining half is given over the next 16 hours.
         (3) Lactated Ringers is used to avoid hyperchloremic metabolic acidosis, associated with large infusions of 0.9% normal saline.
      b. Brooke formula: uses colloid; question if increased ARDS
      c. In children, the Galveston formula is used because children require more resuscitation fluid per kilogram.
         (1) Dextrose is not used in adults for initial burn resuscitation. However, it should be used in the children weighing less than 20 kg due to inadequate hepatic glycogen reserves.
         (2) Maintenance fluid for children should consist of D5 0.45% half normal saline at a rate of 3 to 4 mL/kg/hr.
      d. Colloid can be used after the initial 24 hours because less capillary leak occurs.
   2. Transfer criteria to burn center (Table 3-5).
G. Burn healing and management
   1. Stages of wound healing
      a. Inflammatory phase
         (1) Begins immediately and lasts up to 7 to 10 days
         (2) Infiltration by neutrophils occurs up to 24 hours, followed by macrophage infiltration over the next 2 to 3 days, and completed by lymphocyte recruitment.
      b. Proliferative phase
         (1) Occurs from day 5 through 3 weeks postinjury
         (2) Begins with formation of a provisional matrix consisting of fibrin and fibronectin

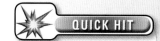

QUICK HIT

Urine output must be maintained at 0.5 mL/kg/hr in adults and 1–2 mL/kg/hr in children; fluid resuscitation should be adjusted accordingly to maintain these goals.

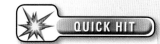

QUICK HIT

Type I collagen predominates throughout the body and is the principal collagen type found in scar tissue.

TABLE 3-5   American Burn Association Criteria for Patient Transfer to a Burn Center

1 Partial-thickness burns greater than 10% total body surface area
2 Burns that involve the face, hands, feet, genitalia, perineum, or major joints
3 Third-degree burns in any age group
4 Electrical burns, including lightning burns
5 Chemical burns
6 Inhalation injury
7 Burn injury in patients with preexisting medical conditions that could increase mortality or morbidity
8 Concomitant burn and trauma in which the burn poses the greatest risk. If the trauma poses the greatest threat, patient may be stabilized initially at a trauma center prior to burn center transport.
9 Burned children at hospitals not equipped to deal with pediatric population
10 Patients who will require special social, emotional, or long-term rehabilitative services

Trauma and Burns

(3) Fibroblasts present by day 3, initiating collagen synthesis.

(4) Macrophages release growth factors inducing angiogenesis.

(5) Vitamin C is necessary for collagen cross-linking and stabilization via hydroxylation of proline and lysine.

c. Remodeling phase

(1) Collagen equilibrium is attained, beginning at approximately 3 weeks and lasting up to 1 year.

(2) Type I collagen predominates type III by a ratio of 4:1.

(3) Collagen remodeling occurs, and wound color changes from purple/pink to pale.

(4) Scarring occurs, in which collagen fibrils align longitudinally along lines of stress with less degree of order than normal skin.

(5) Seventy percent of the strength of unwounded skin is achieved by 84 days.

2. Burn wound management

a. Topical antimicrobials (Table 3-6)

b. Systemic antibiotics should be used for diagnosed infection only, which occurs in approximately 80% of patients with large burns.

c. Tetanus prophylaxis: Tetanus toxoid is given for all patients with burns greater than 10% TBSA. If no prior immunization has been given, or last booster was given more than 10 years prior, immunoglobulin should be administered.

3. Wound closure

a. All eschar or nonviable tissue should be excised as soon as possible, ideally within the first week, and closed with an autograft.

b. Full-thickness grafts are not typically used in burn patients with large TBSA burns.

c. Autograft

(1) The skin graft is harvested from the patient's own tissue.

(2) The patient's own tissue is the preferred coverage material if feasible because of less risk of rejection and poor wound healing.

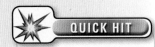

QUICK HIT

Staphylococcus aureus and *Pseudomonas* are common organisms causing burn wound infection.

TABLE 3-6 Topical Antimicrobial Agents for Burns

Antimicrobial Agent	Coverage	Advantages	Disadvantages
For deep wounds or >25% TBSA			
Silver sulfadiazine (Silvadene)	Broad spectrum, especially *Pseudomonas*	Painless	Neutropenia Does not penetrate eschar Discolors skin from silver Inhibits epithelialization
Mafenide acetate (Sulfamylon)	Broad spectrum, including *Clostridium*	Excellent eschar penetration	Painful Carbonic anhydrase inhibitor with secondary metabolic acidosis
Silver nitrate	Broad spectrum	Excellent prophylaxis	Poor eschar penetration Hyponatremia, hypochloremia Methemoglobinemia Stains skin
For superficial wounds or <25% TBSA			
Bacitracin	Gram +/−	Good for shallow facial burns	Decreases colonization, unknown efficacy in treating infected wound
Neosporin	Gram +/−	Painless	Decreases colonization, unknown efficacy in treating infected wound
Polysporin	Gram +/−	Painless	Decreases colonization, unknown efficacy in treating infected wound

TBSA, total body surface area.

FIGURE 3-7 Torso escharotomy can be useful to improve compliance and ventilation. Appropriate lines for torso escharotomy are depicted.

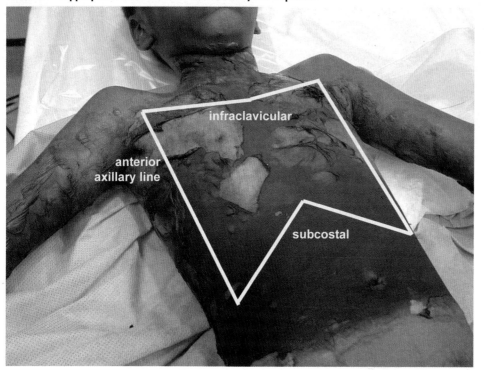

infraclavicular

anterior
axillary line

subcostal

(Reprinted with permission from Mulholland MW, Lillemoe KD, Doherty GM, Maier RV, Upchurch GR, eds. *Greenfield's Surgery: Scientific Principles and Practice.* 4th ed. Philadelphia, PA: Lippincott Williams & Wilkins; 2006.)

  d. Human allograft (cadaveric)
   (1) Graft vascularizes and engrafts, providing coverage for 2 to 4 weeks before rejection.
  e. Xenograft (porcine): will not vascularize or engraft
 H. Systemic complications
  1. Constrictive eschar
   a. These tight, circumferential bands of skin around the extremities and thoracic and abdominal cavities result in neurovascular, respiratory, and end-organ (renal) compromise.
   b. Treatment: escharotomy (Fig. 3-7)
  2. Extremity compartment syndrome
   a. If compartment pressure is greater than 30 mm Hg, perform a fasciotomy.
   b. Suspect extremity compartment syndrome if pain is out of proportion, pain is present with passive movement, or an ischemia time is greater than 6 hours.
  3. Rhabdomyolysis
   a. Rhabdomyolysis may be caused by myoglobinuria, resulting in acute tubular necrosis.
   b. Laboratory values indicative of rhabdomyolysis include positive urine myoglobin, elevated muscle enzymes, and normal serum haptoglobin.
   c. Rhabdomyolysis is treated by maintaining a urine output of 100 mL/hr; urine alkalinization with intravenous $NaHCO_3$ (0.12 to 0.5 mEq/kg/hr osmotic diuresis with mannitol as a last resort).

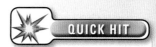

QUICK HIT

There is no benefit to digital escharotomies, and the risk of iatrogenic neurovascular injury is high.

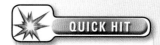

QUICK HIT

The four compartments of the lower extremity are the anterior, lateral, superficial posterior, and deep posterior.

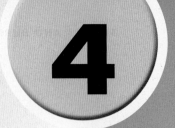

4 Hernias

Cynthia F. Graves, Jason Turner, Patrick Bonasso, and Jessica Partin

I. Abdominal Wall Hernias

A. Anterior abdominal wall anatomy
1. Anterior abdominal wall
   a. Skeletal support includes the lowest ribs, pelvic brim, and lumbar spine.
   b. Compresses and contains abdominal viscera and contributes to support movement of spine and pelvis
   c. Lamination of the muscles and aponeurosis precludes evisceration; hernias most commonly form between laminations (where only peritoneum and fascia exist).
2. Fascial layers
   a. Superficial subcutaneous layer: Camper fascia
      (1) It can contain a significant amount of fat (panniculus adiposis).
      (2) Blood vessels include superficial inferior epigastric and superficial circumflex iliac artery and vein (both arise from femoral vessels).
      (3) Lymphatic drainage to inguinal lymph nodes inferior to inguinal ligament
      (4) This superficial fascial layer fuses with fascia innominata, which invests the external abdominal oblique, binds to inguinal ligament, and continues onto the fascia lata. It includes Hesselbach triangle superiorly and is the weakest part of the groin.
      (5) Not a strength layer. The high adipose content of this layer and the lack of strong fibrinous material usually prevent suture material from holding.
   b. Deep subcutaneous layer: Scarpa fascia
      (1) Compressed fibrous components of superficial fascia where it forms the fundiform ligament of the penis and the superficial perineal fascia
      (2) Has more tensile strength than Camper fascia and more easily identifiable
   c. Rectus sheath: The rectus abdominis muscle is enveloped in a sheath. This sheath is formed from the aponeuroses of the abdominal wall musculature. The aponeurotic fascial layers either completely encircle the rectus sheath or run only on its anterior boarder, depending on its location to the arcuate line. Above the arcuate line, the fascial layers split. Below the arcuate line, the layers all run anterior to the muscle.
      (1) Formed by aponeuroses of external oblique, internal oblique, and transversus abdominis with midline decussation as the linea alba
      (2) Anterior sheath
         (a) Superior to arcuate line: external oblique and anterior division of the internal oblique.
         (b) Inferior to arcuate line: composite of all layers
      (3) Posterior sheath
         (a) Superior to arcuate line: posterior division of the internal oblique, the transversus abdominis aponeurosis, and the transversalis fascia
         (b) Inferior to arcuate line: transversalis fascia
      (4) Arcuate line (of Douglas) is transfer of connective tissue away from the posterior sheath.

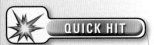

QUICK HIT

Layers of the abdominal wall:
Skin
Subcutaneous fat
Scarpa's fascia
Fat
External Oblique muscle
Internal Oblique muscle
Transversus abdominis
Transversalis fascia
Preperitoneal fat
Peritoneum

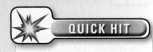

QUICK HIT

A "camper" stays outdoors. Camper fascia is the "outer" most fascial layer.

d. Semilunar line
   (1) Lateral to rectus abdominis
   (2) Site of insertion of lateral abdominal muscle aponeurotic insertions
3. Blood supply
   a. Rectus abdominis
      (1) Superior epigastric (continuation of internal mammary artery)
      (2) Inferior epigastric (off external iliac artery)
      (3) Contribution from lower intercostal arteries near umbilicus
   b. Lateral muscles
      (1) Primarily from 8th to 12th intercostal arteries, deep circumflex iliac arteries, and lumbar arteries
4. Innervation
   a. Dermatome pattern with overlapping fields, so disruption is not normally noticed
   b. Nerves divide into anterior and lateral cutaneous branches of T7 to T12 and Ll to L2 ventral rami.
   c. Lower intercostal and upper lumbar (T7 to T12, Ll, and L2) nerves pass between internal oblique and transversus abdominis and pierce the lateral sheath.
   d. The external oblique receives intercostal branches.
   e. First lumbar nerve divides into ilioinguinal and iliohypogastric.
      (1) Ilioinguinal passes through external ring to run with the spermatic cord.
      (2) Iliohypogastric pierces external abdominal oblique (EAO) to innervate skin above the pubis.
   f. Genitofemoral nerve (L1, L2) innervates cremasteric muscles.
5. Muscles (Table 4-1)

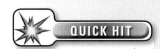

QUICK HIT

Fibers of the EAO run in the same direction as when you put your hands in your coat pockets.

Hernias

TABLE **4-1** **Muscles**			
Muscle	**Origin/Insertion**	**Anatomy**	**Extra Notes**
External abdominal oblique (EAO)	- Posterior lower eight ribs - Inserts on anterior iliac crest - Interdigitates with the serratus and latissimus	- Forms the superficial inguinal ring - Anteroinferior aponeurotic fibers form the inguinal ligament.	Fiber orientation - Above anterior superior iliac crest (ASIC), horizontal orientation - Below ASIC, folds onto self to form inguinal ligament - Fibers insert into the linea alba and anterior rectus sheath.

Internal abdominal oblique (IAO)	- Middle layer of lateral abdominal muscles
	- Arises from iliac fascia along crest and fuses with inguinal ligament
		Internal oblique aponeurosis
		- Superior to umbilicus
		  • Splits and envelops the rectus muscle, reforms in midline to join linea alba
		- Inferior to umbilicus
		  • Anterior to rectus muscle only (do not split)
			- Fibers run obliquely toward lower "floating" ribs and fan out along iliac crest.
			- Lower fibers form the cremaster muscle in males.

Transversus abdominis	- Arises from iliac crest, inguinal ligament, and six costal ribs
	- Interdigitates with lateral diaphragmatic fibers running horizontally to insert on pubic crest
		Aponeurosis
		- Superior to umbilicus
		  • Joins posterior lamina of IAO to form posterior rectus sheath
		- Inferior to umbilicus
		  • Component of anterior rectus sheath
			Termination of aponeurosis is the aponeurotic arch.
			- Area beneath the arch is large and may predispose to direct inguinal hernia.

Rectus abdominis	- Origin from the fifth to seventh costal cartilages - Inserts on the pubic symphysis and xiphoid	Innervation - 7th through 12th intercostal nerves that pierce rectus sheath laterally	Blood supply - Superior and inferior epigastric arteries - Anterior branches of intercostal arteries
Pyramidalis	- Arises from pubic symphysis - Tapers and attaches to linea alba	- Lies within the rectus sheath	

B. Clinical features of hernias
1. All ages, 10% incidence in premature infants, and varies by gender
   a. Inguinal hernias have 7:1 male-to-female ratio.
   b. Femoral hernias have 1.8:1 female predominance. *Femoral hernias are more common in women than in men; however, inguinal hernias are still the most common hernias women experience.*
2. Types of hernias
   a. Inguinal hernias: 80%
   b. Femoral hernias: 5%
   c. Incisional, umbilical, and epigastric hernias: 15%
3. Presentation
   a. Duration of symptoms vary (chronic versus acute).
   b. History of lump or swelling that occurs on straining
4. Complications
   a. Incarceration versus strangulation: Incarcerated hernias are not reducible. They are jailed or "incarcerated." Strangulated hernias are incarcerated hernias that are now being strangled; that is, deprived of blood flow. Strangulated hernias are a surgical emergency.
      (1) Incarceration ("trapped," "jailed," or irreducible hernia)
         (a) Hernia sac contents may vary (omentum, ovary, nonobstructed bowel).
         (b) Irreducible due to chronic adhesions
         (c) Must differentiate between a hydrocele and a hernia (because you will not be able to reduce a hydrocele into the peritoneal cavity)
            i. One can get one's examining fingers above a hydrocele but not a hernia.
            ii. A hydrocele transilluminates, whereas a hernia does not.
         (d) Treatment of incarcerated hernia is surgical.
      (2) Strangulation
         (a) Contents (omentum, bowel, ovary, etc.) of hernia sac are ischemic and/or necrotic.
            i. Pressure on the bowel trapped in the hernia sac produces venous congestion, which leads to edema of the bowel, and subsequent pressures so high that arterial inflow is obstructed and the bowel becomes gangrenous.
         (b) Presentation/physical exam
            i. Strangulated hernias present with tender, irreducible masses and have systemic symptoms such as toxicity, dehydration, and fever.
            ii. The hernia is tense and very tender and may have overlying skin changes (erythematous or bluish discoloration). It may be warm and with induration.
            iii. Bowel sounds are absent in the hernia.
            iv. Leukocytosis is common, and metabolic acidosis may be present.
            v. Lactic acid may be normal because there is no venous outflow to circulate the lactic acid.
            vi. Symptoms of bowel obstruction may be the only sign: obstipation, distension, nausea/vomiting
         (c) Treatment
            i. Strangulated hernias should not be reduced.
            ii. Nasogastric (NG) tube suction, fluid and electrolyte replacement, and antibiotics are started.
            iii. Emergency surgery follows with exposure of the hernia, opening of the sac, and resecting any gangrenous viscera, followed by hernia repair.
            iv. The hernia repair is no longer a sterile field in this setting. Synthetic mesh must NOT be used.
      (3) Intestinal obstruction
         (a) Once the most common cause of obstruction, hernia is now the third most common cause (first is adhesions, second is cancer). ABCs of bowel obstruction: A= adhesions, B= bulge (hernia), C= cancer

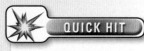

QUICK HIT

Think of incarcerated bowel as being imprisoned (incarcerated): "stuck inside and not able to get out."

Hernias

(b) Presentation/physical exam

    i. An obstructed hernia is tense and irreducible, and the abdomen is distended.

    ii. High-pitched bowel sounds are heard with frequent rushes.

(c) Plain abdominal X-ray

    i. Shows classic dilated loops of bowel with air–fluid levels and paucity of gas distal to obstruction

    ii. Computed tomography may be helpful if clinical diagnosis is uncertain.

(d) Treatment

    i. Patient is sedated and placed in Trendelenburg position. *Flat supine, at 15-30° incline w/ feet elevated above the head.*

    ii. Taxis maneuver elongates neck to allow contents to pass into abdomen.

       (1) Grasping hernia neck with one hand and applying intermittent pressure with other hand on distal neck of hernia

    iii. Abort the attempt at reduction if unsuccessful after two or three tries because reduction of gangrenous bowel or reduction en masse is possible.

    iv. Postreduction

       (1) Reduction of hernia is followed by resuscitation and urgent surgery via a direct approach over the hernia site.

       (2) Viable bowel is reduced back into the abdomen. Nonviable bowel is resected with anastomosis prior to hernia repair.

5. Massive hernia

  a. Large portion of abdominal contents situated in hernia sac; usually chronic

  b. Hernia contents have lost their right of domain; thus, replacement of abdominal contents with fascial closure puts the patient at risk of abdominal compartment syndrome, skin edema, and cellulitis after closure.

  c. Pneumoperitoneum may help when returning contents to the abdominal cavity over 3 weeks prior to repair.

  d. A prosthesis is usually required because of the size of the defect.

II. Groin Hernias

A. Anatomy of the inguinal region

  1. Anatomic connections in the groin

    a. External oblique becomes the inguinal ligament (Poupart ligament).

    b. Internal oblique becomes the cremasteric muscle.

    c. Processes vaginalis evagination of peritoneum that accompanies the testicle and gubernaculums. This forms the hernia sac in an indirect hernia.

    d. Gubernaculum attaches the testicle to the scrotum and is the anatomic equivalent of the round ligament in women.

  2. Spermatic cord contains testicular and cremasteric arteries, pampiniform venous plexus, vas deferens, and processus vaginalis (or hernia sac).

  3. Inguinal canal

    a. The communication between the internal and external inguinal rings

    b. Contains spermatic cord in men and round ligament in women

    c. Anatomic borders

       (1) External oblique aponeurosis is the anterior wall.

       (2) Inguinal ligament is the inferior wall.

       (3) Conjoint tendon (internal oblique and transversus muscles) is the roof.

       (4) Transversalis fascia and aponeurosis are the floor.

  4. Hesselbach triangle (Fig. 4-1) is an area bounded by (a) inferior epigastric vessels, (b) inguinal ligament, and (c) lateral border of the rectus sheath.

  5. The femoral canal contains the femoral nerve, femoral artery, femoral vein, and lymphatics.

B. Types of hernias (Table 4-2)

C. Clinical presentation

  1. Epidemiology

    a. Inguinal hernias are the most common abdominal hernia (80% of total).

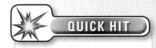

QUICK HIT

The ilioinguinal nerve runs along spermatic cord and must be identified and preserved during an open inguinal hernia repair.

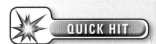

QUICK HIT

Contents of the femoral canal can be remembered from lateral to medial with the mnemonic NAVEL (nerve, artery, vein, empty space [locations of a femoral hernia], and lymphatics).

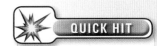

QUICK HIT

A femoral hernia occurs more frequently in women than in men; however, a direct inguinal hernia is the most common hernia in both groups.

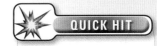

QUICK HIT

One-third of femoral hernias present with incarceration or strangulation due to their narrow neck.

Hernias

Hesselbach triangle.

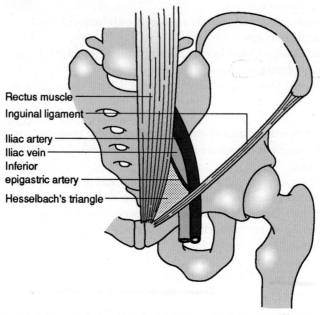

Rectus muscle
Inguinal ligament
Iliac artery
Iliac vein
Inferior
epigastric artery
Hesselbach's triangle

(Reprinted with permission from Mulholland MW, Lillemoe KD, Doherty GM, Maier RV, Upchurch GR, eds. *Greenfield's Surgery: Scientific Principles and Practice.* 4th ed. Philadelphia, PA: Lippincott Williams & Wilkins; 2006.)

TABLE **4-2** **Types of Hernias**

Type of Hernia	Definition	Etiology
Indirect inguinal hernia (Fig. 4-2)	- Hernia lateral to Hesselbach triangle, traveling through the inguinal canal	- Caused by a patent processus vaginalis - Occurs in 5% of men
Direct inguinal hernia (Fig. 4-3).	- Hernia within Hesselbach triangle, directly through abdominal wall without traveling through the inguinal ring	- Acquired defect occurring in 1% of men, increasing with age - Most common hernia in men and women
Femoral hernia	- Hernia under inguinal ligament, medial to the femoral vessels with presentation of swelling below inguinal ligament	- More common in women than men - Account for 5% of hernias
Obturator hernia	- Hernia through obturator canal along with the obturator vessels and nerves, with presentation of swelling on medial thigh - Presents with pain referred to thigh	- More common in women and associated with laxity of pelvic floor
Cooper hernia	- Hernia through the femoral canal, tracking into the scrotum or labia majus	
Pantaloon	- Presence of both direct and indirect inguinal hernias straddling the inferior epigastric vessels	

FIGURE 4-2 Indirect inguinal hernia.

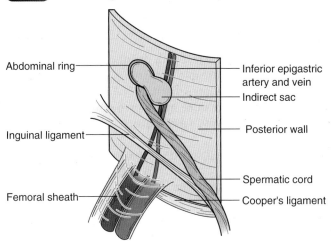

Abdominal ring

Inferior epigastric artery and vein

Indirect sac

Posterior wall

Inguinal ligament

Spermatic cord

Cooper's ligament

Femoral sheath

(Reprinted with permission from Lawrence PF. *Essentials of General Surgery.* 5th ed. Philadelphia, PA: Lippincott Williams & Wilkins; 2012.)

2. Presentation
   a. Groin pain and swelling
   b. Often with sudden onset while lifting or straining
3. Physical examination
   a. Swelling with a cough impulse
   b. During examination, the index finger is used to invaginate the scrotum, thereby placing the finger through the external inguinal ring into the inguinal canal. An indirect hernia pushes against the fingertip, whereas a direct hernia pushes against the side of the finger.
4. Differential diagnosis: hydrocele, varicocele, testicular torsion, undescended or ectopic testis, femoral artery aneurysm, lipoma of the spermatic cord, inguinal lymphadenopathy, and psoas abscess

D. Repair of inguinal hernias
1. Goals of repair are to return contents into peritoneal cavity, ligate the hernia sac, and repair defect to prevent recurrence.
2. Tissue repair includes the Bassini, Shouldice, and McVay procedures.
   a. These repairs use the patient's own tissue to reinforce the weakness in the posterior wall of the inguinal canal.

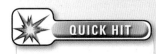

QUICK HIT

An inguinal hernia most commonly contains small intestine in men and ovary or fallopian tube in women.

Hernias

FIGURE 4-3 Direct inguinal hernia.

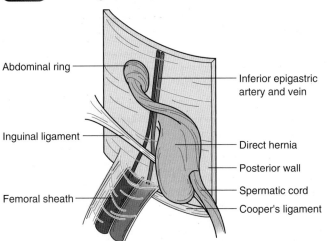

Abdominal ring

Inferior epigastric artery and vein

Inguinal ligament

Direct hernia

Posterior wall

Spermatic cord

Femoral sheath

Cooper's ligament

(Reprinted with permission from Lawrence PF. *Essentials of General Surgery.* 5th ed. Philadelphia, PA: Lippincott Williams & Wilkins; 2012.)

b. These procedures may require a relaxing incision in the rectus sheath to allow approximation of conjoined tendon to inguinal ligament without tension.

c. Tissue repair has a higher incidence of recurrence than repair with prosthesis.

3. Mesh repair

a. Reinforcement of the abdominal wall defect with prosthetic mesh

b. May be done with an open or a laparoscopic approach

c. Laparoscopic options: transabdominal preperitoneal (TAPP) and totally extraperitoneal (TEP). TEP repairs are done in the preperitoneal space, never entering the true peritoneal cavity. TAPP repairs are done through the abdominal/peritoneal cavity.

d. Recurrent and bilateral hernias are well suited to laparoscopic repair.

4. Truss

a. External device that applies pressure over the hernia defect, keeping the space obliterated

b. This may be used when surgery cannot be safely performed or when the patient refuses surgery, but this is not routinely recommended.

III. Common Hernias [Table 4-3]

TABLE 4-3 Common Hernias				
Name	**Definition**	**Epidemiology**	**Presentation**	**Treatment**
Periumbilical	- Improper healing of umbilical scar, leaving a fascial defect covered by skin	Infants - Defect 1–2 cm - 80% close by 2 years Adults - Sudden and underlying cause of increased intra-abdominal pressure must be found.	Differential diagnosis - Caput medusae, metastatic deposits of intra-abdominal tumor, umbilical granulomas, omphalomesenteric duct remnant cysts, and urachal cysts	- Conservative management until age 2 years Small defects - Simple repair via subumbilical semilunar incision Large defects - May require prosthesis in preperitoneal space
Epigastric	- Defect in linea alba - Most contain only preperitoneal fat and are <1 cm	- Incidence 1%–5% - Two to three times more common in men - 10% recurrence	- Painful nodule in the upper midline	- Reduction of preperitoneal fat and simple defect closure
Diastasis recti	- Rectus muscles are widely separated.		- Rarely causes problems with repair for cosmetic reasons	- Removing strip of linea and reapproximating

Incisional	- Complication of any prior surgery with association in patients with morbid obesity, cigarette smoking, steroid use, chemotherapy, pulmonary disease, or hypoalbuminemia	- Highest incidence with midline or transverse incisions
		- 5% incidence of infection with prosthesis
		  • Risks include obesity, overlying skin ulceration, bowel perforation, and seroma.
			- Causes include poor surgical technique, rough handling of tissue, rapidly degradable suture use, closure under tension, and infection.	Repair depends on size
				- Solitary or <3 cm
				  • Primary closure with nonabsorbable suture
				- Large or multiple hernias
				  • Tension-free mesh repair
				  • Omentum to reduce fistula formation

Parastomal	- Etiology due to poor site selection or technical errors (stoma placed lateral to rectus sheath)	- >50% after 5 years - Lower rate for small bowel stomas than colon Contributing factors - Obesity, malnutrition, advanced age, collagen abnormalities, postoperative sepsis, abdominal distention, constipation, obstructive uropathy, steroid use, and chronic lung disease	- Most common complication of stoma formation - Life-threatening complications are few, and less than 20% of parastomal hernias require repair.	**Fascial repair** - Local exploration, primary closure of defect **Stomal relocation** - Indicated for skin excoriation and suboptimal construction - Mesh not recommended **Prosthetic repair** - Exit of stoma must be isolated from surgical field.

IV. Unusual Hernias (Table 4-4)

TABLE 4-4 Unusual Hernias

Hernia Name	Location	Presentation	Treatment	Additional Information
Spigelian	- Weak area lateral to rectus sheath just below semilunar line - Usually intraperitoneal - Rarely penetrates the external oblique (EO) fascia • Dx at laparoscopy	- Lower abdominal swelling lateral to rectus muscle - May present as only pain and tenderness - Elderly female patients	Operative - Transverse incision over mass and split EO - Closure via approximation of transversus and internal oblique (IO)	- May contain omentum or small or large bowel - Approximately 800 cases in literature
Sciatic	- Herniation of peritoneal sac through major or minor sciatic foramen	- Swelling on buttock	Operative - Transperitoneal or transgluteal with mesh	- Can involve sciatic nerve or obstruction of ureter
Littre	- Groin hernia containing Meckel diverticulum		- Resection of diverticulum if symptomatic or strangulated	- May contain the appendix
Perineal	- Laxity of pelvic floor - Anterior or posterior depending on relation to transversus perineal muscle	- Older female patients Anterior - Labial or lateral vaginal wall swelling Posterior - Between rectum and ischial tuberosity	Operative - Transperitoneal approach with mesh depending on size of defect	
Sliding	- Portion of hernia sac is made of an intra-abdominal organ.	Figure 4-4		- Most commonly sigmoid, bladder, cecum, or ovary
Richter	- Any location in which the antimesenteric wall of bowel is partially incarcerated	Figure 4-5		
Perivascular	- Defects between inguinal ligament and iliopubic bone	**Laugier**: through defect in lacunar ligament **Cloquet**: through pectineal fascia **Velpeau**: anterior to femoral vessels and behind the inguinal ligament **Serafini**: posterior to femoral vessels **Hesselbach**: lateral to femoral artery and anterior **Partridge**: lateral to femoral artery and posterior		
Lumbar	- Located in lumbar area with boundaries of 12th rib superiorly and iliac crest inferiorly	**Superior lumbar hernia of Grynfelt**: through space between latissimus dorsi, serratus posterior inferior, and internal oblique posterior border **Inferior lumbar hernia of Petit**: through space between latissimus dorsi, iliac crest, and external oblique posterior border **Secondary lumbar**: from trauma, surgery (renal), or infection. Seen in patients with paraspinal abscesses from spinal tuberculosis.		

FIGURE 4-4 Sliding hernia.

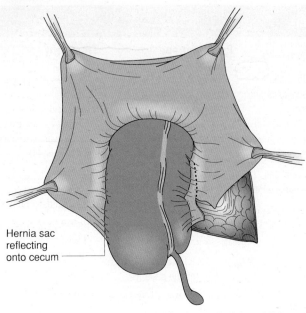

Hernia sac reflecting onto cecum

(Reprinted with permission from Mulholland MW, Lillemoe KD, Doherty GM, Maier RV, Upchurch GR, eds. *Greenfield's Surgery: Scientific Principles and Practice*. 4th ed. Philadelphia, PA: Lippincott Williams & Wilkins; 2006.)

FIGURE 4-5 Richter hernia.

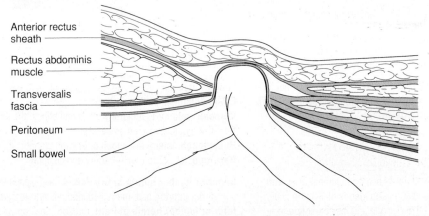

Anterior rectus sheath

Rectus abdominis muscle

Transversalis fascia

Peritoneum

Small bowel

(Reprinted with permission from Mulholland MW, Lillemoe KD, Doherty GM, Maier RV, Upchurch GR, eds. *Greenfield's Surgery: Scientific Principles and Practice*. 4th ed. Philadelphia, PA: Lippincott Williams & Wilkins; 2006.)

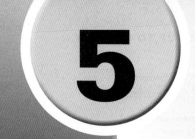

Esophagus and Stomach

Olusola Oduntan, David Michael Fourqurean, Stephen McNatt,
James Longhi, Irfan A. Rizvi, and Antony Joseph

 ## ESOPHAGUS

I. Embryology

A. The esophagus develops from the foregut caudal to the pharynx.

B. The final relative length is established by the seventh gestational week.

C. Separation from the trachea is accomplished by the tracheoesophageal septum. Incomplete fusion of the tracheoesophageal folds to form the tracheoesophageal septum, or deviation of the septum, results in the formation of a tracheoesophageal fistula and esophageal atresia.

D. Initially, the epithelium proliferates and can completely obliterate the lumen of the esophagus. Recanalization then occurs and restores the lumen of the esophagus by the end of eighth week of development.

E. The upper one-third of the esophagus contains striated muscle from the caudal pharyngeal arches.

F. The lower one-third of the esophagus contains smooth muscle derived from splanchnic mesenchyme.

II. Anatomy

A. Segments of the esophagus (~25cm long)

1. The cervical esophagus is approximately 5 cm in length.
   a. It begins below the cricopharyngeus muscle at the level of the sixth cervical vertebra.
   b. It ends at approximately the first thoracic vertebra.
2. The thoracic esophagus is where the esophagus descends from the thoracic inlet to the level of the diaphragm in the posterior mediastinum, lying anterior to the vertebral column.
   a. In the upper chest, it passes behind the trachea and left mainstem bronchus.
   b. At the level of the aortic arch, the esophagus is posterior and to the right of the aorta.
   c. In the lower chest, at the level of the T8 to T10 vertebral bodies, the esophagus is anterior to the aorta.
3. The abdominal esophagus is approximately 1 to 2 cm in length.
   a. It begins as the esophagus traverses the esophageal hiatus.
   b. It ends at the junction of the esophagus with the gastric cardia.

B. Neurovascular supply
1. Arteries
   a. The inferior thyroid artery supplies the cervical esophagus.
   b. The bronchial arterial branches and small unnamed aortoesophageal arteries supply the thoracic esophagus.
   c. The left gastric and phrenic arteries supply the abdominal and lower thoracic esophagus.

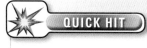

QUICK HIT

Esophageal atresia is associated with a tracheoesophageal fistula in 85% of cases. The most common type of abnormality is a proximal esophageal atresia along with a distal tracheoesophageal fistula.

Esophagus and Stomach

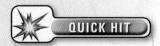

The left gastric or coronary vein drains the lower esophagus and is a source of esophageal varices in patients with portal hypertension.

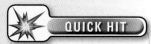

There are three areas of normal anatomic narrowing in the esophagus: the crico-pharyngeus muscle, the area where the left mainstem bronchus crosses, and the diaphragmatic hiatus.

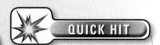

Because of the extensive submucosal lymphatic plexus of the esophagus, cancers of this organ can spread to lymph nodes located significant distances away from the primary tumor along the long axis of the esophagus.

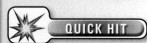

The esophagus lacks a true serosa, which is important in the spread of esophageal cancer.

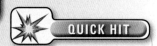

Afferent sensory pain fibers from the esophagus travel in the same pathways as pain fibers from the heart, which explains why heart pain and esophageal pain are at times indistinguishable.

2. Venous drainage parallels the segmental arterial supply, with the cervical esophagus draining to the internal jugular system, the thoracic esophagus draining to the azygous system, and the abdominal esophagus draining to the portal system.
3. Lymphatic drainage of the esophagus, in general, parallels the segmental arterial supply. The esophagus has an extensive network of submucosal lymphatics that interconnect.
   a. Cervical esophageal lymphatics drain to the internal jugular and paratracheal nodes.
   b. Thoracic esophageal lymphatics drain to the paratracheal nodes for the upper thoracic esophagus and to the subcarinal and paraesophageal nodes for the lower thoracic esophagus.
   c. Abdominal esophageal lymphatics drain to the celiac and gastric cardiac nodes.
4. Innervation
   a. Recurrent laryngeal nerves innervate the cervical esophagus and the crico-pharyngeal sphincter.
   b. Vagus nerves supply the thoracic esophagus and synapse with the postganglionic nerves in the myenteric plexus.
   c. Sympathetic innervation of the esophagus arises from the cervical, thoracic, and celiac ganglia.

C. Histology
1. Mucosa: The epithelium of the mucosal layer is composed of nonkeratinized stratified squamous cells. The junction of the stratified squamous epithelium of the esophagus and the columnar epithelium of the stomach is known as the Z-line.
2. Submucosa consists of blood vessels, nerves, lymphatics, and the ganglia of the Meissner plexus.
3. Muscularis consists of inner circular and outer longitudinal muscle layers with the myenteric plexus between.
   a. Skeletal muscle extends from the pharynx and composes the cervical and portions of the upper thoracic esophagus.
   b. Smooth muscle predominates in the thoracic and abdominal esophagus.
4. Adventitia: No consistent serosa surrounds the esophagus.

III. **Physiology.** The esophageal body and two sphincters at either end of the esophagus regulate the passage of a food bolus from the hypopharynx to the stomach.
   A. The upper esophageal sphincter (UES) is a 2- to 4.5-cm region of high pressure located between the cervical esophagus and the hypopharynx.
      1. The UES, a striated muscle sphincter, is closed at rest and relaxes during deglutition to allow the passage of a food bolus into the upper esophagus.
      2. Relaxation of the UES also occurs with belching, vomiting, and regurgitation.
      3. Resting UES pressure varies from 60 to 200 mm Hg.
   B. The lower esophageal sphincter (LES) is a 2- to 4-cm region of high pressure at the gastroesophageal junction that separates the lumen of the stomach from the lumen of the esophagus.
      1. The LES, a smooth muscle sphincter, is tonically contracted at rest with a pressure of 10 to 45 mm Hg.
      2. The LES relaxes to a pressure equal to gastric pressure on deglutition, allowing passage of a food bolus into the stomach.
      3. LES relaxation also occurs with belching, retching, vomiting, and with esophageal distention.
   C. Esophageal body function is when the body of the esophagus acts to propel a food bolus from the hypopharynx to the stomach through peristaltic contractions.
      1. Primary peristaltic contractions are occlusive waves of contraction that follow voluntary swallowing (deglutition).

2. Secondary peristaltic contractions are waves of contraction that occur with esophageal distention from food or refluxed gastric contents.

3. Tertiary contractions are contractions that are not peristaltic, and their significance is a topic of debate.

IV. Disorders of Esophageal Motility

A. Achalasia (Greek for failure to relax): Achalasia is characterized by the failure of the smooth muscle segment of the esophagus. Aperistalsis is noted in the esophageal body along with incomplete relaxation of the LES.

1. Etiology
   a. Idiopathic, where the causes are unknown
   b. Chagasic, which is caused by Chagas disease, a parasitic infection of the esophageal musculature by *Trypanosoma cruzi*
   c. Pseudoachalasia, which is caused by extrinsic compression of the lower esophagus by masses (e.g., tumors, hematoma, and enlarged lymph nodes)

2. Pathophysiology (idiopathic achalasia): Findings are consistent with the failure or loss of neurons of the myenteric plexus.
   a. Loss of myenteric ganglia
   b. Neural fibrosis
   c. Mononuclear inflammatory cell infiltrate surrounding the myenteric plexus
   d. Variable degrees of hypertrophy of the musculature at or surrounding the LES

3. Clinical presentation
   a. Dysphagia occurs in 98% of patients with achalasia and is defined as difficulty in the passage of solids or liquids from the mouth to the stomach. Patients often report that food sticks in their chest.
      (1) They have equal difficulty in eating solids and drinking liquids.
      (2) They tend to try and augment the passage of food by drinking liquids to wash down food. They may also attempt maneuvers such as extending the neck or back, or walking around during a meal to help food pass into the stomach.
   b. Regurgitation occurs in 75% of patients and is defined as the passive return of food to the mouth after eating.
      (1) Often occurs with changes in position (e.g., bending over or lying down)
      (2) May lead to aspiration
   c. Chest pain occurs in 43% of those with achalasia.
      (1) More common in patients with vigorous achalasia
      (2) Heartburn may occur as retained food and liquids in the distal esophagus ferment.
   d. Weight loss occurs in up to 58% of patients.
   e. Pulmonary complications include cough and chronic aspiration. They occur in 10% to 30% of those with achalasia.

4. Diagnostic criteria
   a. Aperistalsis of the smooth muscle segment of the esophagus
   b. Incomplete relaxation of the LES with a residual pressure greater than 8 mm Hg

5. Diagnostic tests
   a. Barium swallow (Fig. 5-1): Classic features include esophageal dilatation, loss of peristalsis, delayed emptying with a column of barium retained within the esophagus, and symmetric narrowing of the distal esophagus (bird-beaking appearance). Uniform dilation of the esophagus is known as "cucumber esophagus" (Fig. 5-2).
   b. Esophagoscopy: Endoscopy is useful in evaluating the mucosa of the esophagus and in excluding neoplasia as a cause of dysphagia. Typical findings on endoscopy include retained food and liquid within the esophagus, a dilated esophagus, and a closed or tight LES on passage of the endoscope into the stomach.

FIGURE 5-1 Esophagogram demonstrating achalasia. The patient has a smooth, abrupt tapering of the distal esophagus and an air–fluid level proximally.

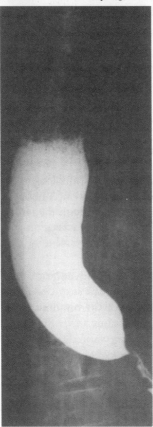

FIGURE 5-2 Esophagogram showing achalasia with "cucumber esophagus."

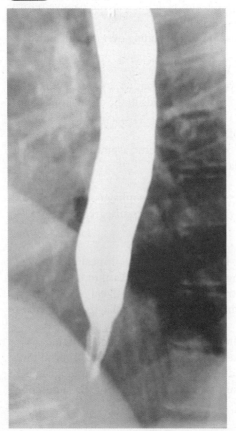

    c. Esophageal manometry: Manometry of the esophagus is the gold standard for diagnosing achalasia. Classic findings include:

      (1) Aperistalsis of the smooth muscle segment of the esophagus, where the contractions are simultaneous and the contractile pressures are usually low

      (2) Abnormal relaxation of the LES, where 70% to 80% have absent or incomplete LES relaxation. Residual LES pressures greater than 8 mm Hg with relaxation strongly suggest achalasia.

      (3) Sixty percent of patients have hypertensive resting LES pressures.

6. Treatment

    a. Medical therapy indicates smooth muscle relaxants.

      (1) Nitrates given sublingually can decrease LES pressure and offer short-term relief of dysphagic symptoms. However, they do not affect LES function, and efficacy decreases over time.

      (2) Calcium-channel blockers can decrease LES pressure and relieve dysphagic symptoms. However, as with nitrates, the function of the LES does not improve, side effects are common, and efficacy is short-lived.

    b. Botulinum toxin A

      (1) Botulinum toxin blocks release of acetylcholine at nerve receptors and, when injected into the LES, leads to relaxation of the LES by inhibiting the function of the unopposed neurons that cause LES contraction.

      (2) Three-fourths of patients respond to an initial injection.

      (3) Response rates vary over time, with approximately half sustaining symptom recurrence after 6 months.

      (4) Efficacy decreases over time with multiple treatments.

    c. Pneumatic dilatation

      (1) Pneumatic dilatation forcefully disrupts the hypertrophied muscle fibers of the LES, leading to decreased LES pressure.

      (2) Response rates typically decline over time.

      (3) Complications include a 1% to 6% risk of esophageal perforation.

      (4) Compared to botulinum toxin and medications, pneumatic dilatation is the most effective nonsurgical therapy.

    d. Esophagogastric myotomy (Heller myotomy)

      (1) The operation consists of splitting the longitudinal muscle fibers and dividing the circular muscle fibers of the distal esophagus at the area of the LES. The myotomy is carried down onto the gastric cardia for 2 to 3 cm, and the operation can be performed through the chest or abdomen and is most commonly done via laparoscopy.

      (2) Myotomy lowers LES pressure more reliably than medication, botulinum toxin, or pneumatic dilatation.

      (3) A fundoplication is usually performed along with the myotomy because 30% to 40% of patients develop symptomatic gastroesophageal reflux disease (GERD).

    e. Esophageal resection is used if there is significant esophageal dilatation and elongation, "sigmoid esophagus" (Fig. 5-3), or a previous failed myotomy.

B. Diffuse esophageal spasm (DES): DES is a problem of uncoordinated esophageal contractions of unknown etiology.

  1. Clinical presentation indicates that the clinical features may be intermittent.

    a. Chest pain commonly mimics angina, and it is not always associated with swallowing.

    b. Dysphagia can occur after the swallowing of either solids or liquids, but it is not consistent with all swallows.

  2. Diagnostic tests: Diagnosis is made by evaluation with esophageal manometry.

    a. Required findings show 10% or more simultaneous contractions, with pressures greater than 30 mm Hg, which are accompanied by intermittent normal peristalsis.

    b. Other findings include spontaneous contractions, contractions of long duration, elevated LES pressure, repetitive contractions, and multiple peaked contractions.

Esophagus and Stomach

FIGURE
5-3 Esophagogram showing "sigmoid esophagus."

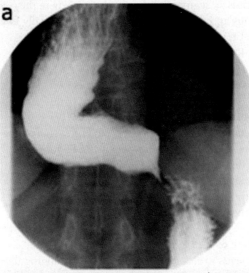

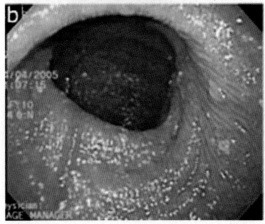

A. Radiographic appearance of sigmoid esophagus on esophagogram. **B.** Gross appearance of sigmoid esophagus during upper GI endoscopy.

     c. Barium swallow studies often show a "corkscrew" appearance of the esophagus (Fig. 5-4).

  3. Treatment: Therapeutic strategies are geared toward relief of symptoms. However, current evidence does not support one predominant treatment.

     a. Medications that relax smooth muscle: nitrates (nitroglycerin and isosorbide dinitrate), calcium-channel blockers (nifedipine and diltiazem), and antimuscarinics (dicyclomine)

     b. Medications that affect the perception of visceral pain: trazodone and imipramine

     c. Botulinum toxin injection into the LES

     d. Long esophagogastric (Heller) myotomy with partial fundoplication to reduce the incidence of gastroesophageal reflux, which frequently occurs following myotomy

V. Gastroesophageal Reflux Disease and Hiatal Hernia

  A. Gastroesophageal reflux disease, or GERD, is the most common disease affecting the esophagus.

    1. Pathophysiology and etiology of GERD are the result of the failure of the LES to be an effective barrier between the esophagus and the duodenogastric contents of the stomach. Exposure of the esophagus to bile as well as gastric acid is injurious to the lining of the esophagus. LES dysfunction, impaired

FIGURE 5-4 Esophagogram showing diffuse esophageal spasm.

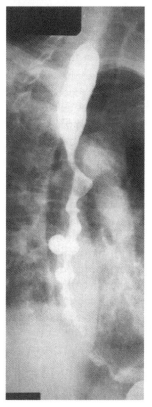

(Reprinted with permission from Castell DO, Richeter JE, eds. *The Esophagus*. 4th ed. New York, NY: Lippincott Williams & Wilkins; 2004:372.)

clearance of reflux from the esophagus, abnormal gastric emptying, and external factors contribute to the development of GERD.

a. Normal LES function is paramount to prevent reflux. A hypocontractile LES and increased transient LES relaxations are the most common causes of GERD. Normal anatomic positioning of the LES is also important because hiatal hernias potentiate GERD by disrupting the influence of the diaphragm on the function of the LES.

b. Impaired esophageal motility leads to poor clearance of duodenogastric refluxate from the distal esophagus. Poor saliva production can also lead to GERD because it normally neutralizes refluxed gastric acid.

c. Delayed gastric emptying leads to an increase in gastric pressure and a large volume of material available for reflux.

d. External factors that can lead to GERD by decreasing LES pressure include dietary factors, such as alcohol, fats, caffeine, smoking, medications, nitrates, and calcium-channel blockers. Hormones like progesterone can also be a factor. Obesity also worsens GERD by increasing abdominal pressure.

2. Clinical presentation

a. Classic esophageal symptoms are heartburn (the most common symptom), regurgitation, and dysphagia. Dysphagia may result from a GERD-induced stricture of the distal esophagus or from impaired esophageal motility.

b. Atypical extraesophageal symptoms are coughing, hoarseness, noncardiac chest pain, and asthma. GERD is a cause of asthma in 45% to 65% of adult onset asthmatics.

3. Diagnostic tests: Various studies are used to evaluate esophageal anatomy and function as well as to provide objective evidence for the presence of GERD.

a. Barium esophagram is useful in delineating esophageal anatomy. Reflux of gastric content, strictures, ulcerations, and hiatal hernias may all be demonstrated with a barium swallow.

Esophagus and Stomach

b. Esophagogastroduodenoscopy (EGD) is an essential study in the evaluation of those with GERD. EGD can provide objective evidence of GERD by identifying esophagitis, peptic strictures, esophageal ulcerations, or Barrett metaplasia within the esophagus. A majority of patients have normal findings on endoscopy (nonerosive esophageal reflux disease). EGD is also useful in evaluating the stomach and duodenum for other non-GERD (gastritis, peptic ulcer) causes of symptoms.

c. Esophageal pH analysis is the gold standard for the diagnosis of GERD. Findings of distal esophageal acid exposure to a pH less than 4 for more than 4.2% of a 24-hour period or exposure of the proximal esophagus (20 cm above the LES) to a pH less than 4 for 1.3% of a 24-hour period are diagnostic for GERD.

d. Esophageal manometry is used to evaluate LES function and the peristaltic function of the esophageal body. It is also useful in eliminating achalasia as a cause of GERD symptoms.

4. Treatment: Therapy consists of controlling the exposure of the esophagus to duodenogastric reflux.

a. Medications are the mainstay of treatment. H_2-receptor antagonists are appropriate for patients with only occasional (once per week) GERD symptoms. Proton pump inhibitors (PPIs) are recommended for those with more frequent or daily symptoms. Both drugs dramatically reduce gastric acid production by the stomach. However, neither class of drug is efficacious against the reflux of bile.

b. Endoscopic therapy for GERD is now FDA-approved and available in some centers. Techniques include endoscopic gastric plication and LES injection.

c. Surgery for GERD consists of constructing an esophagogastric fundoplication to augment the function of the LES and to provide a barrier to duodenogastric reflux into the esophagus.

(1) Efficacy of surgical fundoplication is approximately 90%.

(2) Fundoplications can be total (Nissen 360-degree wrap of the fundus around the distal esophagus) or partial (Toupet 270-degree posterior wrap; Dor 180-degree anterior wrap). However, the Nissen total fundoplication is thought to be the best barrier to reflux.

(3) Most fundoplications are performed as laparoscopic procedures, but they may also be performed through laparotomy or thoracotomy.

(4) The presence of a hiatal hernia often requires surgery for control of GERD symptoms because it signifies a distinct anatomic cause for GERD, which medications do not address.

5. Complications

a. Conditions that may develop include esophageal dysmotility, peptic stricture of the esophagus, erosive esophagitis, asthma, aspiration, recurrent pneumonia, and laryngitis.

b. Barrett esophagus (BE), which develops from a metaplastic process, is the end-stage manifestation of GERD. BE is defined as the replacement of the normal squamous epithelium of the esophagus with intestinal epithelium and stratified columnar epithelium, with the presence of goblet cells.

(1) BE is a premalignant lesion that occurs in up to 10% of patients with GERD.

(2) BE increases the risk of adenocarcinoma of the esophagus by at least 30-fold.

(3) Those with BE should be followed with surveillance endoscopy.

(4) The presence of high-grade dysplasia in BE is an indication for esophagectomy.

B. Hiatal hernias are common, whereas paraesophageal hernias (PEHs) are relatively rare (Figs. 5-5 and 5-6).

1. Etiology: Hiatal hernias and PEHs are thought to arise as an acquired disorder of the diaphragm and the gastroesophageal junction due to chronic elevations in abdominal pressure, weakening of the musculature of the esophageal crura, and possibly shortening of the esophagus from chronic GERD.

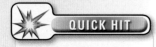

QUICK HIT

Objective evidence for the diagnosis of GERD includes a positive 24-hour pH study or the presence of erosive esophagitis, peptic stricture, or Barrett esophagus on endoscopy.

FIGURE
5-5 CT scan showing stomach located in the chest.

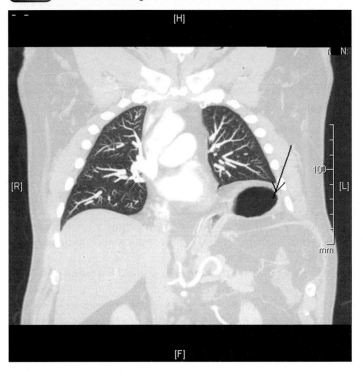

2. Pathophysiology: There are four types of hiatal hernias (Table 5-1).
3. Clinical presentation
   a. The majority of type I hiatal hernias are asymptomatic. However, they may predispose one to GERD and its symptomatology.
   b. Types II, III, and IV hiatal hernias and PEHs account for approximately 5% to 15% of all hiatal hernias. Common symptoms include substernal fullness,

FIGURE
5-6 Chest X-ray demonstrating a retrocardiac air–fluid level of a paraesophageal hernia.

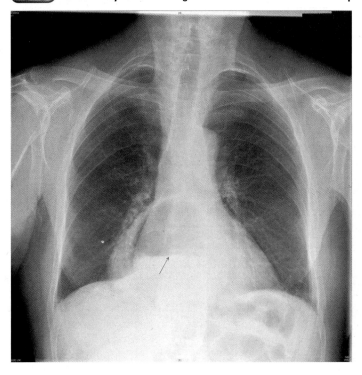

Esophagus and Stomach

TABLE 5-1 Types of Hiatal and Paraesophageal Hernias

Type	Position of Gastroesophageal Junction	Hernia Contents	Volvulus	Spontaneous Reduction
I—Sliding	Variable	Cardia, fundus	None	Common
II—True paraesophageal hernia	Intra-abdominal	Fundus, body	None or organoaxial	Uncommon
III—Mixed	Intrathoracic	Fundus, body	Organoaxial or mesoaxial	None
IV—Mixed + other organ	Intrathoracic	Fundus, body, other abdominal organ	Organoaxial or mesoaxial	None

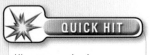

QUICK HIT

Ulcers occurring in a herniated stomach are also known as Cameron ulcers.

regurgitation, dysphagia, chest pain, and respiratory symptoms. GERD occurs infrequently with these types of PEHs.

c. Uncommon complications of PEHs include anemia secondary to ulcers in the herniated stomach (called Cameron ulcers), incarceration and strangulation of the herniated stomach, and perforation.

4. Diagnostic tests: Diagnostic studies are similar to those for the workup of GERD.
   a. Barium esophagram is useful to diagnose hiatal hernia and PEH. The volume of stomach herniated, position of the LES, and presence of mesoaxial (axis of rotation along the mesenteric attachment) or organoaxial (axis of rotation along the long axis of the stomach) volvulus can be determined.
   b. EGD is useful in the diagnosis of hiatal hernia and PEH because the presence of ulceration, ischemia, and rotation of the stomach can be determined.

5. Treatment: Therapy of type I hiatal hernias is straightforward, whereas that of types II, III, and IV PEH is controversial.
   a. Most type I hiatal hernias are asymptomatic and do not require therapy. When symptomatic, therapy parallels that of GERD, with surgery consisting of an esophagogastric fundoplication with hiatal repair.
   b. The morbidity of surgery for patients with types II to IV PEH who are advanced in age and have significant comorbidities makes surgical therapy for asymptomatic patients controversial.
   c. Surgical therapy for types II to IV PEH entails reduction of the herniated stomach, resection of the hernia sac, repair of the diaphragmatic crura with mesh, and esophagogastric fundoplication.

VI. Esophageal diverticula are rare. Classified by the region of the esophagus in which they occur.

A. Hypopharyngeal, or Zenker diverticulum (Fig. 5-7). This is a pulsion (false) diverticulum arising at the junction of the pharynx and the cervical esophagus,

FIGURE 5-7 Barium swallow showing a Zenker diverticulum.

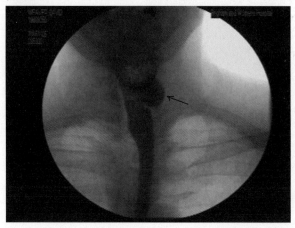

FIGURE
5-8 Triangle of Killian, an area of weakness that allows Zenker diverticulum to develop.

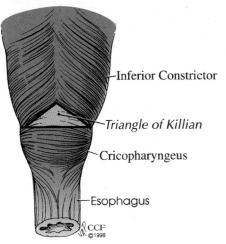

—Inferior Constrictor

—*Triangle of Killian*

—Cricopharyngeus

—Esophagus

CCF
©1998

(Adapted with permission from Castell DO, Richeter JE, eds. *The Esophagus*. 4th ed. New York, NY: Lippincott Williams & Wilkins; 2004:326.)

in the area known as Killian triangle, a relatively weak area in the posterior hypopharynx between the inferior pharyngeal constrictors superiorly and the cricopharyngeus muscle inferiorly (Fig. 5-8).

1. Etiology: The cause of Zenker diverticulum is not completely understood. Two potential causes are increased hyopharyngeal pressure accompanied by poor UES opening or cricopharyngeal incoordination.

2. Clinical presentation: Patients with a Zenker diverticulum are usually advanced in age and present with complaints of cervical dysphagia, regurgitation of food recently chewed, complaints of a "globus" sensation, and a left-sided neck mass. Aspiration and pneumonia are infrequent, and many small diverticula may be asymptomatic.

3. Diagnostic tests
   a. Barium esophagram is the best test to identify the presence of a Zenker diverticulum. Diverticula almost always are demonstrated on the left side of the neck.
   b. Esophagoscopy in general should be avoided because of its challenging nature and for fear of the risk of perforation of the diverticulum. It is indicated only if an esophagram demonstrates findings consistent with neoplasia within the diverticulum, a rare finding.

4. Treatment involves surgery because there is no effective medical therapy, with success rates ranging from 90% to 100%.
   a. Cricopharyngeal myotomy with diverticulectomy or diverticulopexy is classically performed through a left neck incision. The cricopharyngeus muscle is divided, and the diverticulum can either be resected or the fundus of the diverticulum can be sewn to the prevertebral fascia to facilitate its drainage.
   b. Endoscopic myotomy avoids an incision and shortens the hospitalization. An operating laryngoscope is used to expose the neck of the diverticulum, and a myotomy is performed using an endoscopic linear stapler. With this technique, the diverticulum becomes part of a common channel with the cervical esophagus.

B. Mid-esophageal diverticula may result from either traction or pulsion forces.
   1. Traction (true) diverticula are formed when inflammatory or scar tissue adheres to the esophagus, pulling the wall away from its natural course.
   2. Pulsion diverticula arise in the mid-esophagus (Fig. 5-9) as result of esophageal motility disorders that lead to areas of high pressure and diverticular development, with the mucosa protruding through the esophageal wall.
   3. Clinical presentation: Many mid-esophageal diverticula are asymptomatic. Symptoms such as dysphagia and chest pain relate to an underlying motility disorder. Complications are rare.

Esophagus and Stomach

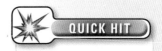

QUICK HIT

Pulsion diverticula are "false" diverticula consisting of only mucosa, whereas diverticula from traction forces are "true" diverticula containing all the layers of the esophageal wall.

FIGURE
5-9 Mid-esophageal traction diverticulum.

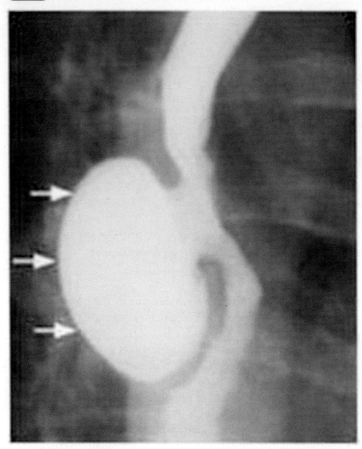

4. Diagnostic tests: Usually, diagnosis is made by a barium esophagram. However, flexible esophagoscopy may also be useful.
5. Treatment: Most mid-esophageal diverticula are asymptomatic and do not require treatment. For those with symptoms and a mid-esophageal diverticulum, treatment consists of a myotomy and a diverticulectomy.
C. Epiphrenic diverticula (Fig. 5-10) are pulsion diverticula that are uncommon and occur in the distal 4 to 10 cm of the thoracic esophagus.
1. Etiology: Almost all epiphrenic diverticula are associated with an underlying motility disorder, such as achalasia or DES. Diverticula have also been seen

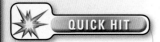
QUICK HIT

Zenker and epiphrenic diverticula are pulsion diverticula whose cause is an underlying esophageal motility disorder. Primary therapy should be directed toward treating the motility disorder, with treatment of the diverticula being a secondary concern.

FIGURE
5-10 Epiphrenic diverticulum.

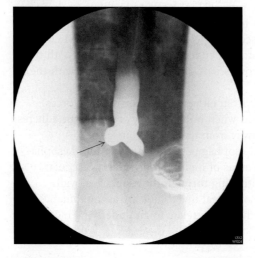

above peptic strictures of the distal esophagus and in association with hiatal hernias.

2. Clinical presentation: Patients with epiphrenic diverticula may be asymptomatic or may have symptoms related to the presence of an associated motility disorder. Dysphagia, regurgitation, and chest pain occur in variable degrees. Esophageal obstruction, perforation, and fistula formation tend to occur rarely.

3. Diagnostic tests
   a. A barium swallow is the best diagnostic test.
   b. Flexible esophagoscopy may be useful in identifying the presence of esophageal inflammation or stricture.
   c. Esophageal manometry is mandatory to rule out the presence of an underlying motility disorder.

4. Treatment: Therapy is directed at the associated motility disorder that is usually present and any complication of the diverticulum.
   a. Small asymptomatic epiphrenic diverticula not associated with a motility disorder may be followed clinically.
   b. Complicated epiphrenic diverticula and those with an associated esophageal motility disorder usually require surgery.
      (1) Esophageal myotomy and diverticulectomy is the initial surgical option.
      (2) Nonsurgical options are reserved for patients with achalasia and an epiphrenic diverticulum. Both botulinum toxin injection and pneumatic balloon dilatation have been used.

VII. Tumors of the Esophagus

A. Benign tumors of the esophagus occur uncommonly and are usually asymptomatic.

1. Leiomyomas arise from the muscular layer of the esophagus and are the most common benign esophageal tumor.
   a. Clinical presentation: Symptoms include dysphagia, chest pain, esophageal obstruction, and bleeding when the overlying mucosa becomes ulcerated.
   b. Diagnostic tests
      (1) On esophagram, these lesions appear as smooth filling defects in the esophageal lumen.
      (2) On endoscopy, the overlying mucosa appears normal, and the mass is firm and nodular.
      (3) On endoscopic ultrasound, the mass is hypoechoic and confirms the layer of origin.
   c. Treatment: Therapy is through surgical resection by enucleation. Surgery is indicated for large (greater than 4 cm) tumors, lesions that are growing, or lesions that are symptomatic. Small asymptomatic lesions may be followed with interval imaging studies.

2. Fibrovascular polyps, or fibrolipomas, originate from the mucosal layer and occur in the proximal cervical esophagus.
   a. Clinical presentation: Dysphagia, regurgitation, and respiratory problems are the main symptoms.
   b. Diagnostic tests: Diagnosis can be made with barium esophagram or endoscopic ultrasound.
   c. Treatment: Therapy is usually reserved for large or symptomatic polyps. Endoscopic resection or open resection via a cervical esophagotomy or thoracic approach is the method of choice.

B. Malignant tumors: Adenocarcinoma and squamous cell carcinoma (SCC) are the two most common malignancies of the esophagus.

1. Adenocarcinoma of the esophagus is increasing in frequency and is the most common malignant esophageal tumor in the United States.
   a. Epidemiology: Adenocarcinoma commonly affects people in their sixth or seventh decade of life, men more than women (at a ratio of 5:1 to 7:1), and Caucasian men more than African-American men.
   b. Etiology: Chronic GERD and BE are causative factors for esophageal adeno-carcinoma.

    c. Pathophysiology: Adenocarcinoma arises from the mucosal layer of the esophagus and spreads by invasion through the wall of the esophagus to contiguous structures (aorta, trachea, and recurrent laryngeal nerve). Lymphatic metastasis occurs to periesophageal, cervical, mediastinal, and celiac lymph nodes. Distant metastasis is usually to the liver, lung, bone, adrenal gland, and brain.

2. SCC is the most common malignant tumor of the esophagus worldwide.

    a. Epidemiology: Like adenocarcinoma, SCC affects people in their sixth and seventh decades of life, and men more than women. However, SCC affects African-American men more than Caucasian men.

    b. Etiology: Chronic exposure of the esophagus to noxious or caustic stimuli such as hot liquids or foods, lye, nitrosamines, alcohol, cigarette smoke, and previous radiation are thought to lead to dysplasia and eventual neoplasia of the squamous-lined esophagus. Rare diseases such as tylosis, Plummer–Vinson syndrome, and achalasia are also linked to the development of SCC.

    c. Pathophysiology: SCC arises from the squamous epithelium of the upper and mid-esophagus. Metastatic sites are similar to those of adenocarcinoma.

3. Clinical presentation: Symptoms are vague and present late in the course of the disease process. They include dysphagia, weight loss, pain, and anemia due to ulceration of the tumor with resultant bleeding.

TABLE 5-2 American Joint Committee on Cancer (AJCC 7th Edition, 2010) TNM Staging of Esophageal Cancer

Primary Tumor (T Stage)	Description
TX	Primary tumor cannot be assessed
T0	No evidence of primary tumor
Tis	High-grade dysplasia. Includes all noninvasive neoplastic epithelia.
T1	Tumor invades lamina propria, muscularis mucosae, or submucosa
T1a	Tumor invades lamina propria or muscularis mucosae
T1b	Tumor invades submucosa
T2	Tumor invades muscularis propria
T3	Tumor invades adventitia
T4	Tumor invades adjacent structures
T4a	Resectable tumor invading pleura, pericardium, or diaphragm
T4b	Unresectable tumor invading other adjacent structures such as the aorta, vertebral body, trachea, etc.
Regional Lymph Nodes (N Stage)	
NX	Regional lymph node(s) cannot be assessed
N0	No regional lymph node involvement
N1	Metastasis in one to two regional lymph nodes
N2	Metastasis in three to six regional lymph nodes
N3	Metastasis in seven or more regional lymph nodes
Distant Metastasis (M Stage)	
M0	No distant metastasis
M1	Distant metastasis

FIGURE
5-11 **Esophageal cancer progression.**

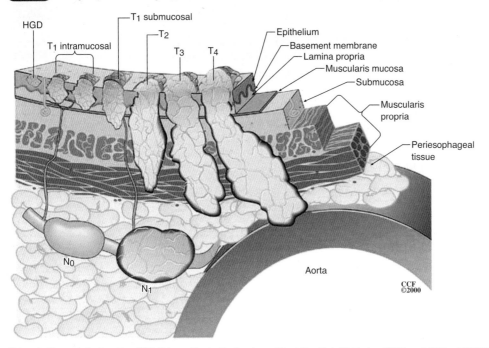

HGD
T₁ intramucosal
T₁ submucosal
T₂
T₃
T₄
Epithelium
Basement membrane
Lamina propria
Muscularis mucosa
Submucosa
Muscularis propria
Periesophageal tissue
N₀
N₁
Aorta
CCF
©2000

(Adapted with permission from Castell DO, Richeter JE, eds. *The Esophagus*. 4th ed. New York, NY: Lippincott Williams & Wilkins; 2004:292.)

4. Diagnostic tests: Certain diagnostic tests are used to determine the stage of the tumor using the tumor-node-metastasis (TNM) system (Table 5-2 and Fig. 5-11).
   a. Flexible esophagoscopy with biopsy for tissue diagnosis
   b. Barium esophagram is useful in the evaluation of obstructive symptoms because it may identify a narrowing or stricture with the characteristic appearance of a tumor.
   c. Endoscopic ultrasound is the most sensitive test to delineate the depth of tumor invasion through the esophageal wall ("T" of the TNM staging system). It may also identify enlarged periesophageal lymph nodes ("N" of TNM staging).
   d. Computed tomography (CT) scanning is important for staging because it is a sensitive method for detecting distant metastasis. It may also be useful for staging both the primary tumor and lymph nodes.
   e. Fluroro-2-deoxy-D-glucose positron emission tomography (FDG PET) scanning may replace CT scans as the modality of choice for determining distant metastases (Fig. 5-12).

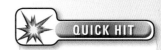

QUICK HIT

Dysphagia is the most common symptom of esophageal cancer. Although not specific for the presence of cancer, dysphagia accompanied by weight loss should prompt evaluation with a barium esophagram and/or flexible esophagoscopy.

FIGURE
5-12 **PET scan showing an esophageal mass with hypermetabolic activity.**

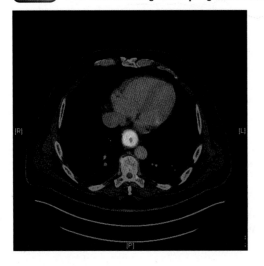

Esophagus and Stomach

TABLE 5-3	Treatment of Esophageal Cancer by Stage. American Joint Committee on Cancer (AJCC) Stage Grouping with Recommended Treatment Strategy and Predicted 5-Year Survival		
Stage	**TNM Designation**	**Recommended Treatment**	**5-Year Survival (%)**
0	Tis, N0, M0	Surgery	95
I	T1, N0, M0	Surgery	75
IIA	T2, N0, M0	Surgery	30
	T3, N0, M0		
IIB	T1, N1, M0	Surgery, or surgery with preoperative chemoradiation	20
	T2, N1, M0		
III	T3, N1, M0	T3 tumors: surgery, or surgery with preoperative chemoradiation	10–15
	T4, any N, M0	Palliation: chemotherapy, radiation therapy, stenting, or combination	
IVa	Any T, any N, M1a	Palliation: chemotherapy, radiation therapy, stenting, or combination	5
IVb	Any T, any N, M1b		1

TMN, tumor-node-metastasis.

5. Treatment: Therapy depends on the stage of the cancer (Table 5-3).
   a. Surgical options consist of esophagectomy by a transhiatal (left cervical incision and laparotomy) or Ivor–Lewis (combined right thoracotomy and laparotomy) technique. Newer, minimally invasive techniques are offered in some centers, and these include laparoscopic/thoracoscopic approaches as well as robotic esophagectomy.
   b. Chemotherapy and radiation therapy are used for unresectable cancers and in combination with surgery in clinical trials of advanced stage cancers.
   c. Endoscopic dilatation and stenting of the esophagus are palliative measures used for obstructing or near-obstructing tumors that are unresectable or are receiving chemotherapy and radiation prior to resection.

VIII. Injury and Bleeding

A. Esophageal perforation is a highly lethal condition.
   1. Etiology
      a. Iatrogenic perforation is now the cause of approximately 60% of esophageal perforations, with esophagoscopy or endoscopic therapies being the most frequent antecedent interventions.
      b. Other causes include spontaneous rupture or Boerhaave syndrome (postemetic rupture of the distal esophagus) 15%, foreign body ingestion 10% to 15%, trauma 10%, and tumor 1%.
   2. Clinical presentation: This depends on the region of perforation and the length of time prior to discovery.
      a. Cervical esophageal perforations cause dysphagia, neck pain, and subcutaneous emphysema. Progression to mediastinitis and sepsis tends to be relatively slow.
      b. Intrathoracic perforations lead to direct mediastinal contamination and symptoms of chest pain, tachypnea, tachycardia, fever, and mediastinal emphysema. Progression to sepsis and shock is rapid.

c. Intra-abdominal perforation of the esophagus causes peritonitis with symptoms of epigastric pain, back pain, tachypnea, tachycardia, and referred pain to the shoulders. Progression to sepsis is usually rapid.

3. Diagnostic tests: A high index of suspicion and early diagnosis are key in effecting early therapy and decreasing mortality. Diagnostic studies include:

   a. Contrast esophagography is the study of choice to evaluate for esophageal perforation. Barium, in general, is avoided because it may cause or worsen mediastinitis. If a water-soluble contrast swallow is negative and suspicion for perforation is high, the test should be repeated with barium or a CT scan should be obtained.

   b. CT scanning of the chest and abdomen is useful for those who cannot undergo esophagography or when the presentation is atypical.

   c. Flexible esophagoscopy is useful in the evaluation of perforations suspected from penetrating trauma and in cases of caustic ingestion.

4. Treatment: Management almost always involves surgery, with the type of surgery depending on the time course of the perforation.

   a. Initial therapy is directed toward volume resuscitation and limiting mediastinal contamination with nasogastric decompression and intravenous antibiotics.

   b. Perforations of the cervical esophagus can be managed by drainage alone through a cervical incision or by primary closure and drainage.

   c. Thoracic and abdominal esophageal perforations of less than 24 hours in duration are usually best managed by primary repair, buttressing of the repair with local vascularized tissue, and drainage of the chest and mediastinum.

   d. Whereas primary repair has traditionally been reserved for perforations presenting in the first 24 hours, primary repair can be considered in patients beyond this time frame. The decision to proceed with primary repair >24 hours after injury is dependent on a multitude of factors including the condition of the patient, the degree of mediastinal contamination, the state of the esophagus prior to the perforation (disease vs. no disease), and whether the perforation is felt to be due to an underlying malignancy. In this case, surgical therapy consists of either diversion of the esophagus above and below the perforation, with exclusion of the perforation from gastrointestinal (GI) secretions, or creation of a controlled fistula with T-tube drainage through the perforation along with wide drainage.

   e. Esophagectomy is reserved for perforations due to cancer or untreatable obstructions.

   f. Nonoperative therapy (antibiotics, cessation of oral intake, intravenous hydration) can be applied to a select group of patients with contained perforations secondary to instrumentation who are clinically stable and have no signs of sepsis.

   g. Another option in patients who are not suitable for other management strategies is the placement of an endoluminal stent to cover the perforation. This can be a good option for a patient with a partial esophageal obstruction due to a tumor.

B. Foreign bodies in the esophagus

   1. The majority of foreign bodies (75% to 90%) pass spontaneously without complication; however, most retained foreign bodies in the GI tract are found in the esophagus.

      a. There is a high morbidity and mortality associated with retained foreign bodies in the esophagus due to the risk of perforation.

      b. Retention times >24 hours are associated with the highest risk of complications.

      c. All foreign bodies should be managed on an urgent basis.

   2. Foreign bodies can be classified into four categories: blunt foreign bodies, sharp foreign bodies, iatrogenic foreign bodies, and food boluses.

FIGURE 5-13 Chest X-ray demonstrating a foreign body in the esophagus (in this case a coin).

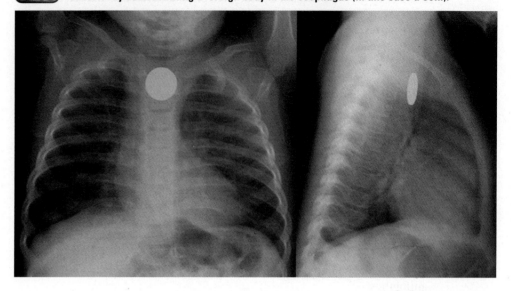

3. Diagnosis and management
   a. Rigid esophagoscopy or direct laryngoscopy are the modalities of choice for initial evaluation of an esophageal foreign body. In addition to direct visualization, foreign bodies can also sometimes be visualized on diagnostic imaging studies (Fig. 5-13).
   b. Flexible gastroscopy can be used to visualize foreign bodies in the distal esophagus.
   c. Endoscopic management of foreign bodies is the preferred modality of treatment with success rates of 90% to 100%.
C. Bleeding from the esophagus can be a significant cause of upper GI blood loss.
   1. Esophagitis is usually secondary to GERD, and therapy is directed at decreasing gastric acid production and controlling duodenogastric reflux.
   2. Esophageal varices are invariably due to portal hypertension and carry a 20% to 30% mortality rate with each episode of bleeding.
      a. Diagnosis is made by endoscopy.
      b. Controlling hemorrhage can be accomplished via therapies directed at sites of hemorrhage or by measures to decrease pressure in the portal system.
         (1) Endoscopic control of bleeding consists of band ligation or sclerosis of individual varices. Efficacy is approximately 80%.
         (2) Surgery is rarely performed for control of life-threatening variceal bleeding. Surgical options focus on decreasing portal venous pressures by shunting blood away from the portal circulation to the systemic circulation. Portocaval, mesocaval, and distal splenorenal shunts are examples of commonly used portosystemic shunts. Mortality for emergency shunting can be up to 20%.
         (3) Transjugular intrahepatic portosystemic shunting (TIPS) has largely replaced emergency surgical shunting as the standard of therapy for bleeding esophagogastric varices that are unresponsive to endoscopic and pharmacologic treatment.
         (4) Temporary control of hemorrhage when endoscopy, surgery, or TIPS are not available can be accomplished by balloon tamponade of bleeding varices with the use of a Sengstaken–Blakemore tube. Definitive therapy is still needed, because bleeding recurs in 50% or more cases.
         (5) Adjuncts to control hemorrhage include the use of the somatostatin analogue octreotide, which decreases bleeding by up to 50% through splanchnic vasoconstriction.

3. Mallory–Weiss syndrome is massive upper GI hemorrhage caused by a tear through the mucosa of the distal esophagus or gastroesophageal junction.
   a. An acute increase in intra-abdominal pressure leading to the development of a pressure gradient across the gastroesophageal junction is thought to be the cause. Examples of causes are forceful retching or vomiting, paroxysms of coughing, blunt abdominal trauma, and straining during a bowel movement.
   b. Hematemesis is the presenting symptom in 80% to 90%.
   c. Upper endoscopy is diagnostic.
   d. Bleeding stops spontaneously in more than 90% of cases.
   e. Endoscopic therapy is effective for those lesions that do not cease bleeding spontaneously. Endoscopic sclerotherapy, banding, hemoclipping, heater probe application, and multipolar electrocoagulation have all been used to control hemorrhage.
   f. Surgery, which consists of suture ligation of the lesion, is rarely used to control bleeding.

STOMACH

I. Embryology
A. The stomach is derived from the embryonic foregut.
B. At the fifth gestational week, a caudal dilation of foregut becomes the future stomach.
C. Ventral mesentery becomes falciform ligament, lesser omentum, gastrohepatic, and hepatoduodenal mesenteries.
D. The celiac artery passes through the dorsal mesentery.
E. Dorsal mesentery forms the gastrocolic, gastrosplenic, and gastrophrenic ligaments.
F. In the sixth to seventh week of gestation, the left gastric wall (the greater curvature) growth is accelerated in comparison to the right gastric wall (the lesser curvature).

II. Anatomy
A. Anatomy of the stomach
   1. Gross anatomy
      a. The gastric cardia is the region just distal to the gastroesophageal junction.
      b. The gastric fundus is the region superior and to the left of the gastroesophageal junction.
      c. The corpus (body) of the stomach encompasses the area between the fundus and antrum.
      d. The antrum compromises the distal stomach and ends at the pylorus.
   2. Vascularization
      a. Arterial supply
         (1) The left gastric artery is a branch of the celiac axis and supplies a large portion of lesser curve and gastroesophageal junction.
         (2) The right gastric artery is a branch of the hepatic artery from the celiac axis and supplies the distal lesser curve.
         (3) The short gastric and left gastroepiploic arteries are branches of the splenic artery and supply the greater curvature and fundus.
         (4) The right gastroepiploic artery is a branch of the gastroduodenal artery and supplies the distal greater curve of the stomach. This artery must be identified and preserved during esophagectomy because it will be the only remaining blood supply to the stomach once the stomach has been mobilized.
      b. Venous drainage of the stomach is to the portal system, and veins parallel the arterial supply.
   3. Innervation
      a. Parasympathetic/vagal
         (1) The vagal trunks pass through the esophageal hiatus along the anterior and posterior esophagus.

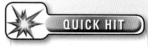
QUICK HIT

Unequal growth at 6 to 7 weeks results in a rotation of the stomach placing the left vagal trunk anteriorly and the right vagal trunk posteriorly.

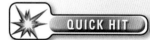
QUICK HIT

Although the distinction of the antrum from the corpus is not apparent externally, it is defined by a line from the incisura angularis on the lesser curve to a point on the greater curve one-fourth the distance from the pylorus to the gastroesophageal junction.

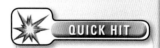
QUICK HIT

The stomach's blood supply is abundant, and it is protected from ischemia with its vast intramural and extramural collaterals. The viability of the stomach can be maintained by preserving only one primary vessel.

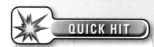
QUICK HIT

The right gastroepiploic artery must be identified and preserved during an esophagectomy because it will be the only remaining blood supply to the stomach.

Esophagus and Stomach

(2) After the gastroesophageal junction, the anterior vagus nerve divides, and the hepatic branch sends fibers to the liver and gallbladder.

(3) Distal to the hepatic branch, the anterior vagus becomes the nerve of Latarjet.

b. Sympathetic

(1) Sympathetic fibers originate from spinal nerve roots T5 to T10 and pass via gray rami communicantes to enter prevertebral ganglia.

(2) Presynaptic fibers then follow the greater splanchnic nerves to the celiac plexus.

(3) Postsynaptic fibers enter the stomach with the blood vessels.

4. Lymphatic drainage

(1) The proximal stomach near the lesser curve initially drains lymph into the superior gastric lymph nodes that surround the left gastric artery.

(2) The distal stomach near the lesser curve drains into the suprapyloric nodes.

(3) The proximal greater curvature drains to the subpyloric and omental lymph nodes.

(4) Secondary drainage from these lymph node basins passes on to the celiac axis nodes.

III. Histology.
The gastric mucosa is composed of simple columnar epithelium with surface mucous cells.

A. Oxyntic glands are located in the fundus and body of the stomach.

1. Glands contain parietal cells that are responsible for acid and intrinsic factor production.

2. They contain chief cells that produce and secrete pepsinogen.

3. Mucous cells produce mucus and bicarbonate that protects the lining of the stomach from damage by luminal acid.

4. Enterochromaffin-like (ECL) cells are also found in oxyntic glands. ECL cells produce histamine and are a major regulator of gastric acid production.

B. Antral glands are located in the distal stomach and pyloric channel.

1. Most secrete mucus, but many also contain G-cells that produce gastrin.

2. D-cells produce the inhibitory hormone somatostatin.

3. Chief cells are also found in pyloric glands.

IV. Physiology

A. Gastric peptides

1. Gastrin

a. Meals stimulate release of gastrin via intragastric breakdown of proteins.

b. Gastric distension contributes to cholinergic activation and subsequent gastrin release.

c. Somatostatin decreases gastrin secretion.

d. Acidification after a meal also inhibits gastrin release when luminal pH falls below 3.0.

2. Somatostatin

a. Inhibits acid secretion and gastrin release

b. A decreased intragastric pH stimulates its release, and an increased pH will inhibit its release.

3. Ghrelin

a. Ghrelin is produced by oxyntic glands.

b. It is an orexigenic hormone, and it stimulates food intake.

4. Pepsins are a group of proteolytic enzymes secreted by gastric chief cells.

a. Cholinergic stimulus is the most important secretagogue.

b. Pepsins initiate protein digestion.

5. Intrinsic factor is secreted by parietal cells. It functions by binding cobalamin (vitamin B_{12}), which is subsequently absorbed in the ileum.

V. Benign Disorders

A. Peptic ulcer disease (PUD)

1. Epidemiology

a. Peak incidence of PUD is in the sixth and seventh decades of life.

b. PUD tends to occur in lower socioeconomic classes.

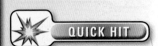

QUICK HIT

Parietal cells contain receptors for histamine, acetylcholine, and gastrin, which are the important stimulants for acid production.

QUICK HIT

A gastrectomy, either partial or total, that removes the oxyntic mucosa and parietal cell mass, or a gastric bypass, can lead to malabsorption of cobalamin and pernicious anemia.

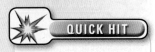

QUICK HIT

Approximately 75% of gastric ulcers and 90% of duodenal ulcers are associated with *H. pylori* infection.

    c. Each year, approximately 300,000 to 500,000 new cases of PUD occur.

    d. Three to four million patients are self-medicating for symptoms of PUD, and 30,000 surgeries are performed annually for PUD.

2. Etiology: Causes of ulceration are multifactorial. Predisposing conditions include:

    a. Age greater than 40

    b. Use of nonsteroidal anti-inflammatories

    c. Pepsin and acid secretion abnormalities

    d. Delayed gastric emptying

    e. Bile reflux

    f. Coexisting duodenal ulceration

    g. *Helicobacter pylori* infection

3. Pathophysiology

    a. Mucosal *H. pylori* infection contributes to ulcer formation in most cases.

        (1) *H. pylori* is a helical gram-negative rod with flagella that resides beneath the mucous layer of stomach.

        (2) Production of the enzyme urease allows *H. pylori* to survive in the acidic environment of the stomach.

    b. There are five types of gastric ulcers (Table 5-4).

    c. The majority of ulcers are type I and are not associated with excessive acid secretion.

4. Clinical presentation

    a. PUD may occur intermittently with relapsing episodes.

    b. Often, it is difficult to differentiate PUD from gastric carcinoma.

    c. Abdominal pain, bleeding, obstruction, and perforation are all symptoms of PUD.

5. Diagnostic tests

    a. Physical examination often reveals epigastric abdominal pain. Peritoneal signs suggest perforation.

    b. Upright chest radiography is useful to evaluate for the presence of free intra-abdominal air, signaling perforation.

    c. Contrast radiography can diagnose PUD, but it may miss some malignant disease presenting as PUD.

    d. Flexible endoscopy is the mainstay in the diagnosis of PUD. Biopsy of all gastric ulcers is mandatory to rule out the presence of a gastric cancer presenting as PUD.

    e. Tests for *H. pylori* include serology, the urea breath test, and biopsy with rapid urease testing (*Campylobacter*-like organism [CLO] test) or histologic analysis.

6. Medical treatment

    a. Eradication of *H. pylori* with regimens that include a PPI in combination with two antibiotics for approximately 14 days

    b. Histamine receptor antagonists

    c. PPIs

    d. Sucralfate (an aluminum salt of sulfated sucrose that polymerizes and becomes viscous to adhere to gastroduodenal mucosa and ulcer bed)

    e. Bismuth compounds for *H. pylori*

TABLE 5-4	**Types of Gastric Ulcers**	
Type	**Location**	**Excessive Acid Secretion**
I	Lesser curve	No
II	Body and duodenum	Yes
III	Prepyloric	Yes
IV	Lesser curve near gastroesophageal junction	No
V	Anywhere, induced by nonsteroidal anti-inflammatory drug	No

7. Surgical treatment
   a. Indications include bleeding, perforation, obstruction, and intractable PUD resistant to medical therapy.
   b. Truncal vagotomy involves the division of vagal trunks at the esophageal hiatus and is usually combined with a pyloroplasty (denervation results in delayed gastric emptying).
   c. Truncal vagotomy and antrectomy have the lowest recurrence rate for PUD.
   d. Proximal gastric vagotomy, where only the nerves to acid-secreting cells are divided. The hepatic and celiac branches, as well as fibers to the antrum and pylorus (nerves of Latarjet), are spared.
   e. Increasingly, treatments have involved addressing the acute problem, such as repairing a perforation, controlling the hemorrhage with nonresective surgical procedures, or managing the PUD medically with acid reduction and *H. pylori* eradication.

VI. Benign Tumors

A. Hyperplastic polyps
   1. Polyps are usually small in size and less than 2 cm in diameter.
   2. Typically, they arise in the setting of chronic atrophic gastritis.
   3. Most resolve with *H. pylori* treatment.
   4. Malignant transformation is unusual to rare, at 1% to 3%.
   5. Endoscopic polypectomy is the treatment of choice.
B. Fundic gland polyps represent hyperplasia of normal fundic glands.
   1. They can be associated with familial polyposis syndromes.
   2. They harbor no malignant potential.
C. Adenomatous polyps
   1. Polyps may be tubular, tubulovillous, or villous.
   2. The risk of malignant transformation increases with larger size and villous type.
   3. Gastric adenocarcinoma may be found in approximately 20% of cases.
   4. Endoscopic polypectomy is effective if the entire polyp is removed and no invasive carcinoma is found on review of the histologic specimen.
   5. Surgical resection is indicated for sessile lesions greater than 2 cm, polyps with invasive tumors, or polyps causing symptoms such as bleeding or obstruction.
D. Ectopic pancreas or pancreatic rests
   1. These occur during embryonic development while the dorsal and ventral fuse.
   2. The majority of cases involve the stomach, duodenum, and jejunum.
   3. Most patients are asymptomatic.
   4. Symptoms include abdominal pain, discomfort, nausea, vomiting, and bleeding.
   5. Diagnosis is made via endoscopy. Endoscopic ultrasound may be helpful for location and biopsy.
   6. Treatment of symptomatic lesions is by surgical resection.

VII. Other Gastric Lesions

A. Hypertrophic gastritis (Ménétrier disease) is an acquired rare premalignant disorder characterized by massive gastric folds involving the fundus and body.
   1. On evaluation, the mucosa has a cobblestone appearance.
   2. Histologic analysis reveals foveolar hyperplasia and the absence of parietal cells.
   3. Ménétrier disease is associated with protein loss from the stomach, excessive mucus production, and achlorhydria. It is linked with cytomegalovirus infection in children and *H. pylori* infection in adults.
   4. Presenting symptoms are epigastric pain, weight loss, vomiting, and peripheral edema.
   5. Medical treatment involves anticholinergics, acid suppression, octreotide, and *H. pylori* eradication.

6. Surgical treatment is via total gastrectomy and is reserved for patients with massive protein loss despite adequate medical therapy or for the development of dysplasia or carcinoma.

B. Dieulafoy gastric lesion
1. Pulsations of an abnormally large artery coursing through the submucosa lead to erosion of the mucosa, followed by exposure to gastric contents and hemorrhage. The vessel is usually located along the lesser curve within 6 cm of the gastroesophageal junction.
2. Peak incidence is in the fifth decade of life and is more common in men.
3. Classic presentation is with sudden recurrent massive hematemesis and hypotension.
4. Endoscopy is used for diagnosis and treatment. Endoscopic control of hemorrhage may be therapeutic.
5. Treatment is surgical and includes laparotomy or laparoscopy with wedge resection that incorporates the offending vessel.

C. Gastric varices
1. These may occur with esophageal varices with portal hypertension or secondary to sinistral (left-sided) hypertension from splenic vein thrombosis.
2. Treatment
   a. Splenectomy is the treatment of choice for splenic vein thrombosis.
   b. Those associated with portal hypertension are treated in a similar manner as esophageal varices.

D. Gastric bezoars are collections of nondigestible substances within the lumen of the stomach.
1. Phytobezoars are made of cellulose from ingestion of vegetables.
   a. Phytobezoars occur as a result of impaired gastric emptying.
   b. Treatment is with enzymatic therapy with papain.
      (1) Papain administration is followed by gastric lavage or endoscopic fragmentation.
      (2) Failure of enzymatic digestion leads to surgical removal.
2. Trichobezoars are formed from the ingestion of hair.
   a. Small lesions can be removed via endoscopy, lavage, or enzyme treatment.
   b. Large casts require surgical removal.

VIII. Malignant Disease

A. Adenocarcinoma of the stomach
1. Epidemiology
   a. The second most common cancer worldwide, adenocarcinoma of the stomach is the 10th most common cancer in the United States.
   b. In the United States, it is more common in black males, and men are more likely to be affected than women, with a ratio of 2:1.
   c. In Japan and in South America, incidence rates are higher.
   d. The site of gastric cancers has shifted from the distal stomach to the more proximal gastric cardia.
2. Risk factors
   a. Diet
      (1) Salted meat or fish
      (2) Nitrate consumption
      (3) Complex carbohydrates
   b. Medical
      (1) *H. pylori* infection
      (2) Adenomatous polyps
      (3) Pernicious anemia
3. Clinical presentation
   a. Symptoms include vague epigastric discomfort and indigestion.
   b. More advanced disease is associated with anemia, anorexia, weight loss, fatigue, or vomiting.
4. For staging, please refer to Table 5-5.

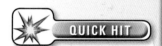

QUICK HIT

In the late stages of gastric adenocarcinoma, patients may have signs of advanced or metastatic disease. These include palpable masses or palpable lymph nodes.
- **Sister Mary Joseph nodes** are located in the periumbilical area.
- **Virchow nodes** are supraclavicular nodes.
- **Krukenberg tumor** is a palpable ovarian mass.
- **Blumer shelf** is peritoneal metastasis palpable by rectal examination.

Esophagus and Stomach

TABLE **5-5**	**American Joint Committee on Cancer (AJCC 7th Edition, 2010) TNM Staging of Gastric Cancer**
Primary Tumor (T Stage)	**Description**
TX	Primary tumor cannot be assessed
T0	No evidence of primary tumor
Tis	Carcinoma in situ; intraepithelial tumor without invasion of the lamina propria
T1	Tumor invades lamina propria, muscularis mucosae, or submucosa
T1a	Tumor invades lamina propria or muscularis mucosae
T1b	Tumor invades submucosa
T2	Tumor invades muscularis propria
T3	Tumor penetrates subserosal connective tissue without invasion of visceral peritoneum or adjacent structures
T4	Tumor invades serosa (visceral peritoneum) or adjacent structures
T4a	Tumor invades serosa (visceral peritoneum)
T4b	Tumor invades adjacent structures
Regional Lymph Nodes (N Stage)	
NX	Regional lymph node(s) cannot be assessed
N0	No regional lymph node involvement
N1	Metastasis in one to two regional lymph nodes
N2	Metastasis in three to six regional lymph nodes
N3	Metastasis in seven or more regional lymph nodes
N3a	Metastasis in 7–15 regional lymph nodes
N3b	Metastasis in 16 or more regional lymph nodes
Distant Metastasis (M Stage)	
M0	No distant metastasis
M1	Distant metastasis
Histologic Grade (G)	
GX	Grade cannot be assessed
G1	Well differentiated
G2	Moderately differentiated
G3	Poorly differentiated
G4	Undifferentiated

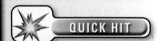

QUICK HIT

Linitis plastica is a form of advanced gastric cancer in which all (or nearly all) of the stomach is involved in a desmoplastic reaction to cancer. It carries a poor prognosis.

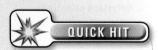

QUICK HIT

H. pylori eradication with antibiotics results in complete regression of low-grade MALTomas in 70% to 100% of cases.

B. Gastric lymphoma
    1. Epidemiology
        a. The stomach is the most common site for lymphoma in the GI tract.
        b. More than 50% of affected patients have anemia.
        c. Peak incidence is in the sixth and seventh decades.
        d. The disease is more common in males.
    2. Mucosa-associated lymphoma tissue (MALT)
        a. Gastric submucosa does not normally contain lymphoid tissue.
        b. *H. pylori* infection is believed to be a causal factor for MALT.
        c. Low-grade MALT resembles Peyer patches.

C. GI stromal tumors of the stomach
  1. These account for 3% of gastric malignancies because these tumors arise in the mesenchymal portion of the gastric wall.
  2. Patients present at a mean age of 60 years and after the sixth decade.
  3. Lesions with more than 5 to 10 mitoses per 10 high-powered fields demonstrate an increased potential for metastasis.
  4. Metastasis occurs via the hematogenous route, and lymphatic involvement is rare.
  5. Surgical resection is the treatment of choice.

D. Carcinoid
  1. Gastric carcinoids are uncommon and account for only 3% to 5% of GI carcinoids.
  2. They appear as reddish-pink to yellow submucosal nodules.
  3. Invasion is rare but occurs more frequently in tumors greater than 2 cm in size.
  4. Curative resection is indicated in most cases.

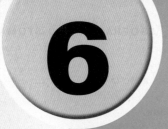

6 Small Bowel

Jennifer Knight, Zachary Baker, and Robert Ferguson

ANATOMY

I. Gross Anatomy

A. Duodenum: extends from the pylorus to the ligament of Treitz
   1. First portion (bulb): from pylorus to an area 5 cm distal and most common site of peptic ulcers
   2. Second portion (descending): 10 cm in length with a retroperitoneal structure bounded by the pancreas medially and Gerota fascia posteriorly. The common bile duct is on the posterior-medial surface of the second portion, and the ampulla of Vater enters about 7 to 10 cm from the pylorus.
   3. Third portion (transverse): almost completely retroperitoneal, except the distal segment
      a. Attached to the uncinate process of the pancreas near L3
      b. Directly posterior to the hepatic flexure of the colon and passes between the superior mesenteric artery and aorta
   4. Fourth portion (ascending): short segment from the aorta to the ligament of Treitz

B. Jejunum and ileum
   1. No clear demarcation between the jejunum and ileum, and the total length ranges from 5 to 10 meters.
   2. Jejunum has thicker mucosa than ileum and more prominent plicae circulares (circular folds of the mucosa).
   3. Ileal diameter decreases as it approaches the ileocecal valve.
      a. The ileocecal valve prevents reflux of fecal material from the colon into the small bowel, leading to different bacterial flora in the colon and terminal ileum.
      b. Distention of the terminal ileum causes relaxation of the ileocecal valve, and distention of the colon increases the tone.

II. Microscopic Anatomy. The small bowel wall has four distinct layers:

A. Mucosa: epithelial layer over lamina propria and muscularis mucosae (smooth muscle)
   1. Cellular turnover of mucosa: 4 to 5 days
   2. Structural unit is villus, a fingerlike projection of mucosa 0.5 to 1 mm high, covered in columnar epithelium
      a. Contains a central lymphatic (lacteal), a small artery and vein, and a capillary network
      b. Columnar epithelial cells make up 90% of cell mass of the villus.
         (1) Apices of cells have microvilli—creating the brush border and increasing absorptive surface area.
         (2) Surface covered with glycocalyx—proteins and glycoproteins
         (3) Maintenance of the brush border is essential for absorption.
         (4) Tight junctions between cells—paracellular route with selective pores for ions and water versus transmembrane transport

3. Crypts of Lieberkühn: contain anchored stem cells of four types:
   a. Absorptive enterocyte: migrates up to the villus tip in 3 to 7 days and sheds shortly after it undergoes apoptosis
   b. Goblet cell: mucus-secreting cell, which also migrates up the villus
   c. Enteroendocrine cell: anchored in crypt and produces enterohormones (including neurotensin, glucagon, motilin, and cholecystokinin). See Table 6-1.
   d. Paneth cell: remains in crypt and is concentrate lysosomal host defense. Has 4-week lifespan.

B. Submucosa
   1. Dense fibroelastic connective tissue with rich blood supply, lymphatic drainage, and Meissner plexus
   2. Strongest layer of the small bowel
   3. Duodenal Brunner glands secrete protective mucus and bicarbonate.
   4. Ileal Peyer patches are collections of lymphoid follicles whose numbers diminish with age.

C. Muscularis: inner circular and outer longitudinal, between which resides the myenteric nervous plexus

D. Serosa
   1. The thin layer of mesothelial cells over loose connective tissue constitutes visceral peritoneum.
   2. Heals by implantation of free-floating mesothelial cells, not by side-to-side epithelialization (e.g., skin)

III. Vascular Anatomy

A. Duodenal bulb: arterial inflow from hepatic artery and gastroduodenal artery
B. Second and third portion of duodenum: dual arterial supply from celiac via gastroduodenal artery (superior pancreaticoduodenal arteries) and from superior mesenteric (inferior pancreaticoduodenal arteries)
C. Fourth portion of duodenum distal: superior mesenteric artery branches

TABLE 6-1 Endocrine Function of the Small Bowel (SB)

Enterohormone	Site of Production	Stimulus to Secretion	Actions
Cholecystokinin (CCK)	Jejunum	Fats, protein in lumen	Increases pancreatic enzyme output, GB contraction; trophic to pancreas and SB mucosa
Enteroglucagon	Ileum	Unknown	Decreases SB motility
Ghrelin	Uncertain	Unknown	Stimulates appetite, increases growth hormone release
Gastric inhibitory peptide (GIP)	Duodenum, jejunum	Fats, glucose	Potentiates insulin release from pancreas, decreases gastric secretion
Motilin	Jejunum	Unknown	Regulates baseline SB motility
Neurotensin	Ileum	Fats	Increases SB motility and pancreatic secretions, decreases gastric secretion, trophic to SB mucosa
Peptide YY	Terminal ileum, colon	Fats	Decreases motility and pan-SB secretions
Secretin	Duodenum, proximal jejunum	Acidification duodenum	Increases water and bicarbonate output from pancreas
Somatostatin	Stomach, entire SB, pancreas	Unknown	Inhibits all gastric, pancreatic, and enterohormone secretion; decreases gastric emptying and SB motility
Vasoactive intestinal peptide (VIP)	SB	Unknown	Splanchnic vasodilatation; increases SB motility, pancreatic and intestinal secretion; decreases gastric acid output

GB, gallbladder.

Small Bowel

D. Vasa recta are the most peripheral arterial branches of the superior mesenteric artery.
   1. They bifurcate as they reach the intestinal wall.
   2. Jejunal vasa recta are long and straight.
   3. Ileal ones are short, with extensive arborization.
E. Venous and lymphatic drainage parallels arterial anatomy.

IV. Innervation

A. Intrinsic nervous system consists of cell bodies in muscular wall.
   1. Mediates reflex activity independent of central nervous system control
   2. Two major plexuses
      a. Myenteric (Auerbach) controls motility and lies between the two muscle layers.
      b. Submucosal (Meissner) primarily is concerned with secretion and absorption.
B. Extrinsic control via vagus and splanchnic nerves
   1. Parasympathetic
      a. Pass through celiac and superior mesenteric ganglia
      b. Postganglionic cell bodies in the enteric ganglia
      c. Efferent fibers increase peristaltic activity and secretions.
      d. Afferents role uncertain, perhaps sensory
      e. Mediates gastrocecal reflex, leading to discharge of ileum into cecum when there is food in the stomach
   2. Sympathetic
      a. Efferent fibers travel in the splanchnic nerves, synapse with vagal fibers in the superior mesenteric ganglia, and inhibit motility and secretion.
      b. Afferent fibers transmit distension as pain.

PHYSIOLOGY

I. Motility

A. Basic electrical rhythm originates in the duodenal pacemaker.
B. Baseline rhythmic fluctuations from slow wave activity of smooth muscle
   1. Eleven to 13 times/minute in duodenum
   2. Eight to 10 times/minute in ileum
C. After a meal, two activity patterns ensue:
   1. Segmentation: Circular muscle contraction divides bowel into segments, churning and circulating chyme to increase local mucosal contact.
   2. Peristalsis: Wavelike propagation of contraction and relaxation propels chyme rapidly over larger surface area.
D. Mean transit time in small bowel is 221 ± 49 minutes.
   1. Meal composition affects transit time.
   2. Ileal transit time prolonged to aid absorption of bile salts and fat
E. Fasting leads to cyclic pattern of migrating motor complexes (housekeeping motor activity).
   1. Starts proximal small bowel and propagates to the terminal ileum with cycles every 90 to 120 minutes
   2. Propels sloughed enterocytes, undigested food particles, and mucus into the colon
   3. Control is from the enteric nervous system and enterohormone release from pancreas and elsewhere.
      a. In periods of stress, central and autonomic control may override.
      b. Cholecystokinin (CCK), gastrin, and motilin increase motility.
      c. Peptide YY and enteroglucagon decrease motility.

II. Digestion and Absorption

A. Water and electrolytes
   1. Eight to 10 L of fluid is presented to small bowel daily, the largest volume being from gastric secretion.

Small Bowel

QUICK HIT

Although bowel motility is a complex interaction of intrinsic myenteric activity, autonomic innervation, and influences of entero-hormones, it appears that the intrinsic activity is the most critical in almost all circumstances.

QUICK HIT

Dumping syndrome results from hyperosmolar solutions quickly entering the small bowel. It may occur as a result of small bowel surgery. Early dumping syndrome starts within 15–30 minutes after eating and has symptoms of nausea, cramps, diaphoresis, and diarrhea. Late dumping syndrome occurs in 2–4 hours with symptoms of hypoglycemia. Treatment is with diet modifications and octreotide or may require surgery.

QUICK HIT

Fat absorption is the most complex of the activities of the small bowel. Abnormalities present as either vitamin deficiencies (e.g., coagulopathy from inability to absorb vitamin K or bone loss from vitamin D) or diarrhea.

2. Eighty percent of water is absorbed in the small bowel, generally passively, via paracellular (proximal small bowel) or transcellular (distal small bowel and colon) routes.

3. Sodium and chloride are absorbed either neutrally or by active transport. Sodium co-transporters aid in the absorption of glucose, amino acids, di- and tripeptides, and bile salts. Electroneutral absorption trades NaCl for H^+ and HCO_3^-.

4. Eighty-five percent of ingested K^+ is passively absorbed in the small bowel.

B. Carbohydrates
   1. Starch digestion starts with salivary amylase and is completed by pancreatic amylase in the distal jejunum.
   2. Brush border enzymes cleave disaccharides (sucrose and lactose) to monosaccharides throughout the jejunum.
   3. Only monosaccharides (glucose, galactose, and fructose) are absorbed by sodium-linked facilitated diffusion.

C. Protein
   1. Digestion initiated in the stomach by pepsin
   2. Most proteolysis occurs in the small bowel, mediated by pancreatic proteases and peptidases (trypsin, chymotrypsin, elastase, carboxypeptidase A and B).
   3. Pancreas secretes inactive precursors, activated in duodenum by enterokinase in the brush border.
   4. Jejunal enterocytes absorb dipeptides and tripeptides as well as single amino acids.

D. Lipids
   1. Entry of fat into the small bowel stimulates release of CCK from the duodenal mucosa, which in turn causes elaboration of lipase and cholesterol esterase from the pancreas.
   2. Fat products combine with bile salts to form water-soluble micelles, which also complex with fat-soluble vitamins.
   3. Micelles diffuse into terminal ileal cells to the Golgi body, are packaged as chylomicrons, and then exit enterocyte by exocytosis into lymphatics.

E. Bile acids
   1. Enterohepatic circulation recovers 95% of secreted bile salts.
   2. A minor amount of reabsorption is passive throughout the small bowel. It is most active and sodium dependent in the terminal ileum.
   3. Loss of terminal ileal function by resection or Crohn disease leads to increased cholelithiasis or bile acid diarrhea due to excess amount bile salts present in the colon.

F. Vitamins and minerals
   1. Fat-soluble vitamins (A, D, E, and K) are absorbed in micelles in the ileum.
   2. Water-soluble vitamins (B and C) are absorbed in the jejunum and ileum.
   3. Vitamin B_{12} absorption in terminal ileum requires intrinsic factor from gastric parietal cells.
   4. Calcium: The stomach solubilizes nonionic calcium salts.
      a. With low calcium intake, ionized calcium is actively absorbed in the duodenum.
      b. With normal or high calcium intake, ionized calcium is absorbed passively throughout the small bowel.
   5. Magnesium: Uptake is not calcium linked and is marginal in all segments of the bowel.
   6. Iron
      a. Need gastric-secreted transfer factor
      b. Taken up in duodenum and proximal jejunum

IMMUNE FUNCTION

I. **Physical Defenses.** These keep bacterial counts low in the upper gastrointestinal (GI) tract.
   A. Most important factor: acidification of the stomach
   B. Other factors that enhance host defense: mucin production, active peristalsis, rapid turnover of mucosal cells, and tight junctions between cells

Small Bowel

II. Gut-Associated Lymphoid Tissue
A. Aggregated: lymph follicles, Peyer patches
B. Nonaggregated

DISEASES OF THE SMALL BOWEL

Crohn Disease

I. Epidemiology
A. Incidence: 4 cases per 100,000 per year
B. Prevalence: 40 to 160 cases per 100,000 persons
C. More common in North America and Europe
  1. Slightly more common in women
  2. Age of onset has bimodal peak: one peak at 15 to 25 years and another at 55 to 65 years
  3. In the United States, more common among whites, and three to four times more common among ethnic Jews. More common in persons of higher socioeconomic status.

II. Pathogenesis and Pathology.
Many theories have been advanced, but none have been validated. An altered immune response may be involved, although no specific defect has been identified.
A. Features of Crohn disease are present anywhere from the mouth to the anus. The most common location is ileocolic (60%).
B. The disease tends to be discontinuous and segmental.
C. Transmural lymphocytic inflammation with noncaseating granulomata is the classic pathology in the bowel. The gross appearance of involved bowel is thickened mesentery with enlarged friable lymph nodes and "fat wrapping" of bowel.

III. Clinical Presentation
A. Extraintestinal manifestations of Crohn disease may antedate the onset of the intestinal changes by months to years.
  1. One-third of patients demonstrate perianal fistulae.
  2. Other findings include oral aphthous ulceration, rashes such as erythema nodosum and pyoderma gangrenosum, uveitis, polyarthralgias or monoarthralgias, and sclerosing cholangitis.
B. Symptoms of Crohn disease generally relate to bowel wall strictures. Characteristic complaints include bloating, abdominal pain, abdominal distention, and postobstructive diarrhea.
  1. Active disease or multiple strictures can result in a "failure to thrive" catabolic state.
  2. Diarrhea may indicate fistula of the proximal bowel to colon.
C. Bowel perforation and clinically evident bleeding are not frequently seen.
D. Other symptoms may result from fistulae to pelvic organs, such as bladder, or to skin, or retroperitoneal fibrosis causing ureteral obstruction.
E. Severe involvement of the terminal ileum leads to gallstone formation and macrocytic anemia due to loss of absorption of bile salts and vitamin B_{12}.

IV. Diagnosis
A. Standard barium small bowel follow-through (or enteroclysis) is very helpful. It shows mucosal ulceration and nodularity, wall thickening, strictures, and fistulae.
B. Colonoscopy is useful in colonic Crohn disease, and intubation of the terminal ileum may confirm ileocolic disease. Biopsies can also be taken to confirm a pathologic diagnosis.
C. Computed tomography (CT) scanning is not as specific as small bowel follow-through but may better demonstrate complications of the disease (e.g., obstruction, abscesses, or fistulae).

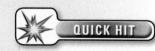

QUICK HIT

Crohn disease, which has a bimodal peak, should always be considered in the differential diagnosis of new-onset GI obstructive symptoms in the late middle-aged patient.

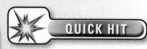

QUICK HIT

Although ulcerative colitis has a more consistent association with sclerosing cholangitis, there remains a notable risk of the same change in patients with Crohn disease.

V. Treatment—Medical

A. Antibiotics are of little value except in anorectal disease where metronidazole has shown some effectiveness.

B. Mildly symptomatic disease should be treated with 5-aminosalicylic acid, especially ileocolic and colonic variants.

C. Moderately active disease mandates use of immunosuppressives.
1. First-line therapy is corticosteroids, which are weaned quickly, if possible, to avoid the significant adverse effects of steroid administration.
2. Steroid-resistant patients are offered azidothymidine or 6-mercaptopurine.
   a. Suppress helper T-cell and natural killer cell activity
   b. Cause myelosuppression, hepatotoxicity, and pancreatitis

D. Failure of immunosuppressive therapy may require a short course of an antitumor necrosis factor agent (infliximab).
1. Chimeric human: mouse monoclonal antibody
2. Primary indication for use is fistula healing.
3. Long-term use is not advisable because of concerns about induction of non-Hodgkin lymphoma.
   a. Medical management should be continued for only as long as the patient with Crohn disease is symptomatic.
   b. There is no evidence for the prophylactic use of immunosuppressives to prevent recurrence of disease.

VI. Treatment—Surgical

A. General principles
1. Up to 90% of patients with Crohn disease eventually need surgery.
2. Crohn disease is the second leading cause of surgically induced short bowel syndrome in adults, and preserving bowel length is critical in surgery for Crohn disease.
3. Guidelines
   a. Do not look for normal bowel to use for anastomoses. Use thickened or fat-wrapped bowel, as long as it can be safely sutured or stapled.
   b. Do not use frozen sections to look for uninvolved margins. You will only waste usable bowel.
   c. Leave the enlarged nodes alone unless you think you are dealing with a Crohn disease–associated cancer. Resection of the mesentery causes devascularization of uninvolved bowel and further loss of bowel length.
   d. Avoid bypass of involved segments because this leaves active disease in place, causing symptoms and extraintestinal manifestations to continue.
4. Laparoscopic approaches to Crohn disease have been shown to be safe and effective, especially at the primary operation.
5. Long side-to-side anastomoses are favored over end-to-end.

B. Indications for surgery
1. Absolute indications include perforation, hemorrhage, suspicion of cancer, and nonresolving bowel obstruction.
2. Relative indications are symptomatic fistula (e.g., enterovesical fistula with recurrent infections), abscess, and "failure to thrive."
3. Resecting the intestinal disease has little impact on most of the extraintestinal manifestations of Crohn disease, and therefore, resection should not be pursued.

C. Operative strategy in Crohn disease
1. To save bowel length in small bowel disease, strictureplasty is favored over resection unless the strictures are all located in a short segment of bowel.
   a. Strictures less than 5 cm are best dealt with by the Heineke–Mikulicz approach of converting a longitudinal enterotomy to a transverse closure.
   b. Strictures up to 10 cm may require a Finney procedure.
   c. Longer strictures can be opened with a sliding type isoperistaltic strictureplasty.
2. Ileocolic disease is generally resected with standard right hemicolectomy, creating a long side-to-side stapled ileocolostomy.

3. Although segmental resection of colonic Crohn is generally pursued, some centers have reported much longer times to disease recurrence by using total abdominal colectomy if the rectum is uninvolved or even total proctocolectomy with end ileostomy creation.

4. Crohn bowel should not knowingly be used for the creation of pouches, such as the J-pouch for the ileoanal pull-through procedure.

VII. Cancer Risk

A. Risk of adenocarcinoma development in the Crohn segment is estimated at 15 to 100 times the risk of small bowel adenocarcinoma.

1. The likelihood of malignant transformation begins after 10 years of active disease. If cancer develops, it is generally after 20 to 30 years of carrying the diagnosis.

2. Experts are uncertain about whether patients with more symptomatic Crohn disease have a greater likelihood of undergoing malignant transformation than those with less symptomatic disease.

B. The prognosis of Crohn-associated small bowel cancer is worse because of its late discovery (symptoms of Crohn disease mimic those of a cancer), not inherent biologic aggressiveness.

Small Bowel Obstruction

I. Pathogenesis: Causes of Mechanical Obstruction

A. Foreign body

1. Can be anything ingested: coins, batteries, undigested plant or food material, hair

2. Treatment: Laxatives may help with a partial obstruction; complete obstruction usually requires surgical removal.

B. Gallstone ileus

1. Generally seen in the elderly and debilitated

2. Symptoms of "tumbling obstruction": pattern of sequential, spontaneously resolving obstructions as gallstone alternately becomes lodged and then passes more distal in small bowel

3. Cause is usually chronic cholecystitis with fistula between gallbladder and second portion of duodenum, through which a large gallstone gains entry into the GI tract.

4. Stone eventually impacts itself in narrow terminal ileum, where complete bowel obstruction results.

5. Abdominal films show high-grade distal small bowel obstruction, calcified gallstone outside the right upper quadrant (possibly), and pneumobilia.

6. Treatment is to first rehydrate patient due to persistent vomiting. At exploration, milk the stone back into the dilated bowel and extract through the enterotomy. Make sure there are no other more proximal stones and close the enterotomy. Due to tenuous patient condition, cholecystectomy and fistula closure are usually not pursued in the acute setting.

C. Intussusception

1. Five percent to 15% of cases occur in adults, representing less than 1% of adult bowel obstruction.

2. Ninety percent of cases are associated with a lead point such as a neoplasm (benign or malignant), diverticulum, old suture line, or adhesion.

3. Diagnosis usually made by contrast study or CT scan

4. Barium column decompression, useful in children, is rarely used in adults.
   a. Presence of lead point makes radiologic reduction unlikely to be successful.
   b. Association with malignancy mandates surgery in most cases.
   c. The increasing risk of perforation and resultant malignant seeding of peritoneal cavity makes this practice questionable.

5. Surgery should be undertaken to decompress the intussusception and evaluate for cause.

D. Malignant obstruction

1. This condition rarely resolves with nonoperative measures.

2. A short trial of decompression may succeed. If this fails, resect or bypass.

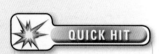

QUICK HIT

Bouveret syndrome is a gallbladder duodenal fistula causing a gastric outlet obstruction. It is treated by pushing the gallstone back into the stomach for removal, taking down the fistula, and performing a cholecystectomy.

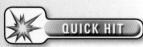

QUICK HIT

The incidence of idiopathic intussusception rapidly decreases with increasing age. From adolescence onward, all intussusceptions should be considered to have a lead point such that most patients should have exploratory surgery.

3. If the obstruction cannot be reduced surgically, somatostatin may reduce cramping pain for palliation.

E. Crohn disease: trial of steroids or other immunosuppressants before exploration

F. Radiation enteritis

    1. Always consider in patients with history of radiation for gynecologic malignancy. It is less common after radiation therapy for colon or prostate cancer.

    2. It usually occurs less than 10 years after radiation therapy.

    3. Signs include obliterative vasculitis and muscular fibrosis.

    4. Surgery is almost always needed and can be daunting due to pelvic fibrosis. In some cases, bypass with venting stomas at the ends of the trapped pelvic bowel segment is all that is possible.

G. Adhesions

    1. More than half of all small bowel obstructions are adhesions in patients with previous surgery.

    2. The vast majority of these occur post abdominal surgery, but occasionally congenital bands are encountered.

    3. Up to 80% of adhesive small bowel obstructions resolve with nasogastric decompression alone.

H. Hernias

    1. Hernias are the second most common cause of obstruction in Western countries and first in the Third World.

    2. In the United States, due to high rate of elective repair of inguinal and umbilical hernias, rare hernias such as femoral, obturator, bowel entrapment in the foramen of Winslow, or congenital defects of the omentum should be considered as causes of adhesions.

    3. Also, consider the very dangerous Richter hernia, where only a portion of the bowel wall is fixed in the hernia sac, leading to a partial obstruction picture with high risk of bowel perforation.

I. Volvulus

    1. Loop of bowel is twisted more than 180 degrees about its axis and is caused by mismatch of bowel length to narrow area of attachment.

    2. Ileocolic most frequent in small bowel but can occur in small bowel alone

    3. Endoscopic decompression is generally not useful (unlike sigmoid volvulus).

    4. Use laparotomy to decompress volvulus and either perform cecopexy or, preferably, resect the involved segment.

II. Functional Obstruction: Ileus. Motility alters without evidence of luminal obstruction.

A. Causes

    1. Neurogenic (e.g., spinal cord injury)

    2. Retroperitoneal process or surgery (e.g., ureteral colic)

    3. Opiates

    4. Metabolic abnormalities, including hypokalemia, uremia, calcium or magnesium imbalance, hypothyroidism, and hyperglycemia

    5. Intra-abdominal or distant infection

    6. Drugs such as anticholinergics and antihistamines

B. Normal return of small bowel function after abdominal surgery is 6 to 24 hours.

C. Ileus is less common after laparoscopic procedures compared with open surgeries.

III. Diagnosis of Small Bowel Obstruction

A. No reliable physical finding or serum laboratory test distinguishes ileus from mechanical obstruction or rules out strangulated obstruction.

B. History is critical.

    1. Prior abdominal surgery

    2. Signs of infection or peritonitis

    3. Prior history of obstructions

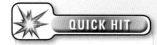

QUICK HIT

Remember that the obturator hernia is much more frequently seen in females and is characterized by the Howship–Romberg sign: bowel obstruction in conjunction with pain in the medial groin/thigh with external rotation of the hip.

4. History of malignancy or inflammatory bowel disease
5. History of abdominal trauma
   a. Splenosis
   b. Diaphragmatic hernia
6. History of endometriosis
C. Radiology of obstruction
   1. Plain films (three-way abdomen): said to be diagnostic in up to 80% of patients
      a. Air–fluid levels may be present in both ileus and mechanical obstruction, although they are more common with latter.
      b. Assess for free air.
   2. Contrast studies
      a. These studies may better delineate both nature and level of obstruction.
      b. Generally, these use water-soluble contrast unless closed loop obstruction is suspected. The hydrophilic activity of water-soluble contrast may cause swelling and perforation of the closed loop.
   3. CT scanning: Most would consider this the preferred test for evaluating small bowel obstruction.
      a. Similar efficacy to contrast studies in terms of luminal findings
      b. More sensitive to secondary signs in obstruction such as presence of malignancy, mesenteric stranding, abscess, vascular compromise, intestinal wall thickening, and pneumatosis (air in the wall of the intestines) (Fig. 6-1).

IV. Treatment of Small Bowel Obstruction

A. Obstructions with low likelihood of resolution with "conservative" measures such as malignancy-associated obstructions, high-grade obstructions, and hernias should be operated on promptly after fluid resuscitation.
B. If an ileus, assess for inciting factors (especially opiate use if fresh postoperative patient) and correct these if possible.
   1. CT is particularly helpful if the cause is uncertain because it confirms the absence or presence of the transition zone associated with a mechanical obstruction and allows assessment for other intra-abdominal processes, such as abscess.
   2. It may be necessary to try to administer an epidural with continuous local anesthesia (not opiates) to allow cessation of intravenous (IV) opiates.
   3. There is some evidence for vagal stimulation through limited oral intake or gum chewing in order to reduce the duration of ileus.

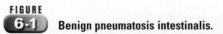

FIGURE 6-1 Benign pneumatosis intestinalis.

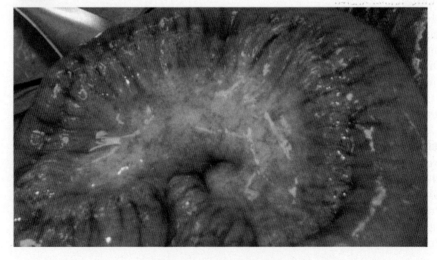

C. Despite the adage that "the sun should not set on a bowel obstruction," what to do with the lower risk obstructions, such as the early postoperative adhesive obstruction, remains problematic.
  1. Most surgeons give a 24- to 48-hour "expectant" trial of nasogastric decompression and bowel rest with close observation of the patient's status and abdominal examination.
  2. There is some evidence for using the time it takes for oral contrast to enter the colon as a predictor of the likelihood of resolution of partial small bowel obstructions.

Meckel Diverticulum

I. Epidemiology and Etiology
A. Meckel diverticulum is the most common congenital abnormality of the GI tract.
B. It is found in 1% to 2% of the population, with slightly higher male incidence. More than 50% of symptomatic cases present in male children younger than 10 years of age. Complications occur disproportionately in males.
C. On average, the location is 60 cm proximal to the ileocecal valve, on the antimesenteric aspect.
D. Factors predictive of symptomatic Meckel diverticulum
  1. Male sex (cause of male predominance unknown)
  2. Diverticular length less than 2 cm (increased length: orifice ratio inclines toward development of diverticulitis)
  3. Presence of ectopic tissue—gastric or pancreatic
  4. Presence of mesodiverticular or vitelloumbilical band
E. It results from failure of the omphalomesenteric (vitelline) duct to close. This should occur around the ninth gestational week.
F. Complete failure to involute results in the infrequently encountered enteroumbilical fistula

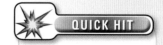

QUICK HIT

Rule of 2's for Meckel diverticulum: M > F × 2, present in 2% of population, 2 inches in size, 2 types of mucosa, 2 symptoms: bleeding or obstruction.

II. Pathology
A. Meckel diverticulum is a true diverticulum of all layers of the intestinal wall.
B. Up to one-third of Meckel diverticula contain heterotropic tissue, with gastric and pancreatic the most frequently found.
C. The majority of symptomatic diverticula are lined with gastric mucosa.

III. Clinical Presentation
A. In children, bleeding from Meckel diverticula is usually occult, manifesting as unexplained anemia, although more brisk hemorrhage presenting as melena or even hematochezia has been seen. Bleeding due to peptic ulceration is the most common presentation, with occasional cases of peptic-induced perforation.
B. In adults, bowel obstruction is most frequent, caused by one of several mechanisms:
  1. Diverticulitis causing fibrous stricture
  2. Ectopic tissue, usually pancreatic, or the diverticulum itself serving as lead point for intussusception
  3. Internal herniation under a mesodiverticular band (remnant of the duct attaching the root of mesentery to diverticulum)
  4. Volvulus of ileum around vitelloumbilical band (bowel suspended from the base of the umbilicus)
C. Obstructive complaints may be partial intermittent type, especially with volvulus, or acute complete small bowel obstruction, as with intussusception.

IV. Diagnostic Workup
A. Rarely diagnosed preoperatively
B. Acute appendicitis is the most common preoperative diagnosis. Meckel diverticulitis is clinically indistinguishable from acute appendicitis.

C. CT scan and ultrasound have low sensitivity in this setting.

D. Barium small-bowel series is more sensitive but generally is not used in the presence of acute abdomen because of concern for perforation.

E. Technetium scan is widely reported to have the highest sensitivity but detects only Meckel diverticula that contain gastric mucosa.

V. Surgical Treatment

A. In the acute setting, limited resection of the ileal segment containing the diverticulum with primary anastomosis is indicated.

B. Controversy persists regarding indications for resection of the incidentally discovered Meckel diverticulum.

1. All incidentally discovered Meckel diverticula in children should be resected.

2. Some advocate the same strategy for adults, whereas others argue that one would have to resect almost 1,000 diverticula to save the life of one adult who would subsequently present with complications of the disease.

3. Factors favoring resection of the asymptomatic Meckel diverticula are palpable ectopic tissue (generally pancreatic, not gastric), diverticular length less than 2 cm, and the presence of an associated band.

   a. Vitelloumbilical bands can simply be divided without diverticulectomy.

   b. Mesodiverticular bands cannot be divided because they are often the sole blood supply to the diverticulum; division of these bands necessitates concomitant diverticulectomy.

C. No incidental diverticulectomy should be pursued in the presence of peritonitis or in the medically unstable patient.

Other Small Bowel Diverticula

I. Epidemiology

A. Eighty percent of small bowel diverticula are in the duodenum; the rest are jejunoileal.

B. Most occur within 2 cm of the ampulla of Vater.

II. Pathogenesis

A. True cause is unknown but likely secondary to abnormal pulsion/peristalsis leading to increased intraluminal pressures (intestinal akinesis).

B. Congenital diverticula are associated with duodenal atresia.

C. Occur at defects in the bowel wall at entrance of large vessels

D. Emerge on the mesenteric boarder of the small bowel

E. Most diverticula are extraluminal.

III. Clinical Presentation

A. Majority are asymptomatic.

1. They are most commonly found at autopsy or on barium swallow.

2. Jejunoileal diverticular are more commonly symptomatic.

B. Can present as small bowel diverticulitis and/or small bowel perforation

C. Chronic iron deficiency anemia secondary to long-standing GI bleeding

D. Biliary/pancreatic duct obstruction from diverticula blocking the ampulla of Vater

E. Nonspecific epigastric pain

IV. Diagnosis

A. Lab tests are nonspecific and of limited value.

1. Complete blood count (CBC) revealing a leukocytosis from diverticulitis/perforation or iron deficiency anemia from a long-standing GI bleed

2. Elevated amylase/lipase and/or hyperbilirubinemia from obstruction of the ampulla of Vater

B. Imaging

1. Diverticula perforation presents as free air under the diaphragm on chest/abdominal X-ray.

2. CT scan: phlegmon/abscess, free air from diverticulitis or perforation
3. Barium swallow/upper GI series
4. Esophagogastroduodenoscopy (EGD) and endoscopic retrograde cholangio-pancreatography (ERCP) can endoscopically visualize the diverticula.

V. Treatment

A. Based on severity of complications
B. Conservative medical management
   1. Nothing by mouth (NPO), maintenance intravenous fluids (MIVFs), broad-spectrum antibiotics in the setting of diverticulitis
C. Surgical management not indicated unless perforation of uncontrolled GI bleed occurs
   1. Diverticulectomy
   2. Exploratory laparotomy with small bowel resection

Benign Small Bowel Tumors

I. General Principles

A. These tumors represent about one-third of all small bowel neoplasms.
B. Growth pattern predicts associated symptoms and signs.
   1. Infiltrative: bleeding
   2. Intraluminal (e.g., polypoid): obstruction either due to lesion or as lead point for intussusception; low-level bleeding
   3. Serosal: pivot point for small bowel volvulus
C. Tend to be slow-growing with long duration, protean symptomatology

II. Hyperplastic Polyps

A. Predilection for distal duodenum and small bowel
B. No malignant potential
C. Rarely symptomatic, except as lead point of intussusception

III. Gastrointestinal Stromal Tumor

A. Gastrointestinal stromal tumor (GIST) is the most common symptomatic small bowel lesion.
B. Benign leiomyomata tend to be smaller in size and firmer than GIST.
C. Differentiating leiomyoma from GIST is difficult but is suggested by lack of cellularity on light microscopy, fewer than two mitoses per 10 high-power fields, and absence of CD34 and CD117 staining on immunohistochemistry.
D. GIST presents with partial obstructive symptoms and minor bleeding from erosion of overlying mucosa.
E. Because intraoperative differentiation between leiomyoma and malignant GIST is difficult, treatment of all smooth muscle tumors of the small bowel is resection, with at least a 2-cm margin in all directions, and avoidance of tumor spillage or rupture.

IV. Lipoma

A. Benign submucosal tumors found anywhere in small bowel
B. If large, may cause bowel obstruction and/or intussusception
C. Occasional bleeding from mucosal erosion
D. Require resection if symptomatic and are highly amenable to laparoscopic resection

V. Hemangiomata

A. These may comprise up to 10% of all small bowel lesions.
B. The cavernous variant is the most common.
C. They are rarely large enough to cause obstruction unless intramural hematoma develops.
D. Bleeding, occasionally massive, is the most common presentation, followed by finding as lead point of intussusception.

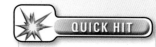
QUICK HIT

Benign tumors of the bowel are GIST, hemangiomas, adenomas, lipomas, and hamartomas and only need surgical treatment if they cause symptoms like obstruction or bleeding. Some do have a malignant potential.

Small Bowel

TABLE 6-2 Unusual Small Bowel Benign Neoplasms	
Neoplasm	**Description**
Amyloidosis	Infiltrative growth may cause obstruction, rarely bleeding
Blue rubber bleb nevus syndrome	Associated with intestinal hemangiomata
Cowden syndrome	Germ-line mutation leads to hamartomas in all three germ layers. Increased risk of thyroid, breast, and endometrial cancer. GI polyps cause obstruction and bleeding.
Endometriosis	Serositis may cause fibrotic obstruction.
Ganglioneuroma	Associated with neurofibromatosis and MEN IIb/III
Inflammatory fibroid polyp	Grossly resembles GI stromal tumors; obstruction/bleeding
Inflammatory myofibroblastic tumor	Generally behaves as benign tumor; obstruction and intussusception
Myxoma	Very rare; may be part of Carney syndrome (myxomas of heart, skin, and breast, and pituitary adenomata), Cushing syndrome

  E. They may be difficult to localize, even using arteriography. Intraoperative enteroscopy has much higher likelihood of success.

  F. Arteriographic embolization can be tried for significant bleeding; otherwise, use surgical resection.

VI. Peutz–Jeghers Syndrome

  A. This autosomal dominant disorder (mutation of 19p2.3 [*LKB1*] gene) is characterized by mucocutaneous pigmentation and myriad benign GI hamartomas.

  B. Ninety percent of affected individuals have small bowel hamartomas.

  C. No nuclear atypia are seen in polyps.

  D. Hamartomas can cause abdominal pain, GI bleeding, and obstruction from intussusception.

  E. There is an increased rate of GI cancers, but not from hamartomas. These arise in synchronous adenomatous lesions.

  F. Surveillance recommendations include the following: starting at age 10 years, biannual esophagogastroduodenoscopy, colonoscopy, and barium small bowel follow-through due to cancer risk.

  G. Multiplicity of polyps makes localization of source of symptoms difficult (Table 6-2).

 SMALL BOWEL MALIGNANCY

I. Epidemiology

  A. Malignancy of the small bowel is very rare in industrialized Western countries (less than 2% of GI cancers in the United States).

  B. Several factors are implicated in low rate of small bowel cancer:

   1. Rapid transit time

   2. Sloughing of mucosal surface cells weekly

   3. Low bacterial counts

   4. Large volume of chyme dilutes carcinogen concentration

   5. High levels of secretory immunoglobulin

  C. Two-thirds of small bowel neoplasms are malignant. About 5,400 cases occur annually, with 40% of malignancies adenocarcinomas, followed by 30% carcinoids, 15% sarcomas, and 15% lymphomas.

D. The mean age of diagnosis is 60 years. Because of protean symptoms, the average delay in diagnosis from symptom onset is 6 months to 1 year.

II. Risk Factors

A. Polyposis syndromes
   1. Patients with familial adenomatous polyposis and Gardner disease have a 300-fold increased risk of duodenal adenocarcinoma but no apparent increase in other small bowel cancers.
   2. Patients with hereditary nonpolyposis colorectal cancer have a 100-fold increased risk of small bowel adenocarcinoma, uniformly distributed throughout the small bowel.
B. Dietary factors: It is suggested that a high intake of animal fat, red meat, and cured foods is associated with a twofold to threefold increase in risk.
C. Crohn disease
D. Celiac disease
   1. Three hundred-fold increased risk of developing lymphoma, 95% of which are T-cell types.
   2. Sixty-seven-fold increased risk of small bowel adenocarcinoma.
E. Male sex (small bowel malignancy has a slight preponderance in men)
F. African-American race

III. Adenocarcinoma

A. Adenocarcinoma has a similar natural history to colorectal carcinoma, with a polyp as premalignant lesion.
B. Genetic changes parallel colon cancer, except the adenomatous polyposis coli mutation is rare in small bowel cancer and SMAD4 tumor suppressor loss of heterozygosity is common.
C. Location: 50% duodenal, 30% jejunal, and 20% ileal
D. Duodenal adenocarcinoma should be considered separately from more distal lesions because it presents earlier at a lower stage and has a much higher 5-year disease-specific survival.
E. Except for tumors with limited or no nodal involvement, more extensive resection does not improve survival.
F. For less advanced tumors, resection with 5-cm luminal margins and modest lymph node resection is indicated.
G. For advanced stage III or IV disease, resection of primary tumors to avoid complications of hemorrhage, perforation, or obstruction as necessary. An extensive mesenteric resection should not be completed.
H. Adjuvant chemotherapy regimen parallels that of colon cancer, but the number of small bowel cancers is so small that no sizeable study has been done to verify any benefit from chemotherapy following surgical resection.

IV. Sarcoma

A. Sarcoma is thought to be derived from the interstitial cells of Cajal.
B. Most of these tumors are not true sarcomas because they do not express muscle-associated antigens such as smooth muscle actin.
C. These tumors are characterized by the generic term GIST.
   1. About two-thirds of GISTs express a growth factor receptor with tyrosine kinase activity that is encoded for by the proto-oncogene *c-kit*.
   2. All suspected small bowel smooth muscle tumors should be tested for *c-kit* expression.
D. The stomach is the primary location for GIST, with about 30% of the tumors occurring in the small bowel.
   1. Small bowel sarcomas are believed to have a worse prognosis.
   2. Due to their propensity for bleeding and perforation, all sarcomas should be resected, even in advanced-stage disease.
   3. As with most sarcomas, lymphatic involvement is rare, so only grossly involved nodes should be excised.

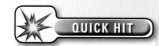

QUICK HIT

Beware of survival statistics that assert a greater than 25% overall 5-year survival in small bowel adenocarcinoma. These are skewed by the inclusion of duodenal cancers that tend to be discovered earlier.

Small Bowel

4. GIST tends to spread hematogenously to liver and lung.
5. Research is ongoing as to the utility of the tyrosine kinase inhibitor as both an adjuvant drug after complete resection and as treatment for advanced disease.
6. Five-year survival prior to the use of tyrosine kinase inhibitors was about 20%.

V. Lymphoma
   A. The GI tract is the most common site of extranodal non-Hodgkin lymphomas.
      1. These account for half of all extranodal lymphomas.
      2. Up to two-thirds of small intestinal lymphomas are diffuse large B-cell type.
      3. Small bowel lymphomas constitute about 25% of GI lymphomas (gastric makes up about 50%).
   B. Up to 50% of patients with GI lymphomas present with an abdominal emergency.
   C. In patients with disease limited to bowel (stage I) or nodal involvement that is infradiaphragmatic (including the spleen, but not the liver; stage II), there is benefit to resecting all disease or debulking it.
      1. This includes mesenteric adenopathy that can be excised without sacrificing large amounts of bowel length.
      2. If the spleen is grossly abnormal, it should be removed.
      3. Nonadjacent adenopathy that cannot be easily resected should be biopsied and marked with clips for possible radiotherapy to these nodal basins.
   D. In stage III (involvement of nodal basins on both sides of the diaphragm) and stage IV (systemic disease including lung, liver, skin, and bone marrow) disease, no resection should be done unless laparotomy is mandated to deal with perforation of, or bleeding from, the primary tumor.
      1. Chemotherapy is the mainstay of treatment in these patients.
      2. Radiotherapy may be added to areas of bulky disease.

VI. Carcinoid
   A. Epidemiology
      1. Over 80% occur in the terminal ileum and appendix.
      2. Increase frequency from duodenum to the ileum
   B. Pathophysiology
      1. Neuroendocrine tumors from Kulchitsky cells in the crypts of Lieberkühn
      2. Secrete numerous vasoactive substances
         a. Serotonin, 5-hydroxytryptophan, substance P, histamine, kallikrein
   C. Clinical presentation
      1. Usually present late—diffuse abdominal pain, obstruction, diarrhea, weight loss
      2. Malignant carcinoid syndrome—from liver metastases
   D. Diagnosis
      1. CT—shows metastases
      2. Somatostatin scan
      3. 5-hydroxyindoleacetic acid (5-HIAA) in urine
   E. Treatment
      1. Surgical resection: Look for synchronous lesions in 30%.
      2. Aggressive resection of metastatic disease
      3. Octreotide, chemotherapy

COMPLICATIONS ASSOCIATED WITH COMMON SMALL BOWEL SURGERIES

I. Ileostomy
   A. Loop ileostomy
      1. Decompressed small bowel but incomplete diversion because contents can enter distal limb
      2. Can be used to protect a more distal anastomosis
      3. Provides for simple closure without having to undergo laparotomy

B. End ileostomy
1. Complete diversion because no distal limb is present
2. Also functions to decompress the small bowel or to protect a more distal anastomosis
3. Commonly requires laparotomy/difficult closure for reversal

C. Complications
1. Complications from ileostomies can include skin irritation, fluid loss, and electrolyte imbalance.
2. Other complications of ostomies include infection, stomal prolapse/retraction, inability to reverse, small bowel obstruction, peristomal hernia, stomal revision, stricture, fistula, and bleeding/hemorrhage.

D. High ostomy output
1. Causes
   a. Intra-abdominal sepsis, obstruction, short gut syndrome, high liquid oral intake
2. Pathophysiology
   a. Small bowel cannot absorb NaCl and therefore water.
   b. Fifty percent stop spontaneously whenever the proximal bowel hypertrophies to compensate.
3. Treatment
   a. Medical treatment is directed at slowing the transit time of the small bowel with proton pump inhibitors (PPIs) or histamine-2 (H2) blockers, Imodium, Lomotil, octreotide
   b. May require IV hydration if output is greater than a liter a day and results in dehydration

II. Short Gut Syndrome (SGS)

A. Commonly occurs whenever you have <200 cm of removal or >50% loss of native small bowel
1. Minimal length required to avoid SGS: 60 cm of small bowel or 45 cm with an intact ileocecal valve
2. Ileum adapts better than the jejunum.

B. Causes
1. Crohn disease
2. Extensive surgical resection: This may occur with one operation or after several operations.
3. Radiation, vascular insufficiency
4. Trauma
5. Recurrent obstruction
6. Necrotizing enterocolitis (NEC; pediatric)
7. Intestinal atresia (pediatric)
8. Volvulus (pediatric)

C. Pathophysiology
1. Loss of GI absorptive surface
2. Adaption may take greater than a year for an adult and greater than 4 years for a child.
3. At risk for kidney stones, gallstones, and peptic ulcer disease due to high gastrin levels: may consider prophylactic cholecystectomy

D. Diagnosis
1. Clinical diagnosis
2. Normal ostomy output should be 10 to 15 mL/kg/hr, usually much higher with short gut.

E. Treatment
1. Most cases will resolve on their own whenever the small bowel hypertrophies to compensate.
2. Total parenteral nutrition for nutritional support
3. Low residue/elemental diet
4. PPIs/H2 blockers
5. Antiperistalsis agents

6. Vitamin supplementation
7. Surgical treatments include stricturoplasty, tapering enteroplasty, artificial valves, segmental interposition, intestinal lengthening, and small bowel transplantation.

 SMALL BOWEL TRAUMA

I. Epidemiology
  A. Twenty percent to 30% blunt versus 70% to 80% penetrating
  B. Jejunum is most commonly injured.
  C. Blunt
    1. Bowel contusion
    2. Mesenteric contusion
    3. Serosal tears
    4. Perforations
  D. Penetrating
    1. Most commonly cause serosal tears and perforation
  E. Small bowel injury scale (Table 6-3)

II. Clinical Presentation
  A. Seatbelt sign, abdominal pain, peritonitis, shock

III. Diagnosis
  A. Clinical diagnosis: based on history and physical exam
  B. Plain film X-ray: Look for free peritoneal air.
  C. FAST exam: low sensitivity and specificity for hallow viscus injury
  D. Diagnostic peritoneal lavage: The presence of white blood cells greater than 500 cells per high-powered field, gram stain positive bilirubin, or amylase may be more indicative of hallow viscus injury.
  E. CT scan: Look for free peritoneal air, bowel wall thickening, or triangles of free fluid within the bowel loops (Figs. 6-2 and 6-3).
  F. Exploration with laparotomy or laparoscopy will provide definitive diagnosis and treatment.

IV. Treatment
  A. Indications for surgery
    1. Peritonitis
    2. Uncontrolled hemorrhage (Fig. 6-4)
    3. Prolong symptoms of abdominal pain
  B. Surgical management
    1. Exploratory laparotomy or laparoscopy
      a. Small bowel resection
      b. Possibility of a second look operation if leaving bowel in discontinuity or if ischemia is a possibility

TABLE 6-3	Small Bowel Injury Scale
I	Laceration, partial thickness, without perforation or hematoma; see also Fig. 6-2
II	Laceration of <50% bowel circumference
III	>50% circumference without transection
IV	Complete transection
V	Transection with segmental tissue loss and/or devascularization

Advance one grade for multiple injuries to the same area.

Small Bowel

FIGURE 6-2 CT of grade I small bowel injury with hematoma.

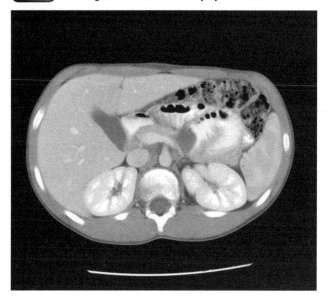

FIGURE 6-3 CT showing small bowel injury with free air and free fluid triangulating in the loops of bowel.

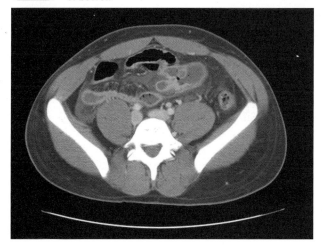

FIGURE 6-4 Hemorrhage control of the small bowel mesentery.

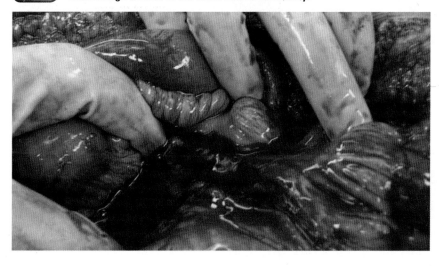

Small Bowel

2. Conservative management: a possibility if low velocity penetrating trauma and no abdominal pain
   a. Serial abdominal exams: should be performed by the same person to detect subtle changes in exam
   b. NPO
   c. CBC

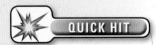

QUICK HIT

The principles of management of an enterocutaneous (EC) fistula are:
1. Resuscitation and stabilization
2. Control of the fistula
3. Convalescence and rehabilitation and nutrition
4. Definitive reconstruction

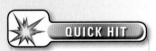

QUICK HIT

Reasons for why a fistula won't close: FRIENDS (Foreign body, radiation, inflammation, ischemia, infection, epithelialization, neoplasm, distal obstruction, sepsis)

SMALL BOWEL POSTSURGICAL ANATOMY

I. Billroth I (Fig. 6-5)

II. Billroth II (see Fig. 6-5)

III. Roux-en-Y Gastric Bypass (Fig. 6-6)

IV. Braun Enteroenterostomy (Fig. 6-7)

FIGURE 6-5 Billroth I (A) and II (B).

A

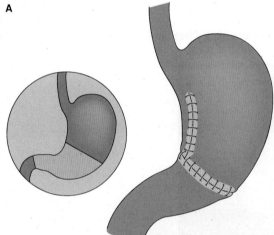

B

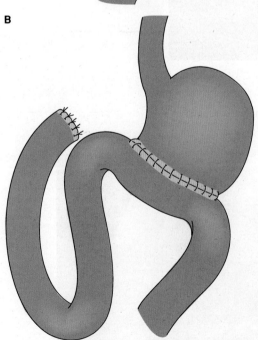

(Reprinted with permission from Mulholland MW, Lillemoe KD, Doherty GM, Maier RV, Upchurch GR, eds. *Greenfield's Surgery: Scientific Principles and Practice*. 4th ed. Philadelphia, PA: Lippincott Williams & Wilkins; 2006.)

Small Bowel

FIGURE
6-6 **Roux-en-Y gastric bypass.**

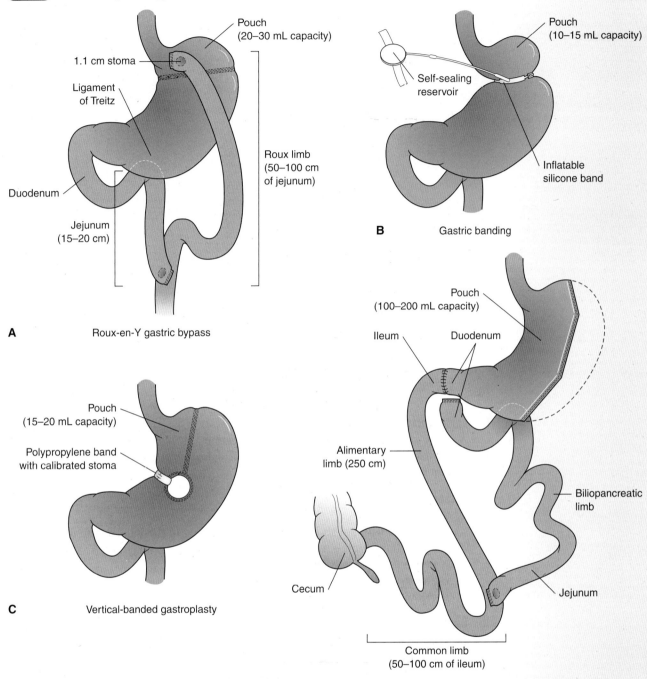

A   Roux-en-Y gastric bypass

B   Gastric banding

C   Vertical-banded gastroplasty

D   Biliopancreatic diversion with duodenal switch

(Reprinted with permission from Smeltzer SC, Bare B, Hinkle JL, Cheever KH, eds. *Brunner & Suddarth's Textbook of Medical-Surgical Nursing.* 12th ed. Philadelphia, PA: Lippincott William & Wilkins; 2010.)

FIGURE
6-7 Braun enteroenterostomy.

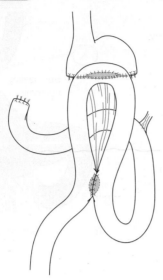

Antrectomy: Billroth II reconstruction (gastrojejunostomy). A Braun enteroenterostomy facilitates decompression of the afferent limb in a Billroth II gastrojejunostomy. It may be done as either a sutured or a stapled anastomosis. An option is to close the afferent limb above the enteroenterostomy with a transverse anastomosis stapler (so that the jejunal lumen is occluded but not divided). This configuration, often referred to as an uncut Roux-en-Y, temporarily discourages but does not prevent reflux of bile into the stomach. (Reprinted with permission from Blackbourne LH. *Advanced Surgical Recall.* 2nd ed. Baltimore, MD: Lippincott Williams & Wilkins; 2004.)

ENTEROCUTANEOUS FISTULA

I. Epidemiology
A. Most commonly a postoperative complication
   1. Inadvertent enterotomies, anastomotic dehiscence, and open abdomen
B. Can be a result of Crohn disease

II. Pathogenesis
A. Complications
   1. Proximal fistulas can have high output leading to fluid/electrolyte imbalance and malnutrition.
   2. Sepsis if drainage is not controlled
   3. Skin irritation similar to that of an ileostomy
   4. Hemorrhage from mesenteric vessel erosion

III. Diagnosis
A. Imaging
   1. Fistulogram/sonogram
   2. CT scan with contrast
   3. Oral methylene blue, charcoal, or congo red serves as a marker.

IV. Treatment
A. Conservative management: Fistula must be controlled with no sign of sepsis and a clear plan for nutritional support.
   1. MIVFs, electrolyte correction, nutritional support, and drainage control
   2. Broad-spectrum antibiotics
   3. Octreotide, H2 blockers/PPIs
   4. Most spontaneously close within 2 to 8 weeks if low output
B. Operative repair: required for uncontrolled fistulas or sepsis
   1. Resection of fistula
   2. Small bowel resection and anastomosis
   3. Fibrin glue therapy, gel foam embolization

Small Bowel

V. Prevention
A. Tension-free anastomosis
B. Accurately placed sutures, staples to avoid a leak
C. Sharp adhesiolysis
D. Resection of bowel defects greater than half the circumference
E. Good bowel prep and preoperative antibiotics
F. Hemostasis but avoiding ischemia
G. Soft drains, if drains are used
H. Avoid hypotension, steroids, and malnutrition.

 ## MESENTERIC ISCHEMIA

I. Epidemiology
A. Rare disease with a high mortality. For acute ischemia, mortality can be as high as 70% to 90%.
B. Can be acute or chronic
C. The key is early diagnosis and treatment.

II. Pathophysiology
A. Decreased intestinal blood flow leading to ischemia and reperfusion injury
B. Can involve superior mesenteric artery (SMA), celiac axis, inferior mesenteric artery (IMA)
C. Acute
  1. Emboli, thrombosis, hypotension, shock, prolonged vasoconstriction/vasospasm, and venous occlusion from thrombosis
D. Chronic
  1. Long-standing atherosclerotic disease

III. Clinical Presentation
A. Acute
  1. Pain out of proportion to exam
  2. Hematochezia and/or melena
B. Chronic
  1. Postprandial pain: usually about 30 minutes
  2. Nausea, vomiting, diarrhea
  3. History of cardiac disease, atrial fibrillation
  4. Weight loss
  5. "Food fear"

IV. Diagnosis
A. Clinical exam
B. Arteriography (most accurate): Look for severe stenosis of two out of three mesenteric vessels.
C. Mesenteric duplex scanning
D. CT angiography
  1. Findings
    a. Atherosclerotic disease
    b. Portal venous gas
    c. Pneumatosis intestinalis (see Fig. 6-1)
    d. Bowel wall thickening
    e. Bowel dilatation
    f. Peri-enteric stranding
    g. Pneumoperitoneum
E. Plain X-ray (portal venous gas)
F. CBC: leukocytosis
G. Lactic acidosis or metabolic acidosis
H. Amylase elevation

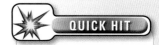

Mesenteric lengthening is accomplished by mobilizing the root of the mesentery at the SMA origin and creating transverse incision in the peritoneum overlying the SMA every 2–3 cm. This technique may be used to facilitate a tension-free bowel anastomosis.

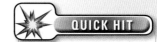

In the setting of mesenteric ischemia caused by venous occlusion, there may not be a lactic or metabolic acidosis because the venous outflow of the bowel is blocked and the acid cannot get into the systemic circulation.

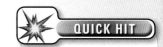

To check for bowel viability the options are:
1. A second-look operation in 24–48 hours
2. Feel for the presence of a pulse in the mesentery
3. Doppler pulses
4. Fluorescence
5. Wood lamp

Small Bowel

V. Treatment

    A. Conservative: if no hard signs for operative intervention, that is, no peritonitis, or low flow state, or patient is too sick for an operation

        1. NPO, nasogastric tube, MIVF, control risk factors

    B. Anticoagulation for venous thrombus

    C. Papaverine infusion for nonocclusive disease

    D. Angioplasty and stenting for chronic ischemia—less invasive but lower long-term success

    E. Endarterectomy for chronic ischemia for occlusion of the ostia of the vessel but no extension into the vessel

    F. Aortomesenteric bypass for chronic ischemia for lesions that are greater than 1 cm into the trunk

    G. Broad-spectrum antibiotics

    H. Surgical bowel resection reserved for severe cases

Colon, Rectum, and Appendix

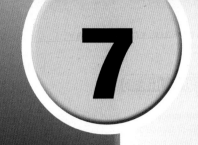

Riaz Cassim, Irfan A. Rizvi, and Farrell Adkins

Dimensions of bowel: Rule 3, 6, 9
Max Normal
Small Bowel = 3cm
Large Bowel = 6cm
Cecum = 9cm

 COLORECTAL AND ANAL DISORDERS

I. **Lower Gastrointestinal Hemorrhage**
   A. Epidemiology: Lower gastrointestinal (GI) bleeding is a common clinical problem with an annual incidence of 20 to 27 cases per 100,000 population.
   B. Etiology (see Clinical Pearl 7-1)
      1. Ischemic colitis, a mostly self-limiting disease, is characterized by the sudden onset of left-sided abdominal pain with bloody diarrhea. Often secondary to other underlying conditions such as hemodialysis, myocardial infarction, postcardiopulmonary bypass, following myocardial infarction, or postaortoiliac surgery. Colitis predominantly affects the mucosa.
         a. Definitive diagnosis is by colonoscopy. Barium enema may outline mucosal ulcers, but its use has generally been replaced by computed tomography (CT), which may reveal colonic wall thickening of the affected segment, or in more severe cases, pneumatosis or portal venous gas.
         b. Treatment includes active observation. Peritonitis with frank gangrene is indication for surgery.
      2. Other causes: radiation proctitis, concealed intussusception (solitary rectal ulcer syndrome)
   C. Diagnosis
      1. Patients with brisk hemorrhage tend to pass bright red blood, whereas patients with slow or proximal colon bleeds tend to pass darker, altered blood mixed with feces.
      2. Recognizing certain common patterns helps facilitate the correct diagnosis. The differential diagnosis includes:
         a. Hemorrhoids: Bright red blood appears on the toilet paper or the bowl and is rarely hemodynamically significant.

Passage of bright red blood per rectum may indicate brisk upper GI bleeding. Whether the source is from the upper or lower GI tract can be easily resolved by passing an NG tube. If clear bilious fluid is aspirated, in most cases, the bleeding source is distal to the ligament of Treitz.

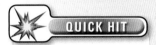

Patients with cecal cancer may not present with an overt bleed but may have iron deficiency anemia instead.

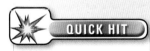

The classical angiographic finding is a slow-emptying, dilated, tortuous vein seen in more than 90% of the cases of arteriovenous malformations.

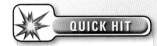

Ninety percent of patients with recurrent or profuse bleeding have either diverticular disease or colonic angiodysplasia.

CLINICAL PEARL 7-1

Common Etiologies of Lower Gastrointestinal Bleeding

- Diverticular disease
- Ischemia
- Anorectal disease (hemorrhoids, anal fissure, rectal ulcer)
- Neoplasm (polyp or cancer)
- Angiodysplasia
- Inflammatory bowel disease
- Radiation colitis
- Small bowel/upper GI bleeding
- Postpolypectomy hemorrhage

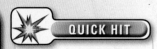

b. Inflammatory bowel disease (IBD): Patients with IBD tend to pass small amounts of blood mixed with mucus and feces.

c. Tumors: The color of defecated blood becomes brighter from proximal to distal colon.

d. Diverticular disease and angiodysplasia: Bleeding is often sudden, brisk, but self-limiting.

   (1) Patients with recurrent or profuse bleeding pose a diagnostic dilemma because the hemorrhage can be difficult to localize.

   (2) In colonic diverticulosis, bleeding occurs when a blood vessel breaks down as it passes through the weakened wall of a diverticulum. Although the disease is more common on the left side, hemorrhages also occur on the right side.

   (3) In colonic angiodysplasia, age-related degeneration of normal submucosal veins occurs. This condition predominantly affects the elderly. Most commonly present in cecum and ascending colon, it can be diagnosed either by colonoscopy or selective mesenteric angiography.

e. Ischemic colitis: Patients are usually elderly and present with left-sided abdominal pain.

D. Management of minor bleeding
   1. History and physical examination
   2. Anorectal examination
   3. Anoscopy, proctosigmoidoscopy
   4. Colonoscopy
   5. Treatment of the cause

E. Management of major bleeding: Regardless of the cause, the initial management in all patients with severe lower GI bleeding is identical.
   1. Resuscitation with nasogastric (NG) tube placement to rule out upper GI source
   2. History
   3. Anorectal examination
   4. Colonoscopy
   5. If the source of the hemorrhage is not revealed by colonoscopy, then consider:
      a. Technetium-99m sulphur colloid isotope red cell scan
         (1) Most sensitive
         (2) Shows extravasation into the gut with bleeding to the order of 0.05 to 0.1 mL/min
         (3) May not precisely localize the site
      b. Selective visceral arteriography
         (1) Localizes bleeding more precisely
         (2) Can be used therapeutically for embolization
         (3) However, it is an invasive test and requires a higher rate of bleeding (0.5 to 1 mL/min) to be diagnostically useful.
   6. Laparotomy
      a. Consider performing concomitant endoscopy to localize bleeding source.
      b. If bleeding continues and cannot be controlled endoscopically, surgery is indicated.
      c. Indicated for patients who require more than 6 units of red blood cells in 24 hours (hemodynamic instability)
   7. Resection
      a. A segmental resection involving the bleeding segment is ideal.
      b. Uncontrolled, nonlocalized bleeding may necessitate a total abdominal colectomy with ileorectal anastomosis.
   8. In colonic diverticulosis:
      a. Because 90% of the patients stop bleeding, nonoperative management is reasonable.
      b. Supportive care in the form of fluid resuscitation and transfusion of blood and blood products is indicated.
      c. Patients who rebleed ultimately need resection of the involved colonic segment.

II. Large Bowel Volvulus

A. General principles

1. In volvulus, the bowel twists on its own mesenteric axis, leading to bowel obstruction.
2. Venous congestion may lead to bowel infarction.

B. Sigmoid volvulus

1. Epidemiology and etiology
   a. Sigmoid volvulus accounts for about 5% of all cases of large bowel obstruction in developed countries. The incidence is higher in the Third World, which has been attributed to fiber-rich diets.
   b. The narrow mesenteric base of the sigmoid colon, along with an elongated floppy loop, makes it particularly susceptible to twisting on its axis.
   c. This condition is seen mostly in elderly, institutionalized patients with chronic medical and neuropsychiatric conditions.
   d. It is postulated that psychotropic drugs affect colonic motility, thus predisposing to volvulus.

2. Clinical features
   a. Patients present with colicky abdominal pain, constipation, nausea, vomiting, and an inability to pass flatus.
   b. The air is able to enter the sigmoid loop but unable to exit. This leads to progressive distention of the sigmoid loop.
   c. The abdomen is usually markedly distended and tympanic on percussion. Severe pain with peritoneal signs is an indicator of underlying bowel ischemia and/or impending perforation.

3. Diagnosis
   a. In most patients, the diagnosis can be made on the combination of history, physical examination, and plain abdominal radiography.
   b. The rectal vault is usually empty on examination.
   c. Plain radiographs show a markedly distended sigmoid loop, which assumes a bent inner tube or inverted U-shaped appearance, with the limbs of the sigmoid loop directed toward the pelvis.
   d. Single-contrast barium enema examination is useful because it demonstrates that the barium readily enters the empty rectum and usually encounters a stenosis, likened to a beak, the so-called *bird beak* or bird-of-prey sign.

4. Management
   a. Patients may be dehydrated and should be fluid resuscitated.
   b. Early decompression via rigid proctoscopy, flexible sigmoidoscopy, or colonoscopy should be attempted. This will allow the mucosa to be visualized for signs of ischemia. The instrument may pass into the obstructed segment. If this maneuver succeeds, there is a sudden, dramatic gush of fluid and feces. It is recommended that a well-lubricated rectal tube be used to prevent early relapse and facilitate continued drainage.
   c. A full colonoscopy should be performed after bowel preparation to rule out an associated neoplasm.
   d. Volvulus can recur in up to 50% of patients; therefore, elective sigmoid resection should be offered to all good-risk surgical patients.
   e. Occasionally, it is not possible to decompress the bowel endoscopically. Alternatively, proctoscopy may reveal mucosal ischemia suggesting sigmoid necrosis. Such a patient should be emergently taken to the operating room.

C. Cecal volvulus

1. Cecal volvulus is uncommon and presents with abdominal pain and distention.
2. Colonoscopic decompression has a high failure rate. Risk of gangrene of the involved bowel segment is also high; therefore, appropriate treatment is cecopexy, cecostomy, or often formal resection, such as right hemicolectomy.
3. A much more common condition is a *cecal bascule,* in which a mobile cecum folds cephalad on a fixed ascending colon. This results in intermittent bowel obstruction.

QUICK HIT

The most common site for volvulus in the large bowel is sigmoid colon (approximately 75% of all cases of volvulus), followed by the cecum and (rarely) the transverse colon.

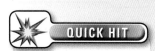

QUICK HIT

The distended cecum comes to lie in the left upper quadrant in most cases and appears on the abdominal radiograph like a "bean" or a "comma."

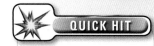

QUICK HIT

Transverse colon volvulus is extremely rare and is associated with congenital bands and other developmental abnormalities. Treatment is similar to cecal volvulus.

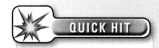

QUICK HIT

Neostigmine is a pathomimetic agent that has been used successfully to treat colonic pseudo-obstruction. An important side effect is bradycardia, and therefore patients should be closely monitored.

D. Pseudo-obstruction
1. This condition is characterized by pronounced abdominal distention, suggestive of a mechanical large bowel obstruction, in the absence of an obstructing lesion.
2. Commonly seen in hospitalized patients with chronic medical conditions
3. The abdomen is distended and tympanic with bowel sounds. There is minimal pain or vomiting.
4. It is important to exclude a mechanical obstruction by water-soluble contrast enema.
5. Management
   a. NG decompression and correction of fluid and electrolyte abnormalities, especially hypokalemia
   b. All medications that inhibit bowel motility, like opiates, should be stopped.
   c. Serial abdominal exams and radiographs are performed.
   d. Neostigmine, an acetylcholinesterase inhibitor, may produce colonic decompression but can be associated with abdominal pain and bradycardia. *use if conservative therapy failed*
6. Colonoscopic decompression may be necessary in patients with marked colonic dilation and impending cecal perforation.

III. Diverticular Disease

A. General principles
1. Colonic diverticula are mucosal outpouchings through the submucosa and the muscular layer of the colon.
2. They occur most commonly in the sigmoid colon, and in 10% of patients, they involve the entire colon.
3. They arise between antimesenteric taenia and the mesenteric taenia at the site of entry of the blood vessels.

B. Epidemiology and etiology
1. Diverticular disease of the colon is an acquired condition.
2. This condition is a disorder of modern civilization and is associated with consumption of refined food products. It is rare in rural African and Asian populations where dietary fiber is high.

C. Clinical features: Most patients are asymptomatic. Occasionally, diverticulosis is associated with lower abdominal colicky pain.

D. Diagnosis of diverticular disease
1. A history of chronic intermittent lower abdominal pain and presence of diverticula on barium enema or colonoscopy are indicative of this condition.
2. In acute diverticulitis, CT may help distinguish a phlegmon from an abscess.
3. Sigmoidoscopy and colonoscopy should be avoided in acute flare-ups of the disease because the risk of perforation is high.

E. Management
1. In acute diverticulitis/phlegmon, intravenous (IV) fluids, antibiotics, and bowel rest are necessary.
2. Abscesses should be drained, usually percutaneously under CT guidance.
3. Fecal peritonitis necessitates exploratory laparotomy. The most commonly performed operation is the *Hartmann procedure,* in which the sigmoid colon is resected, the proximal colon is exteriorized as a stoma, and the rectal stump is oversewn.
4. Patients who develop strictures may need an elective sigmoid colectomy and primary anastomosis.
5. Fistulae are a complex problem. The patient's nutrition should be optimized, and infection should be controlled before surgical repair or resection is attempted.

F. Complications (see Clinical Pearl 7-2)
1. Acute diverticulitis: A diverticulum may become inflamed when a fecalith obstructs its neck. Patients present with left lower quadrant abdominal pain, fever, and leukocytosis.
2. Diverticular abscess: Acute diverticulitis may result in a peridiverticular abscess. Patients experience severe pain, high fever, and white blood

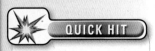

QUICK HIT

Because colonic diverticula do not possess all layers of the bowel wall, they are "false" or "pseudodiverticula."

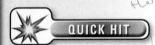

QUICK HIT

The appendix and rectum have a continuous longitudinal muscle layer, rather than taenia, and thus do not have diverticula.

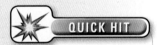

QUICK HIT

Diverticulosis means presence of noninflamed diverticula with or without symptoms. **Diverticulitis** means inflammation of one or more diverticula.

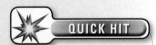

QUICK HIT

Coexisting cancer must be excluded in patients with strictures.

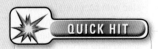

QUICK HIT

Always be mindful of an underlying malignancy as a cause when dealing with presumed diverticular fistulae.

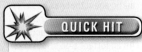

QUICK HIT

Phlegmons do not require drainage because they are semisolid.

CLINICAL PEARL 7-2

Hinchey Classification of Complicated Diverticulitis

- Hinchey I—pericolic or mesenteric abscess
- Hinchey II—contained pelvic abscess
- Hinchey III—generalized purulent peritonitis
- Hinchey IV—generalized feculent peritonitis

cell (WBC) elevation. A CT scan can identify the collection and guide percutaneous drainage.

3. Diverticular phlegmon: The local response to the diverticular inflammation may lead to formation of an inflammatory mass or phlegmon. Such patients need bowel rest and IV antibiotics.

4. Diverticular stricture: Recurrent episodes of inflammation may lead to fibrosis, resulting in luminal narrowing. Patients may present with acute large bowel obstruction.

5. Fecal peritonitis: Perforation of diverticula may lead to fecal peritonitis, which has a mortality rate of about 50%. Patients need emergency exploratory laparotomy.

6. Hemorrhage: Erosion of a peridiverticular vessel can lead to significant bleeding.

7. Fistula: Peridiverticular abscess may erode into adjacent viscera, forming a fistula.

IV. Ulcerative Colitis. This diffuse inflammatory disease affects the mucosa of the colon and rectum.

A. Epidemiology and etiology

1. New cases of ulcerative colitis are seen each year at the rate of 1 to 15 new cases per 100,000 population. The disease has a *bimodal distribution,* with most cases occurring in the teen years followed by a second peak in the 40s.

2. A positive family history is seen in about 10% of patients.

3. Etiology is uncertain. Changes in fecal flora, a history of nonsmoking, appendectomy, milk allergy, and certain genes (12q13, MHC class II genes) have all been considered important in the etiology.

B. Pathology: The primary pathologic process remains unknown.

1. Macroscopic appearance
   a. The disease is limited to the mucosa and submucosa.
   b. The rectum is always involved. The proximal colon may be the site of variable disease.
   c. The mucosal surface is ulcerated with areas of heaped regenerating mucosa called *pseudopolyps*.

2. Microscopic appearance: *Crypt abscesses* form at the base of the mucosa.

C. Clinical features

1. Clinical severity is extremely variable.

2. For most patients, frequent passage of blood-stained stools or diarrhea that contains mucus is the most common initial presentation.

3. Some patients complain of mild lower abdominal pain, fever, and tenesmus but have little in the way of weight loss.

4. In 80% of patients, the disease affects the distal colon.

5. Abdominal examination is usually unremarkable. Rectal examination reveals blood and, on sigmoidoscopy, there is evidence of proctitis. Colonic involvement is continuous, unlike the patchy appearance of Crohn disease.

6. Biopsy of the rectal mucosa is performed to confirm the diagnosis histologically.

7. A minority (20%) of patients with ulcerative colitis present either initially or subsequently with a severe attack, usually with *pancolitis*.
   a. Such patients have unremitting bloody diarrhea (10 to 24 times a day), colicky lower abdominal pain, and weight loss.

Handwritten margin notes:

Incident

Phlegmon Vs Abscess

A Phlegmon is unbounded and can keep spreading out along connective tissue & muscle fibers. An Abscess is walled in and confined to the area of infection.

Proctitis

Inflammation of the Rectum and anus.

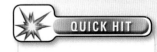

QUICK HIT

Inflammation may extend to terminal ileum, causing backwash ileitis.

   b. On examination, they look pale and ill, and they have tachycardia, fever, and a tender lower abdomen.

  D. Extraintestinal features

   1. Dermatologic

    a. Pyoderma gangrenosum: ulcerated pretibial lesions

    b. Erythema nodosum: symmetric, red, tender papules on extensor surface of limbs

    c. Clubbing

   2. Ocular

    a. Scleritis/episcleritis

    b. Uveitis

    c. Iritis

   3. Rheumatologic

    a. Ankylosing spondylitis

    b. Sacroiliitis

    c. Peripheral arthritis

   4. Hepatobiliary

    a. Sclerosing cholangitis

    b. Fatty liver

    c. Cirrhosis

   5. Vascular

    a. Thromboembolism

    b. Coagulopathy

 E. Diagnosis

  1. History should be taken and a physical examination performed to exclude an infectious cause for diarrhea. Send a stool culture for *Shigella, Salmonella, Campylobacter, Giardia, Escherichia coli,* and *Clostridium difficile.*

  2. Colonoscopy is a definitive imaging technique. A full examination to the cecum is performed. Attempt visualization of the terminal ileum during colonoscopy to rule out Crohn disease, although some patients with ulcerative colitis may demonstrate backwash ileitis.

  3. In many patients, the macroscopic distribution of the colitis is confined to the rectum and part of the sigmoid colon in continuity.

  4. Systemic biopsies throughout the colon enable diagnosis, definition of distribution, and identification of dysplasia.

  5. A barium enema is used less frequently in the imaging of ulcerative colitis but can be used in identifying its characteristic distribution.

  6. In up to 10% of patients, the differentiation between ulcerative colitis and Crohn disease may not be complete, and the colitis is thus labeled *indeterminate.*

 F. Management: The treatment of all patients with IBD is the management of symptoms. This requires an integrated medical and surgical approach that delivers the appropriate therapy consistent with symptom relief.

  1. Medical management of the stable patient consists of drug therapy at a minimum dose that is compatible with good health and fewest side effects. Such a patient may be maintained for months or years on minimal medication, with occasional periods of high-dose steroid therapy for exacerbations.

   a. Steroids: These drugs remain the mainstay of treatment for moderate to severe ulcerative colitis or for patients who have failed aminosalicylate treatment. Their main use is to control symptoms and not to maintain remission.

   b. Aminosalicylic acid compounds: 5-Aminosalicylic acid (5-ASA) is the active compound in different formulations available in the market. Because 5-ASA is disintegrated in the stomach by gastric juices, it is linked to a "stabilizing" compound that facilitates its release at a higher pH in the colon. This drug induces remission and prevents recurrence, and it is the mainstay of medical treatment.

   c. Antidiarrheal drugs may be used to reduce bowel frequency but do not affect the course of the disease. Bowel rest and total parenteral nutrition (TPN) are indicated in severe colitis.

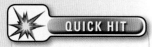

On barium examination, loss of haustra with a flat mucosa and narrow caliber (lead-pipe colon) are indicative of chronic ulcerative colitis.

   d. Immunomodulators

     (1) Calcineurin inhibitors, such as cyclosporine or tacrolimus, are used for refractory colitis.

     (2) The purine antimetabolites (azathioprine and 6-mercaptopurine) are used to facilitate remission induced by cyclosporine. Bone marrow suppression is a serious complication.

   e. Biologic agents

     (1) The antitumor necrosis factor (anti-TNF) antibody infliximab has not seen the same efficacy as it has in Crohn disease.

     (2) Other monoclonal antibodies, such as anti-interleukin-2 receptor antibody or the anti-CD3 antibodies, demonstrated early promise but have not shown efficacy in large-scale trials.

2. Surgical management

   a. Indications for surgery

     (1) The most common indication is intractability of disease and failure of medical management to control symptoms.

     (2) A long history of colitis and a pancolitic distribution of disease are both associated with the potential for malignant change in the colonic mucosa. Mucosal biopsies that show high-grade dysplasia or carcinoma in situ indicate the need for surgical removal of the colon. Colonoscopic surveillance once every 3 years for evidence of mucosal dysplasia is usually started 10 years after diagnosis.

     (3) Other indications for surgical intervention include bleeding, perforation, toxic colonic dilatation, and infection.

   b. Acute severe colitis

     (1) A few patients present with, or develop, an acute exacerbation of colic symptoms that fails to respond to oral high-dose steroids. They require treatment in the hospital.

     (2) IV fluids and hydrocortisone, with bed rest, are the main treatment.

     (3) Combined surgical and medical management from admission is critical because failure to respond quickly to medical measures is an indication for abdominal colectomy.

     (4) Once it is clear that medical therapy has not controlled symptoms within 72 hours of admission, the patient must be apprised of the need for a colectomy. In the acutely ill patient, this comprises abdominal colectomy and ileostomy.

     (5) Subsequent removal of the rectum is necessary in most patients for surgical cure of ulcerative colitis.

   c. From resection to restoration: the pouch

     (1) The elimination of ulcerative colitis and risk of cancer can be done through removal of all colonic mucosa. For many years, total proctocolectomy was the gold standard for curing ulcerative colitis.

     (2) *Total proctocolectomy* involves excising all colon, rectum, and anus with closure of perineal wound. A permanent right lower quadrant spouted (*Brooke*) ileostomy is created.

     (3) The ileal pouch (J, W, or S pouch) or the construction or a new reservoir or neorectum to replace diseased rectum offers the chance of surgical cure without the need for a permanent ileostomy.

     (4) The ileal reservoir most commonly used is the J pouch. Frequency of pouch evacuation usually settles at four to five times daily with good continence.

     (5) Long-term sequelae of restorative proctocolectomy include pouchitis, anastomotic stricture, pouch failure, and sexual dysfunction.

G. Complications: The extraintestinal features complicate 25% to 30% of cases.

  1. Although most respond to treatment of the primary condition, articular and hepatic manifestations do not resolve.

  2. Primary sclerosing cholangitis (PSC) increases the risk of cholangiocarcinoma.

  3. Liver failure secondary to PSC may necessitate a transplant.

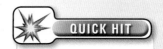

QUICK HIT

The ileoanal pouch is now the reconstructive operation of choice.

V. Crohn Disease

A. Epidemiology and etiology
   1. Crohn disease is a transmural IBD that can affect any part of the GI tract—from the mouth to the anus.
   2. The incidence is about 3 new cases for every 100,000 people, with a prevalence of about 30 cases for every 100,000 people.
   3. Both genetic and environmental factors are implicated.
      a. About 10% of patients give positive family history of IBD. The IBD1 locus on chromosome 16 is strongly associated with Crohn disease.
      b. Infective agents implicated in the pathogenesis include the measles virus and *Mycobacterium paratuberculosis*.
   4. The etiologic factor that could provide a preventative or curative strategy remains elusive.

B. Clinical features (Crohn disease in the small bowel is discussed elsewhere in this text. The following description is confined to the large bowel.)
   1. Three distinct patterns of disease are seen: inflammatory, stricturing, and perforating.
   2. Patients are usually young (peak 15 to 35 years) and present with abdominal pain, weight loss, and diarrhea.
   3. Abdominal pain is colicky. A minority of patients present with the symptoms of colitis: frequent bloody stools with mucus. These patients are indistinguishable from those with ulcerative colitis, including the occasional development of toxic colitis.
   4. Extraintestinal manifestations of Crohn disease include erythema nodosum, pyoderma gangrenosum, uveitis and sacroiliitis, large joint involvement, and clubbing.
   5. Perianal Crohn disease (PCD; see following text), which is often associated with colonic disease, affects about 33% of patients. Perianal pain and suppuration are main symptoms. Rectal examination reveals evidence of ulceration, edematous skin tags, perianal abscess and/or fistulation, and stricture.

C. Diagnosis and imaging
   1. Colonic disease is best diagnosed by colonoscopy. The distribution of colitis is discontinuous with rectal sparing. Often, terminal ileum can be visualized and biopsied to confirm small bowel disease. Barium enema examination is less desirable but may demonstrate Crohn colitis, and reflux of barium into the terminal ileum can be used to diagnose disease at this site. Upper GI series with small bowel follow-through or CT enterography may be useful in identifying small bowel involvement.
   2. Definitive imaging of perineal disease may require examination under anesthesia with endoscopy of the rectum. Other techniques that might help in defining perianal lesions include transrectal ultrasonography and magnetic resonance imaging of the anal canal.

D. Medical management
   1. Aim is symptom relief and maintenance of well-being with minimum side effects.
   2. It is important for the patient to have a well-balanced diet and maintain weight.
   3. An acute flare-up of obstructive symptoms can be managed with a short, high-dose regimen of oral steroids.
      a. In a patient in whom oral steroids cannot be reduced below acceptable levels without symptom reactivation, azathioprine may allow maintenance at a lower steroid dosage.
      b. Budesonide is an enteric-coated steroid that is released into the terminal ileum. It offers means of treating the small bowel without the systemic side effects of oral steroids.
   4. Disease activity can be monitored through measurement of hemoglobin, platelet count, erythrocyte sedimentation rate, and C-reactive protein. In a patient with quiescent colonic disease, sulfasalazine derivatives may also be used (e.g., mesalazine or Pentasa).

CLINICAL PEARL 7-3

Comparison of Ulcerative Colitis and Crohn Disease

- **Ulcerative colitis**
  - Location: colon
  - Lesions: continuous from rectum to more proximal colon
  - Inflammation: limited to mucosa/submucosa
  - Neoplasms: high risk for development
  - Fissures: none
  - Fistulae: none
  - Granulomas: none
- **Crohn disease**
  - Location: entire GI tract
  - Lesions: skip lesions
  - Inflammation: transmural
  - Neoplasms: lower risk
  - Fissures: through submucosa
  - Fistulae: frequent
  - Granulomas: noncaseating

5. PCD: Treatment is conservative because repeated surgical procedures may damage the anal sphincters.
   a. Effective medical therapies include antibiotics such as ciprofloxacin and metronidazole. Immune suppressants such as azathioprine and cyclosporine have been shown to be effective.
   b. The anti-TNF antibody infliximab has been shown to promote healing in complex cases of PCD.
E. Surgical management (see Clinical Pearl 7-3)
   1. Integrated medical and surgical management is required to achieve correct use of surgical resection as treatment.
   2. Surgery is used when drug therapy cannot achieve optimal relief of symptoms with acceptable level of side effects. The presence of a mass in association with the disease is an absolute indication for operation.
   3. Ileocecal disease
      a. The management of ileocecal disease is similar to the management of disease limited to the terminal ileum.
      b. The best option is resection to grossly normal bowel with primary anastomosis. Recurrence tends to occur at the anastomosis and preanastomosis proximal bowel.
   4. Extensive colitis with rectal sparing
      a. Patients with Crohn colitis come to surgery because of chronic ill health but can present acutely with colitis requiring urgent colectomy.
      b. Tendency of Crohn colitis to spare the rectum means that ileorectal anastomosis is the preferred option for subsequent reconstruction.
   5. Segmental Crohn colitis also lends itself to segmental resection and reanastomosis.
   6. Rectal Crohn disease
      a. Many patients with Crohn colitis require panproctocolectomy to eliminate their colonic symptoms.
      b. The ileal pouch is not a generally accepted option after colectomy for Crohn colitis because of the tendency of Crohn disease to affect the pouch, leading to its failure.

VI. Colorectal Polyps
A. General principles
   1. A polyp is a discrete growth that protrudes into the lumen of the colon or rectum.
   2. Polyps may be found throughout the colon and rectum.

B. Epidemiology and etiology
1. Most commonly arise from the mucosa but may be submucosal
2. Mucosal polyps are divided into neoplastic or non-neoplastic.
3. Prevalence parallels that of colorectal cancer, being more common in the developed Western countries such as the United States.
4. From 20% to 40% of asymptomatic patients older than 50 years may have adenomatous polyps identified by colonoscopy.
5. Adenoma prevalence increases with age in all populations.
6. From 30% to 50% of patients with one adenoma have a synchronous adenoma elsewhere in the colon.
7. Adenomas precede carcinomas in a given population by 5 to 10 years. Relatively few adenomas progress to carcinomas.

C. Submucosal polyps
1. Any submucosal growth can expand and push the mucosa into the bowel lumen and appear as a polypoid lesion.
2. Lipomas
   a. Benign fatty tumors mostly seen in the cecum near the ileocecal valve but can be found throughout the colon or rectum
   b. Smooth, yellowish-appearing polyps that are easily deformable
3. Carcinoid tumors (see following section on colorectal cancer)

D. Neoplastic mucosal polyps
1. These are more commonly called adenomatous polyps.
2. Most colorectal cancers arise in preexisting adenomatous polyps.
3. Cancer risk is proportional to the following factors:
   a. The number of adenomas present, synchronously or metachronously
   b. The degree of dysplasia or atypia: The degree of dysplasia correlates with the size of the polyp and degree of villous architecture.
   c. The size of the lesion: Polyps greater than 2 cm have a 30% to 40% risk of harboring a malignancy, whereas polyps less than 1 cm have a risk of 1% to 2%.
   d. The degree of villous component in the polyp.
4. Removal of adenomatous polyps during surveillance proctosigmoidoscopy decreases the risk of subsequent death from colorectal cancer.
5. Adenomatous polyps are characterized according to the following:
   a. Physical structure: sessile, with a broad-based attachment to the colon wall or pedunculated, being attached to the colon wall by a fibrovascular stalk
   b. Glandular structure
      (1) Tubular adenoma characterized by a complex network of branching adenomatous glands (75% of all adenomatous polyps)
      (2) Villous adenomas consist of glands that extend straight down from the surface to the base of the polyp (10% of all adenomatous polyps)
      (3) Mixed tubulovillous adenomas (15% of all adenomatous polyps)

E. Non-neoplastic mucosal polyps
1. Hyperplastic polyps
   a. Small sessile lesions frequently are seen in the distal colon and rectum.
   b. Indistinguishable from small adenomas, they have no malignant potential.
   c. These are found in one-third of the population older than 50 years of age.
2. Juvenile polyps
   a. These growths are also known as retention polyps.
   b. They can occur sporadically or as part of familial adenomatous polyposis (FAP).
   c. Approximately 75% of these polyps occur in children less than 10 years of age and are seen in about 2% of asymptomatic children.
   d. Presenting symptoms include hematochezia. Rectal prolapse and autoamputation may occur with distal lesions, and intussusception may be precipitated by proximal juvenile polyps.
   e. Individually, the polyps have no malignant potential.
3. Inflammatory polyps: seen in idiopathic IBD or severe chronic inflammation of any kind (tuberculosis, amebiasis, schistosomiasis)
4. Peutz–Jeghers hamartomas (see GI polyposis syndromes)

F. Clinical features
1. Most polyps are asymptomatic and are discovered on routine screening colonoscopy.
2. Overt bleeding may be seen as hematochezia, with larger polyps located distally. More commonly, blood loss is clinically occult.
3. Very large polyps may be associated with alterations in bowel habits.
4. Secretory diarrhea with accompanying hypokalemia and hypochlorhydria is associated with large villous adenomas of the rectum and distal colon.

G. Management
1. Polyps must be removed once detected. This can be easily accomplished for pedunculated and small polyps, endoscopically using a biopsy forceps or a snare.
2. Colonoscopy is the most accurate means of detecting polyps and allows biopsy and removal of suspicious lesions.
3. If the polyps cannot be removed via the endoscope, then segmental colon resection is required.
4. Endoscopic polypectomy is adequate for polyps with carcinoma in situ (not invading the basement membrane) and confined to the head of the polyp.
5. There is a 30% to 40% cumulative recurrence rate after index polypectomy in patients over 60 years of age, for multiple adenomas, and for large polyps.

H. Gastrointestinal polyposis syndromes
1. FAP
   a. General principles: FAP is characterized by the development of multiple adenomatous polyps throughout the colon and rectum. Polyps first appear in adolescence (mean age about 16 years). If the polyps go untreated, 100% of affected patients will develop colorectal carcinoma by the third decade of life.
   b. Epidemiology and etiology: This is an autosomal dominant disease with 100% penetrance.
      (1) A germ-line mutation in the adenomatous polyposis coli (APC) gene is located on chromosome 5q.
      (2) Each first-degree relative of an affected individual has a 50% likelihood of inheriting the mutation, and 25% of patients have a germ-line mutation in the APC gene that is not present in either parent.
      (3) The incidence of FAP in the United States is 1 in 10,000 persons.
   c. Pathophysiology: Polyps develop in the stomach and small bowel in 90% of patients. Gastric polyps are primarily fundic gland hyperplasia and not premalignant.
      (1) Periampullary neoplasia: Ninety percent of patients with FAP develop adenomas in the duodenum close to the ampulla of Vater. With time, carcinoma develops in 5% of these patients; this area needs surveillance. Adenomas and carcinomas rarely occur in the jejunum and ileum.
   d. Extraintestinal features: These include osteomas of the mandible, skull, and long bones, as well as soft-tissue tumors such as lipomas and fibromas.
   e. Desmoid tumors: These develop in 10% to 15% of patients with FAP, benign but aggressive tumors of mesenteric fibroblasts; they can obstruct the GI tract, vessels, or ureters.
   f. Attenuated FAP
      (1) Associated with specific codon mutations in APC that result in formation of fewer polyps
      (2) Less than 100 polyps
      (3) Later development of polyps and cancer
   g. *MYH* polyposis
      (1) Autosomal recessive form of FAP
      (2) Associated with mutation in *MYH* gene and no association with APC mutation
      (3) Polyps range from few to hundreds with later development of cancer.

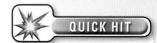

QUICK HIT

The entire colon must be screened because 30% to 50% of patients may have synchronous polyps.

Colon, Rectum, and Appendix

h. Diagnosis and management

(1) At-risk relatives of patients with known FAP should undergo surveillance sigmoidoscopy on an annual basis, beginning after puberty. It is prudent to wait until patient reaches full maturity before planning surgery

(2) Goal of treatment is to remove entire large bowel mucosa, which is at risk for developing colorectal carcinoma.

(3) This is accomplished by total proctocolectomy with end ileostomy or total proctocolectomy with ileoanal pouch anastomosis.

(4) Esophagogastroduodenoscopy is performed every 2 to 3 years for surveillance and removal of gastric and duodenal mucosal polyps.

(5) Surgical management of desmoid tumors is avoided unless simple local excision of abdominal wall or localized lesions is possible. Postoperative recurrences are common. A combination of sulindac and tamoxifen has been successful in some patients.

2. Peutz–Jeghers syndrome

a. Autosomal dominant familial syndrome that is associated with mutations of the *LKB1* gene. Mutations in this gene are only seen in approximately 50% of cases, however.

b. Multiple GI polyps are seen in the stomach, small intestine, and colon. Polyps are non-neoplastic hamartomas consisting of a supportive framework of smooth muscle tissue covered by hyperplastic epithelium. No inflammatory cell infiltrate is present.

c. Rectal bleeding is the most common presentation. Intussusception may also occur. Characteristic skin pigmentation is seen from birth as dark, macular lesions on the mouth (skin and buccal mucosa), nose, lips, hands, feet, genitalia, and anus. This becomes less obvious by puberty.

d. There is no increased risk of colorectal cancer. However, affected individuals are at increased risk of other GI tumors; gonadal tumors (ovarian cysts and sex cord tumors in females and Sertoli cell testicular tumors in males); and breast, pancreatic, and biliary cancers.

e. Management consists of endoscopic polyp removal. Patients presenting with intussusception caused by small bowel polyps require bowel resection.

3. Juvenile polyposis

a. These polyps are the most common solitary lesions seen in the rectum of children. They can be multiple in the entire GI tract.

b. Manifestations can vary but are limited to bleeding, obstruction, and intussusception.

c. Patients are at risk for colorectal cancer if they harbor mixed juvenile and adenomatous polyps. When mixed lesions are found, regular colonoscopic surveillance is recommended.

4. Cowden syndrome

a. Patients with Cowden syndrome, which is associated with mutations of the *PTEN* gene, develop multiple GI hamartomas. Polyps are usually asymptomatic and may be hyperplastic or ganglioneuromas of the colon.

b. There is an increased risk of development of breast tumors and benign and malignant tumors of the thyroid gland.

c. No therapy needs to be directed toward the polyps.

d. This condition is complicated by lesions of the face that arise from follicular epithelium (pathologically trichilemmomas).

VII. Colorectal Cancer

A. Epidemiology and etiology

1. Colorectal cancer is the second most common malignancy in the United States, with more the 155,000 new cases diagnosed annually. Incidence is highest in industrialized countries and is age specific, increasing steadily from the second to the ninth decades.

2. It is the second leading cause of all cancer-related deaths.

3. Rates of colon and rectal cancer are the same in men and women.

4. Animal fats play an etiologic role. They cause an increase in total fecal bile acids that stimulate the generation of reactive oxygen metabolites, enhancing conversion of unsaturated fatty acids to compounds that promote cellular proliferation.

5. Fiber (cereal products, vegetables, and fruits) plays a protective role. Its exact effect is not known, but binding to carcinogens and thus reducing their contact with colonic epithelium and increasing their transit time may be important.

6. Increased calcium intake inhibits colonic proliferation and is associated with decreased risk of colorectal cancer.

7. Clinical risk factors
   a. Familial
      (1) FAP accounts for less than 1% of all colorectal cancers.
      (2) Hereditary nonpolyposis colorectal cancer (HNPCC) accounts for 5% to 10% of all cancers.
      (3) IBD: Risk with chronic ulcerative colitis increases after 10 years of active disease by 1% cumulative/year. It is less in Crohn colitis.
      (4) Adenomatous polyps
   b. General: age greater than 40 years
      (1) Family history of colon cancer
      (2) Personal history of colon polyps or cancer (threefold increase)
      (3) Pelvic radiation for gynecologic cancer (two- to threefold increase)

B. Pathogenesis
   1. Development is a multistep process wherein carcinomas arise from benign adenomas.
   2. The mucosal epithelium progresses through a series of molecular and cellular events that lead to altered proliferation, cellular accumulation, and glandular disarray leading to the formation of adenomatous polyps. Further genetic alteration results in higher degrees of cellular atypia and glandular disorganization (dysplasia), which may evolve to a carcinoma.
   3. The adenoma-to-carcinoma sequence is always associated with genetic changes, even in sporadic colon cancers. Sporadic polyps and cancers are associated with multiple somatic mutations contributed by environmental insults.
   4. Genetic changes that lead to development of adenomas include:
      a. Alteration in proto-oncogenes
      b. Loss of tumor suppressor gene: In more than 75% of cases, stepwise tumor progression is associated with loss of tumor suppressor gene designated DCC (deleted in colorectal cancer) on chromosome 18q– (maintains normal cell–cell adhesive interactions).
      c. Deletions of chromosome 17p involving the p-53 tumor suppressor gene
      d. Abnormalities of genes involved in DNA repair

C. Clinical features
   1. Patients may have intermittent abdominal pain, bleeding, nausea, vomiting, and iron deficiency anemia.
   2. Changes in bowel habits such as constipation and decreased stool caliber are found in constricting rectal cancers. With locally advanced rectal cancers, symptoms of tenesmus, urgency, and perineal pain can occur.

D. Diagnosis
   1. Presence of nonspecific symptoms
   2. In fecal occult blood test in the asymptomatic population, results are positive in 2.5% of patients, and among those, only 10% to 15% have colorectal cancer. The test is not specific because not all polyps and tumors bleed or may bleed intermittently. False-positive results may occur with high-peroxidase diets with rare beef. False-negative results may occur with oral intake of iron, cimetidine, antacids, and ascorbic acids.
   3. Screening is necessary in the following instances:
      a. Every 5 to 10 years in asymptomatic individuals starting at age 50 years
      b. Yearly in first-degree relatives of individuals with known hereditary colon cancer syndromes starting at age 20 years

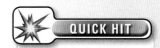

QUICK HIT

Right colon cancer presents with anemia and occult blood, and left colon cancer presents with an obstructive picture.

      c. Every 3 to 5 years in patients who have had a single adenomatous polyp removed, or sooner (6 to 12 months) if multiple or dysplastic polyps are identified

      d. Eight to 10 years after disease activity in patients who have had chronic ulcerative colitis, and then yearly

E. Staging

   1. Ninety-five percent of all colorectal cancers are adenocarcinomas.

   2. Ten percent to 20% of adenocarcinomas are described as mucinous or colloid based on abundant production of mucin. These tumors are associated with a poorer 5-year survival.

   3. Staging is based on the tumor-node-metastasis (TNM) classification.

F. Modes of spread

   1. Colorectal cancer spreads by direct invasion, lymphatic spread, and hematogenous spread. Most commonly, the cancer spreads to the liver, lungs, and bone.

   2. Another mode of spread is via intraluminal or extraluminal exfoliation of tumor cells with subsequent implantation, which may occur during surgical resection with tumor spillage, leading to recurrences in bowel anastomosis, abdominal incisions, or other intra-abdominal sites. Tumors penetrating the intestinal wall can shed cells intraperitoneally and cause carcinomatosis.

G. Management

   1. Surgical therapy is the mainstay of treatment. If colorectal cancer is diagnosed in the early stages, it is curable by surgery.

   2. Surgical goal is resection of the primary colorectal cancer with adequate normal proximal and distal margin (generally obtain 5 cm margins proximally and distally), lateral margin, and regional lymph nodes.

   3. Evaluation for metastasis is important. Careful physical examination is essential, looking for hepatomegaly, ascites, or adenopathy. For rectal tumors, assessing the distance of the tumor from the anal verge and mobility are important in determining resectability and the type of operation required.

   4. Laboratory studies should include a complete blood count, liver function tests (LFTs), and a carcinoembryonic antigen (CEA) assay. A CT scan helps delineate distal metastases. Colonoscopy is essential to look for synchronous lesions.

   5. Adjuvant radiation therapy is used for rectal tumors in which the incidence of local recurrence is significant, including those extending through the bowel wall or with lymph node involvement. Radiation can be given preoperatively or postoperatively. Preoperative therapy prevents radiation to the small bowel and neorectum, and it improves survival.

   6. Adjuvant chemotherapy: Despite local–regional control, patients who die from colon cancer die from disseminated disease: 25% of patients with stage II disease and 50% with stage III disease die from growth of micrometastatic disease present at the time of primary resection. Chemotherapy is offered to patients with stage III colon cancer to improve survival as well as to patients with stages II and III rectal cancer.

H. Follow-up

   1. A subset of colon cancer patients can be cured. Comprehensive follow-up program in patients is appropriate.

   2. Recurrences are likely, with 50% evident within 18 months of surgery, and 90% evident by 3 years. Metachronous primary tumors develop in 5% of patients.

   3. CEA is not helpful as a screening or diagnostic test but as a tumor marker. Concentrations are elevated in 90% of patients with disseminated disease and 20% with localized disease. In two-thirds of patients with recurrence, an increased CEA level is the first marker of disease.

   4. Follow up with periodic physical examinations, CEA assay, LFTs, CT yearly, endoscopy, and chest X-ray.

   5. Hepatic metastasis is the most common site of spread. A subset is resectable.

   6. Pulmonary metastasis: Ten percent of patients with colorectal cancer usually have widespread metastatic disease. If the pulmonary metastasis is solitary, it can be resected with a 20% 5-year survival rate.

7. Prognostic factors
  a. Patients younger than 40 years of age present with more advanced stages than do symptomatic patients.
  b. Prognosis is poorer when obstruction and perforation are present.
  c. Exophytic tumors are associated with less advanced stage compared with ulcerative tumors.
  d. Prognosis is poorer when blood vessel invasion, lymphatic vessel invasion, perineural invasion, and aneuploid tumors are present.

I. Other types of colorectal cancer
  1. HNPCC
    a. HNPCC is also known as Lynch syndrome I. Lynch syndrome II is the same as Lynch syndrome I but with a predisposition to other cancers (e.g., endometrial, ovary, and stomach).
    b. It is responsible for approximately 4% to 6% of all colorectal carcinomas.
    c. It is inherited in an autosomal dominant pattern. The genetic mutation is seen in the DNA mismatch repair genes (*hMSH2, hMLH1, hPMS1*).
    d. Cancers arise in adenomas, but polyposis does not occur. Adenomas and carcinomas occur at an early age (adenomas in the 20- to 30-year range, and carcinomas in the 40- to 45-year range). Tumors are often proximal and multiple.
    e. HNPCC is defined by the Amsterdam criteria:
      (1) Three relatives with colorectal cancer, one of whom is a first-degree relative of the other two
      (2) Colorectal cancer must involve at least two generations.
      (3) At least one cancer must occur before the age of 50 years.
  2. Carcinoid tumors
    a. Most GI carcinoids are found in the ileum. Other potential sites are the appendix, rectum, and colon.
    b. Most rectal tumors are less than 2 cm, submucosal, yellow-gray nodules. Patients are asymptomatic but may present with hematochezia.
    c. Many are less than 1 cm in diameter and can be removed by local excision. Transanal local excision is the treatment of choice because small tumors rarely metastasize.
    d. Tumor size is a prognostic factor. Lesions greater than 2 cm are more commonly malignant but seldom give rise to metastases.
    e. Carcinoid syndrome can arise in patients with metastatic disease to the liver.
  3. Lymphomas
    a. These rare tumors account for less than 0.5% of all colorectal malignancies.
    b. In most cases, widespread disease is documented.
    c. Treatment is chemotherapy and radiation therapy.

VIII. Anal Cancer
  A. General principles
    1. Anal cancer is uncommon and accounts for 2% of large bowel cancers.
  B. Carcinoma of the anal margin
    1. Squamous cell carcinoma (SCC)
      a. SCC grows slowly and has rolled edges with central ulceration.
      b. It is usually well differentiated, and diagnosis is delayed.
      c. All anal ulcers should be biopsied to disprove SCC.
      d. Lymphatic drainage is to the inguinal lymph nodes. SCC is slow-growing and late to metastasize. Surgical therapy involves local excision. If the cancer has invaded the underlying sphincter muscle, metastases can occur proximally along the superior and middle rectal nodes.
      e. Overall, 5-year survival is 34% to 82% depending on stage.
    2. Basal cell carcinoma
      a. This rare cancer occurs 3 times more frequently in men than women.
      b. Lesions are centrally ulcerated and irregular with raised edges.

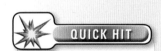

QUICK HIT

The anal canal above and below the dentate line has different lymphatic drainage. The anal margin begins at the hair bearing perianal skin (anal verge).

    c. Local excision is treatment of choice.

    d. Overall, 5-year survival is 73%.

C. Bowen disease (Squamous Cell Carcinoma In-Situ)

  1. In this rare, slow-growing, intraepidermal SCC, lesions are scaly or crusted plaque. Biopsy is confirmatory.

  2. From 70% to 80% of patients eventually develop primary internal malignancy or skin cancer.

  3. Wide local excision is the treatment of choice.

D. Perianal Paget disease

  1. Perianal Paget disease is a rare malignant neoplasm of the intraepidermal portion of apocrine glands, with or without dermal involvement. Lesions are erythematous, scaly, or eczematoid and plaque-like.

  2. It has a long preinvasive course, but invasive adenocarcinoma may develop.

  3. The disease occurs in more women than men, with the highest incidence in the seventh decade.

  4. Eighty percent of patients develop a second primary carcinoma (e.g., breast or rectum).

  5. Biopsy reveals Paget cells—large pale, vacuolated cells with hyperchromatic eccentric nuclei.

  6. Wide local excision is the treatment of choice.

  7. Metastasis to the inguinal nodes, pelvic lymph nodes, liver, bone, lung, brain, or bladder may occur. Once metastasis has occurred, prognosis is poor.

IX. Carcinoma of the Anal Canal

A. General principles

  1. The carcinomas arise from the ducts of the anal glands.

  2. They present with pain, bleeding, and a perianal mass.

  3. Diagnosis is usually made at an advanced stage, when disease has spread beyond hope for cure.

  4. Combination chemo-radiation therapy is the treatment of choice.

  5. This includes SCC, basaloid (cloacogenic arising from the anal transition zone), and mucoepidermoid carcinoma.

  6. Metastasis may occur, with 40% of tumors metastasizing to the superior rectal nodes and 33% to the inguinal nodes.

  7. Overall, 5-year survival is 50%.

B. Management

  1. Local excision: reserved for small, well-differentiated lesions that involve the submucosa only, or for poor-risk patients

  2. Recurrence rates are high after local excision.

  3. Abdominoperineal resection: Five-year survival averages 50%, with 25% to 30% local recurrence after surgery.

  4. Combination chemoradiation therapy (Nigro protocol for SCC: 5-FU and mitomycin C combined with external beam radiation): If the lesion disappears grossly and is microscopically absent, no further therapy is needed. If there is residual disease or recurrence, then proceed to surgery.

  5. Cure rates are between 70% and 90%.

⬤ ANORECTAL DISORDERS

I. Hemorrhoids

A. General principles

  1. In the upper anal canal, there are three cushions of submucosal tissue composed of connective tissue containing venules and smooth muscle fibers. Usually, there are three cushions: left lateral, right anterior, and right posterior.

  2. Their function is to aid anal continence. During defecation, they become engorged with blood, cushion the anal canal, and support the lining of the canal.

3. Muscles that arise partly from the internal sphincter and partly from the conjoint longitudinal muscle support the anal cushions.
4. Hemorrhoid is the term used to describe the downward displacement of the anal cushions, causing dilatation of the contained venules, and they develop when the supportive tissues of the anal cushions deteriorate.

B. Classification
1. External hemorrhoids are dilated venules of the inferior hemorrhoidal plexuses below the dentate line. Thrombosed external hemorrhoids are intravascular clots in the venules.
2. Internal hemorrhoids are the anal cushions located above the dentate line that have become prolapsed. These are graded according to the degree of prolapse.
   a. First degree: The anal cushions protrude into the anal canal but do not prolapse.
   b. Second degree: The anal cushions prolapse through the anus on straining but spontaneously reduce.
   c. Third degree: The anal cushions prolapse through the anus on straining or exertion and require manual replacement into the anal canal.
   d. Fourth degree: The prolapse is not manually reducible.

C. Clinical features
1. The most common manifestation is painless, bright red rectal bleeding associated with bowel movements.
2. The common complaints of burning, itching, swelling, and pain are usually not from hemorrhoids but from pruritus ani, anal abrasion, fissure, thrombosed external hemorrhoids, or prolapsed anal papilla. Patients with thrombosed external hemorrhoids present with abrupt onset of a mass and pain. The pain usually becomes minimal after the fourth day.
3. Patients may also have a feeling of incomplete evacuation. Most patients with thrombosed external hemorrhoids do not give a history of straining, physical exertion, or hemorrhoids.
4. In chronic prolapse, exposed rectal mucosa often causes perianal irritation and mucus staining on the underwear.
5. Congestion of external hemorrhoids or skin tags can cause pain. Symptoms are aggravated by diarrhea or constipation.

D. Diagnosis
1. Diagnosis of hemorrhoids is by careful examination.
2. Internal hemorrhoids cannot be palpated.
3. Anoscopy is used to look for vascular engorgement.

E. Management
1. According to modern concepts, prolapse of the anal cushions is initiated by the shearing effect of the passage of a large, hard stool, or by the precipitous act of defecation, as in urgent diarrhea. If prolapse of the vascular cushion can be prevented, the anal cushions return to their normal state, and symptoms are ameliorated.
2. A high-fiber diet is ideal for first-degree and second-degree hemorrhoids.
3. Rubber band ligation is suitable for first-degree and second-degree hemorrhoids that do not respond to bulk-forming agents. This technique is also suitable for some third-degree hemorrhoids.
4. Infrared photocoagulation coagulates tissue protein or evaporates water in the cells. This technique can be used for first-degree and second-degree hemorrhoids.
5. Hemorrhoidectomy is considered when hemorrhoids are severely prolapsed, requiring manual reduction, or when they are complicated by associated pathology such as ulceration, fissures, fistulas, large hypertrophied papilla, or excessive skin tags.
6. Stapled hemorrhoidopexy can be attempted for second- or third-degree hemorrhoids; however, this procedure has been associated with the development of pelvic sepsis in rare cases.
7. Treatment of thrombosed external hemorrhoids is aimed at prevention of recurrent clot, relief of severe pain, and prevention of residual skin tags. It involves excision of the hemorrhoid or evacuation of the clot.

8. If pain is subsiding, conservative treatment is with sitz baths, proper anal hygiene, and bulk-forming agents.
9. If strangulated hemorrhoids are untreated, they progress to ulceration and necrosis. Pain is severe, and urinary retention is common. Proper treatment requires urgent or emergent hemorrhoidectomy.

II. Anal Fissure

A. General principles
   1. An anal fissure is an ulcer in the lower portion of the anal canal.
   2. It may be acute or chronic.
   3. The primary fissure occurs without association with other local or systemic diseases.
   4. The secondary fissure occurs in association with Crohn disease, leukemia, or aplastic anemia.
   5. Most tears of the anal canal can be traced to the passage of large, hard stool or explosive diarrhea, trauma to the anus, or a tear during vaginal delivery.
   6. In men, almost all fissures are located in the posterior midline, whereas in women, 10% are in the anterior midline.
B. Clinical features
   1. Patients have increased anal resting pressure caused by the increased tone of the internal sphincter muscle. This results in ischemia and ulceration to the overlying anal skin.
   2. Anal pain during and after defecation is the most prominent symptom. The pain is described as burning, throbbing, or dull aching.
   3. Bleeding is common and stains the toilet paper.
C. Diagnosis: Physical examination confirms the diagnosis. Chronic fissures have a triad of a fissure, sentinel skin tag, and hypertrophied anal papilla. The sentinel skin tag is the fibrotic or edematous skin adjacent to the fissure.
D. Management
   1. Initial treatment of acute anal fissure is pain relief with proper anal hygiene and warm sitz baths to relax the anal canal. Bulk-forming agents are used to relieve constipation. Nitroglycerin ointment or calcium-channel blockers applied topically help by decreasing sphincter resting tone. Anal fissures usually heal within 6 weeks.
   2. Surgery is not usually required unless the fissure fails conservative therapy.
   3. Lateral internal sphincterotomy is the surgical procedure of choice.
   4. Fissures or ulcers in Crohn disease are larger and deeper than primary anal fissures. The surrounding skin is macerated and edematous. Treatment consists of proper anal hygiene and treatment of the underlying inflammatory disease.

III. Anorectal Abscesses

A. Etiology
   1. In the wall of the anal canal, a variable number of anal glands (4 to 10) lined by stratified columnar epithelium have direct openings into the anal crypts at the dentate line.
   2. Infection of the glands leads to perianal abscess.
   3. Because the glands lie between the internal and external sphincter, an intersphincteric abscess is formed. Infection then spreads to various spaces: perianal, ischiorectal, intersphincteric, and supralevator.
   4. Supralevator abscesses, which are uncommon, can arise from upward extension of an intersphincteric abscess.
B. Clinical features
   1. Presenting features include pain and fever. Depending on the location, a swollen mass may be felt.
   2. Intersphincteric abscesses do not present with overt perianal swelling.
C. Diagnosis
   1. An anorectal abscess is suspected when anorectal pain is so severe that rectal examination is not possible.

    2. A supralevator abscess is difficult to diagnose. Examination reveals a bulging tender mass on either side of the lower rectum or posteriorly above the ano-rectal ring.

  D. Management

    1. Treatment is primary incision and drainage. Antibiotics after drainage are given to patients with cardiac valvular abnormalities or to patients who are immunodeficient.

    2. Perianal abscesses are the most superficial and easiest to treat. A cruciate incision is made on the most prominent part of the skin and subcutaneous tissue overlying the abscess cavity.

    3. Ischiorectal abscess causes diffuse swelling of the ischioanal fossa. Drainage is the same as in perianal abscess.

IV. Fistula-in-Ano

  A. Etiology: In this chronic form of perianal abscess, the abscess cavity does not heal completely but becomes an inflammatory tract with the primary internal opening in the anal crypt at the dentate line and the secondary opening in the perianal skin.

  B. Classification: The four main types are based on the relation of the fistula to the sphincter muscle:

    1. Intersphincteric: Fistula tract traverses through the internal sphincter.

    2. Transsphincteric: Fistula tract traverses through the external sphincter.

    3. Suprasphincteric: Fistula starts in the intersphincteric plane and then passes upward to a point above the puborectalis muscle, and then laterally over this muscle and downward between the puborectal and levator muscles into the ischiorectal fossa.

    4. Extrasphincteric: The fistula passes from the perineal skin through the ischiorectal fossa and levator ani muscle, and finally penetrates the rectal wall. This may arise from trauma, foreign body, pelvic abscess, or cryptoglandular abscess.

  C. Clinical features

    1. Most patients have a history of anorectal abscess subsequently associated with subsequent drainage.

    2. Low rectal or anal canal carcinomas may present as fistulas.

    3. A superficial tract may be palpable. The external opening is usually visible as a red elevation of granulation tissue with purulent or serosanguineous drainage.

  D. Management: Principles of fistula surgery include unroofing the fistula, eliminating the primary opening, and establishing adequate drainage. Open the entire fistula tract with a guide in place.

V. Pilonidal Sinus

  A. Epidemiology and etiology

    1. Pilonidal sinus is more likely to occur in hirsute patients.

    2. Incidence is highest in the second and third decades of life.

    3. The cause is an infected hair follicle in the sacrococcygeal area.

  B. Clinical features

    1. Pilonidal sinus may present with an acute abscess that ruptures spontaneously, leaving unhealed sinuses with chronic drainage.

    2. Most sinus tracts run cephalad (93%).

  C. Diagnosis

    1. Physical examination may reveal pits in the intergluteal folds.

    2. The differential diagnosis includes furuncles of the skin, anal fistula, syphilitic or tuberculous granulomas, and osteomyelitis with multiple draining sinuses.

  D. Management: Drainage of an acute abscess may be performed under local anesthesia. There may be tufts of hair in the abscess cavity that must be removed. Definitive treatment is by local excision.

VI. Rectal Prolapse

  A. Epidemiology and etiology

    1. Procidentia is an uncommon condition in which the full thickness of the rectal wall turns inside out into or through the anal canal. The extruded rectum is

seen as concentric rings of mucosa. The cause is poorly understood, and the disorder is a form of intussusception. Most patients have a history of straining with intractable constipation or chronic diarrhea. There is a high incidence in patients with mental retardation. Patients have impaired resting and voluntary sphincter activity and impaired continence.

2. Predominates in females with a female:male ratio of 5:1 to 6:1
3. Classification
   a. Partial: prolapse of rectal mucosa only
   b. Complete: First degree with an occult prolapse: Several anatomic defects are constantly demonstrated in patients with chronic rectal prolapse.
   c. Complete: second-degree; prolapse to, but not through, the anus
   d. Complete: third-degree; protrusion through the anus for a variable distance

B. Clinical features: Early symptoms include anorectal discomfort during defecation. Feeling of incomplete evacuation is common. In overt prolapse, protrusion occurs only during or after defecation. As the problem becomes more pronounced, the prolapse may be precipitated by coughing, walking, and exertion. Bleeding from ulcerated mucosa.

C. Diagnosis: Demonstrated on clinical exam by asking the patient to strain or in the bathroom asking the patient to defecate. Occult prolapse by defecography.

D. Management
   1. The goal is to repair the prolapse and prevent intussusception from recurring.
   2. The most reliable repair is via the abdomen involving anterior resection with rectopexy.
   3. For elderly or unfit patients, a transperineal rectosigmoidectomy is more appropriate.
   4. Incontinence is due to mechanical stretch of the sphincter as well as pudendal nerve dysfunction. 50% of patients improve after repair.

 APPENDIX AND APPENDICITIS

I. Appendicitis

A. Etiology: The cause of appendicitis is unclear.
   1. However, luminal obstruction resulting from lymphoid hyperplasia, secondary to bacterial (*Salmonella, Shigella*) or viral (infectious mononucleosis), has been postulated.
   2. Fecaliths (literally fecal stones, or hard stool pellets) can also cause luminal obstruction and may be responsible for up to 30% of cases.

B. Clinical features
   1. Typically, patients present with vague periumbilical pain, fever, anorexia, nausea and/or vomiting, right lower quadrant pain, and tenderness.
   2. Occasionally, patients present with urinary or other complaints.

C. Diagnosis
   1. Dunphy sign: increased pain with coughing or other movement
   2. Rovsing sign: Left lower quadrant palpation induces right lower quadrant pain.
   3. Obturator sign: pain on internal rotation of the right hip
   4. Psoas sign: pain on extension of the right hip

D. Laboratory
   1. Leukocytosis with a moderate elevation in WBC count; less than 20,000/mL is seen
   2. Pyuria (WBCs in the urine) may be present.

E. Radiology
   1. Plain film may show a calcified fecalith.
   2. Ultrasound shows thick-walled, noncompressible luminal lesion (target lesion). This image may be helpful in ruling out other pathologies.
   3. CT allows for prompt diagnosis and obviates the need and consequent costs of in-hospital observation.

F. Management: open or laparoscopic appendectomy
G. Unusual presentations
1. Variants in certain patient populations
a. Children: Higher perforation rates may occur. CT is helpful.
b. Elderly: Higher perforation rates may occur. Be sure to rule out cecal neoplasia.
c. Immunocompromised patients: Cytomegalovirus-related bowel perforation and neutropenic colitis may masquerade as appendicitis.
d. Pregnant women: Confusion may arise due to normal elevations in WBC counts and the presence of nausea and vomiting. Be aggressive, because perforated appendix has a high fetal mortality rate (greater than 30%).
2. Appendiceal masses: Form an average of 5 days after symptom onset and usually represent a phlegmon or abscess. These should be managed nonoperatively with percutaneous drainage with or without IV antibiotics.
H. Appendiceal neoplasms
1. Carcinoids
a. Fifty percent of GI carcinoids arise in the appendix. They have a firm yellow appearance.
b. Most are found incidentally.
c. Size is prognostic. Neoplasms less than 1.5 cm are curative by appendectomy, and those 2 cm or greater require right hemicolectomy.
2. Mucoceles
a. These neoplasms are either cystadenomas or cystadenocarcinomas.
b. Cystadenomas: Appendectomy is curative.
c. Cystadenocarcinomas: An association with peritoneal implantation leads to pseudomyxoma peritonei, which has no effective cure, and may need several debulking operations.
3. Adenocarcinoma
a. These neoplasms are rare.
b. T1 lesions are cured by appendectomy, and more advanced lesions require right hemicolectomy.
c. There is a high incidence of secondary GI tumors.
I. Appendiceal cancer
1. This form of cancer is rare (1.3% of all appendectomy specimens).
2. Carcinoids
a. Appendiceal carcinoids represent two-thirds of all appendiceal neoplasms. Half of all GI carcinoids are in the appendix.
b. These are usually seen as an incidental finding after an appendectomy. The mean age of patients is 41 years.
c. The majority are small, less than 2 cm, and have minimal metastatic potential. Those greater than 2 cm have metastatic potential. Appendectomy is sufficient. If larger lesion, or close to the base, they need right hemicolectomy.
d. Overall, 5-year survival is 99%.
3. Appendectomy for benign disease is sufficient, even if in cases of perforation that result in mucinous ascites.
4. In the malignant form of the disease, the neoplastic mucosa invades the wall of the appendix and may implant in the peritoneum, causing pseudomyxoma peritonei. The 5-year survival is 50%.

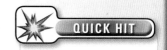

QUICK HIT

Interval appendectomy, performed 6 to 8 weeks after resolution of the appendiceal mass, is generally recommended.

Colon, Rectum, and Appendix

8 Hepatobiliary System

Santosh Shenoy, Amanda Palmer, and Magesh Sundaram

 HEPATIC SYSTEM

I. General Principles

A. Surface anatomy (Fig. 8-1)
1. The liver is the largest solid organ in the body, weighing 1,500 g. It is smooth, reddish brown, and covered by a fibrous sheath known as Glisson capsule.
2. It is an intraperitoneal organ lying predominantly in the right upper quadrant (RUQ) of the abdominal cavity. It is anatomically related to the diaphragm, the stomach, the duodenum, the right kidney and adrenal gland, and the right colon. It is fixated in the RUQ by a number of ligamentous attachments, which include the falciform ligament, the round ligament (obliterated umbilical vein), the right and left coronary, and the right and left triangular ligaments.
3. The contents of the hepatic hilum are contained in the hepatoduodenal ligament. These include the bile duct, the hepatic artery, and the portal vein. The bile duct and hepatic artery lie anterior to the portal vein, with the bile duct lying lateral to the more medially situated hepatic artery.
4. The space behind the hepatoduodenal ligament is known as the (epiploic) foramen of Winslow. It communicates directly with the lesser sac and can be occluded to control the vascular inflow to the liver in what is known as the Pringle maneuver.

B. Segmental anatomy (Fig. 8-2)
1. The liver has a segmental anatomy that was first described in the early 1950s by a French anatomist and surgeon named Claude Couinaud. He described eight distinct liver segments, which are distributed between the right and left lobes of the liver. The anatomic boundary between the right and left lobes of the liver is an imaginary line between the gallbladder anteriorly and the inferior vena cava (IVC) posteriorly. This is known as the Cantlie line.
2. The left lobe of the liver is comprised of segments II to IV. Segments II and III make up the lateral segments of the left lobe of the liver and lie to the left of the falciform ligament. Segments IVA and IVB make up the medial segment(s) of the left lobe of the liver. These lie to the right of the falciform ligament and to the left of the Cantlie line.
3. The right lobe of the liver is comprised of segments V to VIII. Segments V and VIII make up the anterior segments of the right lobe of the liver, and segments VI and VII make up the posterior segments of the right lobe of the liver.
4. Segment I of the liver is known as the caudate lobe. It belongs to neither the right or left lobes because it has a blood supply and venous drainage pattern that are distinct from either the right or left systems.

C. Vascular anatomy
1. The vascular anatomy of the liver is best thought of in terms of the inflow to and the outflow from the liver. The liver has a unique dual blood supply. Eighty percent of the blood flowing into the liver comes via the portal venous circulation. The portal vein is formed by the confluence of the superior

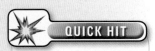

QUICK HIT

The portal vein carries the venous drainage from the entire capillary system of the small and large intestine, pancreas, and spleen to the liver for further digestive processing.

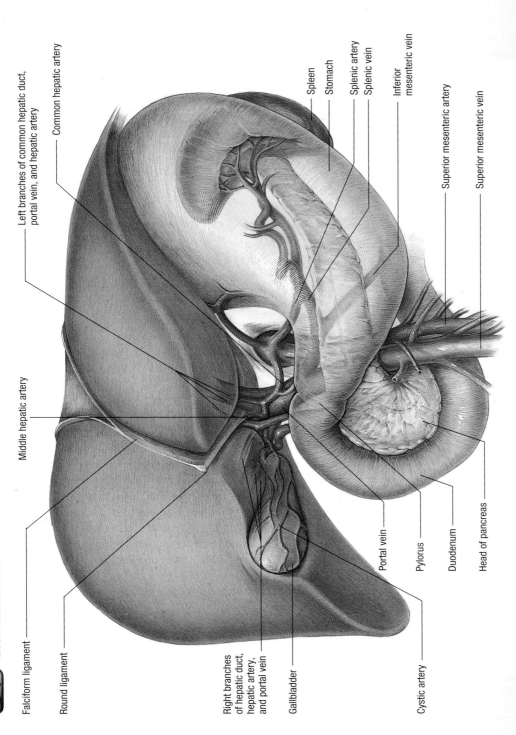

FIGURE 8-1 Liver. Anterior view.

Falciform ligament

Round ligament

Middle hepatic artery

Left branches of common hepatic duct, portal vein, and hepatic artery

Common hepatic artery

Right branches of hepatic duct, hepatic artery, and portal vein

Gallbladder

Cystic artery

Portal vein

Pylorus

Duodenum

Head of pancreas

Spleen

Stomach

Splenic artery

Splenic vein

Inferior mesenteric vein

Superior mesenteric artery

Superior mesenteric vein

(With permission from Anatomical Chart Company, General Anatomy, 2008-05-14 0614, 2008-07-13 1449, Hepatic Tutorial, Spleen.)

Hepatobiliary System

FIGURE
8-2 Functional divisions of the liver and liver segments according to Couinaud nomenclature.

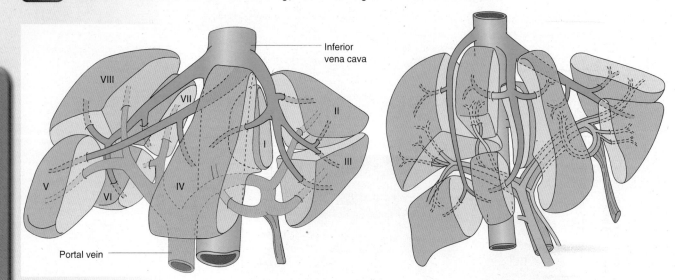

Inferior vena cava

Portal vein

(With permission from Mulholland MW, Lillemoe KD, Doherty GM, Maier RV, Upchurch GR, eds. *Greenfield's Surgery: Scientific Principles and Practice*. 4th ed. Philadelphia, PA: Lippincott Williams & Wilkins; 2006.)

mesenteric vein and the splenic vein. The portal vein bifurcates in the hepatic hilum into the right and left portal veins (see Fig. 8-1).

2. There are a number of potential connections between the portal venous system and the systemic venous system. Under conditions of high portal venous pressure (cirrhosis, hepatic vein thrombosis, right heart failure, splenic vein thrombosis), these portosystemic connections may enlarge and clinically manifest portal hypertension.

3. The more significant locations are:
   a. The coronary vein, draining the stomach and the distal esophagus
   b. Umbilical and abdominal wall veins, which recanalize from flow through the umbilical vein in the ligamentum teres, resulting in caput medusae
   c. The superior hemorrhoidal plexus, which receives portal flow from the inferior mesenteric vein tributaries and may cause large hemorrhoids
   d. Retroperitoneal collaterals, ultimately leading back to the vena cava

4. The remaining 20% of the blood flowing into the liver comes via the hepatic arterial circulation. The common hepatic artery is a branch of the celiac axis. After the takeoff of the gastroduodenal artery, the common hepatic artery becomes the proper hepatic artery, which gives off branches to the right and left lobes of the liver.

   Anatomic variants of the hepatic arterial circulation are legion, with the following being the most common:
   a. Accessory/completely replaced right hepatic artery (RHA; 22%) arising from the superior mesenteric artery: This aberrant artery runs behind the portal vein and the bile duct and, when present, should be identified and preserved during upper gastrointestinal (GI) operations involving the bile duct, duodenum, or pancreas (Fig. 8-3).
   b. Accessory/completely replaced left hepatic artery (18%) arising from the left gastric artery: This aberrant artery runs in the gastrohepatic ligament into the umbilical fissure of the liver and should be identified and preserved during operations in which the gastrohepatic ligament is being opened widely (Fig. 8-4).

5. The venous drainage, or outflow from the liver, is via three main hepatic veins: right, middle, and left. These drain directly into the IVC. The right vein has its own insertion into the IVC, whereas in 95% of patients, the middle and left veins form a common trunk prior to entering into the IVC.

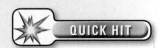
QUICK HIT

The coronary vein drains the lesser curvature of the stomach and the distal esophagus. In portal hypertension, this important tributary of the portal vein enlarges and leads to esophageal varices.

FIGURE
8-3 Example of right hepatic artery arising from SMA. The artery runs behind the portal vein and bile duct.

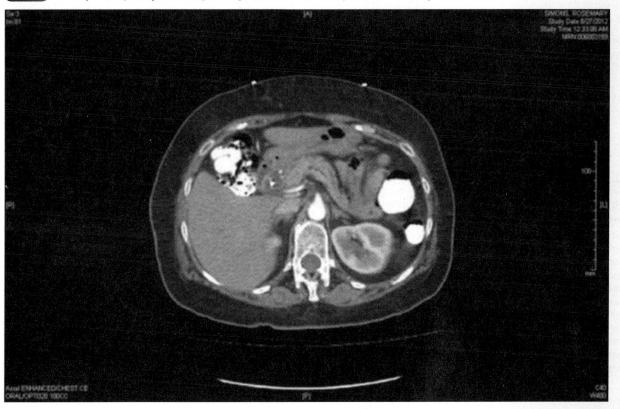

FIGURE
8-4 Example of left hepatic artery arising from the left gastric artery.

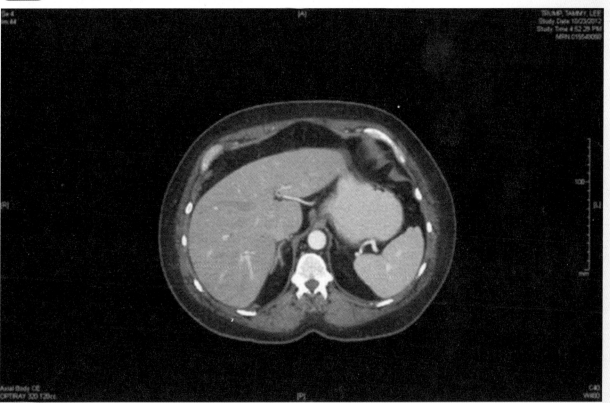

D. Nerves and lymphatics
1. Lymphatic channels in the liver may be deep and found adjacent to the portal and hepatic veins or superficial and found along the liver capsule. The superficial lymphatic channels drain the liver to the coronary and falciform ligaments, to the diaphragm, and to periesophageal nodes. The deep lymphatic channels drain into nodes at the hepatic hilum, in the porta hepatis, and adjacent to the IVC.
2. The liver has a rich parasympathetic and sympathetic innervation.
   a. Vagal innervation adjacent to the bile ducts stimulates the digestive metabolic functions of the liver as well as increases hepatic glycogen synthesis.
   b. Sympathetic innervation from the lower thoracic and celiac ganglia to the liver runs adjacent to the hepatic arteries and monitors intrahepatic sinusoidal pressure. Afferent nerves to the liver register pain when the liver capsule is distended through the right phrenic nerve.

E. Physiology
1. The liver is a truly vital organ. Unlike the lungs (mechanical ventilation), kidneys (hemodialysis), and even the heart (inotropic agents and/or ventricular assist devices), there is no machine or any drug that can replace the function(s) of the liver, which can broadly be thought of in terms of the following: synthetic, metabolic, secretory, and storage.
2. Bile formation and secretion
   a. The liver makes 1 to 1.5 L of bile a day. The main constituents of bile are water, electrolytes, and a variety of organic molecules including bile pigments, bile salts, phospholipids (lecithin), and cholesterol. The primary bile salts are chenodeoxycholic acid and cholic acid, which are produced from cholesterol and then conjugated with glycine and taurine within the hepatocytes. The primary bile acids, when exposed to intestinal bacteria, are converted to the secondary bile acids, deoxycholic acid and lithocholic acid.
   b. The two fundamental roles of bile are:
      (1) Aid in the digestion and absorption of lipids and lipid-soluble vitamins (A, D, E, and K).
      (2) Eliminate waste products (bilirubin and cholesterol) through secretion into bile and elimination in feces.
   c. Approximately 90% to 95% of the secreted bile salts are absorbed at the terminal ileum. The absorbed bile salts are transported back to the liver in the portal vein and re-excreted in the bile. This process is known as the enterohepatic circulation.
3. Bilirubin metabolism
   a. Bilirubin is derived from heme, which is formed from the breakdown of red blood cells.
   b. It is initially bound to serum albumin and circulates as the bilirubin-albumin complex. This complex then enters the hepatic circulation, where it is dissociated. Here, the bilirubin is conjugated to glucuronic acid in a reaction catalyzed by the enzyme glucuronyl transferase and is eventually secreted into bile.
   c. Enteric bacteria then deconjugates the bilirubin to urobilinogens. Most of this urobilinogen is further oxidized and reabsorbed into the enterohepatic circulation. A small portion is excreted into the urine and excreted into the stool, which imparts the yellow color to the urine and the brown color to the stool.
4. Carbohydrate metabolism
   a. In the postprandial state, absorbed carbohydrates are circulated systemically and reach the liver, where most of them are converted to the glucose storage form: glycogen. A smaller amount of excess circulating glucose is removed by the liver via glycolysis or lipogenesis.
   b. In the fasting state, the liver can increase circulating glucose levels by converting glycogen to glucose in a process known as glycogenolysis or by de novo synthesis of glucose from noncarbohydrate precursors such as lactate, amino acids, and glycerol in a process known as gluconeogenesis.

QUICK HIT

About 1,500 mL of bile is secreted daily by the liver. The bile acids are reabsorbed in the ileum to circulate back to the liver via the superior mesenteric vein. This highly efficient process, which extracts up to 90% of the bile acids produced daily, is called the enterohepatic circulation.

5. Lipid metabolism
   a. Fatty acids are synthesized in the liver during states of glucose excess when the ability of the liver to store glycogen has been exceeded.
   b. Excess fatty deposition leads to steatosis, or diffuse fatty infiltration of the liver.
6. Protein metabolism
   a. Ingested protein is broken down into the amino acids and circulated throughout the body. Here, they are used as the building blocks for proteins, enzymes, hormones, and nucleotides.
   b. Excess amino acids are transported to the liver to be converted to glucose, ketone bodies, or fats.
   c. The end product of amino acid catabolism is ammonia (NH_3), which is converted into urea by the liver.
7. Protein synthesis: The liver is the main site of synthesis of various other proteins, such as the coagulation factors, iron-binding proteins, alpha 1-antitrypsin, ceruloplasmin, albumin, and acute-phase proteins.

II. Evaluation of the Liver

A. History and physical examination
   1. Jaundice and icterus refer to the yellow appearance to the skin, sclera, and mucous membranes as a result of retention and systemic deposition of bilirubin. Jaundice typically does not develop until the serum bilirubin level exceeds 2.5 to 3. Jaundice or icterus is a reflection of liver disease, including obstruction of the biliary tract, acute hepatic injury from drugs and toxins, and the chronic loss of hepatic reserve from cirrhosis due to alcohol, the hepatitis virus(es), iron or copper, and parasitic infection.
   2. The triad of splenomegaly, ascites, and caput medusae (dilated abdominal wall veins) indicates portal hypertension. Other signs/symptoms of cirrhosis and/or portal hypertension can include a history of upper GI bleeding from esophageal varices or hepatic encephalopathy from excessive NH_3 levels, testicular atrophy, spider angiomata, pain, and fatigue.
   3. A history of pruritus suggests cholestasis, either intrahepatic or extrahepatic. Causes may be at the hepatocellular level (viral hepatitis), canalicular level (drugs, total parenteral nutrition, amyloidosis), or biliary ductal level (primary biliary cirrhosis [PBC], primary sclerosing cholangitis [PSC]).

B. Diagnostic laboratory testing
   1. Serum bilirubin levels, both conjugated (direct) and unconjugated (indirect), are affected in a number of disease processes and are related to the metabolism of the bilirubin.
      a. Unconjugated bilirubin is generally elevated in hemolysis, drug hepatotoxicity, inherited enzymatic disorders (Gilbert disease, Crigler-Najjar), and the physiologic disorders of the newborn.
      b. Conjugated bilirubin is usually elevated in hepatocellular diseases, cholestasis, or biliary obstruction.
   2. The serum transaminases alanine aminotransferase (ALT) and aspartate aminotransferase (AST) are nonspecific indicators of acute hepatocellular injury. However, an AST:ALT ratio greater than 2:1 is more suggestive of alcoholic liver disease.
   3. Alkaline phosphatase can be used as a marker of cholestasis. Alkaline phosphatase is released by damaged hepatocytes as a consequence of cholestasis, but other organ and tissue production of alkaline phosphatase (e.g., bone, placenta, kidneys, and leukocytes) make it a nonspecific indicator in the evaluation of liver disease. The heat-stable fraction of alkaline phosphatase is more suggestive of liver pathology.
   4. The synthetic function of the liver is measured by the serum albumin level and the prothrombin time (PT), the latter of which is reflective of the vitamin K–dependent clotting factors II, VII, IX, and X. The most sensitive indicator of deficiency of hepatic synthetic function is an abnormal (prolonged) PT. No improvement in the PT despite vitamin K administration reflects severe hepatic functional loss.

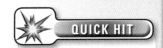

QUICK HIT

Unknown metastatic cancer to the liver rarely presents as new-onset jaundice, unless liver cell mass and hepatic reserve are almost totally replaced by tumor.

Hepatobiliary System

TABLE 8-1 Child-Pugh Classification System

Parameter	1 Point	2 Points	3 Points
Bilirubin	<2 mg/dL	2–3 mg/dL	>3 mg/dL
Albumin	>3.5 g/dL	2.8–3.5 g/dL	<2.8 g/dL
INR	<1.7	1.7–2.2	>2.2
Encephalopathy	None	Controlled	Controlled
Ascites	None	Controlled	Controlled

Child's Class
Class A = 5–6 points
Class B = 7–9 points
Class C = 10–15 points

INR, international normalized ratio.

5. The Child-Pugh classification system (Table 8-1) is a prognostic scoring system that was initially developed to predict mortality during surgery in patients with liver cirrhosis. It consists of measures of the following five parameters: serum bilirubin level, albumin level, PT/international normalized ratio (INR), degree of ascites, and degree of encephalopathy. It had been used in the past to determine a patient's need for liver transplantation (LT), but recently, this scoring system has been replaced with the Model for End-Stage Liver Disease (MELD), which takes into account the serum bilirubin level, the INR, and the serum creatinine level.

C. Imaging and diagnostic tests
   1. Ultrasound
      a. This quick, easy-to-perform, noninvasive test involves no radiation.
      b. It is the primary modality to identify cholelithiasis. Focal and diffuse liver disease can be identified.
      c. Doppler ultrasound allows for evaluation of vascular anatomy and pressures.
   2. Computed tomography (CT) scan
      a. To evaluate the liver for tumors and other pathology, a triple-phase, liver protocol-contrasted CT scan should be obtained (noncontrasted phase, hepatic arterial phase, portal venous phase).
      b. It demonstrates hepatic segmental anatomy, focal disease such as tumors, or diffuse liver disease such as cirrhosis or steatosis.
      c. Various benign and malignant tumors of the liver have characteristic features on triple-phase contrasted CT scans that can help aid in the diagnosis of liver masses (Fig. 8-5).
   3. Hepatobiliary iminodiacetic acid (HIDA) scan shows excretion of tracer along the biliary tract and thus is useful for detecting bile leaks or obstruction.
   4. Magnetic resonance imaging (MRI) scan
      a. MRI provides exquisite detail of hepatic parenchyma and finer detail of tumors to differentiate benign (hemangiomas) from malignant.
      b. Reconstruction of the biliary tree with great detail is possible, including recognition of ductal stone disease, biliary damage, or tumors, through magnetic resonance cholangiopancreatography (MRCP).
   5. Nuclear medicine studies such as sulfur colloid scan or technetium 99 scans can help differentiate hepatic tumors such as focal nodular hyperplasia (FNH) and hemangioma, respectively, when other imaging modalities are nondiagnostic/equivocal.

III. Benign Disorders
A. Infection
   1. Pyogenic abscesses
      a. Most pyogenic hepatic abscesses are caused by infection originating from the GI tract or the biliary tract.

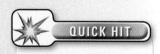

QUICK HIT

The majority of pyogenic abscesses are solitary and involve the right lobe of the liver due to preferential laminar flow of blood to the right lobe. Multiple pyogenic abscesses lead to almost twice the mortality of a solitary abscess.

FIGURE 8-5 Computed tomography scans showing classic appearance of benign liver masses.

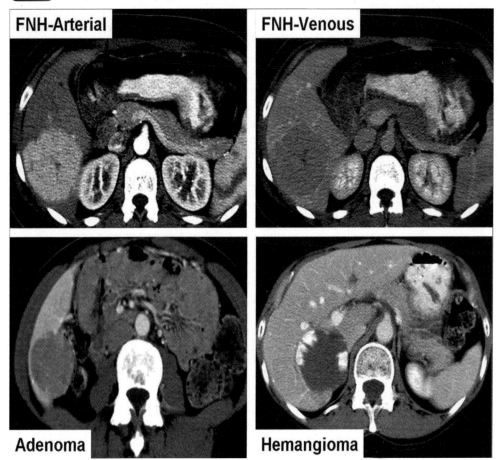

Focal nodular hyperplasia (FNH) is hypervascular on arterial phase, isodense to liver on venous phase, and has a central scar (upper panels). Adenoma is hypodense on venous phase (lower left panel). Hemangioma shows asymmetrical peripheral enhancement (lower right panel).

(1) In the pre-antibiotic era, the most common cause of pyogenic liver abscess was appendicitis.

(2) Now, the more common causes are related to malignancy or stone disease.

b. The potential routes of hepatic exposure to bacteria are the biliary tree, portal vein, hepatic artery, direct extension from nearby foci of infection (gallbladder, kidney), and trauma.

c. Common intra-abdominal sources of pyogenic abscesses include appendicitis, diverticulitis, cholecystitis, infected pancreatitis/pancreatic abscess, and perinephric abscess.

d. Pyogenic abscesses with no identifiable primary infection are called cryptogenic hepatic abscesses.

e. Signs and symptoms may include fever (90%), malaise, rigors, and RUQ pain. Chills and weight loss may be seen in 50% of patients. Symptom duration is typically less than 2 weeks. Jaundice is uncommon, unless biliary tract obstruction is also present. At the time of presentation, 50% of patients have positive blood cultures.

f. Diagnosis is made most commonly with CT scan (93% accurate).

g. Organisms cultured include gram-negative aerobes, which are found 68% of the time. *Escherichia coli* and *Klebsiella* species are most commonly isolated. Aerobic *Streptococcus* and *Staphylococcus* are seen in 20% and 12% of pyogenic abscesses, respectively. Increased use of indwelling biliary stents and broad-spectrum antibiotics has led to an increased prevalence of *Pseudomonas,* anaerobic *Streptococcus,* and fungi.

   h. Management

     (1) Percutaneous abscess aspiration and drainage and selective antibiotics.

     (2) Treatment of the primary intra-abdominal source of infection is mandatory (e.g., surgical management of appendicitis, diverticulitis). Surgical co-drainage of hepatic abscess during laparotomy is still required in up to one-third of patients.

   i. Changing trends involve increased incidence, decreased mortality, better identification (CT), etiology (more likely caused by biliary tract manipulation, such as stents, or malignant biliary obstruction), and better treatment (percutaneous drainage, selective antibiotics).

2. Amebic liver abscess

   a. Amebic liver abscess is the most frequent complication of invasive amebiasis.

   b. *Entamoeba histolytica* is the causative agent of dysentery, colitis, and amebic liver abscess. Infection is endemic in the tropics and in poor communities with inadequate sanitation. The greatest risk is from healthy carriers, who may eliminate up to 1.5×10^9 cysts daily in stools.

   c. Positive serology to *E. histolytica* is indicative of tissue invasion. Higher antibody titers are seen in initial stages of disease, but elevated levels are seen up to 3 years after infection occurred.

   d. Parasitic trophozoites penetrate the bowel and progress to the liver via the portal vein. Solitary space-occupying echogenic lesion or abscess is seen most commonly in the right lobe of the liver.

   e. Liver parenchyma is replaced by necrotic yellowish material with a ring of congested liver tissue, often 5 to 15 cm in size.

   f. Treatment is oral metronidazole up to 1 g PO bid for 10 days in adults. Drainage of abscess is not part of initial therapy but may be needed if a rapid response does not occur (antibiotic therapy fails).

   g. Complications include extension of the amebic abscess to the peritoneum, pericardium, diaphragm, abdominal organs, great vessels (IVC, aorta), and rupture into pleural space with amebic empyema.

3. Hydatid cysts

   a. Hydatid cysts are caused by echinococcal tapeworms. Tapeworms are commonly found in sheep-herding dogs and transferred to humans in contact with the dogs. This infection has a worldwide distribution, but species (*Echinococcus vogeli*) that cause human polycystic hydatid disease are limited to Central and South America.

   b. The cysts are often asymptomatic, fluid-filled structures in the liver, which are associated with daughter cysts. This infection is the most common cystic lesion of the liver outside the United States. Cyst wall calcification is seen on a CT scan along with compression and fibrous reaction of adjacent liver tissue.

   c. The most common presenting symptom is RUQ pain and palpable hepatomegaly. Eosinophilia and positive serology with indirect hemagglutination or enzyme-linked immunosorbent assay is positive in 90% of cases. Casoni skin test is 85% sensitive. Parasitic eggs are not seen in human stool.

   d. Management

     (1) The cysts should not be aspirated to avoid spillage of the organisms and development of new cysts.

     (2) Antihelminthic therapy with mebendazole, praziquantel, or albendazole is given three times daily for up to 16 weeks. Toxicity results in alopecia, leucopenia, and elevated transaminases.

     (3) Surgical therapy includes isolation of the cyst from the rest of abdomen with packs, careful cyst fluid aspiration, and instillation of hypertonic saline to kill the parasitic scolices. This is followed by simple excision of the cyst from the liver.

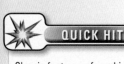

QUICK HIT

Classic features of amebic liver abscess are residence or travel in endemic areas, symptoms of 2-week duration, RUQ pain, abrupt onset of fever (38° to 40° C), tender hepatomegaly, solitary hypoechoic or mixed echogenic liver lesion, leukocytosis with greater than 15,000/μL, and positive serology.

B. Benign tumors and cysts
1. General principles: Solid tumors of the liver can be incidentally found on imaging of asymptomatic patients or for symptoms of abdominal pain. A single imaging study is often nondiagnostic, leading to other studies and even biopsy to confirm the diagnosis. However, biopsy of vascular liver lesions may have serious consequences.
2. Hemangioma
   a. Hemangioma is the most common benign mesenchymal tumor. These tumors vary in size from 1 to 20 cm, and if they are greater than 4 cm, they are called giant hemangiomas. Sixty percent to 80% of these are found in women in the third to fifth decade of life. If greater than 10 cm, 90% present with symptoms of liver capsule distension and pain.
   b. On triple-phase CT scan, hemangiomas are not hypervascular on arterial phase and show asymmetric, centripetal filling on portal venous phase.
   c. MRI is the most accurate noninvasive test, with sensitivity greater than 90%. Hemangiomas have a low T1 signal and a high T2 signal. Technetium pertechnetate liver scans are also useful in identifying hemangiomas. Percutaneous biopsy is potentially dangerous, inaccurate, and not recommended.
   d. Hemangiomas do not require treatment and may be left alone. Spontaneous rupture of even giant hemangiomas is very rare, even in pregnancy. Surgical enucleation of the hemangioma is preferred to surgical resection, yielding less blood loss and fewer transfusion requirements.
3. Hepatic adenoma
   a. Hepatic adenomas are uncommon solid lesions seen in women of childbearing age, usually with antecedent use of more than 5 years of high-dose estrogen oral contraceptives. Ninety-three percent of adenomas occur in this segment of the population.
   b. Grossly, adenomas are soft fleshy tumors with smooth surfaces, and microscopically, they consist of monotonous sheets of hepatocytes containing glycogen. Because portal triads are absent, Kupffer cells are usually absent in hepatic adenomas, and thus, these tumors will be found to be "cold" spots on nuclear liver scan with 99-Tc sulfur colloid, an agent that selectively demonstrates Kupffer cell distribution in the liver.
   c. On triple-phase CT scan, hepatic adenomas are hypervascular tumors on arterial phase that become isodense or even hypodense to the background liver on portal venous phase.
   d. Most patients (52%) present with right upper abdominal pain due to local compression, but they rarely hemorrhage into the tumor, or rupture leads to an acute presentation with hypotension and shock from bleeding.
   e. Management
      (1) Spontaneous regression is observed in smaller adenomas with withdrawal of oral contraceptives. Asymptomatic smaller adenomas may also be observed.
      (2) Increasing alpha-fetoprotein (AFP), an enlarging mass, or one with irregular borders should prompt surgical resection because malignant transformation is associated with these characteristics in hepatic adenomas. Furthermore, size greater than 4 cm is associated with increased rates of malignant degeneration as well as spontaneous rupture and should be used as a criterion for surgical resection in and of itself.
      (3) If a larger hepatic adenoma is not resected, pregnancy should be avoided due to an increased risk of tumor growth, hemorrhage, or rupture during pregnancy.
4. FNH
   a. FNH is the second most common benign solid tumor of the liver. Seen in all ages and both sexes, it is slightly more common in women from age 20 to 50 years. The incidence of FNH is not increased with prolonged oral contraceptive use; however, it tends to be seen slightly more frequently in women who take oral contraceptives.

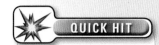

QUICK HIT

Kasabach–Merritt syndrome is consumptive coagulopathy of platelets and red blood cells occurring inside a giant hemangioma.

Hepatobiliary System

Hepatobiliary System

b. FNHs are non-neoplastic solid tumors characterized by a central fibrous scar with radiating septa, often lobulated, and sharply demarcated from adjacent liver, without a capsule. The central scar often contains a large artery that branches out in a spoke-wheel pattern. These tumors arise as a hyperplastic, hepatocellular response to either hyperperfusion or vascular injury from the anomalous central artery in the lesion, which is not accompanied by a portal vein or bile duct branch. Their average size is 5 cm, and they rarely exceed 10 cm.

c. Regenerative nodules resembling FNH tumors may be seen in chronic advanced liver disease. These nodules have the hallmark of vascular inflow reduction, liver cell atrophy centrally in the nodule, and regeneration around the intrahepatic portal triads.

d. Patients with FNH are usually asymptomatic, but those who do present with pain are more commonly women who take oral contraceptives.

e. Physical examination and liver function tests are normal. Liver nuclear scan with 99-Tc sulfur colloid shows FNH tumors to be "hot," with increased presence of Kupffer cells. Both CT and MRI may accurately demonstrate the classic central scar in a solid liver tumor as the characteristic finding of an FNH tumor. Another hallmark of FNH on cross-sectional imaging studies (CT or MRI) is a hypertrophied feeding artery supplying the tumor.

f. Management
Because rupture and malignant transformation are not seen with FNH tumors, they may be left alone. Rarely, the enlarging FNH tumor or a patient with severe pain from liver capsule distension should be taken for surgical resection.

5. Cystic diseases of the liver
a. Specific types
(1) Simple hepatic (nonparasitic) cysts may be observed unless they become symptomatic, in which case, laparoscopic cyst unroofing (fenestration) may be indicated. Sclerotherapy using 95% EtOH is another therapeutic option for large symptomatic cysts, but both methods are equally effective. Simple attempts at aspiration may provide temporary symptomatic relief; however, the cyst reaccumulates fluid and symptoms may recur.

(2) Adult polycystic disease: Surgical approaches to treatment include sclerotherapy, laparoscopic cyst unroofing, hepatic resection, or LT. The goal of treatment is to decompress and reduce the size of the entire liver or remove as many cysts as possible.

(3) Biliary cystadenoma: Radiographically, these appear as a complex cystic lesion with internal septations. It may serve as a precursor to cystadenocarcinoma. Treatment includes complete surgical resection.

(4) Caroli disease is characterized by congenital segmental cystic dilatation of the intrahepatic biliary radicals without other hepatic abnormalities.
(a) This disease is usually accompanied by autosomal recessive polycystic kidney disease.
(b) There is increased incidence of biliary lithiasis, cholangitis, and biliary abscess formation.
(c) Antibiotic therapy is indicated for episodes of cholangitis. LT may be necessary, but only if there is no evidence of persistence of cholangitis infections.

(5) Caroli syndrome is a combination of Caroli disease and cholangitic congenital hepatic fibrosis.

(6) Choledochal cyst is a dilation of the common bile duct (CBD) or biliary tree. Possible causes include anomalous pancreaticobiliary ductal system, allowing for the reflux of pancreatic enzymes into the developing biliary tract. There are five types of choledochal cysts (Fig. 8-6).

b. Management
(1) Radical complete excision of all cystic parts of the biliary tract with hepaticojejunostomy is essential. Anastomosis of any part of the cystic biliary tree leads to complications of cholangitis and stricturing.

(2) Carcinoma is a risk of untreated or incompletely excised choledochal cysts.

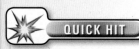

QUICK HIT

Portal hypertension is defined as free portal vein pressure above the normal of 5–10 mm Hg. However, direct portal pressure measurement is difficult. Hepatic vein catheterization with measurement of wedged and free pressures is the simplest and safest indirect means of estimating portal pressure. Complications develop with pressures greater than 12 mm Hg.

FIGURE 8-6 Classification of choledochal cyst.

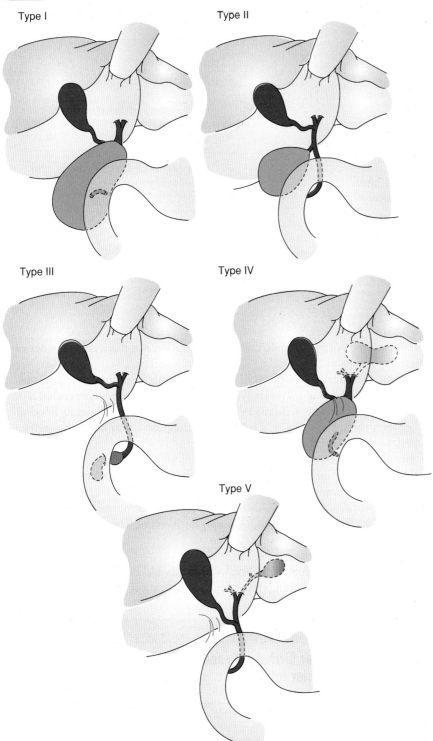

Type I

Type II

Type III

Type IV

Type V

(With permission from Mulholland MW, Lillemoe KD, Doherty GM, Maier RV, Upchurch GR, eds. *Greenfield's Surgery: Scientific Principles and Practice.* 4th ed. Philadelphia, PA: Lippincott Williams & Wilkins; 2006.)

C. Portal hypertension

1. Portal hypertension is the most common and lethal complication of chronic liver disease (i.e., cirrhosis). It is the result of increases in both the vascular resistance to portal flow and the blood flow entering the portal system (see Clinical Pearl 8-1).

2. Cirrhosis is classified based on the site of increased resistance to hepatic vascular inflow (see Clinical Pearl 8-2).

CLINICAL PEARL 8-1

Clinical History and Physical Examination Findings Associated with Cirrhosis

History
- Life-limiting fatigue or weight loss
- Jaundice (icterus; skin, urine, and stool color)
- Anorexia and cachexia
- Abdominal pain
- Peripheral edema
- Ascites
- GI bleeding, hemorrhoids
- Loss of libido
- Loss of menstrual cycle
- Hepatic encephalopathy

Physical examination
- Malnutrition
- Fetor hepaticus
- Jaundiced skin, icteric sclera
- Spider angiomata
- Finger clubbing, white nail beds palmar erythema
- Dupuytren contracture
- Gynecomastia, testicular atrophy
- Hyperdynamic cardiovascular status
- Parotid enlargement
- Ascites, pleural effusion
- Abdominal hernia
- Caput medusa
- Abnormal liver size
- Splenomegaly
- Temporal muscle wasting
- Asterixis

---

3. Complications: Portal-systemic collateral formation is a main consequence of portal hypertension.
   a. The most clinically significant of these collaterals is gastroesophageal varices. Risk of bleeding increases with variceal size but can be prevented if the portal pressure is reduced below 12 mm Hg. These collaterals develop between the coronary vein; a tributary to the portal; and the short gastric, periesophageal, and azygos veins.
   b. Anorectal varices, or hemorrhoids, are seen when collaterals develop between the superior hemorrhoidal vein of the portal system and the middle and inferior hemorrhoidal veins of the caval system.
   c. The umbilical vein may dilate and allow portal decompression to the abdominal wall, draining through the epigastric veins. The characteristic finding is caput medusae.
4. Management
   a. Acute hemorrhage from esophageal varices should be managed with fluid and/or blood resuscitation, endoscopic identification followed by sclero-

---

CLINICAL PEARL 8-2

Diagnostic Considerations for Cirrhosis Based on the Site of Increased Resistance to Hepatic Vascular Inflow

Presinusoidal
- Sinistral/extrahepatic
- Splenic vein thrombosis
- Splenomegaly
- Splenic arteriovenous fistula
- Intrahepatic
- Schistosomiasis
- Congenital hepatic fibrosis
- Nodular regenerative hyperplasia
- Idiopathic portal fibrosis
- Myeloproliferative disorder
- Sarcoid
- Graft-versus-host disease

Sinusoidal
- Intrahepatic
- Cirrhosis
- Viral infection
- Alcohol abuse
- Primary biliary cirrhosis
- Autoimmune hepatitis
- Primary sclerosing cholangitis
- Metabolic abnormality

Postsinusoidal
- Intrahepatic
- Vascular occlusive disease
- Posthepatic
- Budd-Chiari syndrome
- Congestive heart failure
- Inferior vena caval web
- Constrictive pericarditis

therapy or balloon tamponade, and pharmacotherapy. Pharmacotherapy is directed at reducing portal pressure with vasoconstrictors or reducing intrahepatic vascular resistance with vasodilators.

(1) Vasopressin causes splanchnic vasoconstriction, reducing portal pressure. Toxic effects include reduction of cardiac output.

(2) Octreotide is the synthetic analogue of somatostatin. It selectively reduces splanchnic blood flow without producing the systemic cardiac effects of vasopressin.

(3) Propranolol is a nonselective beta-blocker that reduces the portal pressure. It limits portal venous inflow by dual effect of reducing cardiac output and splanchnic vasoconstriction. It is used for the prevention of the first variceal hemorrhage.

b. Emergency endoscopic therapy
(1) Injection sclerotherapy
(2) Endoscopic banding ligation
(3) Variceal obturation

c. Balloon tamponade
(1) The Sengstaken–Blakemore tube is a large, triple-lumen tube with esophageal and gastric balloon and is used to provide temporary mechanical occlusion against the bleeding varix.
(2) This tube has no role in long-term control of bleeding but is used when endoscopic or pharmacotherapy is unable to control bleeding. It should not be used for more than 24 hours because of risks such as esophageal rupture, gastric necrosis, and aspiration pneumonia.

d. Transjugular intrahepatic portosystemic shunt (TIPS)
(1) TIPS can provide definitive control of bleeding varices by reducing portal pressures at the intrahepatic level.
(2) Interventional radiology access of the right hepatic vein is via the jugular approach, with deployment of an expansile metal stent across liver parenchyma from a hepatic vein branch to a portal vein branch.

e. Surgical shunts
(1) All surgical shunts—total, partial, or selective—are designed to control variceal bleeding in up to 90% of patients. However, these shunts are not effective in cases of extensive portal vein thrombosis.
(2) Existing liver failure and reduction/loss of portal inflow in shunt procedures determines the consequences of encephalopathy and fulminant hepatic failure.
(3) Total portal systemic shunts decompress all sites of portal hypertension.
   (a) End-to-side portocaval shunt
   (b) Side-to-side portocaval shunt
(4) Partial portal systemic shunts are designed to reduce portal hypertension to less than 12 mm Hg.
(5) Selective shunts are designed to decompress esophageal varices but not treat the underlying portal hypertension.
   (a) The distal splenorenal shunt (DSRS) or Warren shunt is the most commonly used surgical shunt worldwide over the past 15 years.
   (b) It is used by surgeons to treat the episode of variceal bleeding and also to preserve central venous anatomy of the liver in hopes of a potential liver transplant.

f. Devascularization procedures
(1) Sugiura procedure involves splenectomy, gastric and esophageal devascularization, and, occasionally, esophageal in-line transection/anastomosis.
(2) It may control variceal bleeding in patients who are not candidates for surgical shunts.
(3) Current management algorithm of bleeding esophageal varices from portal hypertension include:
   (a) Beta blockade
   (b) Endoscopic sclerotherapy and pharmacotherapy

      (c) Temporary balloon tamponade

      (d) TIPS

      (e) DSRS or Sugiura procedure, if still bleeding despite (b) and (c), and TIPS is not available

      (f) Also, consider 8-mm partial portocaval H-shunt as a bridge to liver transplant.

      (g) Liver transplant

g. LT

  (1) Liver transplants are one therapy that significantly improves survival in Child's Class C patients with bleeding varices.

  (2) It removes the cirrhotic liver, replacing it with a normal, low-resistance liver, and is the ultimate shunt treatment for portal hypertension.

  (3) The initial 6-month mortality is 10% to 15%, with a long-term risk of major morbidity or mortality of 2% to 5% per year.

  (4) Major complications include rejection, recurrent viral hepatitis in the transplanted liver leading to liver failure, immunosuppression-related infections, and malignancies.

h. Long-term management

  (1) Patients surviving an episode of variceal hemorrhage are at high risk of rebleeding in the following 6 months, with a progressive rise in episodic mortality.

  (2) Long-term management of portal hypertension in such patients includes:

    (a) Selective devascularization surgical procedures

    (b) Surgical shunts

    (c) Liver transplant, which has significantly improved the survival of Child's Class C patients with history of variceal bleeding

IV. Malignant Disorders

A. Hepatocellular carcinoma (HCC)

1. HCC is one of the most common malignancies worldwide and is the number one cause of cancer mortality worldwide. Among the few cancers that can be clearly traced to an antecedent etiology, HCC is almost always linked to the background state of chronic liver disease (i.e., cirrhosis); however, 10% to 15% of HCC cases develop in the setting of a noncirrhotic background liver.

2. Etiology

a. Any process that causes chronic liver damage or cirrhosis may eventually result in HCC, but the most notable conditions are chronic viral hepatitis, alcoholism, nonalcoholic fatty liver disease (NAFLD), hemochromatosis, intrinsic liver diseases, and parasitic diseases.

b. In the Far East and Africa, HCC is more commonly associated with chronic hepatitis B virus (HBV) and appears in the third or fourth decade of life. In the West, HCC is more often associated with hepatitis C virus (HCV) and appears later in life. Worldwide, chronic HBV is the most common etiologic cause of HCC.

c. Chronic HBV infection leads to repeated liver injury through episodes of inflammation, regeneration, and fibrosis. Although HCV alone can lead to HCC, synergistic risk is created when alcoholism, HBV coinfection, and porphyria cutanea tarda are also present. The mechanism underlying the development of HCC from chronic HCV infection is not as clearly understood as is that from chronic HBV disease.

d. Other etiologic factors include smoking, exposure to thorium dioxide (Thorotrast), aflatoxin, estrogens, and androgens. Aflatoxin is a fungal mycotoxin released by *Aspergillus* species that typically contaminates damp, warm foods such as corn and peanuts.

e. Premalignant lesions that lead to HCC include dysplastic nodules that are seen in the regenerative phase of cirrhosis as well as hepatic adenomas.

3. Presentation includes weight loss, abdominal swelling, and RUQ abdominal pain. In a patient known to have stable cirrhosis, sudden hepatic decompensa-

tion may be an indicator of HCC development. HCC may also present with paraneoplastic syndromes caused by ectopic hormonal production (sexual changes, hypercalcemia, carcinoid-like syndrome), metabolic changes (hypoglycemia, hypercholesterolemia, acute porphyria), skin changes (vitiligo, pityriasis, thrombophlebitis migrans), as well as fever, leukocytosis, and cachexia.

4. Diagnosis

   a. Imaging (ultrasound, CT [arterial phase of CT shows HCC lesion to be hypervascular while the portal venous phase demonstrates washout of the lesion compared to the background liver], and MRI) is used for diagnosis. Because of the abnormal appearance of the cirrhotic liver on imaging, diagnostic tissue biopsy confirming HCC may sometimes be required.

   b. Serum AFP level can be a useful tumor marker for HCC; however, it is elevated in only 50% of patients with HCC. It may also be elevated in benign conditions such as chronic active hepatitis, cirrhosis, and pregnancy. An AFP level greater than 400 ng/mL, however, is considered diagnostic for HCC.

5. Management

   One of the keys to treatment of HCC is prevention, because the reduction or improvement of chronic liver damage by treatment of the underlying etiology reduces the risk of HCC development. For example, HBV infection can be prevented by vaccination. Screening in the Far East has been successful in identifying HCC earlier by screening patients with cirrhosis, a family history of HCC, chronic active hepatitis with elevated viral loads, or increasing AFP. For HCV infection, treatment options and guidelines for their initiation exist (*Am J Gastroenterol. 2012 May;107(5):669–689*).

   a. Treatment options for HCC include the following: LT, surgical resection, ablative techniques, regional liver-directed therapies, or systemic treatments. The specific type of treatment chosen is influenced in a large part by the stage of the disease as well as the health of the background liver.

   b. LT is the optimal curative treatment for HCC because it removes the cancer as well as the underlying background liver. Candidacy for LT in patients with HCC is defined by the Milan criteria shown in Table 8-2. LT for HCC outside of Milan criteria typically requires approval through a regional review board.

   c. Surgical resection is the next best curative treatment option for HCC but is often not possible due to excessive postoperative morbidity and mortality associated with liver insufficiency/failure in patients with cirrhotic background livers.

   d. Unfortunately, 75% of patients with HCC are not candidates for either LT or surgical resection at the time of their diagnosis. Untreated, unresectable HCC carries with it a grim prognosis (median survival of 6 to 12 months). Therefore, local ablative therapy (most commonly radiofrequency ablation or microwave ablation) can provide acceptable local control under certain circumstances. The utility of this method is limited in large tumors (>5 cm) or in those that are centrally located and near important hilar structures (particularly the main or segmental right and left bile ducts). Ablation can also be used as a "bridge to transplantation" to avoid having patients drop off of the LT waiting list due to progression of the disease.

TABLE **8-2** **Milan Criteria**
One lesion smaller than 5 cm
Up to three lesions smaller than 3 cm
No extrahepatic spread
No vascular invasion

e. Regional liver-directed therapy for HCC includes transhepatic arterial chemoembolization (TACE) or selective internal radiotherapy (SIR) spheres. These techniques take advantage of the unique dual blood supply to the liver (hepatic arterial and portal venous) as well as the fact that HCCs derive their blood supply predominantly from the arterial circulation while the background liver derives its predominantly from the portal venous system. In TACE, chemotherapy (given in higher doses than that which can be delivered systemically) is injected into the hepatic arterial system in combination with embolization of the feeding vessel(s) to the tumor(s). In SIR spheres, 32 micron in diameter, Yytrium-90 containing beads are injected into the hepatic arterial circulation and eventually get lodged in the capillary network supplying the tumor(s), where they emit local radiation. Response rates to each approach are roughly 50% to 60% and can extend patients' life expectancy by years. Candidates for these approaches must have enough hepatic reserve to tolerate the associated toxicity. These treatments can also be used as a "bridge to transplantation."

f. Systemic treatment for HCC is limited with only one FDA-approved drug (sorafenib, an anti-vascular endothelial growth factor [anti-VEGF] antibody that inhibits angiogenesis). Median survival for patients with unresectable HCC was significantly improved in sorafenib-treated patients compared to placebo (Study of Heart and Renal Protection [SHARP] trial); however, the benefit was minimal (3 months).

6. Unusual forms of HCC include the fibrolamellar variant of HCC. This variant is rarely associated with cirrhosis and presents in young adults (ages 20 to 30 years) in the Western population. There is no association with HBV or HCV infection. AFP levels are rarely elevated. Fibrolamellar HCC usually carries a better prognosis than regular HCC because the patients are younger and do not usually have liver dysfunction.

B. Metastatic cancer in the liver
  1. The liver is the most common site of metastatic disease for a variety of cancers.
    a. Isolated liver metastases are more commonly seen in association with colorectal cancer, neuroendocrine tumors of the GI tract, stromal tumors of the GI tract, and ocular melanomas.
    b. Hepatic metastases from colorectal cancer are often asymptomatic and rarely yield jaundice or liver function derangement at presentation.
  2. Colorectal cancer with liver metastases: management
    a. Sixty percent of patients diagnosed with colorectal cancer will at some point in their disease course develop liver metastases. In selected patients, surgical resection of colorectal liver metastases offers 5-year survival rates of up to 40%.
    b. Systemic multidrug chemotherapy regimens show promising ability to significantly reduce liver tumor volume and/or prevent the development of extrahepatic disease. Chemotherapy alone, however, is not a cure, and therefore, surgical resection should be offered to all patients who are candidates. Unfortunately, only 25% of patients with liver metastases from colorectal cancer are operative candidates. Evaluation by a trained liver surgeon at the time of the diagnosis of the liver metastases to determine their resectability is critical.
    c. Management of hepatic metastases from neuroendocrine tumors, ocular melanomas, and specific GI tract stromal tumors is individualized and based on the patient's clinical course, extent of disease, and symptoms.
    d. Local tumor ablation with cryoablation or radiofrequency ablation achieves local destruction of active cancer tissue and is useful in palliative disease control but does not improve overall survival.
    e. Aggressive surgical or ablative management of liver metastases from gastric, pancreatic, or small intestine adenocarcinomas; soft-tissue sarcomas; and skin melanomas has no oncologic benefit. Patients should be managed with palliative systemic chemotherapy.

BILIARY SYSTEM

I. General Principles

A. Anatomy

  1. Hepatic ducts

    a. The left hepatic duct is formed from the union of the three segmental ducts draining segments 2, 3, and 4.

    b. The right hepatic duct is formed from the union of segmental ducts draining 5, 6, 7, and 8.

    c. Segment 1, the caudate lobe, drains most commonly into both the right and left hepatic ducts.

    d. Both the right and left hepatic ducts join to form the common hepatic duct.

  2. Gallbladder

    a. The gallbladder is a pear-shaped, distensible reservoir structure with an average capacity of 30 to 50 mL.

    b. The inferior and lateral surface is covered by peritoneum, and the superior surface is associated with the hepatic fossa.

    c. This organ has four anatomic portions: the fundus, body, infundibulum, and neck.

    d. It is supplied by the cystic artery, which is most commonly a branch of the RHA.

  3. Cystic duct

    a. This arises from the gallbladder and drains into the common hepatic duct to form the common bile duct (CBD).

    b. Its average length is 2 to 4 cm.

  4. CBD

    a. The CBD is formed by the union of the cystic duct and the common hepatic duct.

    b. It is approximately 8 cm in length, with an average diameter of 4 to 9 mm in adults and 3 to 5 mm in children. After cholecystectomy, it may dilate an additional 2 to 3 mm in size.

    c. It most commonly joins the pancreatic duct to open into the second portion of the duodenum at the ampulla of Vater. The opening is regulated by the sphincter of Oddi.

  5. Triangle of Calot: This region is bordered by the common hepatic duct medially, the cystic duct laterally, and the liver edge superiorly.

  6. Sphincter of Oddi

    a. Located at the ampulla of Vater

    b. Length of 4 to 6 mm

    c. The basal resting pressure is 13 mm Hg.

    d. Regulates the flow of bile and pancreatic juice

    e. Relaxation occurs with cholecystokinin and vagal stimulation. Sympathetic stimulation causes increased pressure and sphincter constriction.

  7. Anatomic variants of biliary anatomy (Fig. 8-7)

B. Physiology

  1. The gallbladder absorbs water and solute from bile, thereby concentrating the solute components.

  2. It acts as a storage organ for bile.

  3. In addition, it secretes mucus and glycoproteins.

  4. Gallbladder contractility is controlled by enteric hormones and autonomic nervous system. Primarily, these stimulants are cholecystokinin and vagal firing.

II. Gallstone Disease

A. Types

Gallstones are classified according to their cholesterol content as either pigment or cholesterol stones. Most of the gallstones are mixed, containing calcium salts in their center.

  1. Pure cholesterol stones constitute only 10% of all gallstones. However, 70% to 80% of the gallstones are considered to be cholesterol stones.

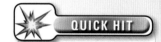

A dilation of the CBD greater than 10 mm in adults who have not had a cholecystectomy is considered abnormal.

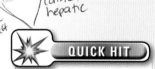

The cystic artery crosses the triangle of Calot. Identification of the triangle, and visualization of any structures within, is very important during a cholecystectomy to avoid injury to the RHA.

FIGURE
8-7 Variations in the origin and course of the cystic artery.

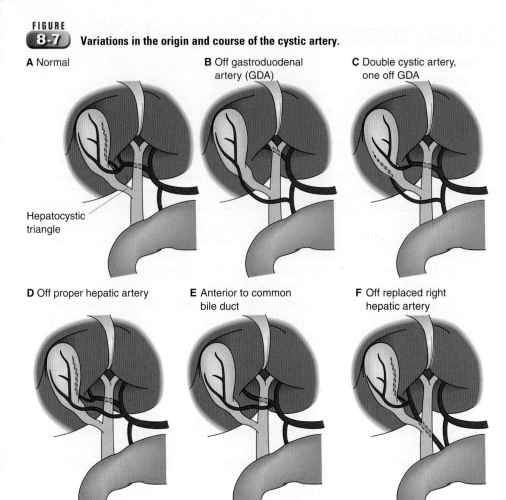

A Normal
B Off gastroduodenal
artery (GDA)
C Double cystic artery,
one off GDA

Hepatocystic
triangle

D Off proper hepatic artery
E Anterior to common
bile duct
F Off replaced right
hepatic artery

(With permission from Mulholland MW, Lillemoe KD, Doherty GM, Maier RV, Upchurch GR, eds. *Greenfield's Surgery: Scientific Principles and Practice.* 4th ed. Philadelphia, PA: Lippincott Williams & Wilkins; 2006.)

2. Approximately 20% to 30% gallstones are pigment stones. There are two types of pigment gallstones:
   a. Black stones consist of calcium bilirubinate and calcium palmitate. They are frequently small and multiple and tend to occur almost exclusively in the gallbladder. Risk factors for black stones are hemolytic anemia and cirrhosis.
   b. Brown stones are more common in the Asian population, in the setting of biliary dysmotility and chronic bacterial and parasitic infections. These may also occur as primary common bile duct stones.
B. Pathogenesis: A combination of the following factors favor the development of the stones:
   1. Cholesterol supersaturation in the bile
   2. Crystal nucleation due to aggregation and precipitation of the cholesterol-rich vesicles
   3. Gallbladder dysmotility
   4. Gallbladder absorptive dysfunction
   5. Percentages of saturation of three elements in bile lead to precipitation and cholesterol stone formation. These three elements are lecithin, cholesterol, and bile salt. Normally, a delicate balance exists between the levels of bile acids, phospholipids, and cholesterol (see Admirand triangle). When this balance is disrupted, especially when there is supersaturation with cholesterol, there is predisposition for the formation of lithogenic bile and the consequent develop-

ment of cholesterol-type gallstones. This is because when cholesterol supersaturates, it tends to crystallize, and in the presence of enucleating factors, it can be a nidus for stone formation. The small, purple-shaded area is the only area where cholesterol remains entirely soluble.

C. Clinical presentation

1. Asymptomatic
   a. The vast majority of patients with gallstones are asymptomatic.
   b. Twenty percent of these patients become symptomatic in 20 years.
   c. Of this group of patients, 1% to 2% develop serious symptoms or complications related to their gallstones.

2. Symptomatic
   a. Biliary colic
      (1) This condition is due to intermittent obstruction of the cystic duct with passage of small stones.
      (2) There is intermittent, spasmodic RUQ pain that occurs most commonly after a fatty meal and may last for a few hours. It is associated with nausea, vomiting, and bloating.
   b. Acute cholecystitis
      (1) This condition is due to occlusion of the cystic duct, and this incites an inflammatory response. Bile may become infected with gram-negative bacteria, most commonly *E. coli*.
      (2) Patients present with RUQ pain, which is usually longer lasting, and they may have constitutional signs of fever and tachycardia. Abdominal examination usually reveals RUQ tenderness.
      (3) Laboratory findings include an elevated white blood cell count and mild hyperbilirubinemia.

D. Diagnosis

1. RUQ ultrasound is the most useful diagnostic test. Ultrasound has 85% specificity and 95% sensitivity in diagnosing acute cholecystitis. Findings suggestive of acute cholecystitis are:
   a. Presence of gallstones
   b. Thickening of the gallbladder wall greater than 4 mm
   c. Pericholecystic fluid

2. Radionucleotide scanning or a HIDA scan may also be helpful.
   a. The radionucleotide is administered intravenously, and the patient is scanned in 30 minutes.
   b. Nonfilling of the gallbladder with the radiotracer but filling of the CBD and the duodenum indicates an obstructed cystic duct and acute cholecystitis.
   c. Highly sensitive and specific, about 95% for each, for acute cholecystitis

E. Management of symptomatic gallstones

Medical management of severe acute cholecystitis includes hospital admission, no oral intake, intravenous (IV) fluids, and use of broad-spectrum antibiotics.

1. Surgical management
   a. Early cholecystectomy, within 3 days of presentation, is advocated by some authors and may be accomplished before onset of second phase of acute inflammatory response. Initial phase often includes pericholecystic fluid or tissue edema, which makes surgical removal easier.
   b. Relative indications for prophylactic cholecystectomy are:
      (1) Pediatric gallstone disease
      (2) Congenital hemolytic anemias (e.g., sickle-cell disease)
      (3) Gallstones greater than 2.5 cm, which increases the incidence of cancer of gallbladder and acute cholecystitis
      (4) Porcelain gallbladder, which increases the incidence of gallbladder cancer
      (5) Bariatric surgery
      (6) Note: Asymptomatic gallstone disease in diabetics is no longer considered an indication for prophylactic cholecystectomy.

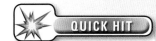

QUICK HIT

Murphy sign, or inspiratory arrest during deep palpation of the RUQ, is the classical finding in acute cholecystitis.

Hepatobiliary System

    c. If patients present with symptoms of more than 3 days duration, it may be prudent to treat the gallbladder disease conservatively (medical management as described earlier) and perform cholecystectomy electively in 4 to 6 weeks.

    d. In certain high-risk patients, or in severely ill patients in the intensive care unit whose conditions do not permit cholecystectomy, percutaneous cholecystostomy may be performed to relieve obstruction and decompress the gallbladder.

    e. Cholecystectomy could be performed either with the laparoscope or in an open fashion. Laparoscopic cholecystectomy has the advantage of short hospital stay and less morbidity associated due to smaller wounds.

F. Complications

    a. Empyema of the gallbladder

    b. Emphysematous cholecystitis: This is more commonly seen in patients with diabetes mellitus. Patients present with RUQ pain and sepsis. Abdominal films or CT scan may show air in the gallbladder wall or lumen. Infection is generally due to *Escherichia coli, Enterococcus, Klebsiella,* or *Clostridia* species.

    c. Gangrene and perforation: The gallbladder may perforate into adjacent viscera such as the duodenum and hepatic flexure of the colon (two most common sites).

    d. Small bowel obstruction: Chronic erosion of the gallbladder wall by a 2-cm or larger gallstone can also form the cholecystenteric fistula. This is seen in up to 2% of patients with acute cholecystitis. Following fistula formation, the large stone may tumble through the GI tract until it reaches the ileum, with the narrowest luminal size. Here, the stone may cause small bowel obstruction, which is termed gallstone ileus. This occurs in up to 15% of patients with cholecystenteric fistulas. The obstruction is described as episodic and recurrent because the impacted stone temporarily impacts in the gut lumen and then dislodges and moves forward. This is known as tumbling obstruction. Abdominal imaging may show evidence of small bowel obstruction and presence of pneumobilia. Surgical management focuses on relieving the acute bowel obstruction and includes proximal enterotomy with stone removal. Takedown and repair of the biliary enteric fistula and cholecystectomy are best deferred to a later date after the patient recovers from the acute obstruction.

G. Acute cholangitis

    1. Acute cholangitis is a bacterial infection of the biliary ductal system due to ductal obstruction and significant bacterial concentration in the bile. The most common causes of biliary obstruction are choledocholithiasis, benign strictures, and tumors.

    2. Patient may present with fever, RUQ pain, and jaundice (Charcot triad) and later with mental status changes and hypotension (Reynolds pentad). Initial management is resuscitative with IV antibiotics, fluids, and systemic support. Urgent clearance of the infected and obstructed biliary tract is paramount. Options for biliary decompression include endoscopic retrograde cholangiopancreatography (ERCP), percutaneous transhepatic cholangiogram (PTC), or surgical decompression. Once the patient is stabilized, surgical removal of the gallbladder (during the same hospitalization) is recommended to prevent recurrent obstructions and episodes of cholangitis.

H. Inflammatory lesions of biliary tract: PSC

    1. PSC is a chronic progressive cholestatic disease in which the inflammatory process involves the bile ducts, resulting in intrahepatic or extrahepatic strictures.

    2. This autoimmune disease is associated with other inflammatory bowel disease, with 85% of the patients having ulcerative colitis and 15% patients having Crohn disease. Males are more commonly affected than females, and PSC tends to present in the fourth decade of life. Prevalence is 10 per 100,000 population.

    3. Patients present with signs and symptoms of biliary obstruction, jaundice, pruritus, weight loss, and fatigue.

4. Diagnosis is based on liver biopsy, which may show presence of cholestasis and cirrhosis. ERCP or MRCP shows the characteristic beaded appearance of the ductal system from the areas of strictures and dilatation.

5. Management: The only definitive cure is liver transplant. Medical management with immunosuppressives and bile acids, such as ursodeoxycholic acid, has shown some temporary benefit.

6. Complications may be secondary to:
   a. Choledocholithiasis
   b. Postoperative biliary strictures
   c. Infections such as ascending cholangitis and parasitic infections
   d. Iatrogenic operative ischemia of the bile ducts
   e. Drugs, chemotherapy with intra-arterial 5-fluorouracil
   f. AIDS-associated cholangiopathy

I. Malignant biliary disease

1. Gallbladder cancer
   a. Incidence
      (1) Women are affected more than men, in part due to their higher incidence of gallstones. The overall incidence of cancer is 2.5 cases per a population of 100,000.
      (2) The disease is more common in Native Americans.
      (3) The highest incidence occurs in residents of Chile.
   b. Etiology
      (1) Risk factors include gallstones greater than 2.5 cm, porcelain gallbladder, choledochal cysts, PSC, and cholecystenteric fistula.
      (2) Approximately 1% of all elective cholecystectomies performed for cholelithiasis harbor an occult gallbladder cancer.
   c. Pathology
      (1) Ninety percent of the cancers of the gallbladder are adenocarcinoma.
      (2) At diagnosis, 25% of the cancers are localized to the gallbladder wall, 35% have associated metastases to the regional lymph nodes or extension into adjacent organs, and 40% have already metastasized to distant sites.
   d. Presentation
      (1) Most often, patients present with RUQ abdominal pain, often mimicking other common biliary and nonbiliary disease.
      (2) Other symptoms may include weight loss, jaundice, and abdominal mass.
   e. Diagnosis: Ultrasound or CT usually demonstrates a mass in the gallbladder. In addition, a CT scan shows the extension into the surrounding structures and the vascular anatomy.
   f. Management
      (1) Patients with a preoperatively suspected cancer of the gallbladder should undergo open cholecystectomy to minimize the chance of bile spillage and tumor dissemination.
      (2) If cancer of the gallbladder is diagnosed after a cholecystectomy, and on pathologic examination of the specimen the lesion is confined to the mucosa, submucosa, or the muscularis (T1), then cholecystectomy is adequate therapy. These patients have an 85% to 100% 5-year survival rate.
      (3) Cancer of the gallbladder with invasion beyond the muscularis is associated with an increasing incidence of regional lymph node metastases and needs an extended cholecystectomy with a 2-cm margin of the adjacent liver tissue with lymphadenectomy.
      (4) Palliative care
          (a) In patients with an unresectable tumor, the obstructive jaundice can be managed with biliary decompression through either percutaneous or endoscopically placed biliary stents.
          (b) Pain should be aggressively treated.

2. Cholangiocarcinoma
   a. This uncommon cancer is located commonly at the hepatic duct bifurcation.
   b. Incidence
      (1) Each year, 2,500 to 3,000 new cases are diagnosed.
      (2) The carcinoma occurs with equal frequency in men and women, and the incidence increases with age.
   c. Etiology
      (1) Risk factors include PSC, choledochal cysts, hepatolithiasis, and previous biliary enteric anastomosis. Other risk factors include parasitic disease, liver flukes, dietary nitrosamines, dioxin, and thorium dioxide (Thorotrast).
      (2) Common factors in all cases are bile stasis, infection, stones, and chronic inflammation.
   d. Classification consists of three broad groups:
      (1) Intrahepatic: 6%
      (2) Perihilar: 67%
      (3) Distal: 27%
   e. Clinical presentation: Ninety percent of patients present with jaundice, pruritus, fever, and abdominal pain. In addition, they may present with acute cholangitis.
   f. Diagnosis
      (1) CT is the initial diagnostic test of choice. This reveals dilated bile ducts, lymph nodes, and vascular anatomy.
      (2) A cholangiogram obtained through either the percutaneous transhepatic route or the endoscopic retrograde route further defines the biliary anatomy.
   g. Management
      (1) For the intrahepatic group, a partial hepatectomy is indicated.
      (2) For the perihilar group, a resection and hepaticojejunostomy is indicated.
      (3) For the distal group, a pancreaticoduodenectomy is indicated.

Pancreas and Spleen

Uzer Khan, Irfan A. Rizvi, and David W. McFadden

9

PANCREAS

I. Anatomy and Physiology (Fig. 9-1)

A. Two endodermal **outpouchings** (buds) of foregut origin fuse to form the pancreas.

1. A **dorsal bud** originating from the dorsum of the embryologic duodenum forms the bulk of the gland.

2. A **ventral bud** originating from the ventral embryologic duodenum forms the inferior part of the pancreatic head and uncinate process. The ventral bud rotates to the right and dorsally along with the bile duct to fuse with the dorsal bud.

B. The main pancreatic duct (**of Wirsung**) is formed by the duct of the distal part of the dorsal bud fusing with the duct of the ventral bud. It joins the common bile duct and opens in a globular cavity (**ampulla of Vater**) in the posteromedial wall of the second part of the duodenum. Sphincteric muscles surround this ampulla and the ends of the two ducts. The entire complex is called the sphincter of Oddi. The remaining proximal part of the dorsal bud duct forms the accessory pancreatic duct (**of Santorini**).

FIGURE 9-1 Relation of the pancreas to the duodenum and extrahepatic biliary system.

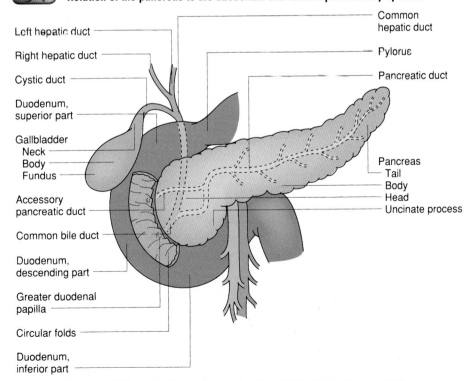

(Adapted from Woodburne RT. *Essentials of Human Anatomy*. New York, NY: Oxford University Press; 1973.)

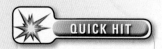

C. The ampulla drains into the duodenal lumen through a nipple-shaped orifice called the **major duodenal papilla.**
   1. The proximal part of the dorsal pancreatic duct (of Santorini) drains into the duodenum through a minor papilla that opens approximately 2 cm proximal to the major papilla.
   2. Successful cannulation of the major papilla allows an endoscopist to perform an endoscopic retrograde cholangiopancreatography (ERCP) (Fig. 9-2).
D. In **pancreas divisum**, the pancreatic duct systems fail to fuse, resulting in the accessory duct (of Santorini) draining the majority of pancreatic exocrine secretions through the minor papilla. Some experts believe that this predisposes to acute

Pancreas and Spleen

FIGURE 9-2 Anatomic configuration of the intrapancreatic ductal system. A lack of communication between the two ducts, which occurs in 10% of cases, is referred to as pancreas divisum.

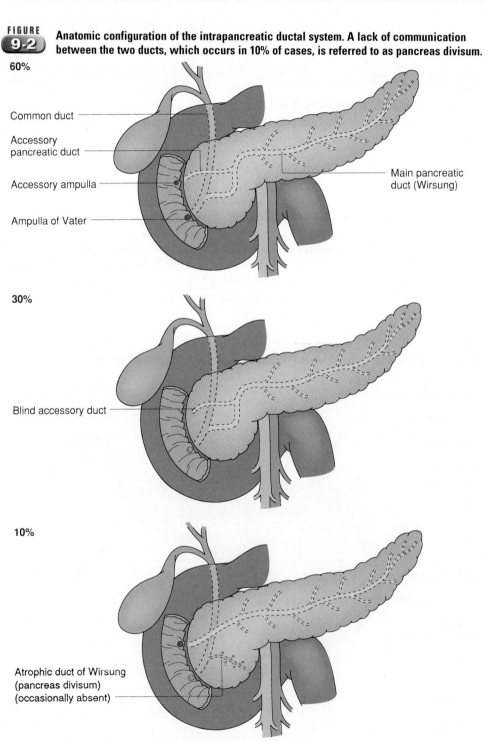

60%

Common duct

Accessory pancreatic duct

Accessory ampulla

Ampulla of Vater

Main pancreatic duct (Wirsung)

30%

Blind accessory duct

10%

Atrophic duct of Wirsung (pancreas divisum) (occasionally absent)

(Adapted from Silen W. Surgical anatomy of the pancreas. *Surg Clin North Am.* 1964;44:1253.)

FIGURE 9-3 The ring of pancreatic tissue contains a large duct and may be heavily fixed to the duodenal musculature. The duodenum beneath the annulus is often stenosed. Thus, cutting the ring may not provide relief from symptoms of obstruction. There is also the danger of creating a pancreatic fistula or duodenal perforation. Duodenojejunostomy bypassing the annulus is the accepted procedure. Annular pancreas usually produces symptoms in the first year of life, but where the stenosis is mild or absent, it may remain silent for many years.

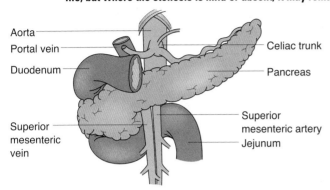

(Adapted from Gray SW, Skandalakis JE. *Atlas of Surgical Anatomy for General Surgeons.* Baltimore, MD: Lippincott Williams & Wilkins; 1985.)

pancreatitis (AP). This congenital anomaly reportedly occurs in approximately 10% of cases, although its incidence is increasing with increased endoscopy.

E. **Annular pancreas** is a rare malformation in which an aberrant migration of the ventral bud results in the second part of the duodenum being encircled by a band of normal pancreatic tissue. Complete duodenal obstruction may result. It is often associated with other congenital anomalies. Treatment is bypass, not resection (Fig. 9-3).

F. The pancreas derives its blood supply from branches of the celiac and superior mesenteric arteries. The superior mesenteric vessels lie posterior to the neck of the pancreas (portal vein forms behind the neck). Invasion of pancreatic head cancer into these vessels is the single most important factor precluding a successful resection (Fig. 9-4).

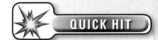

QUICK HIT

Pancreas divisum results from failure of fusion of the pancreatic ductal system, whereas annular pancreas results from aberrant migration and fusion of the ventral pancreatic bud.

FIGURE 9-4 Cross-sectional relation of the pancreas to other abdominal structures in an oblique plane through the long axis of the pancreas extending from the level of L2 on the right to T10 on the left.

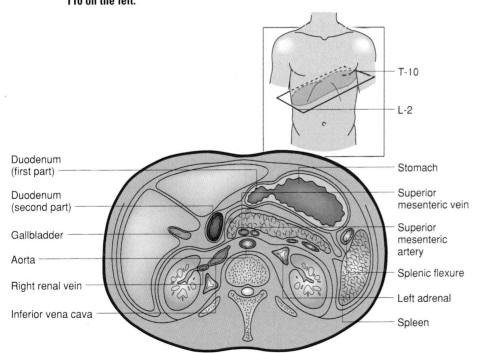

(Adapted from Mackie CR, Moossa AR. Surgical anatomy of the pancreas. In: Moossa AR, ed. *Tumors of the Pancreas.* Baltimore, MD: Lippincott Williams & Wilkins; 1980.)

FIGURE 9-5 Relation of pancreatic secretion and concentration of electrolytes.

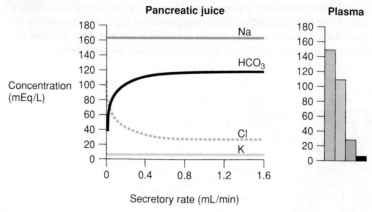

(Reprinted with permission from Bro-Rasmussen F, Kilmann SA, Thaysen JH. The composition of pancreatic juice as compared to sweat, parotid saliva, and tears. *Acta Physiol Scand.* 1956;37(2–3):97–113.)

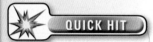

QUICK HIT

Although functionally important, the endocrine pancreas accounts for less than 5% of the pancreatic mass.

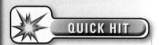

QUICK HIT

CCK, secretin, and the vagus nerve are the major stimulants responsible for the approximately 2 L of pancreatic juice secreted into the duodenum.

G. Physiology of the exocrine pancreas
1. The pancreas releases approximately 2 L of pancreatic juice into the duodenum. Daily secretion of pancreatic juice is under control of the vagus nerve and the two enteric hormones cholecystokinin (CCK) and secretin.
   a. Secretin stimulates the pancreas to secrete a high-volume, bicarbonate-rich juice in response to acid in the duodenum.
   b. CCK is stimulated by dietary fat and increases the enzyme content of pancreatic juice (Fig. 9-5).
2. The proteolytic enzymes are secreted as inactive precursors trypsinogen and chymotrypsinogen, which are activated to trypsin and chymotrypsin in the duodenum by enterokinase.
3. Pancreatic amylase and lipase break down carbohydrate and lipids, respectively, and their serum levels are also useful clinical tools in the diagnosis of pancreatitis.
H. Physiology of the endocrine pancreas: The islets of Langerhans develop in the third month of fetal life. The following types of cells have been described. Their percentage and products are listed below:
1. Alpha cells (15%): glucagon
2. Beta cells (65%): insulin
3. Delta cells (5%): somatostatin
4. PP cells (15%): pancreatic polypeptide
5. Others: D2 cells (vasoactive intestinal peptide), enterochromaffin (EC) cells (substance P and serotonin)

II. Acute Pancreatitis

A. General principles
1. AP encompasses a wide spectrum of clinical presentations, ranging from a mild and self-limited entity in 80% to 85% of patients to a serious illness complicated by shock, sepsis, and multisystem organ failure in the remaining 15% to 20%.
2. AP is a disorder whose pathogenesis remains obscure and for which treatment is largely supportive.
3. Clinically, the overall mortality for AP is approximately 10%, but in its most severe form, which is characterized by pancreatic hemorrhage and necrosis, it induces a systemic inflammatory response whose severity can increase the mortality to 20% to 30%.
B. Etiology (Table 9-1)
1. Common causes include gallstones and alcohol, which are implicated in 80% to 90% of the cases of AP. The "common channel reflux" mechanism is a popular explanation, implicating gallstones as the precipitator of AP.

TABLE 9-1 Etiology of Acute Pancreatitis
Gallstones
Ethanol
Iatrogenic causes 　ERCP 　Abdominal and nonabdominal operations 　Cardiopulmonary bypass
Trauma
Neoplasms (e.g., pancreatic cancer)
Pancreas divisum
Sphincter of Oddi spasm
Medications
Toxins 　Parathion 　Scorpion venom
Hyperlipidemia
Hypercalcemia
Infectious agents 　Viruses (e.g., mumps and coxsackie B viruses; HIV) 　Bacteria (e.g., *Salmonella* and *Shigella* species; hemorrhagic *E. coli*) 　Biliary parasites (e.g., *Ascaris lumbricoides*)
Genetic causes 　Hereditary pancreatitis 　Cystic fibrosis
Vasculitis (e.g., systemic lupus erythematosus and polyarteritis nodosa)
Ischemia
Pregnancy

ERCP, endoscopic retrograde cholangiopancreatography.
(Reprinted with permission from Mulholland MW, Lillemoe KD, Doherty GM, Maier RV, Upchurch GR, eds. *Greenfield's Surgery: Scientific Principles and Practice.* 4th ed. Philadelphia, PA: Lippincott Williams & Wilkins; 2006:641.)

It suggests migration of either gallstones or sludge through the distal bile duct. This results in damage to the common "biliary-pancreatic channel" with resultant edema and blockage of the pancreatic duct. This leads to the pooling of enzymes and their activation within the gland (Fig. 9-6).

2. Rare causes include trauma, hypercalcemia, hyperlipidemia (Fredrickson types 1 and 5), infections (viral and parasitic), drugs (more than 100 drugs, including Imuran, valproate, steroids, sulfonamides, and hydrochlorothiazide), hereditary causes (locus 7q35), and scorpion venom. Medications usually cause pancreatitis as an idiosyncratic reaction, whereas hyperlipidemic pancreatitis has an unknown etiology. After the exclusion of surreptitious alcohol abuse and microlithiasis (i.e., tiny stones, invisible on imaging, that pass into the biliary system and cause pancreatic ductal obstruction), about 5% to 10% of episodes are deemed idiopathic.

3. Only 3% to 8% of symptomatic gallstone disease results in AP. However, the incidence increases to 30% when microlithiasis is involved.

C. Clinical presentation

1. Abdominal pain is by far the most common complaint. Typically, it is epigastric, with radiation to the back.

2. Vomiting and retching are prominent associated symptoms.

FIGURE 9-6 Illustration of the common channel concept. A gallstone lodged at the ampulla of Vater can cause reflux of bile into the pancreatic duct.

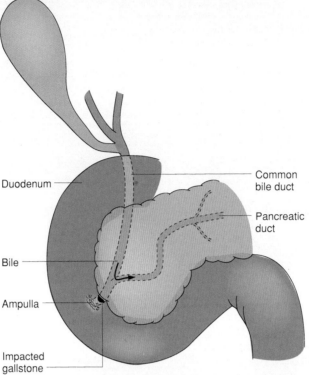

Duodenum

Common bile duct

Pancreatic duct

Bile

Ampulla

Impacted gallstone

(Reprinted with permission from Mulholland MW, Lillemoe KD, Doherty GM, Maier RV, Upchurch GR, eds. *Greenfield's Surgery: Scientific Principles and Practice.* 4th ed. Philadelphia, PA: Lippincott Williams & Wilkins; 2006.)

3. Because the signs and symptoms of AP mimic many acute intra-abdominal and extra-abdominal pathologies, a thorough history and physical examination are extremely important.
   a. Depending on the etiology of the AP, patients may give a history of an inciting factor (e.g., recent ingestion of a fatty meal or alcohol, trauma to the abdomen).
   b. A complete drug and family history is mandatory because this may give vital clues to the etiology.
4. Patients with severe AP may present in shock, multisystem organ failure, or coma.
   a. On physical examination, these patients are usually tachycardic and may have a fever.
   b. Signs of dehydration from vomiting and excessive fluid sequestration in the abdomen are evident. The abdomen is markedly tender and may have obvious guarding and distention.
   c. Severe AP with resultant bleeding in the retroperitoneum and abdominal cavity may reveal ecchymosis in the flanks called Grey Turner sign and in the periumbilical region called Cullen sign, respectively.
D. Laboratory findings
   1. Serum amylase and lipase are the most commonly accepted blood tests for diagnosing AP.
      a. Serum amylase has a sensitivity of 75% to 90% but falls short in specificity (20% to 60%) because virtually, any intra-abdominal pathology can elevate its level in the blood. Perforated duodenal ulcers, mesenteric ischemia, intestinal obstruction, salivary gland pathology, and renal failure can all give false-positive results.
      b. Serum lipase levels are more specific (50% to 99%) and sensitive (80% to 100%) for AP. Studies have shown that serum lipase levels preferentially rise higher in alcoholic AP. Therefore, the lipase:amylase ratio is higher in AP secondary to alcohol than gallstones.
   2. C-reactive protein level of greater than 150 mg/L at **48 hours** has been shown to be associated with a poor prognosis.

E. Radiology

1. A plain chest radiograph rules out pneumonia as a possible etiology for the acute abdomen. It also may show signs of acute respiratory distress syndrome (ARDS) in severe AP.

2. A dilated loop of duodenum (sentinel loop), or transverse colon (colon cutoff sign), secondary to a localized ileus from the inflammatory process in the neighboring pancreas may be evident on plain abdominal films.

3. Ultrasound is good for imaging the edematous pancreas. However, its sensitivity is marred (60%) if intraluminal gas obscures the view. Ultrasound remains the imaging modality of choice for visualizing the gallbladder and biliary system.

4. Computed tomography (CT) scan with intravenous contrast remains the gold standard for diagnosing AP and its complications. It reaches a sensitivity of greater than 90% in diagnosing pancreatitis and is excellent in showing pancreatic necrosis by nonenhancement of the affected area. A sensitivity of 100% is attained if more than 30% of the gland is involved. It also has the added advantage of ruling out other potential causes of acute abdominal presentation and is a means of guidance for sampling pancreatic tissue (Fig. 9-7).

F. Treatment

1. The management of all critically ill patients should proceed in a logical manner. Confirm the presence and adequacy of an airway and intubate with an endotracheal tube for mechanical ventilation as needed. Fluid sequestration and lack of fluid intake leads to dehydration and shock. **Fluid resuscitation to euvolemia and hemodynamic normalcy is one of the few interventions shown to improve outcomes.**

2. Adequate analgesia is also paramount. Morphine is relatively contraindicated in this setting because of its stimulatory effect on the sphincter of Oddi, and therefore, hydromorphone is recommended as an alternative. Stress ulcer prophylaxis is an important adjunct to therapy.

3. Patients who have intractable nausea and vomiting should be treated with parenteral antiemetics (such as promethazine and ondansetron) and have a nasogastric (NG) tube placed. A diet may be initiated as soon as nausea has resolved and pancreatic enzymes have normalized.

4. Certain patients may have such severe disease that they are unable to take meals orally on their own (e.g., multi-organ dysfunction and need for mechanical ventilation). In these situations, enteral feeding should be initiated as soon as possible. Enteral feeds have the advantage of maintaining the integrity of the intestinal mucosa and decreasing bacterial translocation while precluding

FIGURE 9-7 Computed tomography scan of acute pancreatitis.

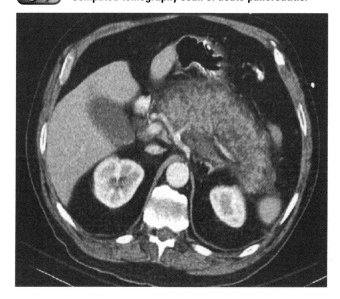

the complications of total parenteral nutrition such as central line infections, cholestasis and hyperglycemia. Nasojejunal feeding (i.e., feeding beyond the pancreas) has not been shown to be superior to NG feeding.

5. Inhibition of pancreatic secretions using H_2-blockers, somatostatin, octreotide, glucagons, calcitonin, and atropine, although theoretically sound, has had no impact on the course of AP. Similarly, cytokine inhibitors, platelet-activating factor antagonists, and gastrointestinal (GI) inhibitory hormones such as peptide YY (PYY) have so far only been effective in experimental models.

6. Although the subject of much debate, antibiotic use is not indicated in mild, AP or in sterile, necrotizing pancreatitis according to the latest guidelines published by the American College of Gastroenterology. In necrotizing pancreatitis that has a proven infection based on Gram stain and culture after fine-needle aspiration, antibiotics can be used in association with surgical debridement. When used, antibiotics should be of the variety that penetrate pancreatic tissue well such as imipenem or a combination of ciprofloxacin and metronidazole. The duration of therapy should not exceed more than 7 to 10 days in light of the risk of fungal superinfection.

7. ERCP is useful in disimpacting common bile duct stones.
   a. ERCP is the therapeutic modality of choice when the biliary system is dilated and/or liver function tests are elevated in the setting of AP. Studies have shown that it also decreases the morbidity and mortality of severe biliary AP if performed within 24 to 72 hours.
   b. In addition, ERCP is useful when the etiology of the AP is unclear.

8. Visualizing common bile duct stones, sampling bile for sludge, and inspecting the anatomy of the region can help identify biliary causes for the AP.

9. Occasionally, tumors or strictures may be diagnosed.

10. Early cholecystectomy, once the clinical pancreatitis has resolved, is currently recommended for almost all patients after the first attack of biliary pancreatitis. Most surgeons favor cholecystectomy during the same hospitalization because of the 25% to 40% incidence of recurrent attacks if the traditional 6-week "cooling off" period is observed.

G. Complications
   1. Pancreatic pseudocysts
      a. A pseudocyst is defined as fluid collection over 4 weeks old that is surrounded by a defined wall made up of fibrous tissue and surrounding organs. It occurs as a consequence of a ductal leak or as a complication of severe inflammation and, therefore, consists mostly of pancreatic secretions. They are known as pseudocysts because they lack the discrete epithelial lining definitive of true cysts.
      b. Pseudocysts develop as a complication in 10% of patients who suffer an attack of AP.
      c. More than half of all pseudocysts resolve within 4 to 6 weeks. After 6 weeks, spontaneous resolution is less likely and surgical intervention is indicated, usually in the form of a cystogastrostomy or cystojejunostomy.
   2. Pancreatic necrosis
      a. Pancreatic necrosis is defined as diffuse or focal area(s) of nonviable pancreatic parenchyma, often associated with peripancreatic fat necrosis.
      b. CT is diagnostic in more than 90% of the cases. Focal or diffuse well-circumscribed areas of nonenhanced pancreatic parenchyma larger than 3 cm, or involving more than 30% of the gland, are required for CT diagnosis.
      c. Infected pancreatic necrosis is an indication for surgical debridement. Therefore, the clinical differentiation between sterile and infected pancreatic necrosis is essential.
      d. Because clinical and laboratory findings in these two groups can be identical, the distinction is best made by cultures and Gram stains from percutaneously attained needle aspirates (Fig. 9-8).
   3. Pancreatic abscesses
      a. Pancreatic abscesses are defined as a circumscribed, intra-abdominal collection of pus in proximity to the pancreas, containing little or no

FIGURE
9-8 Computed tomography scan of acute necrotizing pancreatitis.

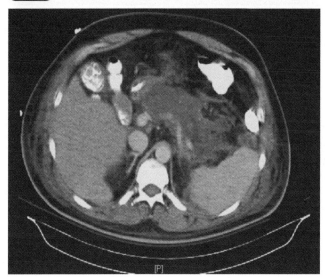

pancreatic necrosis. They can be insidious; are frequently multiple; and are evenly divided among head, body, and tail of the gland.

    b. Abscesses are frequently polymicrobial, containing *Candida* species as well as enteric bacteria such as *Escherichia coli, Klebsiella pneumoniae, Pseudomonas aeruginosa,* and *Proteus mirabilis.*

    c. For both pancreatic abscess and infected necrosis, the treatment consists of adequate drainage. Without it, virtually all patients die. Drainage can be achieved either by image-guided placement of percutaneous drains or a formal surgical debridement.

    d. Aggressive wide debridement is necessary.

    e. Most surgeons prefer to leave large-caliber sump drains in the pancreatic abscess cavity or cavities with closure of the abdomen.

    f. Irrigation of the pancreatic bed may be performed with saline or antibiotic-containing saline for prolonged periods (3 to 21 days).

  4. Pancreatic fistulas

    a. Both internal and external fistulas may result from inflammation and pancreatic duct disruption.

    b. Fluid may track into the left pleural cavity through the retroperitoneum, causing an effusion.

    c. Other complications include splenic vein thrombosis and false aneurysms, which may lead either to bleeding into the pancreatic duct (hemosuccus pancreaticus) or free rupture leading to hemoperitoneum.

 H. Prognosis

  1. C-reactive protein and polymorphonuclear-elastase have been used clinically as predictors of disease severity.

  2. Several scoring systems have been applied to AP.

    a. Ranson reported the first, and most commonly used, in 1974. This system uses 11 clinical and biochemical measurements available within the first 48 hours of disease onset. These were tabulated on a cohort of patients with alcohol-induced pancreatitis (Table 9-2).

    b. The Acute Physiology and Chronic Health Evaluation, or APACHE II, score has had much recent support.

     (1) This system is based on the evaluation of clinical data such as blood pressure, pulse, and temperature; biochemical data such as urea and electrolytes; and renal and pulmonary functional parameters.

     (2) Within 24 hours of hospital admission, this system has an approximate 70% sensitivity in the detection of severe AP, with a specificity of 80% to 90%.

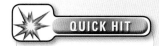

QUICK HIT

The only indication for surgical intervention in the acute stage of AP is infected pancreatic necrosis or a pancreatic abscess.

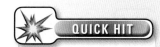

QUICK HIT

Pancreatic enzyme measurements do not form part of any of the severity scoring systems.

Pancreas and Spleen

TABLE 9-2 Ranson Criteria for Assessing Severity of Pancreatitis
At Admission
Age
WBC count
Glucose
LDH
AST
Within 48 Hours
Hematocrit decrease
BUN increase
Calcium
PaO$_2$
Base deficit
Fluid requirement

AST, aspartate aminotransferase; BUN, blood urea nitrogen; LDH, lactate dehydrogenase; PaO$_2$, arterial oxygen pressure; WBC, white blood cell. (Reprinted with permission from Mulholland MW, Lillemoe KD, Doherty GM, Maier RV, Upchurch GR, eds. *Greenfield's Surgery: Scientific Principles and Practice*. 4th ed. Philadelphia, PA: Lippincott Williams & Wilkins; 2006:845.)

III. Chronic Pancreatitis

A. General principles

1. Chronic pancreatitis is an inflammatory disease of the pancreas that is marked by the gradual destruction of pancreatic exocrine and endocrine tissues. Fibrous scar replaces the pancreatic parenchyma.
2. Pancreatic calcifications are seen in one-third of patients with alcoholic chronic pancreatitis.
3. Significant degrees of weight loss are common because food tends to worsen the pain. Narcotic addiction is common.
4. The usual age of onset is in the mid-30s, and men are affected more commonly than women.

B. Etiology

1. Alcoholism is the cause of 75% of the cases of chronic pancreatitis in the United States.
2. Less common causes include cystic fibrosis, pancreas divisum, hyperparathyroidism, tropical pancreatitis, familial pancreatitis, and idiopathic pancreatitis.
3. Another kind of chronic pancreatitis, possibly related to malnutrition, occurs only in certain tropical areas.

C. Clinical presentation

1. The presenting symptom in up to 95% of patients with chronic pancreatitis is abdominal pain.
2. Malabsorption (steatorrhea) and/or diabetes mellitus are hallmarks of significant pancreatic insufficiency.

D. Laboratory findings: No laboratory test is diagnostic of chronic pancreatitis.

1. CT scanning provides the most reliable overall assessment of the pancreas and peripancreatic area. The most common CT findings in chronic pancreatitis include duct dilatation, calcifications, and cystic lesions (Fig. 9-9).
2. ERCP should be done in most patients with chronic pancreatitis who are being evaluated for operation. The radiologic appearance of the ductal system may show ductal filling defects consistent with stones, areas of stricture alternating with segments of dilatation ("chain of lakes" appearance; Fig. 9-10).

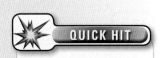

QUICK HIT

Symptoms of malabsorption (diarrhea, steatorrhea) do not occur until 90% of the secretory capacity of the pancreas is lost.

FIGURE
9-9

Abdominal computed tomography in a patient with chronic pancreatitis shows dilatation of the main pancreatic duct (*arrows*).

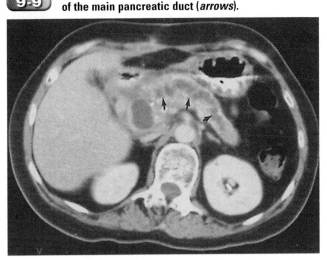

E. Treatment
1. Medical management
a. This includes total abstinence from alcohol, pancreatic enzyme supplements, and optimal nutrition (high-calorie, high-protein diet).
b. Patients are very sensitive to exogenous insulin, which is the only option because oral hypoglycemics are rarely effective.
c. Oral opioids are useful, although dependence is common.
d. Neuroablative procedures such as celiac plexus block have produced inconsistent results.
2. Surgical treatment: The aims of surgery in chronic pancreatitis are to relieve intractable pain, to treat complications, and to preserve as much functioning pancreatic tissue as possible. Three approaches have been used with mixed success:
a. Ductal drainage: When the diameter in the head and body enlarges to 7 to 8 mm or more, an anastomosis between the pancreatic duct and the jejunum, also known as a pancreaticojejunostomy or Puestow procedure, is technically feasible and has a good chance of producing lasting pain relief (Fig. 9-11).
b. Resection
(1) Resection is the treatment of choice when operation is indicated in patients whose ducts are normal or narrow in diameter.

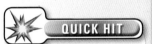

QUICK HIT

In chronic pancreatitis, the head of the gland is usually the source of the developing pancreatitis (from any source). Therefore, surgical procedures addressing the head of the pancreas are usually the most successful in inducing long-term remission (e.g., the Whipple, Beger, and Frey procedures).

FIGURE
9-10

Endoscopic retrograde cholangiopancreatography (ERCP) illustrates moderate dilation of the main pancreatic duct and ectasia of the secondary ducts associated with moderately advanced chronic pancreatitis. Arrows indicate intraductal pancreatic stones.

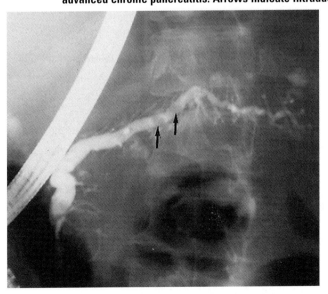

FIGURE 9-11 Lateral pancreaticojejunostomy.

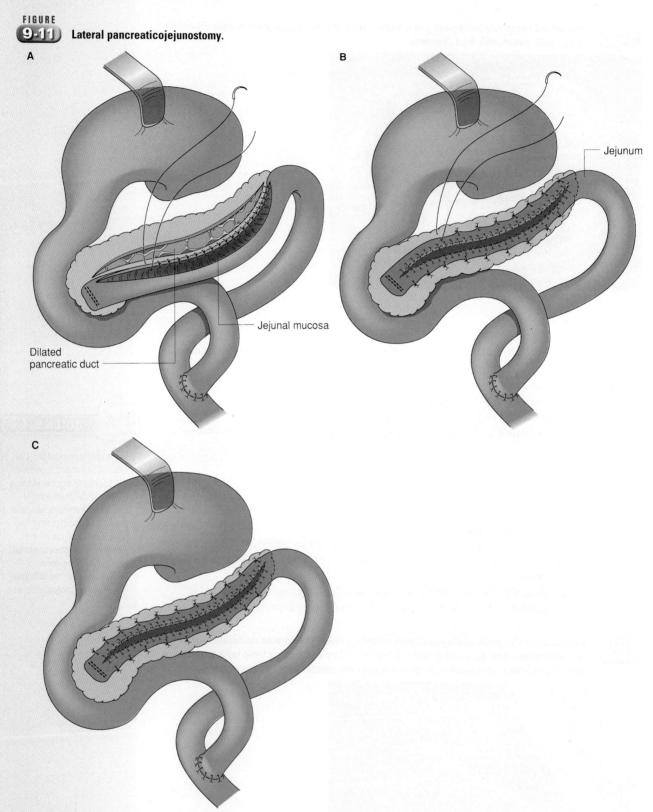

A

B

Jejunum

Jejunal mucosa

Dilated pancreatic duct

C

(Reprinted with permission from Mulholland MW, Lillemoe KD, Doherty GM, Maier RV, Upchurch GR, eds. *Greenfield's Surgery: Scientific Principles and Practice*. 4th ed. Philadelphia, PA: Lippincott Williams & Wilkins; 2006.)

(2) The type of operation depends on the area of the pancreas affected the most. Therefore, a pancreaticoduodenectomy (Whipple procedure) is performed for disease affecting pancreatic head.
   (a) Beger, who advocates a duodenum sparing resection of the head of pancreas, has described alternatives to the Whipple operation.

(b) Frey described an operation that involves coring out the involved pancreatic head without resection and draining the ductal system into a loop of small bowel.

(3) Distal pancreatectomy is performed for extensive distal disease.

(4) Total pancreatectomy is hardly ever performed because it guarantees diabetes mellitus and pancreatic exocrine insufficiency.

(5) Pancreatic autotransplant and islet cell transplants have been attempted postpancreatic resection to preserve glandular function but are only offered at a few centers worldwide.

c. Pancreatic denervation

(1) Surgical sympathectomy and celiac ganglionectomy have relieved pain effectively in many patients.

(2) Transthoracic splanchnicectomy and bilateral truncal vagotomy have also been reported to alleviate pain from chronic pancreatitis.

IV. Tumors

A. Types

1. Exocrine pancreatic neoplasms

a. These tumors, which are either cystic or solid, are the most common "cystic lesions" in the pancreas and are inflammatory pseudocysts that are obviously non-neoplastic.

b. Although many of the cystic lesions are small and benign, they do have malignant potential.

c. The common types of cystic pancreatic lesions with their characteristic features are given in Table 9-3.

d. Remember that the overall postresection survival for malignant cystic lesions is markedly better than for pancreatic ductal adenocarcinoma, which unfortunately is the most common pancreatic neoplasm.

2. Malignant pancreatic neoplasms

a. Ductal adenocarcinomas account for 90% of all malignant pancreatic cancers, and these will be discussed here. Approximately 65% arise in the pancreatic head and uncinate process, and 15% arise in the body and tail. Twenty percent are diffuse. Uncommon malignant conditions include acinar cell carcinoma, nonepithelial tumors, and lymphomas.

b. Every year, 30,000 new cases of malignant pancreatic cancers are diagnosed in the United States.

c. This form of cancer is more common in African-Americans and men and occurs mostly in the sixth to eighth decades.

d. Risk factors include hereditary or chronic pancreatitis, smoking, and Peutz–Jeghers syndrome.

e. Genetic alterations include overexpression of K-ras oncogene and inactivation of p16 and p53.

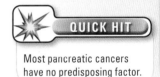

QUICK HIT

Most pancreatic cancers have no predisposing factor.

TABLE 9-3	**Cystic Pancreatic Neoplasms**	
	Serous Cystic Neoplasm	**Mucinous Cystic Neoplasm**
Age (years)	60–70	60–70
Gender	F > M	F > M
Location	Anywhere	Body/tail
Communication with pancreatic duct	No	No
Malignant potential	Low	High
"High yield"	Honeycomb septation with central calcification on computed tomography scan	Cyst wall has ovarian-type stroma.

Pancreas and Spleen

TABLE **9-4** **Pancreatic Endocrine Neoplasms**

Cells	Content	Tumor Syndromes	Clinical Features	Diagnostic Test	% Malignant
A	Glucagon	Glucagonoma	Necrolytic migratory erythema, stomatitis, diabetes, weight loss	Elevated glucagon levels (>200 pg/mL) Hyperglycemia	Nearly all
B	Insulin	Insulinoma	Hypoglycemic symptoms (cate-cholamine release), confusion Whipple triad[a] 10% multiple, 10% associated with multiple endo-crine neoplasia type 1 (MEN-1), 10% malignant	Monitored fast Insulin-to-glucose ratio >0.4 after fasting Elevated C-peptide levels	10
D	Somatostatin	Somatostatinoma	Diabetes, gallstones, steatorrhea	Elevated somatostatin levels (>100 pg/mL)	Nearly all
D2	Vasoactive intestinal peptide (VIP)	VIPoma (watery diarrhea, hypokalemia, achlorhy-dria [Verner–Morrison])	High-volume secretory diarrhea, hypokalemia, metabolic acidosis, hypochlorhydria	Elevated VIP levels (>200 pg/mL)	50
G	Gastrin	Gastrinoma (Zollinger–Ellison syndrome)	Abdominal pain with severe peptic ulcer disease, diarrhea, esophagitis 25% associated with MEN-1 syndrome	Gastrin level >1,000 pg/mL diagnostic; secretin stimulation test increase >200 pg/mL is diagnostic	70

[a]Whipple triad: fasting hypoglycemia (<50 mg/dL), symptoms of hypoglycemia, and symptoms of hypoglycemia relieved by glucose administration.

3. Endocrine tumors
   a. Pancreatic endocrine tumors are rare, with an annual collective incidence of about five cases per million population.
   b. Salient features of important pancreatic endocrine cells and their associated tumors are listed in Table 9-4.
B. Clinical presentation
   1. Early symptoms are nonspecific and include anorexia, nausea, abdominal discomfort, and weight loss. Unlike the liver or the kidney, the pancreas does not have a strong capsule, and consequently, the tumor may advance locally to involve the celiac plexus of nerves, with intractable abdominal and back pain being the first sign.
   2. Jaundice is the most common physical sign. Certain physical findings have been historically associated with advanced pancreatic cancer.
      a. Sister Mary Joseph node: periumbilical adenopathy
      b. Virchow node: left supraclavicular lymphadenopathy
      c. Blumer shelf: pelvic drop metastases
      d. Courvoisier sign: a palpable gallbladder in the presence of obstructive jaundice, which indicates noncalculous biliary obstruction (may result from cancer of the pancreatic head)
   3. Cancer involving the pancreatic head may cause painless obstructive jaundice with pale stools, dark urine, and pruritus.
   4. Unusual presentations may include diabetes or steatorrhea.
C. Laboratory findings
   1. Cancer of the pancreatic head may lead to elevation of ductal enzymes, such as alkaline phosphatase and gamma glutamyl transferase, in addition to total bilirubin.
   2. Fat malabsorption may result in an abnormally prolonged prothrombin time.
   3. Cancer antigen (CA) 19-9 is a tumor marker whose normal upper limit is 37 U/mL. Levels greater than 200 U/mL, when combined with ultrasound, CT, or ERCP, improve the diagnostic accuracy for pancreatic cancer to nearly 100%. Like carcinoembryonic antigen for colon cancer, CA 19-9 can be followed serially as a tool for monitoring response to adjuvant treatment and tumor recurrence.

FIGURE
9-12 **Computed tomography of the abdomen of a patient with adenocarcinoma of the pancreas.**

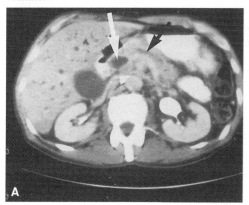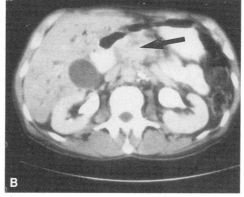

A. The obstructed and dilated common bile duct (*light arrow*) and pancreatic duct (*dark arrow*) can be seen. In the adjacent cross-section (**B**), a large mass is present in the head of the pancreas (*arrow*).

D. Radiology
   1. Transabdominal ultrasound, although useful in detecting gallstones, offers little else.
   2. A spiral CT scan with both arterial and portal venous phase is very sensitive in identifying the typical hypodense lesion along with invasion into important local structures such as the superior mesentric vein (SMV)/portal vein, which would preclude surgical resection (Fig. 9-12).
   3. Traditional MRI has not been shown to be superior to CT scan. However, magnetic resonance cholangiopancreatography provides useful information on the biliary and pancreatic ducts and has the added advantage of being noninvasive, unlike ERCP.
   4. ERCP is highly sensitive for detecting pancreatic cancer. However, it is an invasive test and should not be done routinely.
      a. Diagnostic ERCP should be done selectively in patients with presumed pancreatic cancer and obstructive jaundice without an obvious mass.
      b. Therapeutic ERCP should, of course, be done for palliation of symptomatic obstructive jaundice (Fig. 9-13).
   5. Endoluminal ultrasound and diagnostic laparoscopy are useful tools for staging the tumor in order to establish resectability.

FIGURE
9-13 **Endoscopic retrograde cholangiopancreatography in a patient with adenocarcinoma of the pancreas demonstrates a stricture of both the distal common bile duct and the pancreatic duct (*arrow*).**

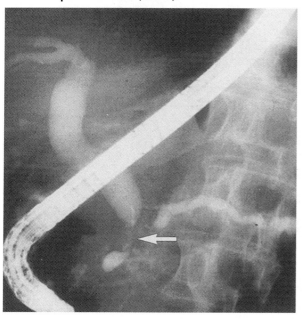

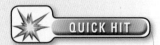

The 5-year survival for patients undergoing pancreaticoduodenectomy for pancreatic cancer is approximately 20% in the best centers.

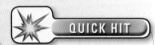

The most common complication after pancreatico-duodenectomy is pancreatic fistula.

E. Treatment
1. Resection of pancreatic carcinoma: Only 10% to 20% of all patients diagnosed with adenocarcinoma of the pancreas are candidates for pancreatic resection.
   a. The principles of operative management of pancreatic cancer are quite simple:
      (1) Assess tumor resectability and determine whether tumor is resectable.
      (2) Do a pancreaticoduodenectomy in case of tumors arising from head, neck, or uncinate process (Fig. 9-14).
      (3) Do a distal pancreatectomy, with or without splenectomy, for tumors arising from the body and tail.

FIGURE 9-14 **Pancreaticoduodenectomy.**

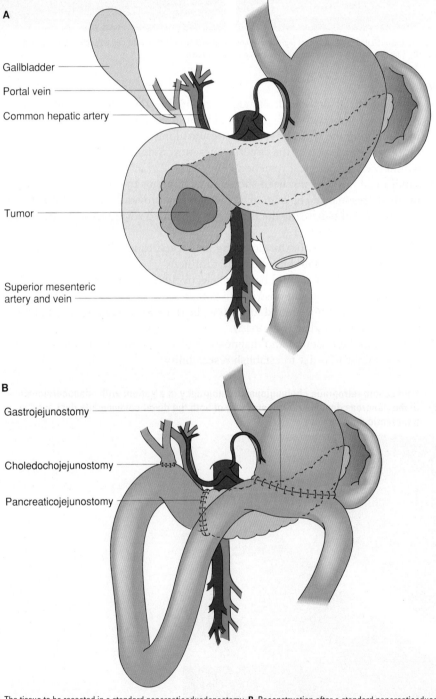

A. The tissue to be resected in a standard pancreaticoduodenectomy. **B.** Reconstruction after a standard pancreaticoduodenectomy. (Reprinted with permission from Mulholland MW, Lillemoe KD, Doherty GM, Maier RV, Upchurch GR, eds. *Greenfield's Surgery: Scientific Principles and Practice.* 4th ed. Philadelphia, PA: Lippincott Williams & Wilkins; 2006.)

b. The additional consideration in the pancreatic head/neck/uncinate tumors is reestablishment of GI continuity after resection.

c. In cases of advanced malignancy with limited life expectancy, palliative biliary or duodenal bypass can help alleviate symptoms. Preoperative and postoperative chemoradiation have been used with mixed success.

d. For advanced unresectable pancreatic cancer, the deoxycytidine analogue gemcitabine has shown some benefit in reducing pain, inducing weight gain, and improving performance status. The overall survival benefit has been modest.

SPLEEN

I. Anatomy and Physiology

A. Anatomy

1. The spleen develops in the left leaf of the dorsal mesogastrium during the fifth intrauterine week.

2. The odd numbers 1, 3, 5, 7, 9, and 11 summarize certain statistical features of the spleen. It measures $1 \times 3 \times 5$ inches, weighs 7 oz, and lies between the 9th and 11th ribs.

3. In order to be palpable below the left costal margin, the spleen has to be at least double in size.

4. The spleen is enveloped in parietal peritoneum, which extends from it in different directions, creating folds that form the suspensory ligaments of the spleen. Two important folds are the splenorenal ligament and the gastrosplenic ligament.

   a. The former extends between the anterior surface of the left kidney to the splenic hilum and invests splenic vessels and the tail of the pancreas.

   b. The latter is a conduit for the short gastric vessels.

5. The splenocolic and splenophrenic ligaments are short and usually avascular. Wandering spleens result from the absence of normal ligamentous attachments.

6. The splenic artery is one of the main branches of the celiac axis and runs a serpentine course over the pancreas to the splenic hilum. The splenic vein joins the inferior mesenteric vein along its course, until it reaches behind the neck of the pancreas, to join the superior mesenteric artery and form the portal vein.

7. Accessory spleens are tiny nodules of splenic tissue completely separate from the gland yet most commonly found in the splenic hilum. Their importance arises in disease processes such as immune thrombocytopenic purpura (ITP), where a total splenectomy is mandatory for cure (Figs. 9-15 and 9-16).

8. The splenic parenchyma is divided by trabeculae, which are inward extensions of the fibroelastic splenic capsule. The trabeculae carry branches of the splenic vessels in the parenchyma.

   a. The central mass of red pulp makes up the bulk of the splenic parenchyma.

   b. The rim of lymphatic tissue around the vessels forms the white pulp.

   c. The marginal zone separates white and red pulps (Fig. 9-17).

B. Physiology: Functions of the spleen include:

1. Hematopiesis in fetal life or later in conditions associated with bone marrow destruction

2. Reservoir for platelets and granulocytes

3. Lymphocyte stimulation and antibody production

4. Production of opsonins: tuftsin and properdin

5. Mechanical filtration of senescent erythrocytes and circulating antigens/pathogens

II. Indications for Splenectomy

A. General principles

1. Despite a move toward nonoperative management, blunt trauma remains the most common indication for splenectomy or a splenic salvage procedure in the United States. It is discussed in another section of this book.

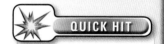

QUICK HIT

The important suspensory ligaments of the spleen include the splenorenal and gastrosplenic, which are conduits for important vascular structures. Laterally, the phrenicocolic is significant. Inferiorly, this ligament is known as the colicosplenic ligament.

Pancreas and Spleen

164 ● STEP-UP TO SURGERY

Pancreas and Spleen

FIGURE 9-15 The relations of the spleen to the abdominal and retroperitoneal viscera are seen in a cross-section of the left-facing torso.

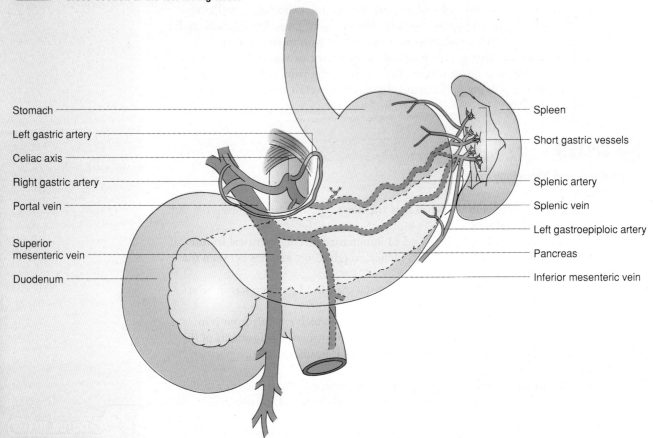

- Stomach
- Left gastric artery
- Celiac axis
- Right gastric artery
- Portal vein
- Superior mesenteric vein
- Duodenum
- Spleen
- Short gastric vessels
- Splenic artery
- Splenic vein
- Left gastroepiploic artery
- Pancreas
- Inferior mesenteric vein

(Reprinted with permission from Mulholland MW, Lillemoe KD, Doherty GM, Maier RV, Upchurch GR, eds. *Greenfield's Surgery: Scientific Principles and Practice.* 4th ed. Philadelphia, PA: Lippincott Williams & Wilkins; 2006.)

2. To better understand the indications for elective surgical removal of the spleen, it helps to categorize them conceptually.

B. Hypersplenism

1. This syndrome is characterized by a decrease in circulating cell count of erythrocytes, platelets, and leukocytes in any combination.
2. The bone marrow shows normal compensatory hematopoietic response.
3. The spleen itself is enlarged as a result of infiltration of stored products of metabolism or neoplastic tissue.

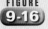

FIGURE 9-16 The arterial blood flow to the spleen is derived from the splenic artery, the left gastroepiploic artery, and the short gastric arteries (vasa brevia). The venous drainage into this portal vein is also shown.

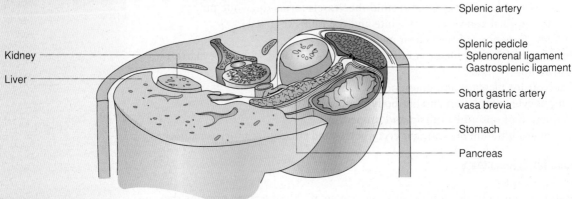

- Splenic artery
- Kidney
- Liver
- Splenic pedicle
- Splenorenal ligament
- Gastrosplenic ligament
- Short gastric artery vasa brevia
- Stomach
- Pancreas

(Reprinted with permission from Mulholland MW, Lillemoe KD, Doherty GM, Maier RV, Upchurch GR, eds. *Greenfield's Surgery: Scientific Principles and Practice.* 4th ed. Philadelphia, PA: Lippincott Williams & Wilkins; 2006.)

FIGURE
9-17 **The splenic microanatomy is shown with depictions of both the open and closed circulations.**

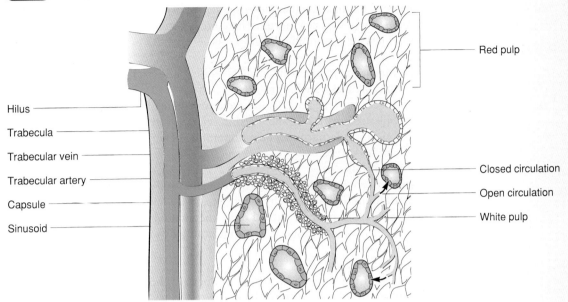

(Reprinted with permission from Mulholland MW, Lillemoe KD, Doherty GM, Maier RV, Upchurch GR, eds. *Greenfield's Surgery: Scientific Principles and Practice.* 4th ed. Philadelphia, PA: Lippincott Williams & Wilkins; 2006.)

4. Examples include:
   a. Chronic lymphocytic leukemia
      (1) Most common of all chronic leukemias
      (2) Patients develop splenomegaly, anemia, and thrombocytopenia.
      (3) Splenectomy is highly successful in relieving these symptoms.
   b. Chronic myelogenous leukemia: Splenectomy is indicated in a select group of patients in advanced stages of chronic myelogenous leukemia, who either have severe transfusion requirements or symptoms due to mass effect.
   c. Other neoplastic conditions in which splenectomy might be indicated, either for relief of pressure-related symptoms or decreased-transfusion requirements, are non-Hodgkin lymphoma, myelodysplastic syndrome, and hairy cell leukemia.
   d. Immunologic disorders such as Chediak–Higashi syndrome and mastocytosis may in rare cases benefit from splenectomy.
   e. Metabolic diseases: Gaucher disease is an autosomal recessive lipid storage disorder. It is the only metabolic disorder where partial splenectomy is the operation of choice.
C. Autoimmune/erythrocyte disorders
   1. In these conditions, the abnormality does not lie with the spleen but results from antibodies against platelets, erythrocytes, or leukocytes. Alternatively, there may be structural changes in the erythrocytes that make them susceptible to destruction by spleen.
   2. ITP
      a. This autoimmune disorder is classified as either acute or chronic.
         (1) Acute ITP occurs mostly in children, secondary to a viral illness, and is self-limiting.
         (2) Chronic ITP is seen almost exclusively in adults.
      b. Disease results from an antibody production (IgG) against platelet antigen.
         (1) The spleen is the site of antibody production. Most patients with ITP have spleens that are either normal in size or slightly smaller than normal.
         (2) Assays are now available for detection of antiplatelet IgG antibody.

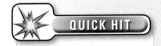

QUICK HIT

ITP is the most common reason for nontrauma, elective splenectomy in the United States.

c. The platelet count drops to less than 100,000, but patients do not become symptomatic until it drops to considerably less than 50,000.

d. The bone marrow compensates for systemic platelet destruction by increasing production of megakaryocytes. Therefore, a bone marrow aspiration is a useful test for confirming the diagnosis.

e. Treatment

(1) Management is mostly medical and includes steroids, gammaglobulins, and platelet transfusion.

(2) Elective splenectomy is indicated in patients who fail medical therapy.

(3) Splenectomy is also indicated in selected cases of thrombotic thrombocytopenic purpura and autoimmune hemolytic anemia of the warm antibody type.

3. Autoimmune anemia

a. A triad of rheumatoid arthritis, neutropenia, and splenomegaly characterizes autoimmune anemia or Felty syndrome.

b. It affects 1% of patients with chronic rheumatoid arthritis.

c. The neutropenia is induced by an IgG antibody and responds effectively to splenectomy.

4. Hereditary spherocytosis

a. This condition is the most common congenital hemolytic anemia and has an autosomal dominant transmission.

b. The defect lies in the cytoskeleton of erythrocytes and results in decreased plasticity of red blood cells. Erythrocyte proteins spectrin and ankyrin are primarily affected.

c. The spleen is the site of destruction of red cells, and splenectomy is indicated in all patients. However, in children younger than 6 years of age, the procedure should be avoided because of the risks of overwhelming postsplenectomy sepsis infection (OPSI).

5. Hereditary elliptocytosis

a. This condition is related to hereditary spherocytosis but is much less severe.

b. Symptomatic patients respond to splenectomy.

D. Incidental splenectomy

1. This involves removal of a spleen as part of a major operation on an adjacent organ (e.g., distal pancreatectomy [with splenectomy] or proximal gastric resection for cancer [with splenectomy]).

2. Removal of the spleen is necessary in these instances, either for completeness of resection or technical reasons.

E. Iatrogenic splenectomy: When the spleen is traumatized during surgery in an adjacent area and cannot be salvaged (e.g., left adrenalectomy, mobilization of splenic flexure of the colon), it is necessary to remove it.

F. Vascular conditions

1. The splenic artery is the second most common intra-abdominal artery to undergo aneurysmal changes.

a. Splenic artery aneurysms are twice as common in women.

b. They are asymptomatic but may undergo spontaneous rupture, especially during pregnancy.

c. Treatment involves catheter-directed embolization or stent placement. Ligation and resection can also be performed. Splenic aneurysms at the distal end of the splenic artery will usually be treated with concomitant splenectomy.

2. Splenic vein thrombosis results from a pancreatic or gastric pathology and is an uncommon cause of upper GI bleed curable by splenectomy.

G. Miscellaneous

1. Staging laparotomies to diagnose Hodgkin lymphoma have decreased considerably over the last decade.

2. Parasitic infection such as *Echinococcus granulosus* can form hydatid cysts in the spleen, and the treatment is a splenectomy.

III. Technique of Splenectomy (Fig. 9-18)

FIGURE 9-18 Technique for elective splenectomy.

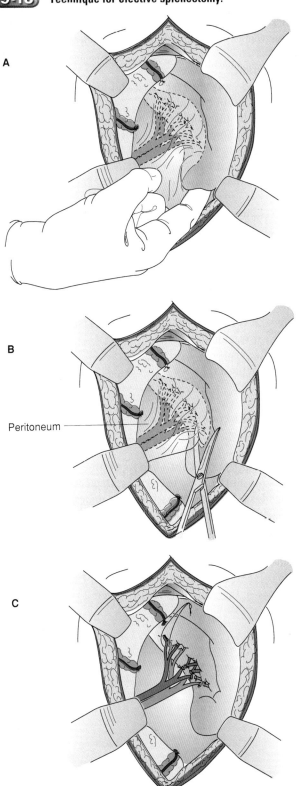

Peritoneum

A. The inferior pole is reflected laterally by the assistant's fingers, exposing the lower edge of the hilar peritoneal envelope. **B.** The hilar peritoneum is opened, here shown progressing from inferior to superior. **C.** Individual vessels are identified and suture-ligated. (Reprinted with permission from Mulholland MW, Lillemoe KD, Doherty GM, Maier RV, Upchurch GR, eds. *Greenfield's Surgery: Scientific Principles and Practice.* 4th ed. Philadelphia, PA: Lippincott Williams & Wilkins; 2006.)

Pancreas and Spleen

IV. Surgical Technique of Splenectomy

Technique can be divided based on indications. Although splenectomy can be accomplished through either a midline or subcostal incision approach, the indication for the splenectomy usually dictates the incision made. Trauma patients who are unstable usually require a midline laparotomy incision to ideally evaluate both the spleen and other concomitant injuries. Elective splenectomies can be accomplished more simply via a left subcostal approach.

- A. Open approach
  1. Make midline or subcostal incision.
  2. In trauma cases, all the blood and clots are evacuated and four quadrants of the abdomen are packed with laparotomy pads.
  3. Deliver the spleen in the wound by placing the left hand on its convex surface and cutting the lateral attachments while slowly mobilizing the spleen anteromedially.
  4. Ligate and divide the short gastric and left gastroepiploic vessels.
  5. Dissect the pancreatic tail free of the splenic artery and vein. Separately ligate and cut those vessels.
  6. Remove spleen. Look for accessory spleens.
- B. Laparoscopic splenectomy
  1. This can be performed via either an anterior or a lateral approach.
  2. It is increasingly being used for elective splenectomies, mostly ITP.

V. Changes after Splenectomy

- A. Changes in peripheral smear
  1. Intraerythrocytic inclusions and cells make an appearance postsplenectomy.
     a. Howell–Jolly bodies (nuclear fragments)
     b. Heinz bodies (hemoglobin deposits)
     c. Pappenheimer bodies (iron deposits)
     d. Target cells
     e. Spur cells (acanthocytes)
  2. Additionally, platelet and leukocyte counts show a transient increase postsplenectomy.
- B. Immunologic changes
  1. OPSI is a phenomenon that results from uncontrolled sepsis due to encapsulated microorganisms. The most significant of these bacteria is *Streptococcus pneumoniae*, followed by *Haemophilus influenzae, Neisseria meningitides,* beta-hemolytic *Streptococcus, Staphylococcus aureus, E. coli,* and *Pseudomonas* species.
  2. OPSI is more severe in children, and the risks of developing it are the highest in the first 2 years postsplenectomy.
  3. To prevent this dreaded complication, patients are vaccinated with pneumococcal, meningococcal, and *Haemophilus* vaccines prior to elective splenectomy. For emergent cases, the vaccine is ideally given 2 weeks postsurgery.

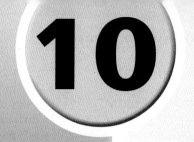

Endocrine Surgery

Fawad J. Khan and Robert Roddenberry

 THYROID

I. Anatomy and Physiology

A. Anatomy

1. Arterial blood supply

   a. The superior thyroid artery originates from the external carotid artery, which is the first branch beyond bifurcation of the common carotid artery.

   b. The inferior thyroid artery is a branch of the thyrocervical trunk of the subclavian artery.

2. Venous blood supply

   a. The superior and inferior thyroid veins are paired with the superior and inferior thyroid arteries.

   b. All venous drainage is to the internal jugular vein.

3. Nerve supply

   a. Recurrent laryngeal nerve (RLN)

   (1) A branch of the vagus nerve that descends along the internal carotid artery, the RLN is located in close proximity to the inferior thyroid artery branches.

      (a) The right RLN loops around the subclavian artery.

      (b) The left RLN loops around the aortic arch.

   (2) The RLN innervates all intrinsic muscles of the larynx except the cricothyroideus.

   (3) The tubercle of Zuckerkandl (pyramidal extension of superior thyroid tissue) and the notch of the cricothyroid membrane are landmarks for RLN insertion.

   b. External branch of superior laryngeal nerve (EBSLN)

   (1) The superior laryngeal nerve is a branch of the vagus nerve and divides into external and internal branches.

   (2) The EBSLN innervates the cricothyroideus muscle and inferior pharyngeal constrictor.

   (3) The internal branch provides sensation to the larynx above the vocal cords. Injury results in the inability to phonate in high-pitched sound, yelling, and "voice fatigue." This is described as the voice becoming softer at the end of the day or with prolonged use.

4. Anomalies of thyroid development

   a. Lingual thyroid: Thyroid tissue at the base of the tongue may require resection.

   b. Thyroglossal duct cyst: This is located in the midline between the base of the tongue and the isthmus, and resection may require removal of the central portion of the hyoid bone.

   c. Pyramidal lobe: should be excised during operation to avoid excess tissue as antigenic stimulus in Graves disease, hindrance to remnant ablation in cancer, or persistent hormone production in hyperthyroidism

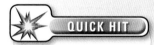

QUICK HIT

The RLN controls the vocal cords. Unilateral injury results in hoarseness with paralysis of the ipsilateral vocal cord and carries risk of aspiration. Bilateral injury results in inability to protect the airway, with paralysis of bilateral vocal cords, and may require tracheostomy.

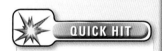

QUICK HIT

The thyroid ima artery is a direct branch of the aorta that, if present, enters the inferior midline of the thyroid.

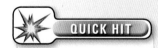

QUICK HIT

Venous drainage is important to venous sampling of PTH for parathyroid adenoma localization.

B. Physiology
 1. Makes thyroid hormones—triiodothyronine (T3) and thyroxine (T4) from iodine and tyrosine. T3 and T4 are stored in the gland when bound to thyroglobulin.
   a. The secretion of T3 and T4 is under the control of thyrotropin-releasing hormone (TRH) secreted by the hypothalamus, which regulates thyroid-stimulating hormone (TSH) from the anterior pituitary.
   b. Increased plasma levels of T3 and T4 result in negative feedback on TRH and TSH.
 2. Calcitonin is secreted by parafollicular or C-cells, which are involved in medullary thyroid cancer.

II. Hyperthyroidism (Table 10-1)
A. Causes
 1. Graves disease (diffuse toxic goiter)
   a. Autoimmune disorder with development of antibodies that stimulate thyroid hormone production or secretion
   b. Hyperthyroid symptoms include nervousness, irritability, heat intolerance, involuntary weight loss, palpitations, sweating, and tachycardia secondary to enhanced effect of catecholamines. It is also associated with exophthalmos, edema of the eyelids, pretibial edema, hypertension, arrhythmias, osteoporosis, and amenorrhea.
   c. The TSH level is suppressed, and T3 and T4 levels are elevated.
   d. Radioactive iodine (RAI) scan and tracer uptake are diagnostic.
 2. Hashimoto thyroiditis (hashitoxicosis)
   a. Five percent of patients with Hashimoto thyroiditis are hyperthyroid.
   b. This is generally a transient process, and eventually, hypothyroidism ensues.
 3. Toxic multinodular goiter
   a. This is adenomatous hyperplasia of the thyroid gland.
   b. The most common type of multinodular goiter is usually euthyroid.
 4. Toxic adenoma: Treatment is RAI ablation or lobectomy for control of hyperthyroidism.
B. Medical management
 1. Antithyroid drugs: propylthiouracil (PTU), methimazole, and Tapazole
   a. Block organification of iodine and formation of thyroid hormone.
   b. Prevent peripheral conversion of T4 to T3 by deiodinase (PTU).
 2. Complications include aplastic anemia and liver function abnormalities.
 3. Failure also occurs with noncompliance.
 4. Beta-blockers control symptoms mediated by catecholamines.
C. RAI
 1. I-131 destroys the thyrocytes with minimal effect to surrounding structures. Its therapeutic effect is not immediate. Sometimes, it requires repeat treatment.

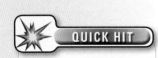

QUICK HIT

T4 is secreted exclusively by the thyroid gland. T3 is mainly produced by peripheral conversion of T4 by deiodinase in the liver, muscle, and kidney.

Endocrine Surgery

TABLE **10-1** Management of Causes of Hyperthyroidism			
	Medical Management	**Radioactive Iodine (RAI)**	**Surgical Resection**
Graves disease	Treatment of choice Rare but serious side-effect is aplastic anemia	Second-line; some advocate this as first-line due to low risk and complications of medical treatment.	For patients who fail RAI or who cannot receive RAI, or failure/complication of antithyroid drug or if tracheoesophageal compressive symptoms of goiter
Hashimoto thyroiditis	Transient phenomenon		Reserved for those with symptoms of goiter
Multinodular goiter			First option for symptomatic goiters due to size of the disease, which limits medical therapy
Toxic adenoma		Treatment of choice	If RAI fails

2. Relative contraindications include large gland, Graves ophthalmopathy, concerns for radiation exposure in the pregnant patient or the patient considering pregnancy in the near future, and the risk of hyperparathyroidism.

D. Surgical management: near-total thyroidectomy
   1. Preoperative preparation for surgery
   2. This most often includes beta-blockers to prevent thyroid storm and control symptoms. It may be necessary to taper these drugs postoperatively.
   3. Lugol solution (iodine solution) orally to decrease vascularity of the thyroid gland and decrease hyperthyroidism

III. Goiter

A. Iodine deficiency is a major cause of goiter.
B. Classification is by function or anatomy (toxic, nontoxic, diffuse, focal, and smooth).
   1. Primary
      a. Intrathoracic location (substernal)
      b. Intrathoracic blood supply
      c. Venous drainage into the chest
      d. No connection to the cervical thyroid gland
   2. Secondary
      a. Direct extension of normally located tissue in the neck
      b. Normal blood supply
   3. Intrathoracic or substernal goiters
      a. From 10% to 15% of these goiters are primary.
      b. If located in a posterior position, they are associated with symptoms of compression of esophagus and displacement of trachea. This location is most likely at the thoracic inlet at the level of the sternal notch secondary to bony confinement.
      c. Diagnosis of airway compromise involves a flow-loop spirogram on pulmonary function test.
C. Treatment
   1. Near-total thyroidectomy is the mainstay when symptoms arise.
   2. Most can be done through a cervical incision, rarely require median sternotomy.
D. Symptomatic goiters
   1. Most goiters are multinodular and benign, and patients are euthyroid. The presence of cancer within a goiter is less than 1%, and within a multinodular goiter 2% to 4%.
   2. Symptoms of aerodigestive obstruction should be sought.
   3. Dysphagia, odynophagia, dyspnea, orthopnea, and changes in these symptoms related to position of head, neck, and arms should be assessed.
   4. Persistent and consistent hoarseness warrants further evaluation to exclude nerve involvement by tumor.

IV. Thyroid Nodule

A. This discrete lesion within the thyroid gland is palpably and/or ultrasonographically distinct from the surrounding parenchyma. These nodules are palpable in 5% of the population.
B. In the United States, approximately 50% of individuals older than 50 years have thyroid nodules by ultrasonic evaluation (more in women than in men).
C. Less than 5% of nodules prove to be malignant. The risk of malignancy is related to history of radiation, age (extremes of age lead to greater malignancy), number of nodules (solitary more worrisome), and sex (men are more likely to have malignant nodules).
D. Diagnosis
   1. Fine-needle aspiration (FNA) biopsy: The most accurate, cost-effective method for evaluating thyroid nodules, this is the procedure of choice.
      a. FNA is safe, minimally invasive, and accurate. The false-negative rate for a benign finding is less than 5%.
      b. FNA should be performed in any nodule greater than 1.0 cm.

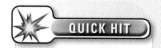

Hürthle cell change in follicular nodules is more likely to be malignant and should be surgically resected.

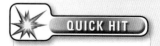

FNAs have a higher false-negative rate in patients with prior head or neck radiation; thus, these patients should have a surgical resection if they develop a thyroid nodule.

c. Diagnostic categories
   (1) Nondiagnostic or inadequate: Repeat FNA. If first attempt not done under ultrasound guidance, do so now (more than two repetitions is of limited benefit).
   (2) Indeterminate: Consider repeat FNA or follow with serial ultrasound. If there is an increase in size, consider repeat FNA, or total thyroidectomy or lobectomy.
   (3) Malignant: Perform surgical excision.
   (4) Benign: No further diagnostic studies or treatment is necessary.
2. Ultrasound
   a. Accurate at determining size, number, and character (solid vs. cystic) of nodules
   b. Used to diagnose multinodular goiter
   c. Used to assess malignant features: calcifications, irregular borders, increased blood flow
3. Radionuclide scanning
   a. Done with radioiodine or technetium-99m pertechnetate
   b. Rarely useful for evaluation of nodular disease (ultrasound and TSH allow accurate prediction of what scan will show)
4. Measurement of TSH and a history of symptoms (mobility, firmness, solitary nodule, adenopathy, voice changes) are used to exclude toxic adenoma.
5. Thyroid function tests are of little value because most nodules are nonfunctional.
E. Treatment: Indications for surgical removal without use of ultrasound or FNA include:
   1. Tracheoesophageal compressive symptoms of a nodule
   2. History of significant radiation exposure or radiation therapy to head and neck or mediastinum (nodule in this setting has a 30% risk of malignancy)
   3. Large nodule (solid or cystic) greater than 4 cm with or without symptoms, which carries high risk of malignancy (FNA may have sampling error due to size)

V. Thyroid Cancer
A. The incidence is 1/10,000 per year, with deaths occurring in 1/200,000 individuals per year (Table 10-2).
B. Well-differentiated cancers (approximately 95% of all; papillary 80% and follicular 15%)
   1. Ten percent are associated with a history of radiation exposure (typically papillary variant).
   2. These cancers most commonly present as asymptomatic thyroid nodules.

TABLE 10-2 Histologic Types of Thyroid Cancer and Their Treatment

Histologic Type	Characteristics	Lymph Node Metastases	Distant Metastases	Treatment
Papillary	X-ray therapy, "psammoma bodies," multicentric	Common	Uncommon	Thyroidectomy and I-131 therapy
Follicular	See invasion of capsule, unifocal, thickly encapsulated	Uncommon	Occasional	Thyroidectomy and I-131 therapy
Hürthle cell	Intermed differentiation, variants of follicular, multicentric, and bilateral	Common	Occasional	Thyroidectomy and I-131 therapy
Anaplastic	Aggressive, older population	Common	Common	Palliative
Medullary thyroid	Arise from C-cells, associated with multiple endocrine neoplasia (MEN) syndromes, contain amyloid RET proto-oncogene	Common	Common	Thyroidectomy and functional neck dissection on the side of the cancer and central node dissection on contralateral side

3. Treatment involves surgery. Lobectomy versus total thyroidectomy:
   a. Advantages of lobectomy
      (1) Eliminates possibility of permanent hypoparathyroidism
      (2) Decreases the risk of nerve injury
      (3) Does not require thyroid hormone replacement
   b. Disadvantages of lobectomy
      (1) Most physicians would recommend thyroid hormone suppression for prevention of recurrence of benign or malignant nodule in the remaining lobe.
      (2) Thyroglobulin cannot be used as a tumor marker as evidence of recurrence of cancer.
      (3) Whole-body RAI scanning cannot be performed to look for recurrent or metastatic disease.
4. Follow-up involves serial neck examinations and ultrasound, thyroglobulin, and RAI scans if total thyroidectomy was performed in patients at moderate to high risk of recurrence.
5. Prognosis makes use of prognostic scoring indices to stratify patients into three risk groups—low-, intermediate-, and high-risk. AMES/AGES and MACIS age is 40 years for men and 50 years for women (45 years for both in tumor-node-metastases system).
   a. AMES: age, metastases, extent, and size
   b. AGES: age, grade, extent, and size (limitation is subjective interpretation of pathologic grade)
   c. MACIS: metastases, age, completeness of resection, invasion, and size
C. Medullary thyroid carcinoma (approximately 4%)
   1. Total thyroidectomy with ipsilateral functional neck dissection is indicated.
   2. No sex or age predilection: This form of thyroid carcinoma is sporadic in 60% to 70% of cases and familial in the rest.
      a. Sporadic cases typically have a single focus with spread to the lymphatics.
      b. Familial cases are typically multifocal and more aggressive.
         (1) These cases carry a worse prognosis. However, even in the face of metastatic disease (miliary liver metastases), patients can live for more than 10 years.
         (2) They can also be associated with multiple endocrine neoplasia (MEN) type II syndrome.
         (3) Spread occurs through the lymphatics and bloodstream.
   3. The tumors secrete calcitonin, so calcitonin is followed as a tumor marker.
   4. Serial ultrasounds are followed to look for recurrence. If there is no evidence of neck disease and consistently rising calcitonin levels, multiple small liver metastases should be considered.
   5. Medullary thyroid carcinoma has a parafollicular C-cell origin, and therefore, RAI and thyroglobulin are not effective in following or treating disease.
   6. Medullary thyroid cancer has a poorer prognosis than well-differentiated thyroid cancer.
D. Lymphoma, anaplastic, and metastatic thyroid carcinoma are rare (1%).
   1. Lymphoma: may present like thyroiditis with rapidly enlarging tender gland
      a. A rare condition, it affects mainly older women (aged 50 to 70 years).
      b. Open biopsy may be required to distinguish from thyroiditis. FNA shows lymphocytes and thyroid follicles.
      c. If focal, it can be treated with radiation therapy.
      d. If diffuse, it can be treated with chemotherapy.
      e. The prognosis is variable and depends on the type and extent of disease.
   2. Anaplastic thyroid cancer: one of the most aggressive cancers; usually presents with advanced disease
      a. This form of cancer affects the older population (aged 50 to 70 years), and it has no sex predilection.
      b. It is rapidly growing, with early invasion of adjacent structures.
      c. Metastasis occurs early via lymphatics and bloodstream.

d. It is usually incurable with a poor prognosis.
   (1) Surgical resection is usually palliative and for control of respiratory compressive symptoms.
   (2) Radiation therapy may have limited benefit.

PARATHYROID GLANDS AND HYPERPARATHYROIDISM

I. **Embryology and Anatomy**
   A. Embryology
      1. The superior gland comes from the fourth brachial cleft.
      2. The inferior gland comes from the third brachial cleft, with the thymus derived from the same source.
   B. Anatomy
      1. Blood supply: The inferior thyroid artery and its branches carry the blood to the glands.
      2. Location: Both glands are usually located within 1 cm of the insertion of the RLN at the cricothyroid membrane. The superior gland is posterior and superior to the nerve, and the inferior gland is anterior to the nerve and inferior to the insertion (Fig. 10-1).
      3. Size and color: Normal glands are less than 8 mm in length, 2 to 4 mm in width, and 0.5 to 2 mm in depth. They are described as mustard-colored and may have a slight purple-to-gray hue when adenomatous or hyperplastic. They are difficult to distinguish from blood-stained fat or small lymph nodes. Normal glands weigh 30 to 50 mg.

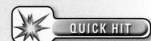

QUICK HIT

Knowledge of parathyroid gland embryology is essential when searching for an ectopic gland. If the inferior gland is not in the usual location, it is most often found in the fat along the thyrothymic ligament or in the thymus.

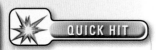

QUICK HIT

Surgical localization of the parathyroid glands can be aided by following the arterial supply from the inferior thyroid artery. Ligation of the main trunk can cause ischemia of the parathyroids.

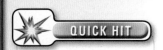

QUICK HIT

Symptoms of hyperparathyroidism have been associated with the mnemonic "stones, bones, intestinal groans, and psychic overtones."

FIGURE 10-1 Ectopic parathyroid gland locations secondary to aberrant migration found on reoperation for persistent hyperparathyroidism.

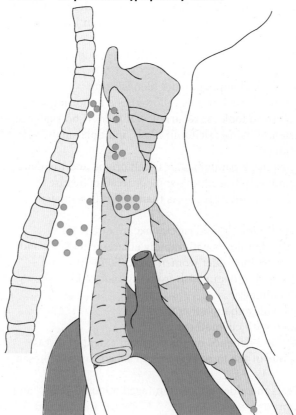

(Reprinted with permission from Karp SJ, Morris JP, Zaslau S. *Blueprints Surgery: Principles and Methods*. 4th ed. Philadelphia: Lippincott Williams & Wilkins; 2006:123.)

II. Hyperparathyroidism and Hypercalcemia

A. Hyperparathyroidism

1. Symptoms are subtle and are often attributed to aging or another medical condition. Hypertension, osteoporosis, heart dysfunction, and premature cardiac death not from atherosclerosis have all been associated with hyperparathyroidism.

2. Diagnosis

   a. Most often, the diagnosis is not suspected. The condition is found when elevated calcium is noted on routine testing.

      (1) Elevated calcium level should not be ignored, and evaluation should begin with parathyroid hormone (PTH) level.

      (2) Low total calcium may be the result of low protein, and serum albumin is first test of choice.

   b. In addition to elevated calcium, elevated PTH is also found.

   c. To exclude familial hypocalciuric hypercalcemia, use normal or elevated 24-hour urine calcium.

3. Secondary and tertiary hyperparathyroidism

   a. Mechanism

      (1) Low serum calcium is secondary to low vitamin D and elevated phosphorus levels.

      (2) With aggressive calcium and vitamin D supplements and phosphate binders, this is less common today.

   b. Treatment

      (1) Calcimimetic (Sensipar) is approved to treat refractory secondary hyperparathyroidism and parathyroid carcinoma; mimics calcium at the calcium-sensing receptor and causes reduction of PTH excretion (and calcium levels in parathyroid carcinoma)

      (2) Surgery is indicated when medications have failed to control the hyperparathyroidism.

         (a) Indications: patients with renal osteodystrophy, bone pain, pruritus, soft-tissue calcification, and necrosis, as well as renal transplant candidates

         (b) Purpose: to avoid tertiary hyperparathyroidism (severe hypercalcemia and hyperparathyroidism occurring following transplant, when calcium and vitamin D mechanisms are restored in patients with hyperplasia from secondary hyperparathyroidism)

      (3) Surgical treatment: subtotal parathyroidectomy or total parathyroidectomy with autotransplantation and cervical thymectomy to minimize risk of recurrence

B. Hypercalcemia

1. Differential diagnosis

   a. Hyperparathyroidism

   b. Malignancy/multiple myeloma

   c. Thiazide diuretics

   d. Hyperthyroidism

   e. Excess of vitamins A or D

   f. Sarcoidosis

   g. Miscellaneous conditions: milk-alkali syndrome, familial hypocalciuric hypercalcemia, immobilization, Paget disease, addisonian crisis

2. Routine (cost-effective) testing for hypercalcemia

   a. Based on frequency of these diagnoses, a reasonable approach would include a careful history and physical examination, chest X-ray, urinalysis with attention to protein and red blood cells, and a PTH level.

   b. Based on the results, consider ordering PTHrP, serum protein electrophoresis, and 24-hour urine calcium level.

3. Treatment for severe or symptomatic hypercalcemia: The mainstay of acute therapy is hydration followed by furosemide after the patient is adequately rehydrated.

III. Parathyroid Surgery

A. Localization studies

1. These are all limited by the difficulty in locating ectopic glands and by the expertise and experience of surgeons performing the studies.

2. Recently, many studies have shown potential cost savings with preoperative localization by decreasing time of exploration when limited explorations are performed.

3. The lack of numbers and prospective randomized controls is the main limitation of all studies of parathyroid localization.

B. Considerations for surgery

1. Risks: recurrence, persistence, nerve injuries

   a. Increased risks in reoperation

      (1) Prior thyroid, parathyroid, carotid surgery, or anterior cervical fusion mandates formal vocal cord evaluation and preoperative localization studies to minimize unnecessary exploration.

      (2) Nerve monitoring is adjunct with possible benefit of preventing injury.

   b. Recurrence and persistence of hyperparathyroidism is best avoided by:

      (1) Recognition of familial disease by careful history preoperatively

      (2) Suspicion of multigland disease or double adenomas based on change in intraoperative PTH assay

   c. Rough handling of parathyroid tissue can lead to implantation of fragments of viable parathyroid tissue. Parathyromatosis (implantation of significant volume of spilled benign tissue) can behave like parathyroid carcinoma.

   d. This ability of implantation with subsequent functional hormonal production is exploited in the care of patients with hyperplasia to allow for autotransplantation and cryopreservation and subsequent implantation to prevent or treat hypoparathyroidism.

IV. Parathyroid Carcinoma

A. Fewer than 1% of cases of primary hyperparathyroidism are cancerous.

B. This form of carcinoma is usually associated with a three- to ten-fold elevation of PTH and higher calcium levels than adenomatous disease (>14 vs. 10.5 to 11.5). There is a palpable nodule in 50% of patients.

C. Treatment is excision, ipsilateral thyroid lobectomy, and ipsilateral lymph node dissection.

1. Sensipar may significantly lower calcium levels and control growth.

2. Reoperation for carcinoma requires use of all the previously mentioned adjuncts and may offer significant duration of control of calcium.

D. Prognosis is poor.

 ## ADRENAL GLANDS

I. Embryology and Anatomy

A. Embryology

1. Adrenal cortex

   a. Derived from mesodermal cells near urogenital ridge

   b. Occasionally form adrenocortical rests (ectopic location), most commonly in the ovary, testis, or kidney

2. Adrenal medulla

   a. Derived from ectodermal cells of neural crest origin, which migrate from the sympathetic ganglion

   b. Occasionally, ectopic locations include the paraganglia, the organ of Zuckerkandl (just below bifurcation of the aorta), and the mediastinum.

B. Anatomy

1. Location: These glands lie on medial aspect of superior pole of each kidney.

   a. The right gland is just posterior to the inferior vena cava, adjacent to the liver and the right diaphragmatic crus.

   b. The left gland is near the aorta, tail of the pancreas, and the spleen.

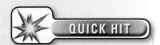

QUICK HIT

PTH levels at 5 and 10 minutes post-excision are anticipated to fall to 50% of pre-excision or baseline peak levels and/or into the normal range in adenomatous disease.

2. Arterial supply: Blood is supplied by the phrenic artery, the aorta, and the renal artery.
3. Venous drainage
   a. A single vein drains into the inferior vena cava on the right and into the renal vein on the left.
   b. The adrenal portal system allows blood from the cortex to drain directly to the medulla.
4. Histology
   a. Zona glomerulosa: outer zone, which produces aldosterone
   b. Zona fasciculata: middle zone, which produces cortisol and other glucocorticoids
   c. Zona reticularis: inner zone, which produces sex hormones
   d. Medulla: produces catecholamines (epinephrine, norepinephrine, and dopamine)
5. For details about the adrenal hormones, see Table 10-3.

II. Adrenal Medullary Tumor: Pheochromocytoma

A. Epidemiology
   1. There are 400 cases per year in the United States.
   2. This tumor follows the 10% rule: 10% are bilateral, 10% are familial, 10% are extra-adrenal, 10% are malignant, 10% are multiple, and 10% occur in children.
   3. This tumor occurs rarely during pregnancy, but if it is unrecognized, very high infant and maternal mortality results.
B. Etiology
   1. Adrenal tumors (90%)
   2. Extra-adrenal tumors (10% are paraganglia, organ of Zuckerkandl, urinary bladder, or mediastinum)
C. Signs and symptoms include palpitations, tachycardia, flushing, headache, and "sense of impending doom."
D. Diagnosis
   1. A 24-hour urine catecholamines and venous assay
      a. Limited by episodic nature of secretion and sensitivity of assay
      b. Vanillylmandelic acid (VMA) and total metanephrines
      c. Other cautions: Monoamine oxidase inhibitor agents, stresses for other reasons, and angiographic dyes may give false-positive results. Aldomet may falsely raise plasma levels.

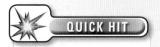

QUICK HIT

Each adrenal gland is supplied by three arteries and drains into a single vein.

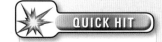

QUICK HIT

Pheochromocytoma symptoms: palpitations, tachycardia, flushing, headache, and "sense of impending doom."

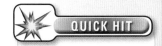

QUICK HIT

Adrenal medullary tumor can be part of MEN II (Sipple syndrome), von Hippel–Lindau disease, and von Recklinghausen neurofibromatosis.

Endocrine Surgery

TABLE 10-3 Adrenal Hormones

Hormone	Stimulated By	Inhibited By	Actions	Diagnostic Tests
Cortisol	Adrenocorticotropic hormone (ACTH) from pituitary	Negative feedback of cortisol on ACTH	Increases gluconeogenesis, lipolysis, and proteolysis; positive chronotropic and inotropic effects on the heart; immunosuppressive and anti-inflammatory effects	Can measure serum-free cortisol (diurnal variation) or 24-hour urinary 17-hydroxy-corticosteroids
Aldosterone	Decreased blood volume via angiotensin II, hyperkalemia, hyponatremia, slightly by ACTH and sympathetic nervous system	Hypernatremia, hypokalemia, fluid overload	Stimulates sodium and free water resorption, potassium, and hydrogen ion excretion	Serum aldosterone, 24-hour urinary aldosterone
Androgens	ACTH	Negative feedback	Promote development of secondary sexual characteristics	24-hour urine for 17-ketosteroids
Catecholamines	Sympathetic nervous system	Negative feedback	"Fight or flight" response	Serum metanephrines, 24-hour urine for vanillylmandelic acid (VMA), normetanephrines, metanephrines

2. Imaging for localization
   a. CT scan: 90% to 95% accuracy
   b. I-metaiodobenzylguanidine (MIBG) scan: to show absorption by pheochromocytomas and paraganglionomas (sympathetic chain tumors that also secrete catecholamines)

E. Treatment: surgery
   1. Preparation for surgery to avoid hypertensive crisis
      a. Alpha blockade with phenoxybenzamine preoperatively until symptoms resolve in 10 to 14 days
      b. Intravenous (IV) hydration when dehydration is secondary to catecholamine excess
      c. Then, add beta-blockers and continue both until the time of surgery.
      d. Calcium-channel blockers alone may be used.
      e. May require vasopressor management intraoperatively as tumor is manipulated and removed
   2. Surgery can be performed with open or laparoscopic technique: Minimal handling is necessary, with early ligation of vein and avoidance of capsular rupture.

III. Cushing Syndrome and Cushing Disease

A. Hypercortisolism
B. Adrenocorticotropic hormone (ACTH)–secreting pituitary adenoma: Cushing disease
   1. Overproduction of ACTH from pituitary leads to bilateral adrenal hyperplasia.
   2. Treatment involves resection of pituitary adenoma.
C. Hypercortisolism and/or ACTH excess from other source: Cushing syndrome
   1. May have cortisol secreting tumor
      a. Primary adrenal adenoma or hyperplasia
      b. Paraneoplastic syndrome: oat cell lung cancer, bronchial carcinoids, thymomas, and tumors of the pancreas and liver
   2. Iatrogenic from steroid use
D. Signs and symptoms: hyperglycemia, truncal obesity, hypertension, striae, immunocompromise, muscle wasting
E. Diagnosis
   1. Obtain a 24-hour urine cortisol and 24-hour urine creatinine.
   2. Overnight (low dose) 1-mg dexamethasone suppression test
   3. If positive, do high-dose dexamethasone suppression test.
      a. If ACTH is high, look for pituitary causes; if very high, this may indicate an ectopic source. Perform CT, magnetic resonance imaging (MRI), or positron emission tomography of the chest, abdomen, or pelvis.
      b. If ACTH is low, perform imaging of adrenals.

IV. Hyperaldosteronism: Conn Syndrome

A. Signs and symptoms: hypertension, hypokalemia, polyuria, polydipsia, headache
B. Diagnosis
   1. Look for evidence of dehydration.
   2. Plasma renin activity: Look for plasma aldosterone:plasma renin activity ratio greater than 30 and plasma aldosterone greater than 20, which indicates aldosteronoma (90% sensitive).
   3. If CT or MRI does not show a 1-cm or greater tumor, adrenal vein sampling may be used to localize hyperfunctioning adrenal. This involves simultaneous sampling of adrenal veins after ACTH IV injection. Cortisol ratios from adrenal vein/plasma ensure adequacy of adrenal vein cannulation. A 4 × aldosterone ratio gives appropriate lateralization.
C. Treatment
   1. For nodular adrenal hyperplasia or bilateral masses, use spironolactone.
   2. For adenoma, use adrenalectomy.
   3. Secondary hyperaldosteronism: due to renal artery stenosis, congestive heart failure, cirrhosis, and malignant hypertension

V. Incidentaloma

A. Diagnosis: discovery of an asymptomatic adrenal lesion on imaging done for another indication

1. One percent to 10% are found in healthy patients on routine imaging.
2. Most are benign and nonfunctioning tumors.
3. Adrenal masses increase in incidence with age.
4. Patients need thorough physical examination, routine laboratory studies, serum potassium, aldosterone/renin, cortisol, and 24-hour urine for VMA, normetanephrines, and metanephrines. Laboratory studies for assessment purposes should be repeated at 1 year.

B. Treatment

1. If nonfunctional and less than 4 cm, serial imaging every 6 to 12 months × 2
   a. If mass grows, then surgical resection
   b. If stable after 2 years, then stop following
2. If nonfunctional and greater than or equal to 6 cm, adrenalectomy is indicated due to higher chance of malignancy.
3. If functional and of any size, adrenalectomy is required.

VI. Adrenal Cortical Carcinoma

A. There are 0.5 to 2 cases per million per year. Sixty percent have hormone production and may have mixed hormone secretion.
B. Needle biopsies should be avoided.
C. Treated with adrenalectomy, with complete resection as only chance for cure

1. Tumors may be slow growing, and debulking a tumor may eliminate symptoms of hormone excess but will not alter prognosis.
2. Chemotherapy is of limited benefit.

VII. Adrenal Insufficiency

A. Signs and symptoms: lethargy, abdominal pain, nausea, vomiting, confusion, hypotension, hyponatremia, hyperkalemia, fever
B. Diagnosis: serum cortisol and ACTH stimulation test. Then, 250 μg of ACTH is given, and cortisol is checked at 30 and 60 minutes.
C. Treatment: Give 4 mg of dexamethasone to initial treatment and hydrocortisone replacement every 6 to 8 hours, plus IV hydration.

VIII. Multiple Endocrine Neoplasia (Table 10-4)

A. Tumor characteristics: multicentric, benign, or malignant
B. Etiology: autosomal dominant
C. MEN I: pancreatic islet cell tumors 10%, parathyroid hyperplasia 80%, pituitary adenomas 20%

1. Tumor suppressor (*MEN-I*): The first mutation is inherited and requires a second mutation to have evident disease.
2. Careful family history allows detection of MEN I in families.

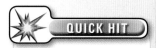

QUICK HIT

All symptoms of adrenal insufficiency are also common symptoms after abdominal surgery and may confuse management of a surgical patient after adrenalectomy.

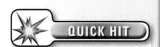

QUICK HIT

Adrenalectomy may result in adrenal insufficiency, even if a nonfunctional adenoma was resected, because contralateral adrenal suppression may occur.

Endocrine Surgery

TABLE 10-4	**Multiple Endocrine Neoplasia Syndromes**	
Syndrome	**Associated Cancers**	**Gene Defect**
MEN I	Pituitary Parathyroid Pancreas (gastrinoma, insulinoma)	MEN-1
MEN II A	Parathyroid Medullary thyroid cancer Pheochromocytoma	RET
MEN II B	Medullary thyroid cancer Pheochromocytoma Neuromas	RET

3. Parathyroid hyperplasia
   a. Treated with 3 1/2 gland resection or total parathyroidectomy with auto-transplantation
   b. Many advocate cervical thymectomy to prevent recurrence.
4. Pancreatic islet cell tumors
   a. Tumors may be isolated, multicentric, or diffuse hyperplasia.
   b. Somatostatin receptor scintigraphy may be helpful to locate tumor.
   c. Gastrinoma
      (1) The most frequent functional tumor of the pancreas
      (2) Diagnosis is indicated by gastrin levels greater than 200 pg/mL.
      (3) The tumor may be in the pancreas or in the submucosa of the duodenal wall.
      (4) The gastrinoma triangle is bounded by the junction of the cystic and common bile duct, the junction of the second and third portions of the duodenum, and the junction of the neck and body of the pancreas.
      (5) Treatment with histamine-₂-receptor antagonists or proton-pump inhibitors is usually successful. Surgical enucleation may be necessary.
   d. Insulinoma
      (1) The second most frequent pancreatic islet cell tumor
      (2) The tumor is small, solitary, and benign.
      (3) Diagnosis involves fasting hypoglycemia and inappropriately elevated insulin.
      (4) The tumor can be localized with CT and angiography, and preoperative and intraoperative ultrasound can be used.
      (5) Enucleation of the tumor is usually successful.
   e. Other pancreatic endocrine tumors are rare.
5. Pituitary adenoma
   a. Prolactin-secreting tumors are most common, but Cushing disease and acromegaly may occur.
   b. Signs and symptoms
      (1) Compression of the optic chiasm produces bitemporal hemianopsia.
      (2) Prolactin excess: amenorrhea, galactorrhea in females or hypogonadism in males

D. MEN IIA medullary thyroid carcinoma, pheochromocytoma, parathyroid hyperplasia
1. Etiology: oncogene RET proto-oncogene on chromosome 10
2. Medullary thyroid carcinoma
   a. This condition occurs in 90% of patients with MEN II.
   b. Early total resection of the thyroid gland by age 2 to 5 years is curative therapy for genetically affected.
   c. This carcinoma is virtually always bilateral and multicentric.
   d. Patients may develop C-cell hyperplasia, a diffuse proliferation of parafollicular C-cells, and elevated stimulated or basal calcitonin without frank invasive carcinoma first.
3. Pheochromocytoma (40%): Eighty percent of these are bilateral and occur in the second or third decade of life.

E. MEN IIB pheochromocytoma, medullary thyroid carcinoma, mucosal neuromas, and a distinctive marfanoid habitus: Medullary thyroid carcinoma usually occurs at an earlier age and is more aggressive.

PANCREAS

I. **Gastrinomas (Zollinger-Ellison syndrome): See Discussion in MEN I**
   A. Sporadic tumors are more likely solitary and benign.
   B. Caution is used in interpreting levels in patients taking acid-blocking medications or prior gastric surgery.
   C. Gastrinomas are sporadic in 75% and familial in 25% of patients (MEN I).

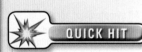

QUICK HIT

Ten percent of pheochromocytomas are located outside of the adrenal gland.

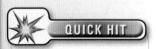

QUICK HIT

Pheochromocytoma must be excluded prior to any surgical resection and, if present, must be treated preoperatively with alpha blockers.

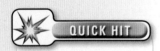

QUICK HIT

Ninety percent of gastrinomas are found in the "gastrinoma triangle."

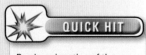

QUICK HIT

Borders: junction of the cystic duct/CBD, second and third portions of the duodenum, and the head and neck of the pancreas medially.

II. Insulinomas: See Discussion in MEN I
A. Sporadic tumors are more likely solitary and benign.
B. Sulfonylurea and C-peptide levels are used to exclude surreptitious hypoglycemia.

III. VIPomas (Verner–Morrison Syndrome)
A. Symptoms are watery diarrhea, hypokalemia, achlorhydria, and flushing.
B. Cell origin is nonbeta.

IV. Somatostatinomas
A. Symptoms are steatorrhea and hyperglycemia.
B. Cell origin is delta.

V. Glucagonoma
A. Symptoms are dermatitis (necrolytic migratory erythema) and hyperglycemia.
B. Cell origin is delta.

VI. Nonfunctioning Islet Cell Tumors
A. Tumors are of islet cell origin but without functional hormone secretion.
B. They are often found at later stage due to lack of secretion.
C. Behavior and treatment are similar to pancreatic adenocarcinoma.
D. Consider octreotide therapy to slow growth.

VII. Localization of Islet Cell Tumors
A. CT and MRI may be used.
B. Nuclear medicine octreotide scanning with possible use of gamma detector intraoperatively may help find occult tumors or metastases.

CARCINOID TUMORS

I. Characteristics
A. Arise from enterochromaffin cells in the crypts of Lieberkühn in the gut. Tumors are composed of multipotential cells with the ability to secrete a variety of hormones, most commonly serotonin and substance P.
B. Most common locations are in the gastrointestinal tract, particularly the appendix (46%), small bowel (28%), and rectum (16%).
 1. Foregut (respiratory tract, thymus) carcinoids secrete low levels of serotonin.
 2. Midgut (jejunum, ileum, right colon, stomach, and proximal duodenum) carcinoids
  a. These tumors secrete high levels of serotonin.
  b. Small bowel carcinoid is multicentric in 20% to 30% of cases.
 3. Hindgut (distal colon and rectum) carcinoids rarely secrete serotonin—usually other hormones such as somatostatin or peptide YY.
C. The majority of tumors (75%) are less than 1 cm and are slow growing.
D. The tumors occur in the fifth decade of life.
E. Invasion into serosa produces an intense desmoplastic reaction in causing fibrosis, intestinal kinking, and obstruction.
F. Tumors have a variable malignant potential and are likely to metastasize, especially ileal carcinoid greater than 1 cm.

II. Signs and Symptoms
A. Eighty percent of tumors are asymptomatic and are found incidentally at the time of surgery.
B. The most common symptoms are abdominal pain, partial or complete small bowel obstruction from intussusception or from a desmoplastic reaction, diarrhea, and weight loss.
C. Carcinoid syndrome is characterized by episodic attacks of cutaneous flushing, bronchospasm, diarrhea, and vasomotor collapse. This condition occurs only in 10% of patients, most commonly with massive hepatic replacement by metastatic disease.

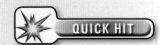

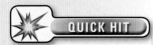

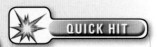

Endocrine Surgery

III. Diagnosis
A. Laboratory tests
1. Elevated urinary levels of 5-hydroxyindoleacetic acid in 24-hour urine
2. Serum chromogranin A: elevated in 80% of carcinoid tumors
B. Localization
1. Barium radiographic studies may show filling defects in the small bowel.
2. Somatostatin receptor scintigraphy 111-in-labeled pentetreotide detects somatostatin receptors.
3. CT or ultrasound may be useful in evaluating metastatic disease.

IV. Treatment
A. Dependent on tumor size, site, and presence of metastatic disease
1. Tumors less than 1 cm without evidence of metastatic disease: segmental intestinal resection
2. Tumors larger than 1 cm, multiple tumors, or lymph node involvement: wide excision of bowel and mesentery
3. Tumors in terminal ileum: right hemicolectomy
4. Small duodenal tumors: local excision
5. Large duodenal tumors: pancreaticoduodenectomy
6. Extensive disease: Surgical debulking can provide symptomatic relief.
B. Anesthetic considerations: carcinoid crisis
1. Symptoms: hypotension, bronchospasm, flushing, tachycardia, and arrhythmias
2. Treatment: octreotide, antihistamine, and hydrocortisone
C. Medical treatment
1. Symptomatic treatment
2. Octreotide: may relieve diarrhea and flushing

Breast

11

Smarika Shrestha, Lisa Jacob, and Hannah Hazard

ANATOMY AND DEVELOPMENT

I. Anatomy

A. Boundaries: sternum, axilla, pectoralis major, serratus anterior

B. Breast tissue: epithelial parenchyma elements (10% to 15%) and stroma

  1. Composition: 15 to 20 lobes of glandular tissue, supported by connective tissue framework with adipose tissue in between

  2. Cooper ligaments: bands of fibrous tissue extending from fascia to dermis that support the breast. Breast size varies depending on the amount of adipose tissue.

  3. Lobes: divided into lobules made up of branched tubuloalveolar glands. Lobes end in 2- to 4-mm lactiferous ducts, which dilate to sinuses beneath the areola and open into a nipple orifice.

  4. Radially arranged smooth muscle fibers with rich sensory innervation below nipple/areola: causes nipple erection

  5. Sebaceous glands, apocrine sweat glands, no hair follicles

  6. Tubercles of Morgagni: nodular elevations formed by Montgomery gland openings at periphery of areola that secrete milk

C. Blood supply

  1. Internal mammary artery (IMA), lateral thoracic artery (branch off the axillary artery), and lateral branches of the intercostal arteries

    a. IMA perforators: supply the medial and central breast

    b. Lateral thoracic: supply the upper outer quadrant

  2. Venous drainage follows arterial supply

D. Lymphatics

  1. Skin and nipple (areolar complex): drain initially to superficial subareolar plexus and then to a deeper plexus

  2. Sites of drainage: 97% to the axilla and 3% to the internal mammary nodes. All quadrants can drain into the internal mammary nodes.

E. Axilla: Borders include the axillary vein (superior), latissimus dorsi (lateral), serratus anterior (medial), pectoralis major (anterior), and subscapularis (posterior).

  1. Nerves: long thoracic nerve (serratus), thoracodorsal bundle (latissimus), and intercostobrachial nerves (sensory upper middle arm)

  2. Node levels

    a. Level I: inferior and lateral to pectoralis minor

    b. Level II: behind pectoralis minor

    c. Level III: medial to pectoralis minor against chest wall

II. Development

A. Role of hormones

  1. Estrogen promotes ductal dilation in primordial breast bud. Androgen causes destruction.

  2. Growth hormone in puberty causes ductal elongation and branching. Estrogen and progesterone are needed as well. During puberty, growth of both glandular

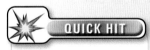

QUICK HIT

Rotter nodes are interpectoral (between the pectoralis major and minor muscles).

and stromal elements occurs. Cyclical increases in menstrual cycle influence breast macroscopic and microscopic structure.

B. Premenstrual period: Patient may feel fullness, nodularity, and sensitivity.

C. Pregnancy

1. Breast enlargement, dilation of superficial veins, and terminal epithelium differentiation lead to development of secretory cells. Lobular-alveolar differentiation produces three types of lobules.

2. Oxytocin causes myoepithelial proliferation and differentiation.

3. Lactation/involution

a. Prolactin, growth hormone, and insulin, which lead to milk production initially colostrums (rich in growth factors)

b. Secretion regulated by oxytocin; release by neuronal reflex

c. Secretory activity decreases gradually after weaning, with gland, duct, and stromal atrophy.

D. Menopause

1. Breast tissue: predominantly fat and stroma

2. Breast regression and predominance of type I lobules

BREAST WORKUP

I. History and Physical Examination

A. History

1. Presenting complaint

a. The most common presenting complaint is breast mass.

b. Other presenting complaints: pain, change in size or shape of breast, nipple discharge, or skin changes

c. Radiographic abnormalities may include calcifications or architectural distortion on mammogram or mass on ultrasound or magnetic resonance imaging (MRI) finding.

2. Baseline menstrual status and breast cancer risk factors (see Breast Cancer discussion)

a. Current menopausal status

b. Risk factor assessment: menstrual history, use of oral contraceptives and hormone replacement therapy, number and age of first pregnancy, family history of breast and/or ovarian cancer, and age of diagnosis

B. Physical examination

1. Inspection

a. Comparison of bilateral chest/breast

b. Check nipple-areola complex for symmetry, retraction, and skin changes.

c. Inspect the skin for erythema, ulceration, dimpling, or eczematous changes.

d. Inspect the breasts in varying arm positions—relaxed, above head, and hands on hips with pectoralis muscles contracted.

2. Palpation

a. Palpate for cervical and supraclavicular lymphadenopathy.

b. Palpate breast for masses/lumps/ridges.

c. Palpate axilla for lymphadenopathy.

d. Examine abdomen for hepatomegaly.

e. Examine extremities for peripheral edema or bone pain.

II. Radiologic Tests

A. Mammography: two types

1. Screening mammogram

a. Performed in asymptomatic women

b. The American Cancer Society (ACS) recommends screening annual mammogram starting at age 40 years.

c. Two views of the breast: craniocaudal and mediolateral oblique projections

d. Research validation of mammography screening

(1) Randomized trials have shown a 20% to 30% reduction in mortality with screening mammograms in women older than 50 years of age.

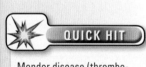

QUICK HIT

Mondor disease (thrombophlebitis of thoracoepigastric vein) is a rare form of breast retraction.

Breast

TABLE 11-1	Breast Imaging Reporting and Data System (BI-RADS) Classification	
Category	Assessment	Recommendations
0	Insufficient data	Additional imaging or clinical correlation
1	Negative	Routine screening
2	Benign finding	Routine screening
3	Probably benign finding	Short-interval follow-up (repeat in 6 months)
4	Suspicious abnormality	Definite probability of malignancy; consider biopsy
5	Highly suggestive of malignancy	High probability of cancer; appropriate action should be taken.

(Modified with permission from Mulholland MW, Lillemoe KD, Doherty GM, Maier RV, Upchurch GR, eds. *Greenfield's Surgery: Scientific Principles and Practice.* 4th ed. Philadelphia, PA: Lippincott Williams & Wilkins; 2006.)

(2) Meta-analysis has suggested a 29% reduction in mortality in 40- to 49-year-old women.

e. Reduction in mortality: a result of detection of nonpalpable abnormalities (e.g., microcalcifications, nodules <1 cm)

f. Sensitive but not specific: Only 20% to 30% of abnormalities found are malignant. For the Breast Imaging and Reporting and Data System (BI-RADS) classification, see Table 11-1.

2. Diagnostic mammogram

a. Performed for women with palpable mass, nipple discharge, breast pain, and so forth or abnormality detected on screening mammogram

b. In addition to the craniocaudal and mediolateral oblique views, lateromedial, mediolateral, magnification views, and spot compression views are performed.

c. BI-RADS 3: less than 2% risk of malignancy

d. BI-RADS 4: 2% to 50% risk of malignancy

B. Ultrasound

1. Performed on all patients with a palpable mass

2. Differentiates cystic from solid mass

3. Benign lesions

a. Simple cysts

b. Solid masses that are oval or round with circumscribed margins

4. Malignant lesions are solid with irregular shape, speculated margins, and posterior acoustic shadowing and are often taller than wide.

C. MRI

1. Useful for screening women with known breast cancer genetic abnormalities (BRCA) or women with a strong family history of breast cancer without a known BRCA mutation

a. ACS recommends screening MRI for women with approximately 20% to 25% lifetime risk of breast cancer regardless of BRCA status, as calculated by the Gail risk model.

2. Diagnostic MRI are for cancer patients or prior cancer patients with uncertain findings on other breast imaging.

3. Aids in detecting capsular leaks in patients with implants

BENIGN BREAST COMPLAINTS AND DISORDERS

I. **Breast Masses**

A. Masses may be cystic or solid.

B. Cysts: a common cause of breast masses

1. Peak in women in their 40s and in perimenopause. Uncommon in postmenopausal women who are not taking hormone replacement therapy.

2. Well-demarcated, mobile, firm, palatable, and may fluctuate with menstrual cycle
3. Simple cysts: no need for long term follow-up
4. Complicated cysts: need 6-month follow-up ultrasound to ensure stability
5. Complex cysts (solid with cystic component): need biopsy
6. Evaluate with needle aspiration or ultrasound.
    a. If fluid is nonbloody on aspiration, discard. Only send bloody fluid for cytology.
    b. If fluid is bloody on aspiration, the mass does not resolve, or the cyst recurs multiple times, then biopsy is necessary (for malignant lesion in cyst wall).
C. Solid masses
1. May be fibrocystic changes, fibroadenoma, and carcinoma
2. History and physical examination
3. Diagnostic imaging
    a. Diagnostic mammogram (vs. screening mammogram) should be obtained before biopsy of palpable mass. This involves placing a marker on an area of palpable concern and includes magnification/compression views of lesion.
    b. Ultrasound is performed on all palpable masses. This can determine cyst from solid lesion and can show characteristics typical of malignancy.
D. Biopsy of palpable breast mass
1. Fine-needle aspiration biopsy (FNA)
    a. Sensitivity: 65% to 98%, with a higher chance of false-negative results with tumors that are small and fibrotic
    b. Advantages: simple, quick, available in office, low cost
    c. Disadvantages: need cytopathologist, poor sample size, and if malignant, cannot distinguish between invasive and noninvasive disease
2. Core needle biopsy
    a. Core of tissue obtained as opposed to individual cells
    b. Preferred method to diagnose breast mass prior to surgery
    c. Advantages: more detailed evaluation of the tissue including receptor status, and invasive versus noninvasive disease
    d. Disadvantages: more labor intensive, increased risk of bleeding
3. Excisional biopsy
    a. Complete removal of the mass
    b. May be performed if patient cannot tolerate core needle biopsy or pathology from core biopsy is indeterminate or discordant with imaging findings.
    c. Outpatient procedure
    d. Specimen should be oriented.
E. Nonpalpable radiographic abnormality
1. Lesions can be sampled by core needle biopsy either via ultrasound guidance if seen on ultrasound or via stereotaxis if only seen on mammogram.
2. For suspicious calcifications or architectural distortion seen on imaging that cannot be biopsied by noninvasive techniques, needle-guided excisional biopsy may be performed, but this is reserved for the most extreme situations.

II. Breast Pain

A. Common condition that is rarely a sign of carcinoma
B. Pain may originate from breast or be referred from other structures (ribs, vertebrae). There are two categories: cyclical and noncyclical.
1. Cyclical: waxes and wanes with menstrual cycle, often bilateral, frequently in upper outer quadrants into axilla; most severe immediately prior to menses
2. Noncyclical: occurs in postmenopausal women, or no relation to menstrual cycle in premenopausal women
C. Hormonally related: more common in premenopausal women and often precipitated by a hormonal change
D. Workup: history, physical examination (fibrocystic changes), mammogram in women age 35 years and older

E. Majority of patients have no breast disease and require only reassurance.

F. About 5% of patients have disabling breast pain. Further treatment includes danazol, bromocriptine, and tamoxifen. Surgery should be avoided.

G. Mondor disease

    1. Tender, subcutaneous cord in lateral breast, with or without skin retraction

        a. The condition can be secondary to trauma, surgery, or irradiation.

        b. Thrombophlebitis of the lateral thoracic or superior thoracoepigastric vein is an uncommon cause.

    2. Anti-inflammatory agents may be necessary.

    3. Because the condition is occasionally seen with nonpalpable breast cancer, a mammogram is indicated if the patient older than 35 years.

III. Nipple Discharge

A. Common complaint, especially in premenopausal women. The cause is benign in 95% of cases.

    1. Patients with nipple discharge that occurs with compression of the breast and is nonbloody need only reassurance.

    2. Except for galactorrhea (nonpuerperal discharge of milky fluid bilateral), nipple discharge is usually not indicative of primary breast disease.

B. Etiology (bloody nipple discharge)

    1. Commonly due to intraductal papilloma (60%) and mostly in subareolar ducts

    2. Peripheral papillomas are usually multiple and less often present with discharge.

    3. Of the women who undergo duct excision, 15% to 20% have duct hyperplasia and 5% to 20% have ductal carcinoma in situ (DCIS).

    4. Single papillomas without atypia carry a three-fold risk factor and a four-fold risk factor when there is atypical hyperplasia (AH) in the papilloma.

    5. Other causes: DCIS or invasive breast cancer

C. Clinical evaluation (spontaneous bloody nipple discharge without breast compression)

    1. History: Determine that symptoms are not side effects of medication (e.g., oral contraceptive pills, phenothiazines, tricyclic antidepressants, metoclopramide, reserpine).

    2. Physical examination

    3. Evaluate for endocrine disorder, pituitary adenoma, and chest trauma.

    4. Measure prolactin level.

    5. Order mammography and ultrasound.

    6. Cytology is often inconclusive and, if sent, should not be aspirated via the breast nipple.

D. Management

    1. Attempt to localize the source (physical examination, ductoscopy). Galactography is controversial.

    2. Perform duct excision with lacrimal duct probe via a circumareolar incision. Visualize the duct and excise.

IV. Breast Infections

A. Infections can occur in lactating and non-lactating breasts.

B. Lactating

    1. Entry of bacteria from nipple into the duct system

    2. Presents as cellulitis with fever, pain, erythema, swelling, and leukocytosis

    3. *Staphylococcus aureus* most common organism involved

    4. Treatment requires antibiotics, and patient may continue breastfeeding.

    5. If antibiotics fail to resolve, consider abscess formation, which will need aspiration or incision and drainage.

C. Nonlactating

    1. Develops in subareolar ducts; also known as periductal mastitis

    2. Occurs in premenopausal women and is associated with smoking and diabetes

    3. Presents as periareolar inflammation and may present as purulent nipple discharge

4. Involves both aerobic and anaerobic skin flora
5. Associated with periareolar abscess and mammary duct fistula
6. Treatment requires antibiotics and drainage of abscess. Recurrent disease requires terminal duct excision.
D. If infection fails to respond to antibiotics and adequate drainage, a biopsy should be considered to rule out underlying breast cancer.

V. Benign Breast Disease

A. Fibrocystic changes
   1. This ambiguous term includes most types of benign breast changes.
   2. Autopsy studies show that more than 50% of women have microscopic changes consistent with fibrocystic breast changes.
   3. Fibrocystic change is not premalignant.
   4. This condition is found in women in their 30s and 40s.
   5. These changes are usually diffuse and ill-defined.
   6. They occur cyclically with menses and are painful and prominent beforehand. They disappear after menopause.
B. Fibroadenomas
   1. These well-defined, palpable, rubbery, mobile masses occur as multiple lesions in 10% to 15% of patients.
   2. They usually present between 20 and 50 years of age.
   3. They involute after menopause, and they may increase in women taking estrogen alone.
   4. On ultrasound, they appear round or oval, well-circumscribed, solid, and homogeneous, with low-level internal echoes and intermediate acoustic attenuation.
C. Pseudoangiomatous hyperplasia
   1. Benign stromal proliferation that simulates a vascular lesion
   2. It is necessary to rule out angiosarcoma by obtaining a larger tissue sample.
D. Mammary duct ectasia
   1. Occurs in perimenopausal and postmenopausal women
   2. Characterized by dilatation of subareolar ducts. Periductal inflammation leads to fibrosis and duct dilatation.
E. Lipoma: benign encapsulated adipose tissue; hard to distinguish by ultrasound from surrounding breast

VI. Gynecomastia

A. Definition: excessive development of male breast tissue; overall incidence is 32% to 36%
B. Etiology: due to a relative or absolute excess of circulating estrogens or a decrease in circulating androgens
   1. Idiopathic: most common
   2. Physiologic: neonatal, pubertal, elderly
   3. Pathologic: cirrhosis, adrenal tumors, hyperthyroidism, testicular tumors, hypogonadism
   4. Pharmacologic: marijuana, calcium-channel blockers, spironolactone, cimetidine, ketoconazole, anabolic steroids
C. Workup
   1. History: age of onset, duration, medications, drug use, medical history
   2. Physical exam: breast, testicular exam, thyroid, feminizing characteristics
   3. Diagnostic tests: B-human chorionic gonadotropin, follicle-stimulating hormone, luteinizing hormone, serum testosterone or estradiol, testicular ultrasound
D. Treatment
   1. Observation: often regresses after 3 to 18 months
   2. Weight reduction if obese
   3. Treatment of testicular tumors
   4. Discontinuation of medication or offending agent
   5. Surgery for persistent gynecomastia >12 months, typically a combination of surgical excision and liposuction for recontouring.

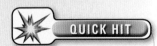

QUICK HIT

Fibroadenomas account for 75% of breast biopsies in women younger than age 20 years.

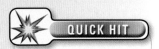

QUICK HIT

Intraductal papilloma is the most common cause of bloody discharge from nipple.

Breast

BREAST CANCER

I. Epidemiology

A. Incidence
1. Estimated number of new invasive breast cancer (2012) is 226,870 females and 2,190 males.
2. Potentially 1 in 8 American women affected
3. Estimated number of deaths (2012) is 39,920, of which 39,510 deaths were women and 410 deaths were men.

B. Risk factors
1. Age: most common risk factor
   a. The risk is 2.5% for women aged 35 to 55 years.
   b. The risk is higher in younger African-American women but becomes higher in Caucasian women after age 40.
2. Family history: Between 20% and 30% of women with breast cancer have a positive family history.
3. Prior personal history of breast cancer
4. Hereditary factors
   a. Of women with breast cancer, 5% to 10% have an inherited mutation in a breast cancer susceptibility gene.
      (1) Most involve *BRCA1* or *BRCA2* autosomal dominant mutations.
      (2) Having either gene gives a 37% to 85% risk of breast cancer, high risk of contralateral breast cancer, and elevated risk of ovarian cancer (greater with *BRCA1*) during life.
      (3) *BRCA2* increases risk of male breast cancer, prostate cancer, and pancreatic cancer; both maternally and paternally inherited.
   b. Chance of mutation varies with ethnicity (higher in Ashkenazi Jews).
   c. Genetic testing is available for patients with suggestive family history, and a counseling session should always precede testing.
   d. Infrequent breast cancer syndromes: Li-Fraumeni syndrome, Cowden syndrome, the Lynch syndrome
5. Hormonal factors
   a. Lifetime exposure to estrogens linked to breast cancer risk
   b. Early age at menarche, late age at first pregnancy, postmenopausal obesity
   c. Relative risk ranges from 1.5 to 2.0 for hormonal factors.
   d. Long duration of lactation reduces risk in premenopausal women.
   e. Small increase in risk with combination postmenopausal hormone replacement but not contraceptive use
6. Environmental factors and diet
   a. Exposure to ionizing radiation (accidental or medical) increases risk, which is greater for childhood and adolescent exposures.
   b. The most commonly encountered group is patients with Hodgkin lymphoma who received treatment with mediastinal irradiation.
7. Diet and weight gain
   a. Diet has not been shown to have a relationship with breast cancer.
   b. There may be a link between weight gain as an adult and the development of breast cancer.
8. Lobular carcinoma in situ (LCIS)
9. Atypical ductal hyperplasia (ADH)

II. Breast Cancer

A. Noninvasive breast cancer
1. DCIS
   a. Pathology
      (1) Proliferation of malignant epithelial cells is confined by the basement membrane of the duct-lobular system.

(2) Classification: comedo, cribriform, micropapillary, papillary, solid
  (a) Up to 60% of mass may be mixed.
  (b) Newer systems use grading of DCIS—high-, intermediate-, and low-grade.
(3) Cannot spread to lymphatics because the disease is confined to the duct

2. Clinical presentation
  a. Nipple discharge, Paget disease of the nipple, mass
3. Mammographic presentation (most common)
  a. Pleomorphic microcalcifications
  b. Frequency of diagnosis of DCIS is increasing because of mammography.
    (1) DCIS represents 30% to 50% of malignancies seen on biopsy of suspicious mammogram abnormalities.
    (2) DCIS may also be an incidental finding when invasive cancer is present.
4. Surgical management
  a. Lumpectomy and radiation: most common treatment (breast conservation therapy)
    (1) NSABP–B17 (randomized trial studying lumpectomy with and without radiation therapy)
      (a) Overall survival rates of lumpectomy both with and without radiation compared favorably with those of mastectomy.
      (b) There was a clear reduction in local recurrence when lumpectomy was combined with radiation, but this did not affect overall survival.
  b. Mastectomy
    (1) Curative in about 98% of patients
    (2) Up to 26% of patients may have invasive cancer not identified preoperatively. Invasive cancer is usually found in larger, high-grade DCIS lesions.
    (3) Mastectomy is usually reserved for diffuse DCIS throughout the breast or because of patient preference.
    (4) In performing mastectomy for DCIS, sentinel lymph node biopsy (SLNB) can be used in the event that incidental invasive cancer is identified on final pathology.
  c. Excision alone
    (1) Silverstein and associates developed the Van Nuys prognostic index (Table 11-2) dependent on certain risk factors: size, surgical margins, nuclear grade, and comedo necrosis.
      (a) Patients with a score of 3 to 4 can be treated with lumpectomy alone.
      (b) Scores of 5 to 7 require the addition of radiation therapy.
    (2) Excision alone may be offered to some patients with small, favorable tumors with wide, negative surgical margins.
  d. Adjuvant therapy for DCIS
    (1) Tamoxifen, as determined by NSABP-B24, was found to reduce the risk of ipsilateral breast cancer recurrence by 38% and contralateral disease by 52%.
      (a) It is recommended for patients with estrogen receptor (ER)–positive tumors.
    (2) Systemic chemotherapy is not needed for DCIS alone.
    (3) Radiation therapy is recommended in most patients undergoing lumpectomy with the possible exception being some patients with small, favorable tumors and widely negative margins.

TABLE 11-2	The Van Nuys Prognostic Index for Ductal Carcinoma In Situ		
Score	**1**	**2**	**3**
Size	<15 mm	16–40 mm	>40 mm
Margin	>10 mm	1–9 mm	<1 mm
Pathology	Low grade, no necrosis	Non-high grade, necrosis	High grade, plus or minus necrosis

B. Invasive cancer
1. Types
    a. Ductal: the most common type (approximately 80%)
    b. Lobular: second most common type
        (1) Can be difficult to detect on mammography
        (2) Consider bilateral breast MRI.
    c. Mammary: tumor with ductal and lobular features
    d. Medullary: less likely to have axillary node involvement
    e. Others (incidence in parenthesis)
        (1) Mucoid or colloid (2.4%)
        (2) Tubular (1.2%)
        (3) Adenoid cystic (0.4%)
        (4) Cribriform (0.3%)
        (5) Carcinosarcoma (0.1%)
        (6) Papillary
2. Pathology
    a. Infiltration of cells across the basement membrane and into surrounding stroma
    b. Final pathology should contain tumor types, histologic grade, and hormonal receptor status.
    c. ERs and progesterone receptors (PRs) are members of a nuclear hormone receptor family that act as transcription factors when bound by their ligands.
        (1) ER-positive tumors account for approximately 70% of breast cancers.
        (2) The greatest numbers of receptor-positive tumors are seen in well-differentiated tumors and in tumors in older postmenopausal women.
    d. HER2/neu protein is a member of the tyrosine kinase receptor family. HER2/neu gene is amplified in almost one-third of breast cancer patients.
        (1) This is associated with a shortened disease-free survival and a decreased overall survival.
3. Diagnosis
    a. History (see earlier)
    b. Physical examination (see earlier)
    c. Imaging
        (1) All patients need bilateral diagnostic mammogram.
        (2) Ultrasound for all palpable masses
        (3) Consider adding bilateral breast MRI in certain circumstances.
    d. Biopsy
        (1) All patients with palpable lesions can undergo core or vacuum-assisted needle biopsy without image guidance, but image guidance decreases false-negative rate.
        (2) All patients with nonpalpable abnormalities need image-guided core biopsy, which can be either ultrasound, stereotactic (mammo), or MRI guided.
        (3) Use image-guided modality that shows lesion best.
    e. Surgical management
        (1) Lumpectomy (also known as partial mastectomy, segmentectomy, or wide local excision)
            (a) Most commonly recommended for stages I/II disease, depending on patient preference
            (b) Surgeon must achieve negative surgical margins.
            (c) If the tissue removed does not have negative margins, additional operations to remove more tissue may be necessary.
            (d) Specimen should be oriented.
            (e) May use neoadjuvant chemotherapy for larger tumors or low breast to rumor ratio to shrink the tumor in order to perform lumpectomy
            (f) Contraindications to lumpectomy (Table 11-3)

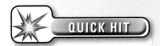

QUICK HIT

Peau d'orange is caused due to dermal lymphatic invasion in inflammatory breast cancer.

Breast

TABLE 11-3	Contraindications to Breast-Conserving Therapy in Invasive Carcinoma
Absolute contraindications	Multicentric breast cancer
	Persistent positive margins after reasonable surgical efforts
	During pregnancy
	History of previous radiation therapy that would result in excessive radiation dose to the breast region
	Diffuse microcalcifications that appear malignant
Relative contraindications	Active systemic lupus erythematosus or history of scleroderma
	Extensive, gross, multifocal disease
	Large tumor in a small breast, resulting in unacceptable cosmesis
	Very large or pendulous breasts (if adequate and reproducible homogeneity of radiation dose is not possible)
Contraindications to sentinel lymph node biopsy	Clinically suspicious axillary lymphadenopathy
	Inflammatory carcinoma or other locally advanced breast cancer
	Patient is pregnant or lactating

(Modified with permission from Mulholland MW, Lillemoe KD, Doherty GM, Maier RV, Upchurch GR, eds. *Greenfield's Surgery: Scientific Principles and Practice.* 4th ed. Philadelphia, PA: Lippincott Williams & Wilkins; 2006.)

(2) Mastectomy (with or without immediate reconstruction)
   (a) Borders: superiorly to inferior border of clavicle, medial to the lateral sternal border, laterally to the latissimus dorsi muscle, and inferiorly to the superior border of the rectus sheath
   (b) Performed for patients with large tumors, all patients with inflammatory breast cancer, and for patient preference
   (c) Skin-sparing mastectomy (removal of nipple-areolar complex only) is used in patients who desire immediate reconstruction.
(3) Lumpectomy versus mastectomy (NSABP–B06)
   (a) Enrolled 1,257 patients who either had total mastectomy, lumpectomy alone, or lumpectomy with radiation therapy
   (b) Incidence of local recurrence was approximately 10% for those with mastectomy, 9% with lumpectomy alone, and 3% for those with lumpectomy with radiation.
   (c) There is no difference in disease-free survival.
f. Axillary staging: required for invasive cancer
   (1) SLNB
      (a) Lymphatics of the breast drain into the axilla and intramammary chain, and the first nodes in either lymphatic basin are the sentinel lymph nodes (SLNs).
      (b) SLNs can be identified in two ways:
         i. Radionucleotide (technetium-labeled sulfur colloid)
            (i) Radioactivity is measured by a handheld gamma probe, and nodes are removed surgically.
         ii. Isosulfan blue dye (peritumoral or subareolar injection)
            (i) Blue lymph nodes are removed surgically.
         iii. SLNs are blue, radioactive, or both.
         iv. Be wary of firm, enlarged lymph nodes in the axilla that are neither blue nor radioactive because they may be completely replaced by tumor and therefore unable to uptake tracers.
      (c) SLNB can be performed with lumpectomy or mastectomy.
      (d) If SLN is negative for tumor, no further axillary surgery is necessary.
      (e) If SLN is positive for tumor, the current recommendation is an axillary lymph node dissection (ALND).

(f) SLNB is not recommended for patients with clinically or histologically involved axillary nodes and in inflammatory cancer, and it is contraindicated in pregnancy.

(g) Ultrasound-guided biopsy of abnormal nodes can help direct surgical intervention.

(2) ALND

(a) Definition: removal of level 1 and 2 axillary nodes

(b) Boundaries of ALND

   i. Superior: axillary vein

   ii. Posterior: latissimus dorsi

   iii. Anterior: pectoralis major and pectoralis minor

   iv. Medial: serratus anterior

(c) Morbidity associated with ALND includes lymphedema (10% to 15%), decreased range of motion at the shoulder, and numbness of the axilla and/or arm.

4. Staging (Tables 11-4 and 11-5)

5. Systemic therapy (www.nccn.org)

a. Chemotherapy

(1) Should be considered for all patients with receptor-negative disease

(2) Should be considered for all patients with positive nodal involvement

(3) Should be considered for all patients with tumors greater than 1 cm

---

TABLE 11-4 Tumor-Node-Metastasis Classification in Breast Cancer

Primary Tumor

Tx	Primary tumor cannot be assessed
T0	No evidence of primary tumor
Tis	Carcinoma in situ; ductal, lobular, or Paget disease of the nipple without tumor
T1	Tumor 2 cm or less
T2	Tumor more than 2 cm and less than 5 cm
T3	Tumor greater than 5 cm
T4	Tumor of any size directly extending into chest wall (not including pectoralis muscle), skin edema or ulceration, satellite skin lesions, or inflammatory carcinoma

Regional Lymph Nodes (Pathologic)

Nx	Lymph nodes cannot be assessed
N0	No histologic evidence for regional node metastases
N1	Metastases in one to three axillary nodes or internal mammary nodes with microscopic disease detected by biopsy
N2	Metastases in four to nine axillary nodes or clinically apparent disease in internal mammary nodes
N3	Metastases in: 1. Ten or more axillary nodes 2. Disease in infraclavicular or supraclavicular nodes 3. Internal mammary nodes with one or more positive axillary nodes 4. More than three axillary nodes with internal mammary metastases

Distant Metastases

Mx	Distant metastases cannot be assessed
M0	No distant metastases
M1	Distant metastases

TABLE 11-5	Stages of Breast Cancer Using the Tumor-Node-Metastasis Classification		
Stage 0	**Tis**	**N0**	**M0**
Stage I	T1	N0	M0
Stage IIA	T0	N1	M0
	T1	N1	M0
	T2	N0	M0
Stage IIB	T2	N1	M0
	T3	N0	M0
Stage IIIA	T0	N2	M0
	T1	N2	M0
	T2	N2	M0
	T3	N1	M0
	T3	N2	M0
Stage IIIB	T4	N0	M0
	T4	N1	M0
	T4	N2	M0
Stage IIIC	Any T	N3	MM0
Stage IV	Any T	Any N	M1

(Reproduced with permission from Mulholland MW, Lillemoe KD, Doherty GM, Maier RV, Upchurch GR, eds. *Greenfield's Surgery: Scientific Principles and Practice.* 4th ed. Philadelphia, PA: Lippincott Williams & Wilkins; 2006.)

(4) Should be considered for HER2/neu-positive patients in conjunction with Herceptin
(5) Most common regimen includes Adriamycin and cyclophosphamide.
   (a) Side effects of Adriamycin include cardiotoxicity, bone marrow suppression, fatigue, and hair loss.
(6) A taxane may be added for tumors with poor prognosis or increased lymph node involvement.
   (a) Side effects of taxanes include neuropathy and arthralgias.
b. Antihormonal therapy: for ER-positive and PR-positive cancers
   (1) Selective estrogen receptor modulators (SERM) (tamoxifen)
      (a) Only antihormonal agent for premenopausal women
      (b) When used for 5 years, it is associated with a significant reduction in the risk of recurrence and the risk of dying from breast cancer in the affected and contralateral breast.
      (c) Side effects include hot flashes, small increase risk of deep vein thrombosis (including pulmonary embolus), and small increase risk of uterine cancer.
      (d) Can be used in premenopausal and postmenopausal women
   (2) Aromatase inhibitors (AI)
      (a) Inhibit the synthesis of estrogens from androgens
      (b) Only used in postmenopausal patients
      (c) The Arimidex or Tamoxifen Alone or in Combination (ATAC) trial showed advantages to Arimidex over tamoxifen for postmenopausal women with early stage, hormone receptor–positive disease.
      (d) AIs have fewer rare but serious side effects in comparison to tamoxifen, but the AIs are associated with more bone loss and fractures.
      (e) ATAC trial showed that Arimidex is better than tamoxifen in:
         i. Preventing or delaying recurrence
         ii. Lowering the risk of contralateral breast cancer

c. Antibody therapy (trastuzumab)
   (1) Trastuzumab (Herceptin) is a murine monoclonal antibody that can be used to treat HER2/neu-positive cancers.
   (2) Clinical studies have confirmed that trastuzumab, in combination with Adriamycin or taxanes, improves survival in patients with HER2/neu overexpression in metastatic disease.
   (3) Used only in patients with HER2/neu overexpression
6. Radiation therapy
   a. High-energy beams of radiation are focused on the affected breast.
   b. In whole-breast radiation, patients receive radiation treatment as an outpatient in daily sessions over 5 to 7 weeks. Delivery is delayed until after chemotherapy if chemotherapy is required.
   c. In partial breast radiation, patients receive focused radiation to the lumpectomy cavity and 1 cm of surrounding tissue twice daily for 5 days.
      (1) This is a newer form of radiation delivery, and long-term trials are still necessary for validation.
   d. Radiation after mastectomy
      (1) Tumor is greater than 5 cm.
      (2) Positive margins of resection
      (3) Four or more lymph nodes with metastatic disease
   e. Radiation after lumpectomy
      (1) Broadly speaking, radiation is necessary after lumpectomy to affect adequate local control.
   f. Radiation is felt to be a contraindication or a relative contraindication in the following cases:
      (1) Prior radiation to the affected area of the body
      (2) Patient with connective tissue disorders like lupus or vasculitis
      (3) Pregnancy
      (4) Unable to commit to the rigorous schedule required to complete treatment

III. Reconstruction

A. Types
   1. Implant-based reconstruction: simplest form of breast reconstruction. Uses a saline or silicone gel implant to recreate breast mound. Carries higher risks in radiated fields.
      a. One-stage reconstruction: performed at the same time as the mastectomy. A permanent implant is placed in the subpectoral plane with or without the use of acellular dermal matrix (ADM).
      b. Two-stage reconstruction: The first stage involves placement of a temporary implant called a tissue expander. The tissue expander is placed in the subpectoral plane with or without the use of ADM. The patient then undergoes weekly tissue expansions with saline injections. Once the skin envelope and muscle are fully expanded, the tissue expander is removed and a permanent implant is placed.
      c. ADM: a biologic product made from acellular cadaveric dermis. It is used as a sling along the lower pole of the pectoralis major muscle to help support the tissue expander/implant, improve lower pole projection, and control position of the inframammary fold. Carries higher risk of seroma formation.
   2. Autologous tissue reconstruction: uses the patient's own tissue to recreate breast mound. Most complex form of reconstruction. Offers the most natural appearance and feel. Recommended in the setting of reconstruction following radiation therapy.
      a. Pedicled transverse rectus abdominis muscle (TRAM) flap: Skin, subcutaneous tissue, and muscle from the lower abdomen are transferred to the chest to recreate a breast mound. Sacrifices rectus abdominis muscle. Carries higher risk of abdominal bulge or hernia formation.
      b. Free tissue transfers: Tissue is harvested from another area of the body with a vascular pedicle attached. The tissue is then transplanted to the breast and

Breast

a microvascular anastomosis is performed under a microscope. Common donor sites include abdominal tissue (deep inferior epigastric perforator [DIEP] flap, superficial inferior epigastric artery [SIEA] flap), buttock tissue (superior gluteal artery perforator [SGAP] flap, inferior gluteal artery perforator [IGAP] flap), and thigh tissue (transverse upper gracilis [TUG] flap, anterolateral thigh [ALT] flap). Usually does not involve muscle sacrifice; therefore, there is less donor site morbidity.

c. Latissimus dorsi flap: Muscle with or without a skin paddle is transferred from the back to the breast. The latissimus is a broad, flat muscle and does not offer significant volume or projection. Therefore, an implant is typically placed beneath the muscle.

3. Nipple areolar reconstruction: Using either the native breast skin or flap skin paddle, a nipple is created from a multilobed skin flap. There are numerous flap designs, including skate flap, star flap, and so forth. The areola can be created using a skin graft. Tattooing is used to give pigment and create color. 3-D tattoos are now being used to recreate the whole nascent polypeptide-associated complex (NAC) without the need for additional surgery.

B. Timing
1. Immediate reconstruction: performed in the same setting as the mastectomy. Offers the best esthetic results.
2. Delayed reconstruction: performed months to years following the mastectomy. Preferable in more advanced-stage cancers or inflammatory breast cancer. More challenging to reconstruct due to loss of skin envelope.
3. Delayed-immediate reconstruction: attempts to convert a patient who is known to require postmastectomy radiation from a traditional delayed reconstruction into an immediate-type reconstruction. The patient undergoes a skin-sparing mastectomy, and a tissue expander is placed. The expander is fully inflated. The patient then undergoes radiation therapy with the expander in place. The patient then undergoes definitive reconstruction with autologous tissue 6 to 12 months following completion of radiation.

PATIENTS AT HIGH RISK FOR BREAST CANCER

A. Definition
1. Hereditary: BRCA-positive status or with a strong family history of breast or ovarian cancer
2. Proliferative disorders: personal history of ADH, atypical lobular hyperplasia (ALH), or LCIS.
B. Increased monitoring
1. Augment screening mammogram with liberal use of ultrasound.
2. Addition of screening bilateral breast MRI alternating every 6 months with screening mammography in BRCA-positive patients
C. Strategies to reduce the risk of breast cancer
1. Tamoxifen, a SERM
a. National Surgical Adjuvant Breast and Bowel Project (NSABP)—P1 showed that women taking tamoxifen had a 49% reduction in risk of invasive breast cancer and a 50% reduction in risk of noninvasive breast cancer in ER-positive tumors.
b. Tamoxifen reduced the risk of breast cancer in women with personal history of LCIS and AH by 65% and 85%, respectively.
2. Raloxifene, a newer SERM, may reduce the risk of breast cancer in ER-positive postmenopausal patients.
a. NSABP P-2 (Study of Tamoxifen and Raloxifene [STAR] trial) showed raloxifene is as effective as tamoxifen in reducing the risk of invasive breast cancer with a lower side-effect profile.
b. Raloxifene does not reduce the risk of noninvasive breast cancers.
3. Oophorectomy
a. Removal of both ovaries can reduce the risk of breast cancer by approximately 50% in high-risk women.

QUICK HIT

Prophylactic mastectomy reduces the risk of breast cancer by only approximately 90% (not 100%).

4. Prophylactic mastectomy
   a. Should be performed only after complete risk assessment and thorough discussion with the patient
   b. Should remove the entire breast using the same boundaries as therapeutic mastectomy
   c. Skin-sparing mastectomy may be used to facilitate immediate reconstruction.

D. Hereditary breast cancer
   1. About 5% to 10% of breast cancers are attributed to inherited mutations, most of which are caused by mutations of *BRCA1* and *BRCA2*.
   2. *BRCA1* and *BRCA2* are tumor suppressor genes that have roles in DNA repair and regulation of gene expression.
   3. Mutations of both genes carry a lifetime risk of breast cancer of 40% to 85% and are associated with an increased risk of ovarian cancer, with 30% to 45% lifetime risk with *BRCA1* and 10% to 20% with *BRCA2* mutation.
   4. There is also an increased risk of male breast cancer in BRCA families, with 1% to 5% lifetime risk with *BRCA1* and 5% to 10% with *BRCA2* mutation.
   5. Other genetic breast cancer syndromes include Li-Fraumeni, Cowden, and Lynch syndromes. Li-Fraumeni syndrome is associated with mutation in the tumor suppressor gene p53.

E. Proliferative lesions
   1. ALH
      a. Composed of cells similar to those found in LCIS but less than half the acini are filled or distorted
      b. Associated with a fivefold relative risk of developing breast cancer
   2. ADH
      a. Marked proliferation and atypia of the epithelium
      b. Found in 3% of benign breast biopsies
      c. Associated with a 13% development of breast cancer (fourfold risk)
      d. Diagnosed by the same criteria as DCIS but does not have all the characteristics necessary to diagnose intraductal cancer
   3. LCIS
      a. An incidental finding or core or excisional biopsy or marker
      b. Patients have an 8 to 10 times risk, or about a 1% per year risk of developing invasive carcinoma in the same or opposite breast.
      c. Treatment may be observation, antihormonal (tamoxifen), or bilateral mastectomies, depending on patient preference.

SPECIAL PROBLEMS

I. Breast Cancer in the Elderly

A. Approximately half of breast cancers in the United States are diagnosed in women 65 years old and over.

B. Either mastectomy or breast conservation therapy may be offered, depending on physiologic (not chronologic) age. Some studies suggest lower failure rates with lumpectomy in older women than in those younger than 65 years.

C. Radiation therapy is fairly well tolerated, but limited mobility may make daily visits difficult. If the tumor is less than 2 cm, radiation therapy may offer only marginal benefit. Wide excision combined with hormonal therapy may be offered.

D. Tamoxifen alone as an alternative to surgical treatment has been studied, and although local recurrence was better controlled in women treated surgically, there was no survival benefit to surgical therapy.

E. Endocrine therapy is a viable alternative for the elderly patient with a limited life span or significant comorbid conditions that may preclude surgery.

II. Breast Cancer in Pregnancy

A. This is a relatively uncommon occurrence, and only 7% to 14% of breast cancer patients of childbearing age are pregnant at diagnosis. Approximately 2.2 breast cancers per 10,000 pregnancies are seen.

Breast

B. Clinical presentation is the same as in patients who are not pregnant, with a palpable mass being the most common presenting symptom.

C. Mammography is indicated, and ultrasound should be performed for all palpable masses.

D. Diagnosis is commonly delayed. Pregnant women may safely undergo core needle biopsy or biopsy under local anesthesia.

E. If the patient wishes to continue the pregnancy, treatment options are limited.
1. Lumpectomy may be performed with delayed radiation, depending on the trimester.
2. Radiation therapy is contraindicated at all times because the fetus cannot be shielded from internal scatter.
3. Mastectomy is recommended if cancer is diagnosed in the early trimester.
4. Staging is performed by axillary dissection because the effects of radiocolloids and blue dyes in SLNB are unknown.
5. Termination of pregnancy has not been shown to confer survival advantage.
6. Chemotherapy may be offered after the first trimester (risk of fetal malformation during first trimester is 20%, and it declines to 2% in the second and third trimesters).
7. Tamoxifen is contraindicated in pregnancy.

III. Inflammatory Breast Cancer

A. Clinical presentation
1. Presents with skin changes of erythema, tenderness, edema, peau d'orange, and induration
2. Peau d' orange resembles the peel of an orange and is caused by blockage of the dermal lymphatics with tumor and subsequent edema of the tissue around hair follicles.
3. There may be a palpable ridge or border to the erythema.

B. Diagnosis
1. Based on clinical presentation and pathology
2. Biopsy may be performed with percutaneous core biopsy of the breast tissue or skin punch biopsy.
3. Ductal histology and dermal lymphatic invasion are common.
4. One-third of patients will have metastatic spread at presentation, and therefore, a thorough evaluation for metastatic disease needs to be performed.
5. Mammography is usually negative except for skin edema.

C. Treatment
1. Neoadjuvant chemotherapy is recommended prior to surgery.
2. Anthracycline-based treatments are currently used, and trastuzumab is added to chemotherapy regimen if the tumor is HER2/neu positive.
3. Restaging PET scan prior to surgery
4. If response is achieved with chemotherapy, surgical treatment is performed with a total mastectomy with ALND. Breast-conserving therapy is contraindicated.
5. If response is not achieved with chemotherapy, additional systemic chemotherapy and radiation therapy are considered prior to surgery.
6. After surgery, radiation therapy is undergone for local control regardless of the response to neoadjuvant chemotherapy.

IV. Paget Disease

A. Eczematoid lesion of the nipple and areolar complex caused by large malignant cells
1. A nonpalpable mass is usually due to DCIS.
2. A palpable mass usually indicates invasive ductal carcinoma.
3. Begins on nipple and can spread onto the areola, not the other direction

B. Diagnosis
1. Tissue is obtained by scrape cytology, epidermal shave biopsy, punch biopsy, wedge incision biopsy, or nipple excision.

Breast

2. Retroareolar spot compression views should be added to the standard bilateral mammogram.

3. MRI is indicated in those with normal mammogram and ultrasound.

C. Management

1. Patients with disease extending beyond the central portion of the breast by physical examination or imaging studies should undergo mastectomy.

2. Patients choosing breast conservation (lumpectomy with excision of nipple-areolar complex) should combine surgery and radiation.

3. SLNB may be performed if invasive breast cancer is present.

V. Occult Primary Tumor Presenting with Nodal Metastases

A. Breast cancer is the most common type of metastatic adenocarcinoma presenting in the axillary lymph nodes.

B. Less than 1% of cases in most large series of patients

C. MRI should be used to detect primary tumor when an ultrasound and a mammogram are negative.

D. If breast cancer is presumed, treatment is mastectomy, as in other patients with similar stage.

E. May use ALND with whole-breast radiation if the patient refuses mastectomy

VI. Male Breast Cancer

A. Uncommon disease, where the mean age at presentation is 10 years more than in women

B. Risk factors

1. Klinefelter syndrome, *BRCA2* mutations, family history, hepatic disorders, radiation exposure

2. There is no clear association with gynecomastia, except in Klinefelter syndrome.

C. Typical presentation is a mass under the nipple-areolar complex with ulceration or retraction of the nipple. Approximately 80% are hormone-receptor positive.

D. Management

1. Mastectomy is the most common treatment; may have to excise some of the pectoralis muscle

2. If the mass is small, can offer lumpectomy and radiation

E. SLNB is used to stage the patient, unless histologically positive axillary lymph-adenopathy is present (mandating axillary dissection).

F. Compared to women of the same stage, survival is similar in men. Axillary nodal status is the major predictor of outcome as it is in women.

G. Largest advantage of systemic adjuvant therapy is seen with hormonal therapy (Table 11-6)

1. Tamoxifen improved 5-year survival to 55% (compared to 20% with no systemic therapy) but may be less well tolerated in men.

2. Orchiectomy is a second-line hormonal therapy in metastatic disease, resulting in an 80% response rate in receptor-positive male breast cancer.

VII. Locally Recurrent Breast Cancer

A. After breast conservation therapy

1. Causal factors: inappropriate patient selection, poor surgical or radiotherapy technique, or tumor biology

2. Frequency

a. Uncommon in the first 2 postoperative years

b. Develops at a constant rate, usually adjacent to site of primary tumor, during years 2 to 6

c. Develops in other quadrants after year 6 and may be new primary tumors (supported by 1% annual risk, which is equal to risk for developing a new contralateral tumor)

3. Most tumors recur in the breast parenchyma (5% to 10% occur in the skin). Evaluation for metastatic disease is mandatory prior to local therapy, which is mastectomy in the absence of metastases.

Breast

TABLE **11-6** Recommendations for Adjuvant Therapy in Breast Cancer	
Node Negative, Low Risk	
Tumor <1 cm Special histologic types 1–2 cm, grade 1, estrogen receptor (ER)-positive	No treatment, or endocrine therapy if tumor is ER-positive
Node Negative, High Risk	
ER positive ER negative	Endocrine therapy or chemotherapy with endocrine therapy Chemotherapy
Node Positive	
ER positive Premenopausal Postmenopausal ER negative	Chemotherapy with endocrine therapy Chemotherapy with endocrine therapy or endocrine therapy alone Chemotherapy

(Reproduced with permission from Mulholland MW, Lillemoe KD, Doherty GM, Maier RV, Upchurch GR, eds. *Greenfield's Surgery: Scientific Principles and Practice.* 4th ed. Philadelphia, PA: Lippincott Williams & Wilkins; 2006.)

    4. Treatment for ipsilateral recurrence is mastectomy because the breast can only be radiated once.

    5. Five-year survival ranges from 60% to 79%.

  B. After mastectomy

    1. Frequency

      a. Different time frame than after breast conservation

      b. About 75% of local recurrences occur in first 3 postoperative years; half of these have distant metastases at the time of recurrence.

    2. Best predictor of chest wall recurrence is the number of axillary nodes with metastases.

    3. Evaluation for distant metastases is mandatory.

      a. Check computed tomography scans of brain, chest, abdomen, and pelvis. Order bone scans.

      b. Locally excise recurrences if possible.

      c. Radiation therapy is indicated to include chest wall. This field includes supraclavicular space (second most frequent site of recurrence).

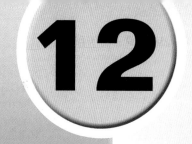

Skin and Soft Tissue

Bruce Freeman, Matthew Loos, Richard Casuccio,
Glen Jacob, and Daven J. Savla

 ANATOMY

See Figure 12-1.

I. Epidermis

A. Layers
1. Stratum corneum: outermost layer consisting of mostly dead keratinocytes, typically 20 to 30 cells thick, and making up approximately 75% of the thickness of the skin
2. Stratum lucidum: few flattened rows of dead keratinocytes
3. Stratum granulosum: three to five layers of cells with increased levels of keratin
4. Stratum spinosum: several rows of mature keratinocytes

 FIGURE 12-1 Anatomy of the skin.

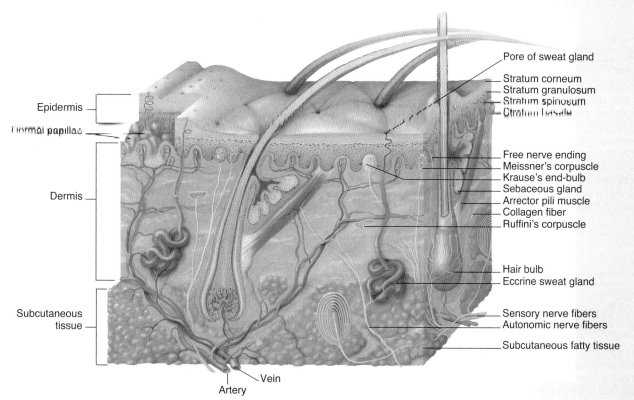

(Reprinted with permission from Eroschenko VP. *DiFiore's Atlas of Histology with Functional Correlations*. 10th ed. Baltimore, MD: Lippincott Williams & Wilkins; 2005:184.)

5. Stratum basale: single row of continuously dividing cells that produce keratin. This layer is attached to the dermis via a basement membrane that acts to selectively filter substances passing up from the dermis.

B. Cell types
1. Melanocytes
   a. Produce melanin, which protects the skin from the harmful effects of ultraviolet (UV) light
   b. Act to pigment the skin so that those individuals with more melanin have darker skin and those with less have lighter skin
2. Merkel cells: mechanoreceptors that provide information of light touch sensation
3. Langerhans cells: act to protect the body by attacking and engulfing foreign material

C. Appendages
1. Hair follicles: regulate body temperature and contain sebaceous glands that produce sebum to aid in lubricating the skin and hair
2. Sudoriferous glands: produce sweat to aid in temperature regulation and fight infection
3. Nails: are hard keratin produced at the tips of the fingers and toes

II. Dermis

A. Thickness: 2 to 4 mm
B. Consists of two layers
1. Papillary dermis: thin and loosely woven fibers that conform to the stratum basale and aid in anchoring the epidermis and protecting the appendages
2. Reticular dermis: dense, irregularly arranged fibers that contribute to the strength of the skin
C. Highly vascular and provides the more superficial layers of skin with nutrient supply
D. Contains lymphatics
E. Cell types
1. Fibroblasts: produce collagen and elastin for strength and flexibility
2. Macrophages and white blood cells (WBCs): for fighting infection
3. Mast cells: for secretion of numerous mediators such as histamine, tumor necrosis factor-alpha (TNF-α), and interleukin-1 (IL-1)
4. Sensory receptors: for touch, pressure, vibration, and temperature

III. Subcutaneous Tissues

A. Adipose tissue
B. Fascia
C. Deep lymphatic tissue

WOUNDS AND SCARS

I. Wounds

A. Phases of wound healing
1. Inflammation
   a. Vascular response
      (1) Injured vessels allow leakage and edema formation.
      (2) Vasoconstriction then reduces further blood loss.
      (3) Platelets arrive and adhere to the exposed endothelial lining (collagen). They release growth factors and chemotactic agents such as vascular endothelial growth factor, prostaglandin E2, platelet-derived growth factor, transforming growth factor alpha (TGF-α), thrombin, and thromboxane A2.
      (4) Vasodilatation then resumes and contributes to the pain, swelling, and redness seen in most acute wounds.

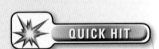

In addition to its other functions, skin plays a vital role in the production of vitamin D.

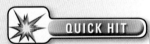

Blisters appear in the junction between the papillary dermis and the stratum basale as the result of friction.

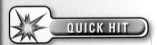

Wounds are classified by the depth of the injury. Superficial wounds involve the epidermis only, partial-thickness wounds involve the epidermis and dermis, and full-thickness wounds are through the dermis and into the subcutaneous tissues or deeper.

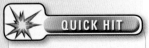

Five signs of inflammation: tumor (swelling), rubor (redness), calor (heat), dolor (pain), and functio laesa (loss of function).

TABLE 12-1 Inflammatory Cytokines

Cytokine	Cellular Source	Action
Proinflammatory		
TNF-α	Macrophages	PMN margination and cytotoxicity, collagen synthesis
IL-1	Macrophages, keratinocytes	Chemotaxis and collagen synthesis
IL2	T-lymphocytes	Fibroblast metabolism and infiltration
IL-6	Macrophages, PMNs, fibroblasts	Fibroblast proliferation, protein synthesis
IL-8	Macrophages, fibroblasts	Chemotaxis
IFN-γ	Macrophages, T-lymphocytes	Activation of macrophages and PMNs increase collagenase action
Anti-Inflammatory		
IL-4	T-lymphocytes, basophils, mast cells	Inhibits TNF, IL-1, IL-6, fibroblast proliferation
IL-10	T-lymphocytes, macrophages, keratinocytes	Inhibits TNF, IL-1, IL-6, inhibits macrophage and PMN activation

PMN, polymorphonuclear leukocyte.

b. Cellular response (Table 12-1)
   (1) Reduced blood flow through the area of injury forces the traveling WBCs to be pushed against the sidewalls of the vessel (margination). These WBCs then migrate through the vessel walls and move toward the zone of injury during the first 24 hours.
      (a) The WBCs are guided by changes in pH, chemotaxins produced by dead or dying cells, and bacterial toxins.
      (b) This begins the process of clearing the wound of foreign material.
   (2) Monocytes arrive next (2 to 3 days) and become macrophages in the interstitium.
      (a) These contribute to wound cleaning not only by direct phagocytosis but also as the source of over 30 growth factors as well as cytokines.
      (b) Mast cells also contribute to the wound clearance at this point
2. Proliferation
   Proliferative cytokines and inflammatory mediators are defined and described in Table 12-2.
   a. Typically begins within about 48 hours of injury
   b. Has four major elements
      (1) Angiogenesis: Endothelial cells adjacent to the zone of injury bud and grow into the wound.
         (a) Led by ischemia and chemical mediators
         (b) Form new capillary beds, thus providing nutrition and avenues for removal of waste products
         (c) Lymphatics also regenerate and aid in lessening the edema within the wound.
      (2) Granulation: temporary connective tissue that fills the wound
         (a) Fibroblasts are important elements in the formation of the extracellular matrix.
         (b) Fibroblasts are drawn into the wound by ischemia.
      (3) Contraction: Fibroblasts are transformed into myofibroblasts and are capable of action similar to smooth muscle. Myofibroblasts are actin-rich and stretch the dermis to attempt to cover the wound.

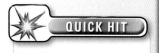

QUICK HIT

Not all wounds heal at the same speed. Linear wounds contract faster, while rectangular and circular wounds close more slowly.

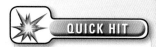

QUICK HIT

Wounds, even when they are completely remodeled, regain only 80% of their initial strength.

Skin and Soft Tissue

TABLE 12-2	Proliferative Cytokines	
Cytokine	**Source**	**Function**
PDGF	Platelets, macrophages, endothelial cells, keratinocytes	Chemotaxis, angiogenesis, wound contraction, remodeling
TGF-β	Platelets, macrophages, endothelial cells, keratinocytes, fibroblasts, T-lymphocytes	Chemotaxis, angiogenesis Inhibits keratinocytes and MMPs Induces TGF-β
EGF	Platelets, macrophages	Mitogenic
TGF-α	Macrophages, T-lymphocytes, keratinocytes	Mitogenic
FGF	Macrophages, endothelial cells, keratinocytes, mast cells, T-lymphocytes, fibroblasts	Chemotaxis, angiogenesis, wound contraction, matrix deposition
KGF	Fibroblasts	Keratinocyte migration, proliferation, differentiation
IGF-1	Macrophages, fibroblasts	Like growth hormone, stimulates collagen, fibroblasts, keratinocytes
VEGF	Keratinocytes	Increases vasopermeability, mitogenic

EGF, epidermal growth factor; FGF, fibroblast growth factor; IGF-1, insulin-like growth factor 1; KGF, keratocyte growth factor; MMPs, matrix metalloproteinases; PDGF, platelet-derived growth factor; TGF-α, transforming growth factor alpha; TGF-β, transforming growth factor beta; VEGF, vascular endothelia growth factor.

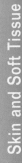

    (4) Epithelialization: Keratinocytes from the wound margins and appendages multiply and migrate across the wound.
        (a) Keratinocytes further debride the wound and require an oxygen-rich environment.
        (b) Thus, if the wound is full of debris or has poor blood supply, reepithelialization is hindered.
  3. Maturation
    a. Collagen within granulation tissue is further remodeled through a process of creation and destruction via collagenases.
      (1) This process can take up to 2 years to complete but is primarily complete by 6 to 12 months.
      (2) The collagenases convert immature collagen (type III) to mature collagen (type I).
    b. The collagen realigns itself through an interaction of forces, both internal and external.
      (1) Internal alignment comes when the collagen attempts to match the collagen found at the wound edges.
      (2) External alignment is based on the forces applied to the wound.
B. Wound closure
  1. Primary intention
    a. Clean wounds in which the edges are approximated either by suture, staples, or other adhesives.
    b. This limits the inflammatory and proliferative phases. In fact, epithelialization begins in as early as 24 hours.
  2. Secondary intention
    a. The wounds are not approximated.
    b. This requires all phases of healing and is therefore longer and requires more energy.
    c. This allows for contaminated wounds to be removed by the physiologic (phagocytic) or mechanical means.
    d. Open wounds are less prone to infection.

3. Tertiary intention: also known as a delayed primary closure
   a. The wound is left open initially for a certain period of time while the wound is cleaned and observed.
   b. The wound edges are then approximated in the usual fashion with stitches or adhesive.

C. Factors that affect wound healing
   1. Cause of wound: Sharply incised wounds heal faster than blunt traumatic wounds.
   2. Time since injury: Delay in presentation and cleaning can prolong the inflammatory phase and thus delay wound healing.
   3. Location: Wounds that occur in areas with reduced vascular supply heal more slowly.
   4. Size: Wounds heal from the periphery; thus, the larger the area affected, the longer it will take for the wound to progress through the phases of healing.
   5. Temperature: Decreased temperature inhibits wound healing.
   6. Hydration: Dry wounds progress through the phases of healing more slowly than those in a moist environment.
   7. Foreign bodies: prolong the inflammatory phase and delay wound healing
   8. Necrotic tissue: impairs wound healing by providing a medium for microbes to exist
   9. Irradiation: causes endothelial cell damage and hypoxia
      a. Inhibits angiogenesis
      b. Impairs keratinocytes and fibroblasts in their G2-phase and S-phase of replication
   10. Diabetes: impaired microcirculation and red cell function, resulting in poor blood flow to the wound
      a. Decreased leukocyte and lymphocyte function
      b. Increased collagen degradation and poor collagen reformation
   11. Infection: prolongs inflammation and slows healing overall
      a. For a wound to be considered infected, the quantitative amount of bacteria is greater than 10^5 microbes per gram of tissue.
      b. Amounts less than this imply colonization and may still impair wound healing through their competition for oxygen within the wound.
   12. Age: As people age, their macrophage and fibroblast functions are reduced. Cellular turnover is decreased, and microvasculature is reduced.
   13. Nutrition: Adequate nutrition is vital to the healing process because all of the phases of wound healing require energy to complete.
      a. Vitamins A and C are especially important.
      b. Zinc deficiency inhibits collagen formation and delays wound healing
   14. Smoking: Nicotine acts to constrict the microvasculature, thereby reducing the blood flow within a wound.
      a. Nicotine causes platelet aggregation and clot, thus impairing blood flow to the wound.
      b. Carbon monoxide binds to the red blood cells and thus limits the amount of oxygen available to the wound bed.
   15. Medications that impair wound healing
      a. Glucocorticosteroids
      b. Doxorubicin
      c. Tamoxifen
      d. High-dose nonsteroidal anti-inflammatory drugs
   16. Oxygen content: Polymorphonuclear neutrophils require PaO_2 levels greater than 50 mm Hg to produce superoxide derivatives.
      a. Typically, oxygen levels at the center of a wound are significantly lower than those in the surrounding tissue. In areas of hypoxia, collagen synthesis is driven by glycolysis, but oxygen is essential for formation of the triple helix and cross-linking.
      b. The role of hyperbaric oxygen in wound healing is to increase the oxygen levels in the bed of the wound and thus stimulate growth.

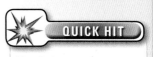

QUICK HIT

Vitamin A acts to reverse steroidal effects on lysosomes and can improve wound healing in patients who require steroids.

Skin and Soft Tissue

D. Wound management
  1. Description of the wound
    a. Depth
      (1) Superficial (stage I)
      (2) Violating the dermis (stage II)
      (3) Violating the subcutaneous tissue (stage III)
      (4) Violating to the deep structures of muscle or bone (stage IV)
    b. Dimension
    c. Location
    d. Presence of infection
      (1) Purulence
      (2) Erythema
      (3) Crepitus
      (4) Induration
  2. Debridement
    a. Benefits
      (1) Reduces bacterial load of a wound
      (2) Increases effectiveness of antibacterials applied to the wound
      (3) Improves action of leukocytes: provides an aerobic environment for the opsonization and phagocytosis of bacteria
      (4) Shortens the inflammatory phase of wound healing
      (5) Decreases the energy required for wound healing
      (6) Decreases the physical barrier to wound healing
    b. Indications for debridement
      (1) Necrotic, devitalized, and dead tissue
      (2) Foreign matter and debris
      (3) Disorganized, violet, and dusky-colored granulation tissue
      (4) Blisters, if they impede function or they contain pus (otherwise, they can be considered sterile biologic dressings)
      (5) Callus (a relative indication based on the clinical presentation of the patient, e.g., associated with a wound or present in the feet of a diabetic patient)
    c. Contraindications for debridement
      (1) Organized, uniform, and brightly pink granulation tissue
      (2) Viable tissue
      (3) Deep tissue injuries
      (4) Healthy deep tissues (e.g., muscle, tendon, ligament, nerve, capsule of joint)
    d. Types of debridement
      (1) Sharp: removal of tissue with scalpel or scissors
        (a) This is commonly performed at the bedside or in the operating room.
        (b) This is the fastest means of debridement but is associated with pain and other complications such as bleeding.
      (2) Autolytic: removal of tissue by providing an environment for the body's own defenses to work
        (a) Application of a moisture-retentive dressing to allow for the body's own collagenases and inflammatory cells to soften and debride the wound
        (b) Principles of topical therapy
          i. Remove necrotic tissue
          ii. Identify and eliminate infection
          iii. Obliterate dead space
          iv. Absorb excess exudates
          v. Maintain moist environment
          vi. Thermal insulation
          vii. Protection from trauma
        (c) Labor intensive and requires more time to clean the wound
        (d) Lower rate of infection than with traditional gauze dressings

(3) Enzymatic: application of enzymes topically to the wound. The U.S. Food and Drug Administration (FDA) has removed fibrinolytics and proteolytics from the market for patient safety reasons, leaving collagenase as the only approved debrider.

    (a) Time consuming: Typical course is daily wound application for 2 weeks.

    (b) Labor intensive and costly

(4) Mechanical

    (a) Wet-to-dry dressings

        i. Inexpensive and work intensive. Such dressings should be changed twice daily.

        ii. Good for removing debris within the wound

        iii. May traumatize the wound and remove viable tissues

        iv. Do not maintain a moist environment.

        v. Promotes granulation tissue formation

    (b) Whirlpool

        i. Nonspecific

        ii. Good for removing debris within the wound

    (c) Scrubbing

        i. Nonspecific

        ii. Cytotoxic: Hydrogen peroxide and Betadine are especially toxic to tissues and should be avoided in open wounds.

        iii. May be painful and traumatic to tissues

II. Scars

A. Keloid

  1. Uncommon, occurs mainly in dark-skinned patients

  2. Extends beyond the boundary of the original scar and invades the surrounding normal tissue

  3. Genetic predisposition

  4. Characterized by an overabundance of collagen. Collagen formation outpaces the actions of collagenases.

  5. Can be considered a benign neoplasm with the potential for recurrence

  6. Treatment

    a. Steroid injection

    b. Re-excision followed by radiation

    c. No single therapy with good results

B. Hypertrophic scars

  1. Overabundance of collagen

  2. Contained within the borders of the original scar

  3. Treatment

    a. Re-excision, especially for wounds allowed to close by secondary intention

    b. Application of silicone sheets

    c. Pressure garments

    d. Steroid injections

NEOPLASMS OF THE SKIN

I. Melanoma

A. Risk factors

  1. Fair skin

  2. UV light exposure

  3. History of precursor lesions

    a. Dysplastic nevi

    b. Xeroderma pigmentosa

    c. Congenital nevi

  4. History of blistering or peeling sunburns

  5. Immunosuppression

6. Family history
   a. Some cases (5% to 10%) of melanoma are familial. Individuals who have one first-degree relative with melanoma have a 70 times increased risk of the disease.
   b. Earlier age of onset
   c. Chromosomes 1p and 9p
7. *CDKN2A*/p16/*MC1R* mutation

B. Diagnosis
   1. The ABCD rule (Figure 12-2)
      Asymmetry
      Border irregularity
      Color (nonuniform, varying shades of brown, black, blue, red, and/or yellow)
      Diameter (greater than 6 mm [the diameter of a pencil eraser] or different from the rest)
   2. Early detection is the key. Monitor precursor lesions for any change in size, shape, color, or persistent itching.
   3. Education of the patient to monitor lesions and report any changing moles can play a vital role in early detection.

C. Types of melanoma (based on histologic and clinical characteristics)
   1. Superficial spreading melanoma
      a. This type accounts for 70% of cases.
      b. The lesions typically arise from a pre-existing nevus.
      c. This type often displays the classic melanoma features of ABCD.
   2. Lentigo maligna melanoma (Hutchinson freckle)
      a. This type accounts for 10% to 15% of cases.
      b. Lesions are usually on sun-exposed areas of the skin, especially the face.

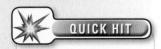

QUICK HIT

The ABCD rule may not effectively screen for nodular melanomas because these do not generally arise in pre-existing nevi.

FIGURE 12-2 ABCD rule for melanoma. Comparison of ABCD rule versus benign moles.

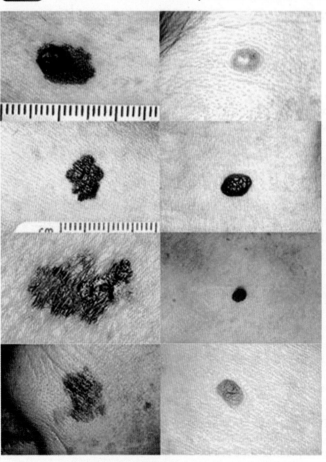

(Courtesy of Public Domain Images from National Cancer Institute Visuals Online.)

Skin and Soft Tissue

     c. Usually seen in the elderly, the disease typically starts as a brown lesion that grows and becomes mottled with black.

     d. The substantial diameter of these lesions makes excision difficult.

  3. Acral lentiginous melanoma

     a. This type accounts for 2% to 8% of cases.

     b. It is the most common melanoma in people of color.

     c. It affects the palms of the hand, the soles of the feet, the fingers, and the toes (including under the nails).

     d. Delay in detection is common because the affected areas are not routinely examined.

  4. Nodular melanoma

     a. This type accounts for 15% to 30% of cases.

     b. The age of onset is lower than that of the superficial spreading variant.

     c. Typically the most aggressive form of melanoma, it does not often display the classic appearance of the disease.

     d. The majority arise de novo in seemingly unaffected skin.

  5. Other: Mucocutaneous and amelanotic melanomas can occur.

D. Staging

  1. Thickness

     a. Clark defined melanoma based on the level of invasion through the layers of the skin. (This is now used to define T1 lesions only.)

       (1) Clark I: in situ

       (2) Clark II: papillary dermis

       (3) Clark III: papillary/reticular dermis junction

       (4) Clark IV: reticular dermis

       (5) Clark V: subcutaneous involvement

     b. Currently, the Breslow method of classification is most used.

       (1) This defines melanoma by its thickness in millimeters.

       (2) Breslow thickness directly correlates with overall survival.

  2. Lymph node status: Involvement of regional lymph nodes is a poor prognostic indicator.

     a. A greater number of involved nodes (especially more than four) and macroscopic involvement of the nodes adversely influences long-term survival.

     b. The 5-year survival rate for persons with involved lymph nodes is 25% to 70%.

  3. Staging using the tumor (thickness), nodal status, and metastasis (TNM) system (Table 12-3)

  4. Other prognostic factors

     a. In stages I to III, ulcerated primary lesions portend a worse prognosis.

     b. The visual presence of mitosis in a field equal to or smaller than 1.0 mm^2 or the presence of regression adversely

     c. These indicators have been shown to be independent prognostic factors.

E. Treatment

  1. Biopsy: Full-thickness biopsy down to subcutaneous fat is required for accurate determination of the Breslow depth.

     a. Remove the entire lesion if possible.

     b. Biopsy the most irregular portion if the lesion is large.

     c. Taking wider margins is not recommended because this may inhibit the ability to perform accurate mapping for sentinel lymph node dissection.

  2. Re-excision is required if the biopsy reveals melanoma. The thickness of the lesion determines if there is a need for sentinel lymph node biopsy at this same surgery.

     a. The re-excision should have margins of 0.5 cm to 2.0 cm, depending on the thickness of the original biopsy, as per the World Health Organization recommendations (Table 12-4).

     b. Studies have shown that there may be higher local recurrence with narrower margins. However, there is no survival advantage with wider margins (e.g., 4 cm vs. 2 cm).

TABLE 12-3	American Joint Committee on Cancer 2009 Revised Melanoma Staging			
			Overall Survival	
Stage	Histologic Features/TNM Classification	1-Year (%)	5-Year (%)	10-Year (%)
0	Intraepithelial/in situ melanoma (TisN0M0)		100	100
IA	≤1 mm without ulceration and mitosis <1/mm^2 (T1aN0M0)		95	88
IB	≤1 mm with ulceration or mitosis ≥1/mm^2 (T1bN0M0)		91	83
	1.01–2 mm without ulceration (T2aN0M0)		89	79
IIA	1.01–2 mm with ulceration (T2bN0M0)		77	64
	2.01–4 mm without ulceration (T3aN0M0)		79	64
IIB	2.01–4 mm with ulceration (T3bN0M0)		63	51
	>4 mm without ulceration (T4aN0M0)		67	54
IIC	>4 mm with ulceration (T4bN0M0)		45	32
IIIA	Single regional nodal micrometastasis, nonulcerated primary (T1-4aN1aM0)		69	63
	Two or three microscopic regional nodes, nonulcerated primary (T1-4aN2aM0)		63	57
IIIB	Single regional nodal micrometastasis, ulcerated primary (T1-4bN1aM0)		53	38
	Two or three microscopic regional nodes, ulcerated primary (T1-4bN2aM0)		50	36
	Single regional nodal macrometastasis, nonulcerated primary (T1-4aN1bM0)		59	48
	Two or three macroscopic regional nodes, nonulcerated primary (T1-4aN2bM0)		46	39
	In-transit met(s)/satellite lesion(s) *without* metastatic lymph nodes (T1-4aN2cM0)		30–50	
IIIC	Single microscopic regional node, ulcerated primary (T1-4bN1bM0)x		29	24
	Two or three macroscopic regional nodes, ulcerated primary (T1-4bN2bM0)		24	15
	Four or more metastatic nodes, matted nodes/gross extracapsular extension, or in-transit met(s)/satellite(s) *and* metastatic nodes (anyTN3M0)		27	18
IV	Distant skin, subcutaneous, or nodal mets with normal LDH (any TanyNM1a)	59	19	16
	Lung mets with normal LDH (anyTanyNM1b)	57	7	3
	All other visceral mets with normal LDH or any distant mets with increased LDH (anyTanyNM1c)	41	9	6

LDH, lactate dehydrogenase.

Below thickness is defined as the thickness of the lesion using an ocular micrometer to measure the total vertical height of the melanoma from the granular layer to the area of deepest penetration. The Clark level refers to levels of invasion according to depth of penetration of the dermis.

(Adapted with permission from Balch CM, Gershenwald JE, Soong SJ, Thompson JF, Atkins MB, Byrd DR, et al. Final version of 2009 AJCC melanoma staging and classification. *J Clin Oncol.* 2009;27(36):6199–6206.)

(Copyright © 2002 The Cleveland Clinic Foundation.)

3. Metastatic evaluation
   a. Determines staging, prognosis, and survival benefit of surgical and adjuvant immunotherapy or chemotherapy and, in conjunction with sentinel lymph node biopsy, prevents unnecessary extensive surgical procedures
      (1) If the lesion is less than 1 mm in depth, current recommendations are to perform no routine testing but to follow the patient with recurrent checkups

TABLE 12-4	Melanoma Thickness and Required Clinical Excision Margin
Melanoma Thickness	**Clinical Excision Margin**
In situ	0.5–1.0 cm
1.0 mm	1.0 cm
1.1–2.0 mm	1.0–2.0 cm
2.1 mm or greater	2.0 cm

Skin and Soft Tissue

(2) For lesions 1 mm or more, no routine tests but may obtain chest X-ray, lactate dehydrogenase, or sentinel lymph node biopsy

(3) For lesions greater than 4 cm, positron emission tomography (PET)/computed tomography (CT) evaluation is recommended. Sentinel lymph node biopsy is controversial.

b. Common sites of metastasis: Melanoma can metastasize anywhere and is one of the few tumors that can cross the placenta and lodge in the fetus.

(1) Liver, skin, gastrointestinal tract

(2) Lung

(a) Observation is indicated to see if further metastasis occurs.

(b) If no further metastasis present, then pulmonary metastasectomy may be considered.

(3) Adrenals: resection if isolated metastases

(4) Bone: radiation for palliation

(5) Brain/central nervous system: some success with resection or "gamma knife"

c. If regional nodes are involved (palpable) at presentation with the primary lesion:

(1) Fine-needle aspiration of the node confirms diagnosis of stage III disease.

(2) CT of the chest/abdomen/pelvis and magnetic resonance imaging of the brain rules out distant disease.

(3) The 5-year survival for patients with palpable nodes at presentation is 40% to 50%.

4. Sentinel lymph node biopsy

a. Two methods for isolating the sentinel lymph node

(1) Lymphazurin: Blue dye injected at the site of the original lesion is seen during surgical exploration of the lymph node bed.

(2) Radiolabeled colloid: This too is injected into the skin near the original lesion and is detected in the lymph node bed by gamma detector probe.

(a) Take the node with the highest count.

(b) Also take all nodes that have counts at least 10% of the "hottest" node removed.

b. These methods have improved the accuracy of finding the sentinel lymph node to over 95%.

c. If the sentinel lymph node is positive for disease, then the patient must undergo a radical lymphadenectomy.

(1) The 5-year survival after lymphadenectomy is 25% to 70%.

(2) Biopsy/removal of the sentinel lymph node has high morbidity, with increased risk of lymphedema, especially in the groin.

d. Follow up

(1) Education of the patient and family for self-examination of the skin

(2) Clinic visits every 3 to 6 months for the first 3 years following a resection to perform skin survey. By this time, 75% of people who are going to have a recurrence have one.

e. Recurrences (local and/or nodal)

(1) Incidence of 0.2% to 13%

(2) Long-term survival is less than 20% in those with a recurrence.

(3) Re-excision is the treatment of choice.

5. Adjuvant therapy: chemotherapy (numerous agents have been tested without demonstration of significant survival advantage)

a. Interferon-alpha has offered some increased survival and is generally indicated for patients with stage III disease and for those with primary tumors greater than 4 mm deep.

b. Limb perfusion with either melphalan or TNF is useful for limb conservation when there are multiple subcutaneous (in-transit metastases) or skin lesions.

(1) No improvement in overall survival

(2) No utility as an adjuvant treatment after surgical resection

c. IL-2 also has shown some survival advantage and is usually combined with dacarbazine-containing chemotherapy regimens.

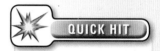

QUICK HIT

If the sentinel lymph node is negative, the patient is 96% likely to have the rest of that nodal basin be negative.

Skin and Soft Tissue

II. Basal Cell Carcinoma

A. Most common form of skin cancer

B. Locally invasive and rarely metastasizes

    1. Main problem is local recurrence due to difficult locations for wide resections such as nose, ear, and periorbital areas.

    2. Those that do metastasize were generally either neglected by patient or have recurred multiple times, and they have a median survival rate of less than 1 year.

C. Types

    1. Nodular

        a. Pearly nodules with central depression

        b. Pruritic

        c. May bleed if irritated (telangiectasias)

    2. Pigmented: dark and often confused with melanoma

    3. Morpheaform, sclerosing, or fibrosing: scar-like, flat, aggressive local invasion

    4. Squamous metaplasia with keratinization: aggressive and may develop lymphatic spread

    5. Ulcerative: raised rolled edges with central ulcer ("rodent")

D. Treatment

    1. Surgical excision with pathologically free margins

        a. Margins are typically only 3 to 4 mm.

        b. Mohs surgery has lowest recurrence rate.

    2. Cryotherapy

    3. Radiation therapy

    4. Electrodesiccation

III. Squamous Cell Carcinoma

A. Derived from the keratinocyte and can deeply invade surrounding structures

B. Appears as a pink, nonhealing sore with ulceration

C. Metastasizes to regional lymph nodes, especially in immunocompromised patients and in those with Marjolin ulcer (Fig. 12-3)

    1. Marjolin ulcer is a squamous cell carcinoma that arises in areas of chronic inflammation, such as old burn scars, hydradenitis, pilonidal cysts, draining osteomyelitis, and skin lesions associated with lupus.

    2. Regional nodal metastases account for 80% to 90% of metastatic squamous cell cancer, whereas metastases to the brain, lung, liver, and bone account for 10% to 20%.

    3. Squamous cell cancers of the mucocutaneous areas, such as the perineum and vulva, as well as those involving the ear or scalp, have highest rates of distant metastatic involvement. Patients with distant metastases have a 10-year survival of 10%.

 FIGURE 12-3 Ulcerative squamous cell carcinoma of the hand. The tumor had eroded through all of the tissues and to the bone. All tissues biopsied (wound base, bone, and skin edge) were positive for squamous cell carcinoma. This patient required forearm amputation.

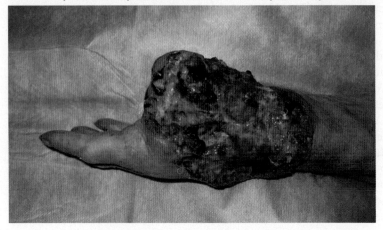

D. Precursor lesions: actinic keratoses, Bowen disease, and erythroplasia of Queyrat
E. Treatment
   1. Surgical excision with pathologically free margins. Margins are typically only 3 to 4 mm for low-risk lesions and 6 mm for high-risk lesions.
   2. Cryotherapy
   3. Radiation therapy
   4. Electrodesiccation
   5. Topical 5-fluorouracil

IV. Merkel Cell Carcinoma
A. Neuroendocrine tumor
B. Aggressive, locally invasive, and high rate of metastasis
C. Five-year survival varies from 88% for stage I disease to 0% for distant metastasis.
D. Order chest X-ray to rule out pulmonary primary tumor because tumor pathology resembles small cell carcinoma of the lung.
E. Appears as a red or purple papulonodule or indurated plaque
F. Has characteristic positive immunocytochemical staining for CK-20. The small round blue cell tumor appears neuroendocrine.
G. Treatment
   1. Wide local excision with 1 to 2 cm margins
   2. Sentinel lymph node biopsy
   3. Radiation to the primary site and nodal bed, if the latter is involved
   4. Use of adjuvant chemotherapy controversial if node-positive disease, with a regimen similar to that used for small cell cancer of the lung

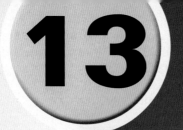

13

Vascular Surgery

Robert Andres, Moungar Cooper, Pamela Zimmerman
and Lakshmikumar Pillai

 INTRODUCTION

Every cell in the human body is critically dependent on oxygen in order to function and maintain homeostasis. Oxygen combined with hemoglobin is carried by the blood and delivered to tissues and cells throughout the body. Waste products of cellular metabolism are then carried to organs that can efficiently excrete them. This vital process is dependent on the heart and the vascular system, the pump, and the tubes.

The vascular tree is composed of the arterial, venous, capillary, and lymphatic systems. The arteries carry oxygenated blood from the heart to the tissue. Gas exchange with oxygen delivery and carbon dioxide takes place at the capillary level, and the blood is then carried back to heart via the venous system. The only exception to this rule is the pulmonary vasculature.

The arterial tree is a high-pressure/low-volume system designed to provide the mechanical and kinetic energy needed to transport blood to peripheral tissues in the body. At any given time, less than one-third of the circulating blood volume is contained within the arterial system. The walls of the arteries are thicker and more adept to elastic recoil during cardiac systole and diastole, hence the pulsatile flow pattern. The only one-way valve in this design is at the origin of the system (i.e., the aortic valve).

The venous side is a low-pressure/high-capacitance multibranched conduit. Veins have a tremendous capacity to accommodate increased or backed-up blood volume. Their walls are thinner and flow is nonpulsatile. The venous system depends on unidirectional valves and the action of peripheral skeletal muscles for continued return of blood back to the heart.

In addition to the body's own natural wear and tear, genetic, environmental, dietary, and iatrogenic factors pose a constant threat to the integrity of the vascular tree. Arterial vascular disease can manifest in the form of narrowing (stenosis, occlusive disease), which impedes blood flow, or enlargement (aneurysm), which risks rupture. Venous disease can take the shape of undue clotting (deep venous thrombosis), valvular incompetency (reflux insufficiency), or localized acute infections (thrombophlebitis). All of these are described in the following text.

 FEMOROPOPLITEAL AND TIBIAL OCCLUSIVE DISEASE

I.   General Principles
   A. This extremely debilitating condition leads to claudication, rest pain, and critical ischemia, resulting in gangrene.
   B. There is an increased risk of cardiovascular and cerebrovascular mortality.
   C. Limb loss rates can be as high as 1% to 5% as a result of infrainguinal disease.

II.   Anatomy
   A. Outflow disease is defined as being distal to the inguinal ligament.
   B. Hunter canal (adductor canal): As the superficial femoral artery courses toward the knee, it passes via the adductor canal. This is the most common site of occlusion below the inguinal ligament.
   C. It is important to identify the collateralization in the lower extremity via the profunda femoris and the geniculate branches at the level of the knee.

TABLE **13-1** Signs of Peripheral Vascular Insufficiency
Progression of Symptoms
Onset, timing, number of events, exercise-induced, alleviation by rest, and rest pain
Reproducibility
Is pain reproducible with stimuli (e.g., walking two blocks, exercise)?
Description of Pain
Burning, paresthesias, severity of pain, loss of activity, and effect on daily living
Skin Changes
Nonhealing ulceration, cyanosis, skin discoloration, gangrene, and muscle wasting

III. Diagnosis (Table 13-1)

A. History: Identify patient symptomatology. Patients often present with exercise-induced lower extremity pain, nonhealing ulcer, and muscle wasting. Eighty percent have a history of smoking.

B. Physical examination: begins with a pulse examination. Identify trophic changes, muscle wasting, thinning of the skin and nails, and loss of hair. Ischemic ulcerations begin as small dry ulcers of the toes or heel and progress to frank gangrene.

C. Noninvasive testing: Check ankle-brachial index (ABI), segmental pressures, and pulse volume recordings. Magnetic resonance angiography and computed tomography (CT) angiography are being increasingly used to identify disease and plan intervention.

D. Diabetes and renal failure make patients more susceptible to arterial insufficiency.

E. In blue toe syndrome, atheroembolic disease moves from an aortoiliac or femoro-popliteal source to the distal microvasculature, resulting in digital ischemia.

IV. Management

A. Risk factor modification: cornerstone for management of lower extremity occlusive disease, which includes blood pressure control, smoking cessation, lipid/diabetes management, weight loss/dietary modifications, and regular exercise (Table 13-2).

B. Medical management: use of HMG CoA reductase inhibitors, aspirin, and pentoxifylline

C. Interventional management options

1. Percutaneous angioplasty: With the advent of low profile balloons and flexible stents, this option is being considered more frequently as a first-line treatment.

   a. It can be performed under local anesthesia, with complications primarily related to the contrast agents (such as renal failure and reaction to the agent) and access site.

   b. Other complications include bleeding, pseudoaneurysm, and distal plaque embolism.

   c. Technical success achieved in 88% to 93% of patients with patency rates up to 60% at 1 year

2. Other operative techniques

   a. Autologous vein bypass: The ipsilateral or contralateral saphenous vein is harvested for bypass around the occluded segments. The vein is reversed to allow flow through the venous valves.

   b. In situ vein bypass: The saphenous vein is identified in its native location. The venous valves are disrupted using a valvulotome, and the bypass is carried out around the occluded segments.

   c. Prosthetic bypass: Cryopreserved vein, Dacron, or PTFE grafts may be utilized to bypass the occlusion. This modality is used primarily for above-the-knee reconstructions when there is well-preserved in continuity popliteal tibial/peroneal artery blood flow distally.

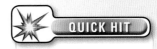

QUICK HIT

Use of preoperative normal saline or sodium bicarbonate hydration prior to using hypo-osmolar/iso-osmolar contrast agents has markedly decreased the incidence of acute renal failure in this population.

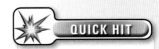

QUICK HIT

Patients with lesions amenable to percutaneous interventions benefit from angiography at the hands of an experienced endovascular surgeon. This ensures the identification of appropriate distal targets, and therapeutic interventions such as angioplasty can be performed with stenting, if possible.

Vascular Surgery

TABLE 13-2 Risk Factors

Established	Recommendations
Hypertension	SBP <140/90
Cigarette smoking	Complete cessation
Hyperlipidemia	Low-density lipoprotein (LDL) <100; high-density lipoprotein (HDL) >35; TG <200
Type 2 diabetes mellitus	HbA1C <7%
Obesity	BMI 18.5–25; waist circumference: women <35 in.; men <40 in.
Exercise	Structured exercise program
Relative	
Age	
Gender	
Lifestyle	
Family history	
Hypercoagulable state	
Homocysteine	

BMI, body mass index; SBP, systolic blood pressure; TG, triglycerides.
With permission from AHA/ACCF Secondary Prevention and Risk Reduction Therapy for Patients with Coronary and Other Atherosclerotic Vascular Disease: 2011 Update.

 ## AORTOILIAC OCCLUSIVE DISEASE

I. General Principles

A. This disease is restricted to the distal aorta and the bilateral common and external iliac arteries.

B. Disease of the aorta and the iliac arteries is referred to as "inflow" disease, and disease distal to the groin is referred to as "outflow" disease.

C. Inflow disease affects the major muscle groups of the pelvis and lower extremities and can result in disabling symptoms.

II. Anatomy

A. The abdominal aorta enters the diaphragmatic hiatus at the level of the 12th thoracic vertebra and bifurcates at the level of the 4th lumbar vertebra.

B. At the level of the bifurcation (approximately the level of the umbilicus) forms the right and left common iliac arteries. The common iliacs curve posteriorly into the sacral hollow and divide into the internal iliac and the external iliac.

C. The internal iliac supplies the pelvic viscera. The external iliac courses anteriorly along the psoas muscle under the inguinal ligament, forming the common femoral artery.

III. Pathophysiology

A. As noted earlier, the disruption in normal laminar flow at the level of the bifurcation results in the formation and organization of plaque. Further plaque deposition results in the augmentation of collaterals around the occlusive segments.

B. These collaterals are not always sufficient to provide flow to the pelvic viscera or lower extremities. When unable to meet the metabolic demands of the lower extremities or pelvis, impotence, buttock claudication, and severe disabling lower extremity pain occurs.

IV. Clinical Features

A. Risk factors (see Table 13-2): Multiple risk factors have been identified in this disease process. These include smoking, hypertension, hyperlipidemia, diabetes mellitus type 2, male sex, older age (age 50 to 60 years), and genetic predisposition.

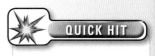

B. Claudication: This denotes an extremely disabling condition with characteristic exercise-induced cramping pain when oxygen supply does not meet demand in active muscles. Pain is relieved by rest.

C. Erectile dysfunction: In men, reduced internal iliac perfusion can lead to erectile dysfunction.

D. Classification
1. Type I: confined to the distal aorta and bilateral iliacs (10%) This often presents in young females with claudication of the buttocks and hips.
2. Type II: most common. More extensive (80%) and involves the aorta, the iliacs, and often the common femoral artery.
3. Type III: involves the femoropopliteal and tibial segments (10%). Patients with type III disease usually present with critical limb ischemia.

QUICK HIT

Disease severity: Type III is greater than type II, which is greater than type I.

V. Diagnosis

A. Physical examination
1. Presence of gangrene
2. Tissue atrophy, especially in the calf
3. Dermal changes such as livedo reticularis suggest proximal occlusive disease with showering of distal microemboli.
4. Presence/absence of pulses in the groin and along the lower extremity
5. Presence of bruits in the abdomen and groin

B. Noninvasive vascular testing
1. Segmental pressure measurements: ABI in a patient with claudication ranges from 0.5 to 0.9, whereas patients with rest pain and tissue loss have ABI less than 0.5 (Table 13-3).
   a. In some scenarios, the ABI at rest may be normal, but with exercise, the ABI may decrease.
   b. A drop of 15% in the ABI after exercise is considered significant.
   c. Also, realize that patients with medial calcinosis (e.g., diabetes mellitus type 2, renal disease) may have falsely elevated ABI.
2. Duplex scanning: Although this can be used to identify occlusion, utility is limited by such factors as the patient's body habitus and operator expertise.

C. Arteriography: This technique involves the use of radiopaque dye to delineate the vascular anatomy/abnormalities of the lower extremity. The patient requires a palpable pulse (either in the femoral artery or an upper extremity artery) to cannulate the vessel for the angiogram (Fig. 13-1).

D. Angiography

E. Leriche syndrome: Classic case of aortoiliac disease that includes claudication, impotence, atrophy, and absent or diminished femoral pulses (Table 13-4).

QUICK HIT

The symptom constellation consisting of lower extremity claudication, gluteal atrophy, impotence, and diminished femoral pulses results in Leriche syndrome.

VI. Management

A. Medical management
1. Smoking cessation: the most important modifiable risk factor that has been shown innumerable times to improve claudicatory symptoms
2. Vigorous exercise program: must be emphasized in patients who are able to exercise. It is thought that exercise increases the anaerobic tolerance in ischemic muscle tissue.

TABLE 13-3 Ankle-Brachial Index

Class	ABI
Normal	1.0
Intermittent claudication	<0.8
Severe claudication	<0.6
Rest pain/tissue loss	<0.3

**FIGURE
13-1** Normal angiogram of a left lower extremity.

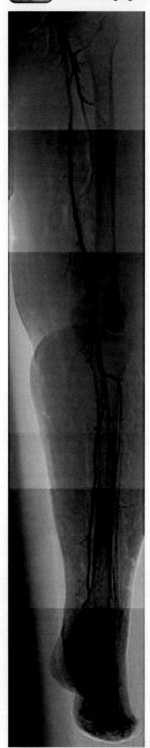

TABLE 13-4   Leriche Syndrome

Claudication	Muscular pain in the calf, buttocks, or groin, usually due to decreased blood flow to these regions
Impotence	Related to decreased flow to the hypogastric
Atrophy	Lower extremities
Absence or diminished	Femoral pulses

3. Aspirin (acetylsalicylic acid [ASA]): Although no specific data support the use of ASA in aorto-occlusive disease, its use must be recommended, considering the benefit in the treatment of occlusive disease in other vascular territories.

4. Pentoxifylline: a phosphodiesterase inhibitor. Its benefit is still unclear; however, trials have shown a small decrease of claudication symptoms with its use.

5. Cilostazol: a phosphodiesterase 3 inhibitor. It results in antiplatelet and vasodilatory effects that are believed to improve walking distance in patients with intermittent claudication. The phosphodiesterase 3 inhibitor properties are detrimental in patients with congestive heart failure and are, therefore, contraindicated in this patient population.

6. Hypertension, diabetes, and hyperlipidemia control: This approach may not reverse the disease but certainly may prevent its progression.

B. Surgical management
1. Endovascular techniques
   a. Percutaneous access followed by balloon angioplasty with a stent has shown some promise for short segment, nonocclusive disease in the iliacs.
   b. Complications include perforation, dissection, thrombosis, and distal embolism.

2. Aortoiliac endarterectomy: usually reserved for focal type I disease in the distal aorta. This operation can provide excellent results provided there is no aneurysmal dilation of the distal aorta. The procedure involves an arteriotomy with careful dissection to remove the plaque from the aortic wall.

3. Arterial reconstruction with anatomically placed prosthesis: involves the use of a Dacron or polytetrafluoroethylene (PTFE) graft from the proximal aorta to the iliacs or femorals. The orientation of the graft is similar to the anatomy of the vasculature.

4. Arterial reconstruction with extra-anatomically placed prosthesis
   a. In patients with a hostile abdomen or in poor-risk patients, inflow can be derived from the axillary artery.
   b. A PTFE graft is used connecting the axillary artery to the femoral artery. A second piece of graft is used connecting the two femoral arteries. This provides blood flow to the extremities using the axillary artery as inflow. The patency rates are lower than aortobifemoral prosthesis.

 ## ANEURYSMAL VASCULAR DISEASE

I. General Principles

- Important definitions/descriptions include:

A. Aneurysm (derived from the Greek word *aneurysma*): a permanent localized enlargement that is 1.5 times or greater than the diameter of the normal proximal artery

B. Arterial ectasia: a localized enlargement less than 1.5 times of normal diameter

C. Arteriomegaly: generalized arterial enlargement in contiguous vessels, less than 1.5 times normal and a well recognized risk factor for progression to aneurysmal proportions

D. True aneurysm: enlargement composed of all three layers (tunics) of the vessel wall

E. False aneurysm: Also known as pseudoaneurysms, they lack at least one and sometimes all three layers of the vessel wall. Blood is contained by perivascular connective tissue and, if present, the tunica adventitia.

F. Aortic dissection: passage of blood from the arterial lumen into the arterial wall, thereby creating a false lumen. The false lumen may reestablish flow back into the main arterial lumen and become a double-barrel system.

G. Dissecting aneurysm: aortic dissection with aneurysmal dilatation of the false lumen. These are prone to rupture.

H. Mycotic aneurysm: refers to any aneurysms that result from direct infectious process resulting in destruction of the supportive tissue in the arterial wall. These compose a small (<5%) proportion of all aneurysms. Bacteria and fungi are the most commonly implicated organisms.

I. Syphilitic aneurysm: Although extremely rare in this day and age, this is characteristic of tertiary syphilis and occurs secondary to inflammatory disease of the ascending thoracic aorta.

The most common cause of false aneurysms is trauma to the blood vessel. This includes iatrogenic insults.

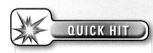

The proximal aorta is distinguished from the distal aorta by presence of the renal vessels.

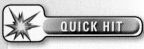

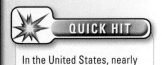

J. Infrarenal aneurysm: aneurysm with a normal-caliber aorta between the renal arteries and the aneurysm

K. Juxtarenal aneurysm: involves the renal arteries or is within 1 cm of the renal arteries

II. Abdominal Aortic Aneurysms (AAAs)

A. Anatomy (Fig. 13-2): The abdominal aorta is a direct continuation of the thoracic aorta as it passes through the aortic hiatus in the diaphragm. It lies in the retroperitoneum and slightly to the left of midline. It bifurcates into the right and left common iliac arteries at the level of L4.

1. The major branches include the celiac axis, superior mesenteric artery, renal artery, and the inferior mesenteric artery.

2. Other named vessels of clinical interest are the inferior phrenic, gonadal, and lumbar arteries.

3. There are two main types of aneurysms: fusiform and saccular (Fig. 13-3).

B. Epidemiology

1. AAAs affect about 1% to 3% of the general population. Aging of the population and increasing use of routine radiographic studies has resulted in an increase in the prevalence of AAA.

FIGURE 13-2 AAA. CT of (A) axial, (B) coronal, and (C) sagittal cross sections.

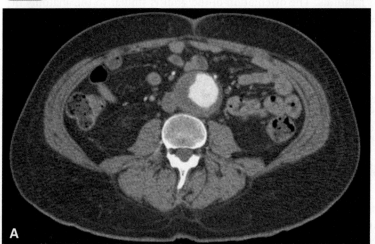

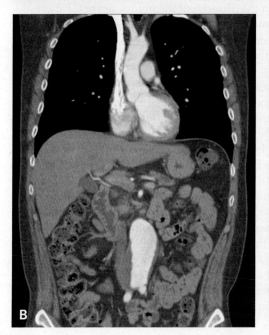

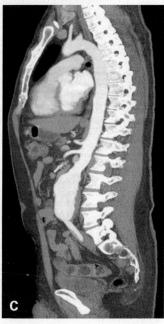

FIGURE 13-3 A. Fusiform and (B) saccular aneurysms.

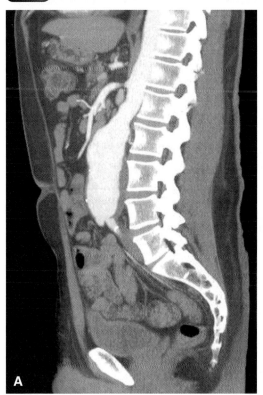
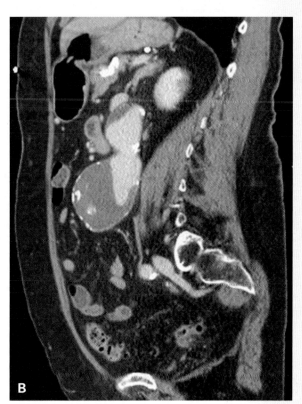

A

B

2. AAAs are the 13th leading cause of death in all age groups.
   a. They are the third leading cause of sudden death in males older than 70 years of age.
   b. Ruptured AAAs account for 15,000 deaths per year in the United States.
C. Risk factors for AAA (Table 13-5)
   1. Smoking: This is by far the single most important environmental risk factor. The prevalence of AAA in smokers is four times that of nonsmokers.
   2. Age: Natural tissue degeneration and atherosclerosis increase with age and predispose to the formation of aneurysms. Most patients are 65 years of age and older.
   3. Gender: Males are at least six times more likely to develop AAA than women

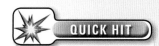

QUICK HIT

Comparison of the relative risks for different diseases in chronic smokers shows that the risk of developing AAA is threefold more than the risk of developing coronary artery disease and nearly fivefold more than the risk for cerebrovascular disease.

TABLE 13-5 **Risk Factors for Abdominal Aortic Aneurysm**
Established
Smoking: accounts for 75% of aneurysms >4 cm
Gender: males six times more common than females; size for size, women three times more likely to rupture
Family history: doubles risk
Hypertension
Relative
Caucasian
Atherosclerosis
Hypertension
Femoral/popliteal aneurysms
Obesity

TABLE **13-6** Risk Factor for Rupture of an Abdominal Aortic Aneurysm
Size: single most important factor; law of Laplace
Hypertension
Smoking
Gender
Family history

4. Infections: Salmonellosis and tuberculosis have been implicated in the formation of certain aneurysms.
5. Connective tissue disorders: Individuals with Marfan syndrome and Ehlers–Danlos type IV have an increased risk of aneurysm.

D. Risk factors for rupture of AAA—which patients need elective surgery (Table 13-6)
1. Size: the single most important factor. According to the Laplace law, the tension on the wall of a fluid-containing structure is a product of the radius and pressure ($T = P \times r$). Increasing size not only results in increasing wall tension but also implies weakening of the aortic wall. Generally, aneurysms 5.5 cm or larger should be repaired.
2. Hypertension: The second variable in the Laplace equation, hypertension (uncontrolled) can result in rapid enlargement of the aneurysm and a higher risk of rupture for any given size of aneurysm.
3. Smoking: Especially if there is associated chronic obstructive pulmonary disease (COPD), smoking is an independent risk factor for rapid enlargement and eventual rupture of AAA.
4. Gender: Although AAA are more common in males, size for size, females are at three times the risk of rupture. The recent increasing popularity of smoking among females is drawing the statistics closer between males and females.
5. Family history: There is a clear association here, as 25% of patients who present with AAA rupture have a first-degree relative with a history of a ruptured AAA.

E. Clinical features and diagnosis
1. Most AAA are asymptomatic and are discovered incidentally.
2. Symptoms can be due to mass effect and irritation of regional sensory nerves (i.e., back and/or abdominal pain) or due to showering of clots distally (thromboembolism).
3. Abdominal sonography is a good screening and surveillance tool. In experienced hands, the accuracy can reach margins of 3 mm.
4. CT scans with intravenous (IV) contrast and high resolution serve as confirmatory evidence and also help with surgical planning and approach.

F. Management (Table 13-7)
1. The decision to electively repair AAA is based on size and associated risk factors. The surgeon needs to weigh risk of rupture versus risks and complications of surgery. In the absence of significant risk factors for rupture, aneurysms smaller than 5 cm can be followed by surveillance sonography or CT scans.

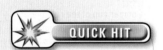

QUICK HIT

Nonspecific back and abdominal pain in older patients warrants thorough investigation with physical examination and radiographic imaging.

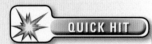

QUICK HIT

Because of its retroperitoneal location, back pain may be the presenting feature of AAA.

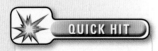

QUICK HIT

Sonography is an excellent screening modality, but it is an operator-dependent test. If there is poor visualization with a sonogram, the results should be adjudicated with a CT scan.

TABLE **13-7** Management of Abdominal Aortic Aneurysms
<5.5 cm
Follow-up screening with either abdominal ultrasound or with CT scan every 6 months.
≥5.5 cm, presence of symptoms or rapidly expanding (>5 mm per 6 months)
Surgical repair

TABLE 13-8	Annual Risk of Rupture
Size (cm)	Risk of Rupture
3–4	<0.5%
4–5	0.5%–5%
5–6	3%–15%
6–7	10%–20%
7–8	20%–40%
>8	30%–50%

2. Symptomatic aneurysm (i.e., aneurysms that are tender to palpation) and those that are rapidly enlarging (more than 5 mm/6 months) should be repaired electively. As shown in Table 13-8, the annual risk of rupture significantly increases with increasing size of the aneurysm.

3. In patients who warrant surgical treatment, there are three different techniques: endovascular aneurysm repair (EVAR), open transperitoneal, and open retroperitoneal. Circulation of pressurized blood through the aneurysm sac is responsible for expansion and eventual rupture of all aneurysms.

   a. The choice of procedure is determined by several factors, most importantly the anatomy of the aneurysm. When trying to decide on the most suitable approach key factors to keep in mind, include previous history, including surgical history; unusual anatomic features on the CT scan; and comorbid conditions. One such memory tool is outlined in Figure 13-4.

   b. The basic principle of all three techniques is to channel blood from the normal-caliber aorta proximally to the normal-caliber aorta or iliacs distally, thereby excluding the aneurysm from the circulation. This is achieved by placing nonexpansile yet durable synthetic tubes (grafts) in the aorta at the two ends of the aneurysm. In the open approach, the graft is sutured to the aorta using a nonabsorbable suture. In EVAR, the graft is attached to the aorta by metallic hooks.

G. Ruptured AAA

   1. Most feared complication of AAA

   2. Carries an overall mortality rate of more than 80%

FIGURE 13-4 Ruptured AAA. CT of (A) axial and (B) coronal views.

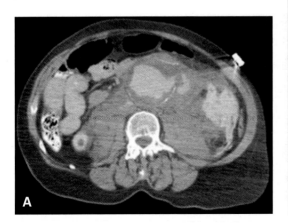
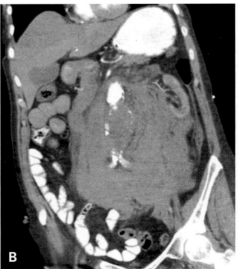

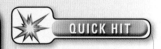

3. Presents with acute abdominal pain, back pain, and hypotension
4. Immediate operative intervention is the only treatment that can offer hope for survival.

H. Inflammatory AAA
1. Inflammatory AAAs represent about 5% of all infrarenal AAAs.
2. There is usually a dense fibroinflammatory tissue that may be adherent to the fourth portion of the duodenum, inferior vena cava, and left renal vein.
3. These aneurysms can also have associated ureteral involvement with renal outflow obstruction.
4. Patients can present with pain, weight loss, and elevated erythrocyte sedimentation rate.
5. CT scan is diagnostic and shows four layers: aortic lumen, luminal clot (thrombus), thickened aortic wall, and adjacent inflammatory tissue.
6. Inflammatory aneurysms are less prone to rupture.
7. This is a technical challenge, and most surgeons prefer either EVAR or the open retroperitoneal approach.

III. Thoracic Aorta: Aneurysms and Dissections

A. Anatomy: Thoracoabdominal aortic aneurysms (TAAs) refer to fixed aortic dilatation, starting anywhere from the descending thoracic aorta from the left subclavian to the aortic bifurcation. The aneurysmal segments of the aorta may involve intercostal arteries, celiac axis, superior and inferior mesenterica, renals, and gonadal vessels.

B. Classification: DeBakey (type I – III) and Stanford (A and B) (Table 13-9 and Fig. 13-5)

C. Etiology: The majority of these aneurysms are due to degenerative changes secondary to abnormal collagen and elastin metabolism. Previous chronic aortic dissections are the second most common cause. Connective tissue disorders, trauma, and vasculitis (especially Takayasu aortitis) make up a small percentage.

D. Clinical features: Most TAAs, like most AAAs, are discovered incidentally. When symptomatic, TAAs can present with pain or signs of distal embolization. Mass effect symptoms include dyspnea and dysphagia from compression of the aerodigestive tract or ascites, visceromegaly, and lower extremity swelling from caval compression.

E. Management: Surgical repair, as with AAAs, comprises replacement of diseased aortic segment by an artificial graft. The approach requires gaining exposure in the thoracic as well as the abdominal cavities. The complex anatomy of TAA makes their repair a surgical challenge.
1. Indications for repair include the presence of symptoms that are attributable to the aneurysm. In the absence of symptoms, size greater than 6 cm or increase in size of more than 0.5 cm per 6-month interval are accepted criteria for elective repair.
2. To the operating team, perfusion of the spinal cord and abdominal viscera during the aortic clamping is of paramount importance. Cerebral spinal fluid (CSF) drainage is necessary to maintain perfusion of spinal cord. This is best achieved by a specialized team approach.

TABLE 13-9 Classification of Thoracoabdominal Aortic Aneurysms		
DeBakey	**Description**	**Percentage**
Type I	Ascending and descending aorta (most common)	60%
Type II	Ascending only	10%–15%
Type III	Descending only	25%–30%
Stanford	**Description**	
A	Proximal (DeBakey type I and II)	
B	Distal (type III)	

FIGURE 13-5 Classification systems for acute aortic dissection. Shown are the DeBakey and Stanford (Daily) classification systems.

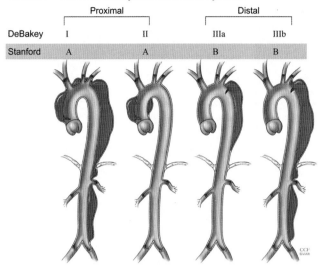

	Proximal		Distal	
DeBakey	I	II	IIIa	IIIb
Stanford	A	A	B	B

(Used with permission from Topol EJ, Califf RM, Prystowski EM, Thomas JD. *Textbook of Cardiovascular Medicine.* 3rd ed. Philadelphia, PA: Lippincott Williams & Wilkins; 2006.)

3. Like AAAs, TAAs are also amenable to thoracic endovascular aortic repair (TEVAR). TEVAR and fenestrated grafts have demonstrated excellent results for treatment of such lesions in patients with suitable or modifiable anatomy. If the subclavian artery is covered by the endograft, the patient may require revascularization of the left subclavian if the patient has a patent left internal mammary artery coronary bypass, the left vertebral artery terminates in the posterior inferior cerebellar artery, an occluded right vertebral, or planned extensive coverage of more than 20 cm of aorta. Open repair and debranching can be undertaken but will result in higher morbidity and mortality.

4. Thoracic aorta injury: TEVAR is considered first-line treatment for thoracic aorta transection (Fig. 13-6).

5. Thoracic aorta dissections: Type A aortic dissections are a surgical emergency. Medical management with blood pressure control is still the standard of care for type B dissections. Invasive intervention is reserved for failure of medical management or the presence of a complication such as malperfusion or rupture.

IV. Femoral and Popliteal Aneurysms

A. Epidemiology and etiology

1. Almost 90% of the peripheral aneurysms are found in the femoral and popliteal arteries.

2. Popliteal aneurysms alone make up about 70% of the peripheral aneurysms. The majority are secondary to degenerative atherosclerotic disease and are predominantly an affliction of men.

B. Clinical features: These aneurysms, although not life threatening, can certainly be limb threatening in a number of ways. Accumulation of thrombus, distal propagation, and limb-threatening ischemia can often be the presenting catastrophic features. Other symptoms include pain secondary to nerve compression or edema and venous thrombosis secondary to venous outflow obstruction.

C. Diagnosis

1. Due to its deep location, the popliteal artery is barely palpable in normal individuals. Prominent pulsation in the popliteal fossa is an indication that the patient may be harboring a popliteal aneurysm. Finding an aneurysm in these vessels should prompt a thorough evaluation because 50% are bilateral and 30% have an aortic aneurysm associated with them.

FIGURE
13-6 **Aortic transection.**

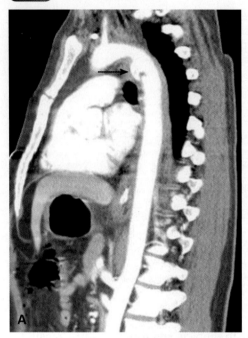

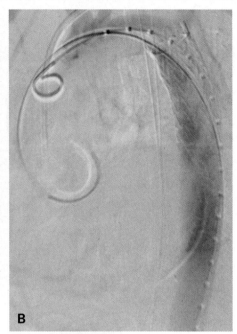

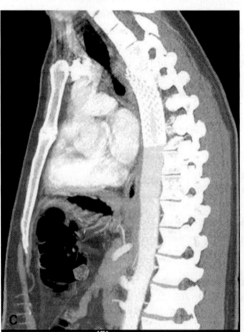

A. Sagittal cross section of computed tomography angiography (CTA) of the chest. Imaging is remarkable for aortic transection as noted by the arrow. **B.** Angiogram after deployment of the thoracic aorta graft (TAG). **C.** Postoperative CTA demonstrating no further evidence of aortic transection.

    2. If suspected by physical examination, duplex ultrasonography can be used to confirm the anatomic configuration as well as the flow dynamics of the aneurysmal segment.

  D. Management: Indications for intervention include thromboembolic complications and size. It is generally agreed that femoral aneurysms of greater than 2.5 cm and popliteal aneurysms of greater than 2.0 cm should be repaired. Here, unlike AAAs, replacement with artificial graft is generally unnecessary, and usage of autogenous vein is feasible. Endovascular treatment with placement of covered stents that can exclude the aneurysm from the circulation is also a popular approach.

V. Splenic Artery Aneurysms

A. Splenic artery aneurysms (SAAs) are the most common of the visceral artery aneurysms. After the aorta and iliacs, they are the third most common intra-abdominal aneurysms.

B. Unlike most aneurysms, SAAs are predominantly a disease of the female sex. Moreover, there is a close association with parity. More than 90% females with SAAs have been pregnant at least once.

C. Like most aneurysms, SAAs are asymptomatic.

D. Indications for treatment are presence of symptoms, documented enlargement, pregnancy or anticipated pregnancy, and diameter of greater than 2.5 cm. SAA discovered during pregnancy should be repaired because pregnancy greatly increases the risk of rupture.

E. All potential surgical candidates should receive preoperative immunizations, similar to splenectomy patients (i.e., *Haemophilus, Pneumococcus, Meningococcus,* influenza). However, aneurysm repair with splenic preservation is the ideal treatment.

F. The main complication of SAA is rupture.

VI. Renal Artery Aneurysms

A. Aneurysms of the renal artery are the second most common visceral aneurysm. Even so, they occur in about 0.09% of the general population. They are more commonly seen in the female multiparous population.

B. They, like other aneurysms, are discovered as incidental lesions. Most are associated with hypertension.

C. Indications for surgery
   1. Difficult-to-control hypertension
   2. Size of greater than 2 cm
   3. In the majority of cases, excellent response with blood pressure control is seen.

VII. Mycotic Aneurysms

A. Mycotic aneurysms result from localized infection, which may be a consequence of periaortic infectious process, or due to aortic intimal seeding from bloodborne pathogens. The most common infectious bacteria are *Staphylococcus aureus* and *Salmonella typhi*, and the most common fungal agents are *Candida albicans* and *Aspergillus fumigatus*. Bacterial infections are more common than fungal infections. The usual sites are the femoral arteries and the aorta.

B. Clinical presentation can be nonspecific but with recurrent bacteremia or fungemia. Fevers, chills, and tenderness not attributable to size alone should prompt the physician to include an infected aneurysm in the differential diagnosis.

C. Management is resection and repair of the aneurysm, thorough debridement of infected tissue, and lifelong antibiotic treatment.

VIII. Pseudoaneurysms

A. Pseudoaneurysms (PSAs) are contained arterial disruptions. The main types are traumatic and postsurgical.
   1. Traumatic PSAs are usually iatrogenic and are a result of arterial punctures for various procedures. Because the femoral artery is the most common site for such procedures, iatrogenic PSAs are predominantly found in this area.
   2. Postsurgical PSAs are due to contained suture line disruptions between the arterial wall and graft material.

B. The diagnosis can be made readily by duplex sonography.

C. Traumatic PSAs greater than 2.5 cm are treated by injection of thrombin, a procoagulant, in the cavity of the PSA under sonographic guidance. Those that do not respond to this approach require open surgery to repair the localized disruption in the vessel wall.
   1. Asymptomatic, traumatic PSAs less than 2.5 cm do not require treatment.
   2. Postsurgical PSAs most often require revision of the surgical site suture line.

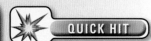

QUICK HIT

In 10% of the population, the left common carotid artery comes off the brachiocephalic trunk.

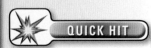

QUICK HIT

The carotid bifurcation is most commonly affected due to increased turbulent flow in this area.

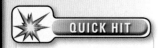

QUICK HIT

In trauma to the cervical vertebrae, the vertebral arteries also need to be studied to prevent any missed injuries.

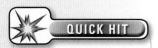

QUICK HIT

There is potential for multiple collaterals in the cerebral vasculature. These collaterals become the source of blood supply when arterial occlusive disease develops in one of the four major arteries supplying the brain.

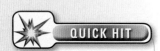

QUICK HIT

There are some recent data implicating the endopeptidase metalloproteinase-9 in plaque disruption and embolization. The clinical significance/utility is yet to be confirmed.

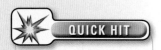

QUICK HIT

The supraclinoid portion of the carotid, intracranially, gives rise to the ophthalmic, posterior communicating, and the anterior choroidal arteries. Ophthalmic artery occlusion is often the initial indicator of carotid occlusive disease (amaurosis fugax).

 CEREBROVASCULAR OCCLUSIVE DISEASE

I. Anatomy
   A. Divisions of the aorta
      1. Ascending aorta courses anteriorly from the left ventricle.
      2. Branches of the ascending aorta
         a. Brachiocephalic trunk (innominate artery): The aorta courses from a right anterior to left posterior position in the upper mediastinum. The first and most anterior branch is the innominate artery. At the right clavicular head, it splits into the right common carotid and the right subclavian artery.
         b. Left common carotid artery: arises 1 cm from the innominate and courses posteriorly into the left base of the neck
         c. Left subclavian artery: located posterior and at the distal end of the aortic arch
   B. Divisions of the common carotid artery
      1. External carotid artery: The common carotid bifurcates at the angle of the mandible to form the internal and external carotid. The external carotid splits to form the ascending pharyngeal artery, superior thyroidal artery, lingual artery, occipital artery, posterior auricular artery, and superficial temporal arteries.
      2. Internal carotid artery: Main divisions of the internal carotid artery are the intrapetrosal, intracavernous, and supraclinoid arteries.
   C. Divisions of the subclavian artery
      1. Vertebral artery: This artery arises from the first portion of the subclavian and enters the foramina transversum at the level of the sixth cervical vertebra. It gains intracerebral access through the foramen magnum.

II. Epidemiology
   A. Each year, 500,000 individuals suffer from stroke. The Framingham study (1975) noted that 62% of all stroke victims exhibit decreased socialization, 71% are dependent on other means of mobility, and 16% are institution bound.
   B. Stroke is the third most common cause of death in the United States. About 200,000 individuals die as a result of stroke annually.
   C. Public health costs for disabilities related to stroke exceed $16 trillion a year.

III. Etiology and Pathophysiology
   A. Atherosclerotic/embolic strokes
      1. Most common cause of cerebrovascular occlusive disease (Fig. 13-7)
      2. Risk factors include advanced age, hypertension, diabetes, hyperlipidemia, positive family history, tobacco use, hypercoagulable state, and elevated homocysteine levels.
      3. Occlusion is thought to occur secondary to focal vessel wall injury in areas of turbulent blood flow. Brownian movement of blood results in particulate deposition and atherosclerotic plaque. An endothelium-lined fibrous cap usually covers this plaque. Disruption of the cap causes platelet deposition. Platelet aggregates or plaque material may embolize, resulting in stroke.

IV. Clinical Features
   A. Transient ischemic attack (TIA): sudden onset of focal neurologic deficit that resolves in 24 hours. Manifestations include hemispheric deficit (e.g., sensory or motor), transient monocular blindness (amaurosis fugax), and drop attacks/falls (from vertebrobasilar TIA).
   B. Hemispheric stroke: An embolic event in the cerebral circulation typically occurs in the watershed area of the brain and is manifested as contralateral sensory or motor loss, a prominent visual field defect, and aphasia or partial inattention. Strokes of the posterior circulation may cause ataxia, vertigo, diplopia, syncope, and nystagmus.

CTA of the head and neck demonstrates a diminutive right internal carotid artery with critical stenosis (*arrow*) when compared to the contralateral side (A). Imaging taken further cranially additionally demonstrates the presence of calcified thrombus/plaques (*arrows*) (B). Sagittal cross-section shows a filling defect in the proximal portion of the right internal carotid (C).

FIGURE 13-7

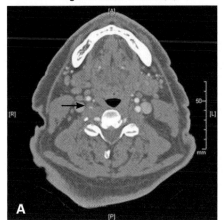

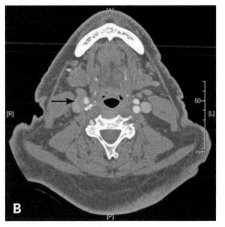

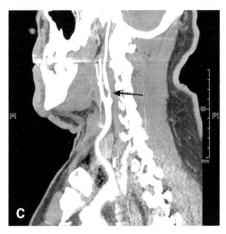

C. Carotid bruits: These are usually detected on routine physical examination and are reported in 5% of the population older than 60 years of age.
   1. There is a poor correlation between the presence of carotid bruit and stenosis.
   2. Less than 23% of patients with a carotid bruit actually have disease greater than 50% stenosis.

V. Management
A. Medical management
   1. Lifestyle modification (e.g., weight loss, smoking cessation)
   2. Control of hypertension and diabetes
   3. Aspirin (ASA): to prevent platelet aggregation. Data support the use of ASA for symptomatic disease with a 22% risk reduction in recurrent TIA when compared to controls. ASA also improves mortality from coronary artery disease.
   4. Clopidogrel (antiplatelet agent): This also has been shown to have a relative risk reduction in the incidence of TIA, myocardial infarction (MI), and death.
   5. Lipid-lowering agents: The 3-hydroxy-3-methylglutaryl coenzyme A (HMG CoA) reductase inhibitors may be of benefit. However, the data are still inconclusive.
   6. Anticoagulation: This treatment is only recommended in patients with embolic stroke from atrial fibrillation (Table 13-10).

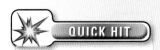

QUICK HIT

A cholesterol crystal in the retinal artery results in the characteristic Hollenhorst plaque. However, an ophthalmologic examination within 24 hours of the episode may not reveal this. Classically, patients describe the occurrence of amaurosis as a shade being pulled down on the affected side.

Vascular Surgery

TABLE **13-10**	**CHADS2 Score (Risk of Stroke in Patients with Nonrheumatic Atrial Fibrillation)**	
	Criteria	**Points**
C	Congestive heart failure	1
H	Hypertension (consistently >140)	1
A	Age >75 years	1
D	Diabetes	1
S2	Stroke or TIA	2

B. Surgical management
  1. Carotid endarterectomy (CEA)
      a. Indications for CEA (Table 13-11): The risk of stroke is substantially increased, irrespective of the degree of stenosis, after a TIA or stroke (10% to 40%). This clearly indicates the need for an intervention in this scenario. In asymptomatic patients, there is a clear risk reduction in stroke if the degree of luminal stenosis is 80% or greater.
      b. Procedure for CEA: anatomy of carotid sheath. Exposure of the carotid artery is achieved by an incision over the medial border of the sternomastoid muscle. It is important to minimize the degree of manipulation in order to prevent embolization of plaque. A temporary plastic shunt may be placed prior to vessel occlusion. Following adequate exposure, the common, internal, and external carotid vessels are clamped. An arteriotomy is performed, and the plaque is gently dissected off the inner vessel wall. The arteriotomy is closed using a vein or synthetic patch. Studies have shown that restenosis rates and thrombosis rates are lower with the use of a patch.
      c. Contraindications for CEA: The main contraindications to repair include an acute profound stroke, a stroke in evolution, or complete occlusion of the internal carotid.
      d. Postoperative/intervention complications: These include perioperative plaque embolization with stroke, injury to the recurrent laryngeal nerve (causes hoarseness), injury to the hypoglossal nerve (causes the tongue to deviate to the side of the injury), and injury to the superior laryngeal nerve (causes voice to fatigue easily) (Table 13-12). Non-neurologic complications can also occur postoperatively. Bleeding can result in neck swelling/hematoma resulting in airway compromise, requiring re-exploration.
  2. Endovascular therapy: The U.S. Food and Drug Administration has approved the use of endovascular therapy for treatment of carotid stenosis in very

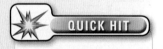

QUICK HIT

The most common postoperative complication after a CEA is MI.

TABLE **13-11**	**Indications and Contraindications for Endarterectomy**

Indications

Previous cerebrovascular accident: Risk is substantially increased (irrespective of degree of stenosis) by 10%–40%.
Asymptomatic with >80% stenosis

Contraindications

Acute profound stroke
Stroke in evolution
100% occlusion

TABLE 13-12 Complications of Carotid Endarterectomy	
Deficit	**Injury**
Hoarseness	Recurrent laryngeal: most common injury, secondary to vascular clamping during procedure
Tongue deviation	Hypoglossal: deviation to side of injury
Difficulty swallowing	Glossopharyngeal: infrequent but most dreaded of complications, occurs with high carotid lesions
Smile (droopy oral commissure)	Facial: marginal mandibular branch

specific instances. For example, it may be used in high-risk patients such as those with recent MI, poor ejection fraction, severe COPD, carotid restenosis, prior neck dissection, radiation to neck, or contralateral recurrent nerve injury (Table 13-13).

3. Aortic root reconstruction: performed in cases of brachiocephalic occlusion via median sternotomy approach
4. Vertebral artery reconstruction: performed for vertebral occlusion. The vertebral artery is usually ligated, and the distal portion is transposed to the ipsilateral carotid.

SPLANCHNIC OCCLUSIVE DISEASE

A. Occlusive disease of the splanchnic circulation is fairly uncommon.
B. Most patients remain asymptomatic, with occlusion of two of three of the following arteries: the celiac, superior mesenteric, and inferior mesenteric arteries, which have a rich collateral network among the three vessels. These arteries supply the gastrointestinal tract. Symptoms begin when the third becomes occluded.
C. Within this large scope of disease, three specific entities will be discussed.
   1. Acute splanchnic ischemia (Table 13-14)
      a. This occurs primarily due to embolus from a cardiac source or due to thrombosis of a partially occluded native vessel.
      b. Patients often present with acute onset of pain that is clearly out of proportion to the clinical examination. This warrants urgent attention before the ischemia results in frank necrosis and perforation of the bowel.
      c. Treatment begins with active resuscitation followed by the administration of heparin and possibly catheter-directed thrombolysis with thrombolytics

TABLE 13-13 Indications for Endovascular Therapy with Angioplasty and Stent Placement
Recent MI
Poor ejection fraction
Severe COPD
Recurrent carotid stenosis
Prior neck dissection
Previous radiation to the head and neck
Contralateral recurrent nerve injury
High or low carotid artery bifurcation

TABLE 13-14	Acute versus Chronic Mesenteric Ischemia	
	Acute Mesenteric Ischemia	**Chronic Mesenteric Ischemia**
Pain	Acute	Acute or chronic
Food fear	No	Yes
Weight loss	No	Yes
A-fib association	Yes	No
Hypertension association	No	Yes

such as tissue plasminogen activator. Alternatively, a surgical embolectomy may be performed.

2. Chronic splanchnic ischemia (see Table 13-14)
   a. This syndrome occurs as a result of arteriosclerosis at the origins of the major vascular supply of the intestine.
   b. Symptoms often involve postprandial pain (intestinal angina) with associated profound weight loss. Patients often develop food fear due to pain.
   c. Workup is often undertaken when there is a strong index of suspicion and involves arterial duplex and possible magnetic resonance angiography or CT angiography.
   d. The treatment is revascularization with vein graft or angioplasty with stent.
3. Renovascular occlusive disease
   a. This is the most common form of surgically correctable hypertension.
   b. Renal artery occlusion causes decreased blood flow to the kidneys with resultant activation of the renin-angiotensin axis. This activation causes hypertension. Occlusion may either result from arteriosclerosis or fibromuscular dysplasia.
   c. Treatment involves angioplasty with stenting or aortorenal bypass.

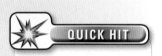

QUICK HIT

Fibromuscular dysplasia often affects young women and is related to increased estrogen production. It is amenable, with excellent results, to angioplasty and stenting.

UPPER EXTREMITY OCCLUSIVE DISEASE

I. General Principles
   A. This debilitating condition is associated with severe pain, and patients often are disabled from occupations and are unable to perform daily activities.
   B. Lesions that are more proximal are more amenable to surgical correction, and the lesions that are more distal require aggressive medical management.

II. Diagnosis
   A. History of pain, exercise-induced fatigue, occupational exposure (such as in cases of thoracic outlet syndrome or vibration syndromes), and medical conditions (e.g., arteritis, fibromuscular dysplasia, azotemic arteritis in end-stage renal disease, postradiation arteritis)
   B. Raynaud phenomenon: This phenomenon is described as episodic color change in the digits secondary to hypothermia and emotional stimuli. It is thought to occur due to vasospasm (causes pallor), followed by cyanosis (as tissue oxygenation is completed), and finally hyperemia from reperfusion.
   C. Examination of the extremity should include palpation of the pulse along the length of the extremity. An Allen test should be performed to evaluate the adequacy of blood flow to the hand.
   D. Noninvasive testing including plethysmography, transcutaneous Doppler, and duplex scanning should be performed to assess for occlusion in the upper extremity.
   E. Thoracic outlet syndrome (Table 13-15) can be a very debilitating condition leading to ischemia and arm pain. This results from compression of nerve, artery,

TABLE **13-15** **Thoracic Duct Components**
Brachial plexus
Subclavian artery
Subclavian vein

or vein at the space between the first thoracic rib and clavicle, between the pectoralis minor and the coracoid process, or the head of the humerus while the patient externally rotates the arm.

III. Management

A. Lifestyle modification includes smoking cessation, avoidance of cold, and avoidance of occupational exposure (vibratory injury in patients with digital ischemia).

B. Short segments of occlusion in the upper extremity may require bypass grafting or angioplasty, with or without stent, to increase blood flow to the arm.

C. Treatment for thoracic outlet syndrome may involve a first rib resection and anterior scalenectomy to relieve pressure.

D. In cases of occlusions in the palmar arch, which are not amenable to surgical therapy, nifedipine may be helpful.

E. Arteritis may be treated with steroids.

VENOUS DISEASE: ACUTE VENOUS THROMBOEMBOLIC DISEASE

I. Acute Lower Extremity Deep Vein Thrombosis: Proximal Vessels

A. Epidemiology

1. Incidence of deep vein thrombosis (DVT): about 250,000 patients per year, with 200,000 patients also with pulmonary embolism (PE)

2. Risk factors: age, malignancy, immobilization, surgery and trauma, oral contraceptives, hormone replacement, pregnancy, neurologic disease (spinal cord injury), cardiac disease, obesity, and genetic hypercoagulable state (Table 13-16)

B. Pathogenesis and clinical features

1. Most thromboses affect the iliac, femoral, or popliteal lower limb veins. The deep venous system includes the common femoral, femoral (or superficial femoral), deep femoral, popliteal, and tibial veins.

2. After thrombus formation, an acute and chronic inflammatory response leads to thrombus amplification, organization, and recanalization, often with vein wall and valve damage.

TABLE **13-16** **Risk Factors for Deep Vein Thrombosis (DVT)**
Established
Age
Malignancy
Prior DVT
Prior PE
Congenital hypercoagulability (factor V Leiden)
Oral contraceptives
Trauma
Obesity

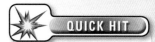

QUICK HIT

Because of the anterior position of the innominate artery, it is accessible for reconstruction by a median sternotomy approach.

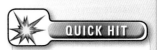

QUICK HIT

Because of the distal and posterior location of the left subclavian artery, its origin is inaccessible by a sternotomy and can be easily approached by a left high anterior or anterolateral thoracotomy.

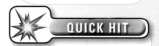

QUICK HIT

Thromboangiitis obliterans (Buerger disease): This unique disease affects the venoarterial plexus, causing digital/distal ischemia that results in pain and gangrene. It is strongly associated with smoking of an addictive nature. Treatment is supportive and includes smoking cessation.

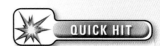

QUICK HIT

DVT prophylaxis should be considered for all hospitalized patients. Pneumatic compression boots and early ambulation should be considered as initial therapy for DVT prevention.

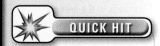

3. Vein wall response is highly dependent on endothelial selectins P- and E-selectin.
4. Presenting symptoms may include unilateral leg pain and swelling, positive Homans sign (pain on passive dorsiflexion of foot—a nonspecific physical finding), or PE.

C. Diagnosis
1. Fifty percent of patients with acute DVT may be asymptomatic.
2. Duplex ultrasound imaging has become the test of choice, with greater than 95% sensitivity and specificity.
3. Differential diagnosis of lower extremity pain and swelling includes muscle strain or contusion, cellulitis, Baker cyst, iliac vein obstruction due to retroperitoneal tumor or mass, and systemic causes of swelling and edema (e.g., congestive heart failure or venous insufficiency).

D. Management
1. Treatment for acute DVT is anticoagulation. Initial therapy is often with IV unfractionated heparin (UFH) or subcutaneous low molecular weight heparin (LMWH), such as enoxaparin.
   a. IV UFH has a narrow therapeutic window and unpredictable dose response. Heparin is administered continuously, requiring inpatient treatment. It is useful for patients with renal failure. The therapeutic response is monitored by following partial thromboplastin time. Patients who do not respond should have antifactor Xa levels measured.
   b. LMWH is more predictable and has greater bioavailability. Administration is daily or twice a day. LMWH should be avoided in patients with renal failure. No routine blood monitoring is required.
2. Vena caval interruption via filter placement should be considered when anticoagulation is contraindicated, PE recurs on anticoagulation, or a complication develops from use of anticoagulation.
   a. Filters may be retrievable.
   b. Contraindications to anticoagulation include evidence of ongoing bleeding, trauma resulting in solid organ injury, intracranial hemorrhage, or spinal hematoma and complication of anticoagulation, such as bleeding.
   c. Anticoagulation should be resumed or initiated, when possible, because a filter alone is not effective treatment of DVT.

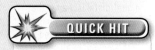

3. Systemic or catheter-directed thrombolysis and surgical extraction or thrombectomy should be used only in patients with massive iliofemoral DVT at risk of limb gangrene secondary to venous occlusion.
4. Patients who present with idiopathic or recurrent DVT should be evaluated for hypercoagulable state.
5. Ambulation with DVT does not increase the risk of PE and does decrease the incidence and severity of chronic venous disease after DVT. Ambulation and sequential compression therapy are encouraged in the management of DVT.
6. Long-term treatment
   a. Between 15% and 50% of patients often develop symptomatic extension or recurrent events.
   b. Long-term treatment involves anticoagulation, usually with vitamin K antagonist (warfarin).
      (1) Patient with a first episode of DVT with underlying reversible risk factor should receive 3 to 6 months of treatment.
      (2) Patients with a first episode of idiopathic DVT should receive treatment for 6 to 12 months and should be considered for indefinite anticoagulant therapy.
      (3) Patients with DVT and malignancy should receive 3 to 6 months of LMWH and indefinite anticoagulation therapy.
      (4) Patients with a first episode of DVT and antiphospholipid antibodies or two or more thrombophilic conditions should receive 12 months of therapy and be considered for indefinite treatment.

    (5) Patients with a first episode of DVT and a documented thrombophilic condition should receive 6 to 12 months of treatment and be considered for indefinite therapy.

    (6) Patients with two or more documented episodes of DVT should receive indefinite treatment.

II. Upper Extremity Deep Venous Thrombosis

A. Thrombotic obstruction of the subclavian, axillary, or brachial vein
1. Usually associated with central venous catheters or other instrumentation
2. Compression in the thoracic outlet, also known as Paget-Schroetter syndrome or "effort thrombosis"

B. Signs and symptoms are edema, dilated collateral circulation, and pain.

C. Diagnosis is clinical with venous duplex.

D. Management is controversial.
1. Generally, removal of foreign body is sufficient.
2. Treatment may be similar to lower extremity DVT. However, the level of evidence for this course is lower than for lower extremity DVT.
3. No reliable evidence is available on superior vena cava interruption.
4. Thrombolysis with 3 to 6 months of anticoagulation is indicated for effort thrombosis with possible rib resection.

III. Distal Lower Extremity Deep Venous Thrombosis

A. Between 10% and 15% of patients will propagate to the proximal venous system and require treatment.

B. DVT of the calf is usually treated expectantly although anticoagulation can be considered if the patient is symptomatic.

IV. Pulmonary Embolism

A. DVT and PE are different manifestations of a similar disease process, and their treatment is therefore similar.

B. The majority of patients with proximal DVT also have symptomatic or asymptomatic PE and vice versa.

C. Patients treated for PE are four times more likely to die of recurrent venous thromboembolic disease in the next year when compared with patients treated for DVT (1.5% vs. 0.4%).

POSTPHLEBITIC SYNDROME AND CHRONIC VENOUS INSUFFICIENCY

I. Incidence

A. Post-thrombotic syndrome (PTS) develops in 20% to 50% of patients after documented DVT. In the absence of DVT, this constellation of symptoms is referred to as chronic venous insufficiency (CVI).

B. CVI affects 50 million Americans, with 500,000 of them developing venous ulcers.

II. Pathology

A. Development of CVI may be related to venous obstruction, valvular insufficiency, or calf muscle pump malfunction.

III. Clinical Features/Symptoms

A. Chronic postural dependent swelling, pain, local discomfort, and venous ulceration at the ankle

B. Superficial venous insufficiency that may appear as spider vein, telangiectasias, or varicosities

C. Pain, hyperpigmentation, stasis dermatitis, or venous ulcers

D. Venous ulcers that tend to form just above the medial malleolus

Vascular Surgery

E. Venous claudication: pain associated with walking from increased swelling and prominence of the superficial venous system, usually observed in the setting of both venous obstruction and venous incompetence

IV. Diagnosis

A. Venous duplex ultrasonography allows imaging of veins as well as analysis of blood flow.
B. Plethysmography uses an air-filled cylinder fitted over the extremity to analyze changes in the extremity with position change and exercise.
C. Venography has no significant role in diagnosis of acute or chronic disease but may be used to complement noninvasive testing when considering intervention in the deep venous system or in research protocols.

V. Management

A. Elastic compression stockings should be used for 2 years following DVT and for symptom improvement in the setting of PTS or CVD.
B. Conservative medical therapy includes using compressive stockings (30 to 40 mm Hg at the ankle), avoiding prolonged periods of standing, elevating legs intermittently through the day, elevating the foot of the bed at night, and exercising.
C. Sclerotherapy is needle injection of a caustic solution directly into superficial veins and is used to treat isolated varicosities, telangiectasias, and varicosities remaining after saphenous stripping.
D. Vein stripping/ablation as well as endovascular laser or radiofrequency ablation act by disrupting the great saphenous vein, usually at the saphenofemoral junction, with removal of the vein to the level of the knee or below. This is indicated for treatment of saphenous vein insufficiency.
E. Perforator vein ligation can be performed for treatment of isolated perforator vein incompetence.

SUPERFICIAL THROMBOPHLEBITIS

I. Incidence

A. This condition may occur spontaneously or be associated with IV lines, trauma, varicose veins, pregnancy, and the postpartum period.
B. Number of cases is 125,000 per year.
C. Migratory superficial thrombophlebitis may suggest abdominal cancer (Trousseau syndrome).
D. PE is rare.

II. Clinical Features/Symptoms

A. Patients present with localized pain, erythema, and induration.
B. No generalized swelling occurs unless DVT develops.
C. Over time, a firm cord forms.
D. Fever and shaking chills may result from septic/suppurative thrombophlebitis with recannulation.

III. Differential Diagnosis

Localization over superficial vein differentiated from cellulitis, ascending lymphangitis, erythema nodosum, erythema induration, and panniculitis

IV. Management

A. Treatment may involve nonsteroidal anti-inflammatory drugs, local heat, elevation, and support with compressive stocking or elastic wrap.
B. Most cases resolve within 7 to 10 days.
C. Recurrence may be treated with surgical excision usually 6 months after acute inflammation.
D. Septic thrombophlebitis requires IV antibiotics, and if the patient becomes septic, surgical excision may be necessary.

VASCULAR NONINVASIVE DIAGNOSTIC STUDIES

I. General Principles

A. Noninvasive testing is a secondary modality, after clinical examination, to help identify vascular disease.

B. The specific indications and the utility in specific scenarios will be described.

II. Arterial Studies

A. Cerebrovascular testing
   1. Carotid duplex: The degree of velocity of blood flow in the carotids (duplex scanning) and the arteries luminal diameter is viewed (B-mode analysis).
   2. Oculoplethysmography: This test measures the flow of blood in the ophthalmic artery (indicator of flow in the internal carotid artery) and compares it to the flow of blood in the ipsilateral ear (indicator of flow in the external carotid artery). Rarely performed.

B. Lower extremity testing (see Table 13-3)
   1. ABI
      a. This test is done by measuring the blood pressure in the ankle and in the arm while the patient is at rest. The measurements may be repeated after 5 minutes of exercise to evaluate for decrease in flow with activity.
      b. The ratio of the ankle pressure to the brachial pressure is a sensitive indicator of degree of peripheral occlusive disease. Normally, the ratio should be 1. Mild arterial disease has an ABI of 0.7 to 0.9. Patients with ABIs of 0.5 to 0.7 may have intermittent claudication, and those with ABIs less than 0.5 may have rest pain and/or severe limb-threatening ischemia.
   2. Segmental pressures
      a. Blood pressure cuffs are placed around the ankle, upper calf, and thigh.
      b. Decreased pressure in relation to the proximal cuff or to the contralateral pressure at the same level is an indicator of occlusion proximal to the measuring site. Pressure considered significant is 20 to 30 mm Hg.
   3. Pulse volume recordings
      a. Doppler waveforms are obtained at the thigh, upper calf, ankle, foot, and toe levels after a pneumatic cuff is inflated to 60 mm Hg. A transducer connected to the cuff records the flow patterns/waveforms at the artery.
      b. Disease is indicated by irregularity within the flow or flattening of the wave.

C. Mesenteric arterial evaluation: utilizes ultrasound technology to examine aneurysmal disease of the abdominal aorta. Flow velocities in the mesenteric vessels are compared with flow velocity in abdominal aorta and define degrees of stenosis in the vessels.

III. Venous Studies

A. Venous duplex: Ultrasound technology is utilized to examine venous patency, obstruction, and reflux. These data are used to diagnose venous thrombosis and treat venous reflux.

B. Vein mapping: This examines the course and location of the vein prior to planning an operation (e.g., saphenous vein mapping prior to coronary bypass or jugular vein identification prior to central line placement).

IV. Computed Tomography and Magnetic Resonance Angiography.
The utility of these modalities is still under review. They offer the benefit of examining the anatomy of the vasculature and its relation to other surrounding structures. The drawback of these techniques is primarily related to the use of contrast. Contrast reactions range from mild (nausea, vomiting, flushing, urticaria, pruritus) to moderate (laryngeal or facial edema) to severe (cardiac or respiratory arrest and anaphylactic shock). Patients with pre-existing kidney disease (GFR <30 mL/min/1.73 m) are at risk for acute kidney injury requiring dialysis or nephrogenic systemic fibrosis (NSF). NSF is an uncommon complication of MRI with gadolinium-based contrast agents. It is a severe condition that causes widespread tissue fibrosis and has only been reported in patients with pre-existing renal disease.

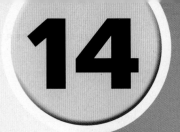

14 Pediatric Surgery

Kevin Day, Richard A. Vaughan, Tarun Kumar, and
Shelley Reynolds Hill

 ## HEAD AND NECK

I. Congenital Torticollis

A. Congenital shortening of the sternocleidomastoid muscle

B. Clinical features

  1. Incompletely understood but thought to arise from one of two causes:

    a. Fixed position in utero leads to shortening and tightening of one sternocleidomastoid.

      (1) Higher incidence in breech infants

      (2) Associated with craniofacial abnormalities such as asymmetric ears and eyes, flattening of the frontal bone, and/or flattening of the mandible

    b. Birth trauma leads to a tear and bleeding of the muscle, with resultant scar formation and contracture.

  2. Distinguished from acquired type, which is due to a variety of causes:

    a. Atlantoaxial subluxation

    b. Brain stem tumors

    c. Infectious causes

      (1) Tonsillitis

      (2) Retropharyngeal abscess

      (3) Cervical adenitis

  3. Spasmodic with gastroesophageal reflux: Sandifer syndrome

C. Diagnosis

  1. Purely clinical diagnosis

  2. History

    a. Fetal positioning

      (1) Breech versus vertex

      (2) Was the infant "stuck" in utero? Did it seem to move much?

    b. Onset of symptoms

      (1) Congenital type presents immediately or within weeks of delivery.

      (2) Acquired type presents later.

    c. Preferred head positioning of the infant

    d. Difficulty with breastfeeding

  3. Physical examination

    a. Head is tilted toward the involved side, with the chin slightly rotated away from the involved muscle.

    b. Test range of motion of the infant's neck.

  4. No imaging required

D. Treatment

  1. Conservative treatment with physical therapy, stretching of the neck muscles, and range-of-motion exercises is the mainstay of treatment.

  2. If condition fails to resolve by 1 year of age despite aggressive physical therapy, surgical division of the involved sternocleidomastoid may be required.

II. Cystic Hygroma

A. General principles

1. This is a benign multiloculated lymphatic malformation.
2. The majority (65%) present at birth; the remainder present within the first 2 years of life.
3. Most (95%) occur in the neck or axilla, but they may occur anywhere in the body.

B. Clinical features

1. Lymphatics begin to develop from mesenchymal clefts in the sixth gestational week. When lymphatics fail to fuse with the venous system, a disorganized collection of blind-ending lymphatics forms, causing a hygroma.
2. Typically asymptomatic, but complications may occur:
   a. Airway obstruction is possible if the hygroma is large enough, and it may be life threatening.
   b. Infection may occur in 16% of hygromas and presents with redness, fever, and pain.
   c. Hemorrhage into the hygroma occurs in 15% of cases and presents with rapidly enlarging, painful mass with evidence for blood loss.

C. Diagnosis

1. History
   a. Onset
   b. Enlarging or stable
   c. Fever
   d. Difficulty breathing
2. Physical examination
   a. Look for signs of airway obstruction: tracheal deviation, stridor, and impingement of the neck by the mass.
   b. Palpate to assess size and extent of the mass.
   c. Look for associated congenital abnormalities because hygromas are associated with chromosomal abnormalities.
3. Diagnosis is typically clinical, with a mass noted in the neck or axilla.
   a. Diagnosis of retroperitoneal or pelvic hygromas may require computed tomography (CT) or magnetic resonance imaging (MRI) scanning.
   b. MRI is essential prior to surgical resection to rule out adjacent neurovascular structures.

D. Treatment

1. Medical treatment with injection of sclerosing agents has been successful in treating large cystic hygromas but is less successful in treating smaller lesions.
   a. Bleomycin should be avoided due to toxicity and the resultant scarring, making later surgical resection difficult.
   b. Pure ethanol may be used.
   c. Picibanil (OK-432), a derivative of penicillin and streptococcus pyogenes, is a trial drug that has shown success in shrinking large, unilocular lesions.
   d. Recurrent disease may respond poorly to repeat sclerosis.
2. Surgical resection is the mainstay of treatment.
   a. Treatment is generally for cosmetic purposes and can proceed at the time of diagnosis, unless adjacent neurovascular structures would make risk of morbidity high for a small infant.
   b. If the mass is asymptomatic, surgery may be delayed until 2 years of age to allow for neurovascular structures to increase in size for better visualization in surgery.
   c. Emergent resection should proceed if there is any airway impingement.
   d. Complications include chylous fistula, chylothorax, hemorrhage, and damage to surrounding neurovascular structures.

III. Brachial Cleft Remnants

A. General principles

1. A congenital anomaly of the neck due to persistence of the fetal branchial clefts. The cause is unknown, but the remnants result from incomplete obliteration of the clefts as the fetal neck develops.

2. Brachial clefts form in the fourth to eighth weeks of gestation, during embryologic segmentation.
    a. Four pairs of branchial arches form in the cervicofacial region of the embryo, with clefts expressed externally and pouches expressed internally.
    b. Branchial clefts and their adult derivatives:
        (1) Cleft I becomes the eustachian tube and a portion of the external auditory canal (EAC).
        (2) Cleft II is obliterated without a distinct adult counterpart.
        (3) Cleft III migrates inferiorly to form the inferior parathyroid glands and the thymus.
        (4) Cleft IV migrates inferiorly but stops above the final level of cleft III and forms the superior parathyroid glands and thyroid C-cells.

B. Clinical features
    1. Although these are congenital anomalies and are thus present at birth, not all are recognized immediately.
    2. Individual cleft remnants may form cysts, sinuses, fistulas, and cartilaginous remnants.
        a. Cleft I remnants occur along the angle of the mandible, and sinuses/fistulas may extend to the EAC.
        b. Cleft II remnants occur along the anterior border of the sternocleidomastoid muscle and may communicate with the tonsillar fossa. They are the most common form.
        c. Cleft III and IV remnants communicate between the piriform sinus and the glands they form or the neck lower than second-cleft remnants. They are rare.
    3. A very small number may harbor malignancy.

C. Diagnosis
    1. Diagnosis is purely clinical typically.
    2. Sinuses, fistulas, and cartilaginous remnants tend to present early, whereas cysts present later as fluid slowly accumulates.

D. Treatment
    1. Complete surgical excision is the only effective treatment.
    2. Tract should be free of infection at time of surgery and, if not, antibiotics should be given and surgery postponed.

IV. Thyroglossal Duct Cysts

A. General principles
    1. A remnant of the thyroglossal duct; the path of downward migration of the thyroid gland from the base of the tongue to its adult location
    2. Found mainly in the midline and may contain nests of thyroid tissue

B. Clinical features
    1. Cysts develop when the thyroglossal duct fails to obliterate following migration of the thyroid gland from the foramen cecum on the base of the tongue to the neck.
    2. Cysts may occur anywhere along the path of the thyroglossal duct.
    3. Ectopic thyroid tissue along the duct may develop into papillary adenocarcinoma.
    4. The duct passes through the central portion of the hyoid bone in its descent.
    5. In rare cases, may contain the patient's only functional thyroid tissue.

C. Diagnosis
    1. Typical clinical diagnosis is by palpation of a mass in the midline between the submental region and the superior aspect of the trachea.
    2. The mass may present as a midline abscess in the neck if there is communication with the base of the tongue, with resultant contamination by oral flora.
    3. Noninfected cysts are soft, smooth, and nontender.
    4. Cysts may move with swallowing or protrusion of the tongue.

D. Treatment
   1. To prevent recurrence or the possibility of ectopic thyroid carcinoma (less than 1%), the entire thyroglossal duct tract should be excised.
      a. Excision should include the cyst, its tract, and the entire central portion of the hyoid bone.
      b. Dissection is carried up to the foramen cecum at the base of the tongue.
   2. If thyroid tissue is present in the resected specimen, thyroid function tests should be performed to rule out postresection hypothyroidism.

CHEST

I. Chest Wall Deformity
A. General principles
   1. Represents deformity in development of the supportive architecture of the chest
   2. Functional impairment
      a. Rarely affects cardiopulmonary function
      b. Frequently causes psychosocial impairment due to being "different," especially during puberty
B. Clinical features
   1. Ribs are formed by segmental somites that advance ventrally toward the sternum. The sternum develops from two mesodermal bands that eventually fuse in the center. The costal cartilages link the developing ribs to the sternum.
   2. A wide variety of deformities exist, most of them rare. They include pectus excavatum, pectus carinatum, and sternal cleft.
      a. Pectus excavatum
         (1) The most common chest wall deformity, this condition is present in 1 of 300 to 400 live births.
         (2) The deformity is due to abnormal growth regulation of the costal cartilages.
         (3) If deformity is severe, with compression of the heart, an echocardiogram should be obtained. CT or plain radiographs may help delineate the defect.
         (4) Surgical correction is typically for cosmetic purposes primarily.
      b. Pectus carinatum
         (1) From the Latin *pectus* for chest and *carina* for keel
         (2) This deformity is characterized by a protrusive appearance with outward displacement of the sternum, which tends to become more pronounced in adolescence.
         (3) Surgical correction is purely cosmetic.
      c. Sternal cleft
         (1) This deformity occurs when the sternal bars of mesoderm fail to completely fuse during development. It may be associated with exstrophy of the heart.
         (2) Part of the pentalogy of Cantrell: sternal cleft, omphalocele, diaphragmatic defect, pericardial defect, and intracardiac defect
         (3) Surgical correction
            (a) Reapproximation of the cleft in the midline is curative.
            (b) If incomplete, the cleft must be divided completely to allow proper healing.

II. Pulmonary Sequestration
A. General principles
   1. This abnormal lung tissue develops without normal communication with the trachea or a bronchus with an aberrant blood supply.
   2. Arterial blood supply is systemic, from the aorta, and venous drainage is either pulmonary or systemic.
   3. Pathogenesis is not completely understood but is thought to arise as a result of an accessory lung bud separate from the main lung, arising from the primitive foregut, with angiogenesis occurring from the aorta instead of the pulmonary circulation.

B. Intralobar and extralobar sequestrations
  1. Intralobar sequestrations are always within the chest and are invested by visceral pleura.
    a. They tend to be located in the medial, posterior segments of the lower lobes.
    b. Majority are fed by vessels arising from the infradiaphragmatic aorta and running through the inferior pulmonary ligament.
  2. Extralobar sequestrations are not invested by pulmonary pleura and may occur within the chest, the diaphragm, or the retroperitoneum.
    a. 4:1 male-to-female predominance
    b. Often associated with other congenital anomalies and discovered incidentally during workup
    c. Rarely may have communication with the foregut
    d. Almost uniformly left-sided
C. Clinical features, diagnosis, and treatment
  1. Intralobar sequestrations
    a. Clinical features: Although no distinct bronchus is present, there are usually microcommunications with the airways that can lead to infection of the sequestrum.
    b. Diagnosis
      (1) Typical history is that of recurrent pneumonias beginning early in childhood.
      (2) Diagnostic "gold standard" is arteriography, but contrast CT or MRI have largely replaced this.
      (3) Chest X-ray may reveal an inferiorly located consolidation.
      (4) Frequently, aeration shows on imaging studies.
      (5) Advanced imaging study is essential to delineate blood supply prior to resection.
      (6) Now more frequently being diagnosed on prenatal ultrasound
    c. Treatment
      (1) Treatment is surgical resection of the sequestrum in symptomatic patients.
      (2) Frequently, complete lobectomy is necessary due to inability to distinguish sequestration from surrounding pulmonary lobe.
  2. Extralobar sequestrations
    a. Clinical features: Aeration is rare unless there is communication with the foregut.
    b. Diagnosis. Typically, diagnosis occurs by CT obtained to evaluate another congenital anomaly.
    c. Treatment
      (1) Typical treatment is observation.
      (2) Surgical resection is indicated if there is communication with the foregut with resultant infection or if there is extrinsic compression of the gastrointestinal (GI) tract.

III. Esophageal Atresia/Tracheoesophageal Fistula
A. General principles
  1. Esophageal atresia: congenital disruption of esophageal development, resulting in blind-ending esophagus with obstruction
  2. Tracheoesophageal (TE) fistula: abnormal fistulous tract between the trachea and esophagus that usually occurs in conjunction with esophageal atresia
  3. Five anatomic variants of esophageal atresia/TE fistula (Fig. 14-1)
    a. Type 1: blind-ending proximal and distal pouches without TE fistula (6%)
    b. Type 2: proximal TE fistula with distal blind pouch (2%)
    c. Type 3: proximal blind pouch with distal TE fistula (85%)
    d. Type 4: proximal and distal pouches with TE fistula (1%)
    e. Type 5: pure TE fistula without esophageal atresia H-type fistula (2%)

FIGURE
14-1 Variants of tracheoesophageal fistula.

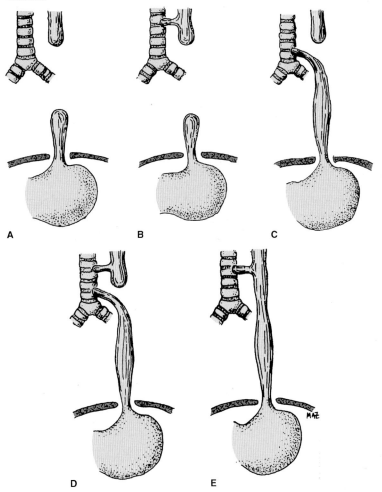

A B C

D E

A. Atresia without fistula (5%–7% of cases). **B.** Proximal fistula and distal pouch (<1% occurrence). **C.** Proximal pouch with distal fistula (85%–90% of cases). **D.** Atresia with proximal and distal fistulas (<1% of cases). **E.** Fistula without atresia (H-type) (2%–6% occurrence). (Reprinted with permission from Washington University School of Medicine Department of Surgery, Meko JB, Olson JA, Doherty GM. *The Washington Manual of Surgery.* 3rd ed. Baltimore, MD: Lippincott Williams & Wilkins; 2002:642.)

4. Frequently occurs with a constellation of other abnormalities known as the VACTERL syndrome:
   a. V = vertebral anomalies
      A = anorectal malformation
      C = cardiac abnormalities
      TE = tracheoesophageal fistula
      R = renal anomalies
      L = limb deformity
   b. One, several, or all anomalous features may be present.
B. Pathogenesis
   1. The trachea and esophagus are derived from a common embryologic tube, the laryngotracheal tube, which forms during the fourth week of gestation.
   2. The lateral walls of the tube invaginate to form the TE septum, which eventually divides the trachea from the esophagus.
   3. Incomplete division of the esophagus and trachea results in esophageal atresia and TE fistula.
C. Diagnosis
   1. The majority are diagnosed at birth by excessive oral secretions and inability to pass a nasogastric (NG) tube.

2. Once diagnosed, patients should also undergo diagnostics to rule out VACTERL syndrome.
   a. Imaging of the chest and spine
   b. Echocardiogram
   c. Renal ultrasonography
   d. Examination of anus and limbs
   e. Genetic workup

D. Treatment
   1. Treatment is surgical division of the TE fistula, with anastomosis of the esophageal pouches.
   2. Surgery may be accomplished as a single procedure for short-gap atresia.
   3. Long-gap atresia may require a staged procedure.
      a. Multiple operations have been described:
         (1) Stretching of upper and lower pouches by serial bougienage
         (2) Fistulization along a surgically placed rod, or suture connecting the pouches
         (3) Circular esophagomyotomy with primary anastomosis
         (4) Cervical spit fistula of proximal pouch, with sequential lengthening down the neck
      b. All staged procedures require a gastrostomy for feeding until anastomosis can be performed.

IV. Congenital Diaphragmatic Hernia

A. General principles
   1. Congenital diaphragmatic hernia (CDH) is a congenital defect in the development of the diaphragm that allows peritoneal contents into the chest, leading to pulmonary hypoplasia.
   2. Left-sided defects are much more common due to earlier closure of the right pleuroperitoneal membrane and the protective mass effect of the liver under the right side.
   3. CDH carries a mortality rate of 30% to 40%.
   4. Two distinct types
      a. Bochdalek: most common type, located in the posterolateral position
      b. Morgagni: rare, located anteromedially behind the sternum

B. Pathogenesis
   1. The primordial diaphragm is formed by the pleuroperitoneal membranes, over which the lateral body wall musculature grows inward to create the muscular diaphragm.
   2. Failure of the pleuroperitoneal membranes to close leads to CDH.

C. Clinical features
   1. Presenting symptoms include marked respiratory distress and cyanosis at birth.
   2. Mild cases may be asymptomatic or present with mild chronic respiratory disease, pneumonia, feeding difficulty, or bowel obstruction.

D. Diagnosis
   1. Presenting symptoms are diagnostic.
   2. CDH is typically diagnosed by prenatal ultrasound.
      a. Polyhydramnios (80%)
      b. Seen as abdominal contents in the thoracic cavity
   3. A chest X-ray usually confirms the diagnosis.

E. Treatment
   1. In utero surgery (fetal surgery) is being performed in select centers but has not shown significant promise in terms of improving mortality.
   2. CDH requires treatment in an advanced neonatal intensive care unit.
   3. Pulmonary support in the immediate postnatal period is critical.
      a. Extracorporeal membrane oxygenation
      b. High oscillation ventilation
      c. Partial liquid ventilation
      d. Inhaled nitric oxide and exogenous surfactant
   4. Reduction of the abdominal contents to the peritoneal cavity with repair of the defect is the mainstay of treatment.

5. Pulmonary hypoplasia may be so extensive as to preclude cure, and thus, survival has not improved significantly despite advanced techniques for cure.
   a. Most deaths are due to the pulmonary disease and hypoplasia and not from the hernia itself. The biggest physiologic consequence is the persistent pulmonary hypertension that results from the hypoplasia.
6. Surgery should be delayed until the pulmonary hypertension has had time to decrease.

ABDOMINAL WALL

I. Gastroschisis

A. General principles
   1. Gastroschisis, or "split stomach," is a misnomer for a condition that is actually a division of the anterior abdominal wall musculature.
   2. Infants are born with their intestine protruding through the abdominal wall defect into the amniotic cavity (Fig. 14-2).
   3. Gastroschisis is more common in males.
   4. The risk of associated congenital or genetic anomalies is low.
   5. Defect is almost uniformly to the right of the umbilical cord. Defects to the left of the cord are associated with much higher rates of other congenital defects.
   6. Malrotation is present.

B. Etiology: No uniform cause known, but environmental and drug exposures are thought to play a role.
   1. The condition becomes much more frequent when the mother is younger than 20 years of age.
   2. Use of cigarettes, alcohol, and recreational drugs increases risk.
   3. Use of aspirin, ibuprofen, and pseudoephedrine increases risk.

C. Clinical features
   The intestine is typically shortened, thickened, and matted or stuck together at birth, which is due to the inflammatory reaction of the bowel wall to exposure to amniotic fluid.
   There is a high rate of associated intestinal atresias due to vascular accidents in utero due to amniotic bands.

D. Diagnosis and treatment
   1. Diagnosis
      a. Gastroschisis is easily diagnosed by prenatal ultrasound.
      b. If it is discovered prenatally, the patient should be referred for delivery at a facility with neonatal intensive care, pediatric surgery, and high-risk obstetrics coverage.

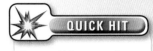

Gastroschisis occurs almost exclusively to the right side of the umbilicus, which is always spared.

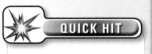

In 15% of infants born with gastroschisis, there is an associated intestinal atresia.

FIGURE 14-2 Gastroschisis. The defect is to the right of the normal umbilicus, and the bowel is thickened and inflamed.

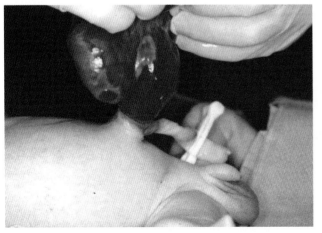

(Courtesy of Douglas Katz, MD.)

    c. Mothers should be followed with serial ultrasounds to assess for continued bowel viability. Bowel edema can be a sign of imminent strangulation.

    d. Most authors agree that cesarean section is not mandatory if mother and infant are able to tolerate vaginal delivery.

2. Treatment

    a. Immediately postdelivery, the intestine should be covered in a moist, sterile dressing; an NG tube should be placed to keep the intestine decompressed; intravenous access should be obtained; and broad-spectrum antibiotics should be initiated and continued until the defect is closed. The infant is usually placed in a sterile "bowel bag" to the level of the chest to lessen insensible fluid losses from exposed intestines.

    b. Reduction of the abdominal contents into the peritoneal cavity and surgical closure of the abdominal defect is curative.

    c. If adequate reduction of the intestine is not possible, placement of a silo bag, with sequential tightening, can be used until intestines are reduced back and abdominal wall closure can be performed without much tension.

    d. Patients will almost uniformly have a prolonged postoperative ileus.

      (1) Patients should be maintained on total parenteral nutrition (TPN) until bowel function is initiated.

      (2) Liver function should be monitored closely while on TPN because cirrhosis, portal hypertension, and liver failure can occur.

II. Omphalocele

A. General principles

1. Abdominal wall defect in which viscera extrude through the umbilicus and are encased in a peritoneal and amniotic sac (Fig. 14-3).

    a. Felt to be an arrest in development of the abdominal wall

    b. Malrotation is present.

2. High association with genetic and congenital abnormalities

    a. Associated with trisomy 13, 18, and 21

    b. Cardiac, musculoskeletal, and GI anomalies are common.

    c. Beckwith–Wiedemann syndrome: *Exomphalos* (omphalocele), *Macroglossia, Gigantism,* and hyperinsulinemia hypoglycemia

3. There are 1 in 5,000 live births with omphalocele and herniation of intestine and 1 in 10,000 live births with omphalocele and herniation of intestine and solid organs.

B. Pathogenesis

1. Between the 6th and 10th weeks of normal gestation, the abdominal contents herniate into the umbilicus and undergo a series of coordinated rotations before returning to the peritoneal cavity, after which the abdominal wall closes.

2. Omphalocele occurs when the intestine fails to return to the abdominal cavity.

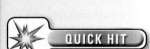

QUICK HIT

The inner lining of the omphalocele sac is peritoneum, whereas the outer covering is epithelium of the umbilical cord, derived from the amniotic sac.

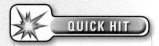

QUICK HIT

Omphalocele is much more likely to be associated with other congenital anomalies than gastroschisis.

FIGURE 14-3 **Omphalocele. The herniated intestines and liver are visible inside the sac. The umbilical cord attaches to the sac.**

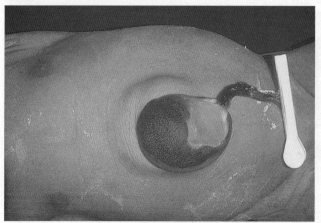

(With permission from Klossner NJ, Hatfield NT. *Introductory Maternity and Pediatric Nursing.* 2nd ed. Philadelphia, PA: Lippincott Williams & Wilkins; 2009.)

CLINICAL PEARL 14-1

Gastroschisis

- Herniation of bowel through the abdominal wall without a peritoneal covering (no sac)
- Higher rate of intestinal atresias
- Low rate of other associated congenital malformations
- Defect to the right of the normal umbilical cord

Omphalocele

- Herniation of abdominal contents through the abdominal wall covered by peritoneum (sac)
- Higher rate of other congenital malformations (cardiac, trisomy 21, etc.)
- Defect is through the umbilical ring.

C. Diagnosis and treatment (see Clinical Pearl 14-1)
1. Typically diagnosed by prenatal ultrasound
2. Pre- and postnatal care is essentially the same for omphalocele as for gastroschisis.
3. Workup for associated anomalies should be undertaken.

III. Exstrophy of the Bladder
A. General principles
1. Defect in the infraumbilical abdominal wall with failure of the median inferior portion to close, resulting in exposure and protrusion of the posterior wall of the urinary bladder through the defect
2. In males, almost uniformly associated with epispadias
3. In females, almost uniformly associated with bifid clitoris
4. Occurs 1 in every 10,000 to 40,000 live births
B. Pathogenesis
1. During the fourth week of gestation, mesenchymal cells migrate into the space between the cloaca and ectoderm of the primitive abdomen.
2. Failure of this migration leads to no development of abdominal musculature in this position.
3. Eventually, the thin epidermis and anterior wall of the bladder rupture, allowing wide exposure of the mucous membrane of the bladder.
C. Diagnosis and treatment
1. Diagnosis is clinical by inspection.
2. Surgical correction consists of closure of the bladder plate and concurrent repair of epispadias in boys. Surgical repair should proceed within 72 hours of birth with favorable outcomes.

IV. Umbilical Hernia
A. General principles
1. A defect in the connective tissue around the umbilicus present at birth
2. The most common abdominal wall defect in the newborn
3. Tends to occur more commonly in African-American infants than in Caucasian infants
B. Pathogenesis
1. Failure of complete closure of the linea alba at the umbilicus
2. The umbilicus is reinforced by the paired umbilical ligaments (umbilical artery remnants), the round ligament (umbilical vein remnant), the urachus (remnant of the primitive allantois), and the transversalis fascia.
3. Weakness or failure of any of the reinforcing structures can predispose to umbilical hernia.
C. Diagnosis and treatment
1. Diagnosis is clinical by inspection and palpation.
2. In most cases of congenital umbilical hernia, the defect will close spontaneously during the first 3 years of life.
3. If the hernia persists at 5 years of age, surgical closure is indicated.

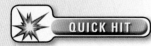

QUICK HIT

Hydrocele may be **communicating**, in which a small opening in the proximal processus vaginalis remains open, which allows fluid passage but not herniation; or **noncommunicating**, in which proximal closure of the processus vaginalis occurs with distal fluid collection.

V. Congenital Inguinal Hernia/Hydrocele

A. General principles
1. Inguinal hernia: due to failure of processus vaginalis to close and allowing herniation of abdominal contents into the inguinal ring, and possibly the scrotum
2. Hydrocele: collection of fluid around the testicle within tunica vaginalis—may be communicating or noncommunicating
3. Predisposing factors include prematurity.
4. More common in male infants
5. Represents the most common indication for surgery in the infant population

B. Pathogenesis
1. The testes develop intra-abdominally and migrate along a path created by gubernaculum.
2. The testis descends into the scrotum through the processus vaginalis, a canal that protrudes through the abdominal wall into the inguinal canal.
3. After descent of the testis, the processus vaginalis closes and is obliterated.
   a. Failure of the processus vaginalis to close, allowing herniation of intra-abdominal contents, results in a congenital inguinal hernia.
   b. Partial closure of the processus vaginalis with resultant collection of fluid results in hydrocele.

C. Diagnosis and treatment
1. Diagnosis is clinical.
   a. Typical history is of a groin bulge that enlarges with crying or straining with hernias, or a stable scrotal or groin swelling for hydrocele.
   b. Most reduce spontaneously or with gentle pressure.
   c. Hydrocele will transilluminate on examination. Noncommunicating hydrocele will not extend to the inguinal ring and will not reduce on exam.
2. Treatment
   a. Surgical treatment is indicated at the time of diagnosis for inguinal hernias and communicating hydrocele, which have a tendency to develop into true hernias.
   b. Noncommunicating hydrocele may be observed because they tend to resolve spontaneously during first 2 years of life.

ABDOMEN

I. Hypertrophic Pyloric Stenosis

A. General principles
1. Obstruction of the gastric outlet due to hypertrophy of the pyloric muscle
2. Results in narrowing of the pyloric lumen
3. Occurs in 1 in 150 live births of males and 1 in 750 live births of females

B. Pathogenesis
1. This is incompletely understood but is now thought to result from a deficiency of nitric oxide synthase in the pylorus, resulting in inability of pyloric muscle to relax, resulting in muscular hypertrophy.
2. Maximum narrowing occurs between the fourth and eighth weeks postpartum.

C. Diagnosis
1. Classic history is of projectile, nonbilious emesis beginning in the second to fourth weeks of life.
2. The diagnostic procedure of choice is pyloric ultrasonography that shows a thickened pyloric muscle (4 mm or more) and pyloric channel length (17 mm or more).
3. Contrast upper GI series can be helpful in cases in which physical examination and ultrasonography is not clear. Features include failure of contrast to pass through the pylorus or very small amount of transit on fluoroscopy, resulting in "string sign."
4. Pathognomonic physical exam finding is a palpable "olive" in the epigastric region. Requires a relaxed infant and a decompressed stomach.
5. Differential diagnosis includes gastroesophageal reflux disease (GERD), pyloric spasm, and malrotation.

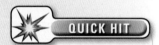

QUICK HIT

Projectile, nonbilious emesis with a palpable abdominal "olive" in the epigastrium is pathognomic for pyloric stenosis, and no further workup is required before surgery.

D. Treatment

1. Treatment is surgical pyloromyotomy (Ramstedt) in which the layers, except mucosa, are divided along the entire hypertrophied segment.
2. Preoperatively, intravenous (IV) hydration and correction of serum electrolytes are advised.
   a. Classic metabolic derangement is a hypokalemic hypochloremic metabolic alkalosis.

II. Duodenal Atresia/Stenosis/Web

A. General principles

1. Obliteration of a segment of duodenum during development that results in a stricture or blind-ending obstruction (atresia)
2. Narrowing of duodenal lumen secondary to annular pancreas (stenosis)
3. Diaphragm, with or without hole, blocking the duodenal lumen (web)
4. Categorized into three types:
   a. Type 1 (92%): intraluminal web or diaphragm with intact mesentery and intact seromuscular layers in the involved intestinal segment
   b. Type 2 (1%): fibromuscular cord replaces intestinal segment on an intact mesentery
   c. Type 3 (7%): complete atretic segment with mesenteric gap and proximal/distal blind-ending intestinal pouches
5. Incidence: 1 in 6,000 to 10,000

B. Pathogenesis

1. Failure of recanalization
2. Atresia occurs with vascular disruptions during development.

C. Clinical presentation

1. Epigastric fullness
2. Bilious emesis

D. Diagnosis

1. Maternal history: polyhydramnios
2. Birth history: prematurity
3. Clinical signs: epigastric fullness, bilious emesis
4. "Double-bubble" sign on X-ray of abdomen (Fig. 14-4)
5. Absence of gas in the small bowel or colon on abdominal X-ray

FIGURE 14-4 Classic radiographic appearance of duodenal atresia. There is a double bubble of gas in the stomach and proximal duodenum, with no gas in the distal intestinal tract.

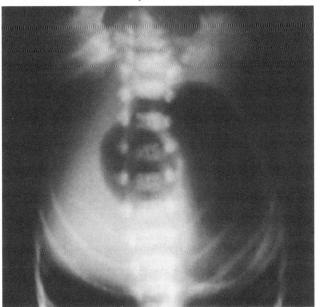

(Reprinted with permission from Mulholland MW, Lillemoe KD, Doherty GM, Maier RV, Upchurch GR, eds. *Greenfield's Surgery: Scientific Principles and Practice.* 4th ed. Philadelphia, PA: Lippincott Williams & Wilkins; 2006.)

E. Treatment
1. IV fluids, antibiotics, and NG or orogastric tube
2. Surgery
a. Duodenoduodenostomy
b. Duodenojejunostomy

III. Intestinal Atresia/Stenosis

A. General principles
1. Obliteration of a segment of intestine during development that results in a stricture or blind-ending obstruction of the intestine
2. Categorized into four types:
a. Type 1: intraluminal web or diaphragm with intact mesentery and intact seromuscular layers in the involved intestinal segment
b. Type 2: fibromuscular cord replaces intestinal segment on an intact mesentery
c. Type 3: two subtypes
(1) Type 3a: complete atretic segment with mesenteric gap and proximal/distal blind-ending intestinal pouches
(2) Type 3b: complete atretic segment with mesenteric gap, with distal pouch corkscrewed around a single mesenteric vessel
d. Type 4: multiple atretic segments in succession with mesenteric gaps (Fig. 14-5)
3. Occurs in about 1 in 500 to 1,500 live births
4. Occurs in about 15% of cases of gastroschisis
B. Pathogenesis
1. Fetal intestine develops from the midgut and undergoes a sequence of elongation, herniation from the coelomic cavity, rotation, return to the coelomic cavity, and fixation to the posterior abdominal wall.
2. Blood supply is derived from the superior mesenteric artery (SMA) that arises off of the dorsal aorta during development.
3. Atresia occurs with vascular disruptions during development.
4. The greater the vascular insult, the more severe the atresia.
C. Clinical features
1. Bilious emesis
2. Abdominal distension
3. Failure to pass meconium
D. Diagnosis
1. Maternal history: polyhydramnios
2. Birth history: prematurity
3. Signs and symptoms: bilious emesis, abdominal distension, failure to pass meconium
4. Plain abdominal films: dilated proximal intestine and a decompressed distal intestine/colon
5. Barium enema: microcolon
E. Treatment
1. NG suction should be initiated upon diagnosis of atresia.
2. Correction of any fluid or electrolyte imbalances should be undertaken before surgery.
3. Surgery may be performed semi-electively after stabilization.
a. Tapering jejunoplasty
b. End-to-end anastomosis
4. TPN until return of bowel function

IV. Necrotizing Enterocolitis

A. General principles
1. Necrotizing enterocolitis (NEC) is an intestinal ischemic injury that begins in the mucosa but may progress to full-thickness necrosis of segments of small bowel and/or colon.
2. NEC occurs most commonly in premature infants.
3. The incidence of NEC is increasing because of neonatal intensive care advances allowing younger gestational age infants to survive past delivery.

FIGURE 14-5 Classification of intestinal atresia. Type I, muscular continuity with a complete web. Type II, mesentery intact, fibrous cord. Type IIIa, muscular and mesenteric discontinuous. Type IIIb, apple-peel deformity. Type IV, multiple atresias.

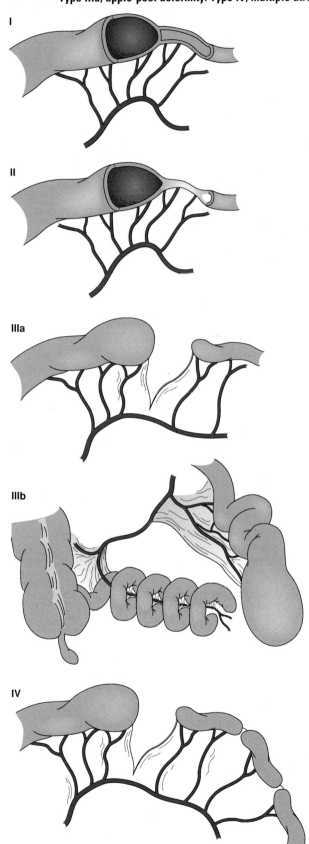

I

II

IIIa

IIIb

IV

(Adapted with permission from Grosfeld JL. Jejunoileal atresia and stenosis. In O'Neill JA Jr., Rowe MI, Grosfeld JL, Fonkalsrud EW, Coran AG, eds. *Pediatric Surgery.* 5th ed. St. Louis: Mosby; 1998:1145–1158.)

B. Etiology
1. The exact cause of NEC is unknown.
2. The cause is most likely multifactorial. NEC is associated with the initiation of enteral feeding.
   a. It is linked with low blood flow states/hypoxia in the intestine.
      (1) Cardiac defects with shunting (ventral septal defect [VSD], tetrology of Fallot [TOF], coarctation with closure of the patent ductus arteriosus [PDA])
      (2) Respiratory failure
      (3) Hypotension
   b. Infectious etiology
      (1) Tends to occur in clusters
      (2) Association with *Clostridium, Pseudomonas, Klebsiella, Enterobacter,* and *Staphylococcus* species
   c. Immunologic factors
      (1) Host inflammatory response and free radical damage play a role.
      (2) May help to propagate and worsen an existing case of NEC

C. Diagnosis
1. Diagnosis and degree of disease is made clinically based on several types of findings.
2. Useful findings
   a. Clinical symptoms include abdominal distention, bloody stools, bilious emesis, and intolerance of feedings.
   b. Physical examination findings include abdominal distention with tenderness, decreased bowel sounds, blood per rectum, and/or abdominal wall erythema.
   c. Laboratory values may show thrombocytopenia, neutropenia, elevated prothrombin time/partial thromboplastin time, metabolic acidosis, and/or hyponatremia.
   d. Imaging may reveal diffuse bowel distention/ileus, pneumatosis intestinalis, fixed loops on serial X-rays, and portal venous air/free air.

D. Treatment
1. Most cases of NEC can be managed medically.
   a. NG decompression and bowel rest with TPN
   b. Broad-spectrum intravenous antibiotics
   c. Close monitoring and correction of fluid and electrolyte abnormalities
   d. Proper ventilation and avoidance of hypoxemia
2. Surgery is indicated in any case of bowel perforation/necrosis with pneumoperitoneum.
   a. Abdominal compartment syndrome becoming worse in spite of maximum medical efforts
   b. Goal of surgery is to resect necrotic segments while maintaining as much viable bowel as possible to avoid short bowel syndrome (SBS).
      (1) Standard of care is to create an ostomy, rather than to perform primary anastomosis, because the disease process may still progress postoperatively.
      (2) Multiple resections and multiple enterostomies may be necessary.
      (3) To help preserve intestinal length, marginal areas may be left and re-evaluated at a second-look procedure.
   c. Some data suggests that in highly unstable neonates with evidence of perforation and sepsis, peritoneal drains and antibiotics may be sufficient for initial treatment and superior to operative management.

V. Meconium Ileus

A. General principles
1. This is an obstructive condition of the distal ileum in newborn infants with cystic fibrosis, due to thicker-than-normal, inspissated meconium.
2. The presenting symptom in 10% to 20% of patients with cystic fibrosis

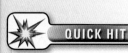

QUICK HIT

During the acute inflammatory phase of NEC, contrast studies can worsen the condition and are contraindicated. If the diagnosis is in question, serial abdominal radiographs should be obtained.

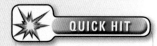

QUICK HIT

If the infant with NEC has a concurrent PDA, surgical closure of the PDA, rather than indomethacin administration, is indicated.

B. Clinical features
   1. Cystic fibrosis is a disorder of chloride channels caused by a single base deletion in the cystic fibrosis transmembrane conductance regulator (CFTR) gene.
   2. GI and pulmonary secretions are abnormally thick due to diminished volume of secretions and increased reabsorption of sodium chloride via normal sodium-potassium pump function, leading to further dehydration of the secretions.
   3. Patients typically present with failure to pass meconium, abdominal distention, and bilious vomiting.
C. Diagnosis
   1. Presence of cystic fibrosis, with a family history of the disease
   2. Abdominal X-ray: dilated loops of small bowel
   3. Contrast enema: a small diameter to the colon
D. Treatment
   1. Treatment of meconium ileus is conservative initially.
      a. Saline enemas/irrigation
      b. Gastrografin enemas
      c. Dilute N-acetylcysteine enemas
      d. Manual stimulation or suppositories
   2. In refractory cases, surgery may be required.
      a. Laparotomy, with enterotomy and manual removal meconium
         (1) Simple enterotomy with primary closure is the procedure of choice.
         (2) If any nonviable or marginal bowel noted, segmental resection with primary anastomosis may be required.
      b. Temporary surgical enterostomy with continued irrigation may be necessary.
      c. T-tube placement into terminal ileum for continued irrigation may also be used.
   3. Complicated cases may involve segmental volvulus, ischemia, stenosis/atresia, or perforation and require segmental resection and anastomosis.
   4. Postoperatively, the continued irrigation of the bowel with dilute N-acetylcysteine via NG tube, or enema to keep meconium and stool soluble for easier passage, may be required.

VI. Malrotation

A. General principles
   1. This abnormal anatomic position of the bowel is due to aberrant or absent embryologic rotation of the gut between the 5th and 10th weeks of gestation.
   2. The result is a malpositioned, shortened intestine with abnormal attachments to the peritoneal wall.
   3. Main types of malrotation
      a. Nonrotation: very shortened small intestine on the right, duodenum does not cross midline, cecum at midline, and colon on left
      b. Incomplete rotation: small intestine mostly on the right, colon on the left with cecum in the left upper quadrant, densely affixed to the right posterior body wall
      c. Mesocolic hernia: incomplete rotation, resulting in essentially normal length of bowel, but with nonfixation of the right or left colon, allowing for potential space for internal herniation of bowel to occur
      d. Nonfixation: normal position of duodenum and cecum and colon without the normal attachments to the retroperitoneum, resulting in potential for volvulus
B. Pathogenesis
   1. Normal midgut rotation occurs along the axis of the SMA with a 270-degree counterclockwise rotation resulting in an anteriorly located colon and posteriorly located small intestine.
   2. Rotation occurs during physiologic herniation outside of the coelomic cavity between weeks 5 and 10 of normal gestation and is associated with a significant lengthening of the jejunoileal segment during this time.
   3. The failure or cessation of rotation and fixation due to unknown causes is the source of malrotation.

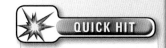

QUICK HIT

A classic finding on abdominal X-ray is Neuhauser or "soap bubble" sign, in which there is a ground-glass appearance meconium mixed with air in the right lower quadrant.

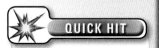

QUICK HIT

60% to 70% of meconium ileus cases resolve with conservative management.

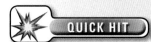

QUICK HIT

The dense attachments between the body wall and cecum in incomplete rotation are known as Ladd bands; they pass anterior to the small intestine and may serve as a point of obstruction.

Pediatric Surgery

C. Clinical features: Patients typically present by 1 month of age with bilious emesis, due to duodenal obstruction due to Ladd bands, or midgut volvulus due to nonfixation.

D. Diagnosis
   1. Many patients remain asymptomatic, and may be discovered incidentally due to studies performed for other reasons.
   2. The diagnostic study of choice is upper GI series with small bowel follow-through.
      a. If the duodenum does not cross the midline, malrotation is the diagnosis.
      b. The appearance will be of a mostly right-sided small bowel and mostly left-sided colon in malrotation.

E. Treatment
   1. Because of the risk for midgut volvulus with complete occlusion of the SMA and full loss of the bowel it supplies, the treatment of choice is emergent laparotomy and repair even in asymptomatic patients.
   2. Surgical repair, known as Ladd procedure, includes:
      a. Detorsion of the midgut
      b. Division of Ladd bands
      c. Placement of the cecum in the left upper quadrant and placement of the small intestine in the right upper quadrant
      d. Passage of a catheter through the duodenum to rule out associated duodenal obstruction
      e. Widening of the mesentery
      f. Appendectomy to prevent future misdiagnosis

VII. Hirschsprung Disease (Congenital Aganglionic Megacolon)

A. General principles
   1. A functional, rather than mechanical, obstruction of the colon due to failure of ganglion development in a segment of the colon
   2. Results in failure of colonic peristalsis and obstruction

B. Pathogenesis
   1. During the fifth to seventh gestational weeks, neural crest cells migrate (craniocaudal migration) into the wall of the colon, forming the Auerbach myenteric plexus and Meissner submucosal plexus.
   2. Failure of the migration of neural crest cells into the colon wall, or subsequent failure of microenvironmental support and development of neural crest cells that have migrated into the colonic wall, leads to Hirschsprung disease.
   3. Exact cause is unknown, but several genes, including the *RET* prow to oncogene, endothelin 3 gene, and endothelin B receptor gene, have been implicated.
   4. Varying degrees of aganglionosis occur, but they always occur in distal to proximal fashion.

C. Clinical features
   1. Patients may present with bilious emesis, abdominal distention, and a history of infrequent bowel movements/constipation.
   2. In neonates, a delayed passage of meconium (greater than 24 hours) may occur.
   3. More mild cases may present later in life and are felt to be due to "super short segment" aganglionosis.

D. Diagnosis: A diagnostic pathway includes:
   1. Anorectal examination to rule out anorectal anomaly
   2. Abdominal X-ray to rule out other sources of obstruction
   3. Barium enema to identify the transition zone—results in a "bird beak" appearance.
   4. Anorectal manometry
   5. Suction-assisted rectal biopsy with absence of ganglion cells confirms the diagnosis.
   6. Full-thickness rectal biopsy

E. Treatment
   1. Surgical correction is curative.
   2. Typically requires temporary colostomy proximal to the transition zone

3. Definitive procedure is performed at age 6 to 12 months.
4. Definitive procedures
   a. Duhame–Martin procedure: resection of aganglionic segment with colorectal anastomosis of normal colon posteriorly to aganglionic remnant of rectum anteriorly (retrorectal colonic pull-through)
   b. Soave procedure: division of the colon at the transition point with transanal mucosal proctectomy and transrectal pull-through (endorectal pull-through) excision of aganglionic segment, with colorectal anastomosis
   c. Laparoscopic-assisted pull-through

VIII. Intussusception

A. General principles
   1. Invagination or "telescoping" of a segment of bowel into itself, resulting in mechanical obstruction
   2. May occur in any segment of intestine, but ileocolic is the most common
B. Etiology
   1. The exact cause is unknown, but it is thought to occur due to a "lead point" at which the intussusceptum initiates and peristalsis propagates.
   2. Lead points may be lymphoid hyperplasia due to viral infections, Meckel diverticulum, polyps, lymphoma, or other space-filling lesions in the intestine.
C. Clinical features
   1. Typical presentation of a young child with severe colicky abdominal pain, alternating with periods free of pain
   2. Other symptoms and signs include bilious vomiting, abdominal distention with a sausage-shaped right lower quadrant mass, and "currant jelly stools" on rectal examination.
D. Diagnosis
   1. The presence of clinical features is diagnostic.
   2. The diagnostic procedure of choice is contrast enema, which is also therapeutic in roughly 60% of cases.
E. Treatment
   1. Hydrostatic reduction with contrast enema is the initial therapeutic procedure.
   2. If hydrostatic reduction fails, pneumatic reduction with air-contrast enema may be attempted.
      a. Pressures are 80 mm Hg for infants and 120 mm Hg for young children.
      b. This is successful in 90% of patients.
   3. Surgery is indicated for peritonitis/shock or with failure of nonoperative means.
      a. Manual reduction on exploratory laparotomy (open or laparoscopic) is usually sufficient in uncomplicated cases.
      b. Resection may be required if bowel necrosis or a worrisome lead point is observed.
      c. Most surgeons perform an appendectomy to prevent future misdiagnosis.
   4. Patients should be kept in the hospital postreduction. Approximately 12% of intussusceptions recur.
   5. Recurrent intussusceptions in older children warrant exploratory surgery to rule out tumors as a causative lead point.

IX. Imperforate Anus

A. General principles
   1. Failure of the anorectal orifice to develop, which can result in communications between the rectum and urogenital systems anywhere in the pelvis
   2. Classified as low or high types
      a. Low: located distal to the puborectalis muscle
         (1) Does not require colostomy
         (2) Frequently presents with perineal meconium fistula
      b. High: located above the puborectalis muscle
         (1) Requires colostomy
         (2) Typically with fistulization to urethra, bladder, or vagina

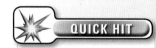

QUICK HIT

Although intussusception may occur in adults, it is overwhelmingly more common in infants and young children. When it occurs in adults, surgical exploration is indicated to rule out a malignant lead point.

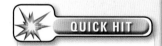

QUICK HIT

Although currant jelly stools (bloody, mucoid stools) are classically described in intussusception, they are only variably present. However, guaiac-positive stools occur in 90% to 95% of cases.

Pediatric Surgery

B. Etiology
1. Imperforate anus occurs due to abnormal development of the urorectal septum, which results in incomplete division of the fetal cloaca into urogenital and anorectal portions.
2. Associated anomalies
   a. VACTERL syndrome
   b. Urogenital abnormalities (in up to 50%) such as vesicoureteric reflux, solitary kidney, pelviureteric junction obstruction, megaureter, and undescended testis, as well as urinary incontinence
   c. Skeletal abnormalities (in up to 40%) such as spinal and vertebral anomalies
   d. Cardiovascular abnormalities (in up to 30%) such as atrial septal defect (ASD), VSD, and PDA
   e. GI abnormalities (in up to 15%) such as TE fistula and duodenal obstruction
C. Diagnosis
1. Diagnosis is by physical examination, with close attention paid for possible fistula.
2. Plain X-ray of the pelvis 24 hours after birth (to allow distal passage of swallowed air), with the infant held head down, helps reveal the level of involvement.
D. Treatment
1. Low type: primary repair with perineal approach and pull-through
2. High type
   a. Colostomy in infancy, followed by posterior sagittal anorectoplasty at age 4 to 8 months
   b. Laparoscopic-assisted anorectoplasty

X. Biliary Atresia

A. General principles
1. Obliteration of the biliary tract in infants, resulting in neonatal cholestasis and jaundice
2. Classified into two types
   a. Intrahepatic: also known as biliary hypoplasia, a rare condition consisting of a patent but narrow-caliber biliary system
   b. Extrahepatic: more common form that involves obliteration of the extrahepatic bile ducts and gallbladder
      (1) Type I: obliteration of the common bile duct
      (2) Type II: obliteration of the proper hepatic duct with cystic dilation of the porta hepatis
      (3) Type III: atresia of the left and right hepatic ducts, extending up to the level of the porta hepatis (most common type)
3. Untreated, this will progress to cirrhosis and hepatic failure.
B. Etiology
1. Etiology is unknown, but biliary atresia is thought to occur as a result of inflammatory process in the biliary ductal system after birth.
2. There is no clear causative factor, but viral infection or toxin exposure in the ductal system may play a role.
3. The condition is extremely rare in premature or stillborn infants, suggesting a postgestational cause.
C. Clinical features: neonatal jaundice lasting greater than 2 to 4 weeks, icteric urine, and acholic, clay-colored stools
D. Diagnosis
1. Clinical symptomatology is suggestive.
2. Elevated direct bilirubin is suggestive.
3. α1-Antitrypsin with PI typing, to rule out deficiency of this enzyme, and sweat chloride test to rule out cystic fibrosis as sources for cholestasis
4. Definitive studies
   a. Hepato-iminodiacetic acid (HIDA) scan showing rapid liver uptake with no excretion of radiotracer into bowel
   b. Liver ultrasound showing increased liver echogenicity and biliary dilation with a small, shrunken gallbladder

c. Liver biopsy
    (1) Considered the most important diagnostic test
    (2) High sensitivity in a suggestive clinical picture
    (3) May perform intraoperative cholangiogram via gallbladder cannulation at time of surgery
d. Endoscopic retrograde cholangiopancreatography (ERCP)
    (1) Until recently, small enough scopes did not exist.
    (2) Likely to be a more utilized diagnostic study in the future

E. Treatment
  1. Intrahepatic form requires orthotopic liver transplant for survival.
  2. Extrahepatic form can be treated with portoenterostomy.
    a. Described by Kasai in the 1950s
    b. Involves resection of the atretic ductal system and anastomosis of a Roux-en-Y limb to the porta hepatis
      (1) Level of resection determined by frozen section to assess duct diameter adequacy
      (2) Cholangitis is a frequent postoperative complication.
    c. From 25% to 35% of patients have a 10-year survival without liver transplant, and the remaining two-thirds require transplant.

XI. Short Bowel Syndrome

A. General principles: SBS is the need for TPN for more than 42 days after bowel resection or a residual small bowel length of less than 25% expected for gestational age.
  1. Anatomic: less than 75% of intestinal resection
  2. Functional: failure to thrive in spite of adequate length
  3. Etiology
    a. NEC: 32%
    b. Atresia: 20%
    c. Volvulus: 17%
    d. Gastroschisis: 17%
    e. Aganglionosis: 6%
    f. Other: 8%

B. Clinical features
  1. Initial period: extreme fluid and electrolyte loss (1 to 2 weeks)
    a. Dehydration secondary to diarrhea
    b. Electrolyte abnormality
    c. Weight loss
  2. Intestinal adaptation (48 hours up to 2 years)
    a. Mucosal hypertrophy: increased villi height and increased crypt depth
    b. By removing specific portions of small bowel, such as in a jejunectomy, the ileum takes over all the absorptive function of jejunum and gastric hypersecretion, due to jejunal resection.
    c. Ileal resection
      (1) Decreased transit time
      (2) Loss of bile salts leads to cholelithiasis and malabsorption of fat, leading to vitamin deficiency (A, D, E).
      (3) Hyperoxaluria leads to nephrolithiasis.

C. Treatment
  1. Medical and nutritional management
    a. TPN is required to maintain nutritional support and continued growth.
    b. Continued enteral feeding is required for the intestinal adaptation.
      (1) Volume should be increased gradually.
      (2) Enteral feeding should be increased and TPN should be reduced relatively as per patient tolerance.
      (3) If fluid losses increase by greater than 50% in 24 hours, do not increase enteral feeds.

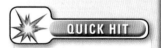

QUICK HIT

Normal length of small intestine in a full-term infant: 200–250 cm.

Pediatric Surgery

(4) Once the balanced combination of enteral and parenteral nutrition is stabilized, TPN should be changed from around the clock to cycling nighttime infusion.
  c. Pharmacotherapy
    (1) Nutritional supplement
      (a) Glutamine: fuel for enterocytes
      (b) Medium-chain fatty acids: fuel for colonocytes
      (c) Pectin
      (d) Soy polysaccharide
    (2) Decrease the gastric secretion.
      (a) H$_2$ blocker
      (b) Protein pump inhibitor
    (3) Increase the intestinal transit time.
      (a) Opioid: codeine
      (b) Diphenoxylate
      (c) Loperamide
      (d) Cholestyramine
      (e) Somatostatin and octreotide (severe refractory diarrhea)
2. Surgical management: functions and options
  a. Increased transit time
    (1) Intestinal valves
    (2) Reverse segments
    (3) Recirculatory loop
    (4) Colon interposition
  b. Functional improvement
    (1) Tapering enteroplasty
    (2) Stricturopathy
  c. Increase in intestinal length (increased mucosa surface area)
    (1) Bianchi procedure: where bowel is cut in half, and each half is closed lengthwise and sewn together end to end
    (2) Serial transverse enteroplasty (STEP): Bowel is stapled serially in a zig-zag pattern.
    (3) Kimura procedure (Iowa): autologous staged reconstruction used in patients with inadequate mesentery for a Bianchi procedure
    (4) Intestinal transplant
3. Complications
  a. TPN-induced liver disease
  b. Bacterial overgrowth leading to sepsis
  c. Secretory diarrhea
  d. Vitamin deficiencies
  e. Failure to thrive
  f. Central line infections

XII. Meckel Diverticulum

A. General principles
  1. A true diverticulum of the small bowel, a remnant of the omphalomesenteric duct
  2. Present in 2% of the population
B. Presentation: in children, can result in brisk lower GI bleeding, intussusception, or diverticulitis with perforation
  1. Bleeding: usually due to gastric tissue located in the diverticulum, which results in an ulcer on the mesenteric border of small bowel
    a. Treatment is with resection of the entire section of small bowel.
  2. Obstruction/intussusception: Meckel diverticulum can act as a lead point for intussusception.
    a. Intussusception caused by Meckel diverticulum is usually recurrent after successful reduction with barium enema, and exploration should be considered.

CLINICAL PEARL 14-2

"Rule of Twos" for Meckel Diverticulum

- Two percent of the population
- Usually present by age 2 years
- Within 2 feet of the ileocecal valve
- Contain two types of tissue: pancreatic and gastric
- Usually 2 inches long
- Two percent are symptomatic.
- Boys are two times more likely to have Meckel diverticulum than girls.

3. Diverticulitis
    a. Can present with similar features as appendicitis
    b. Exploration for appendicitis that reveals a normal appendix warrants further exploration for Meckel diverticulum.
    c. Can be treated with simple diverticulectomy
4. Management of incidentally found Meckel diverticulum during exploration for another pathology is controversial (see Clinical Pearl 14-2).

ABDOMINAL CYSTS

I. Mesenteric Cysts
A. The majority of these cystic intra-abdominal masses involve the short segment of mesentery.
B. Clinical features include pain and vomiting.

II. Duplication Cysts
A. Cyst walls have all three layers of intestine. They can present anywhere along the GI tract.
B. Types
    1. Tubular (communicating)
    2. Cystic (noncommunicating)
C. Diagnosis
    1. X-ray of abdomen
    2. Ultrasonography and CT of abdomen
D. Treatment: Surgical therapy involves excision of cyst with or without bowel resection, depending on extent of lesions.

III. Omental Cysts
A. Cysts are lymph-filled.
B. Symptoms and signs include pain, tenderness, and abdominal distention, depending on size.
C. Treatment involves laparoscopic or open operation.

IV. Hepatic Cysts
A. May be single or multiple
    1. Congenital
    2. Acquired
B. Symptoms include abdominal pain.
C. Diagnosis
    1. Ultrasound of the abdomen
    2. CT scan of the abdomen
    3. HIDA scan to rule out biliary connectors

D. Treatment: surgical
1. Noncommunicating cyst: laparoscopic or open marsupialization
2. Communicating cyst: Roux-en-Y drainage

V. Choledochal Cysts

A. Cystic malformation of biliary tree
B. Types
1. Saccular or diffuse dilatation of extrahepatic bile duct
2. Diverticulum of extrahepatic bile duct
3. Choledochocele
4. Multiple cysts of extrahepatic or intrahepatic bile duct
5. Single or multiple intrahepatic bile duct
C. Clinical features
1. Obstructive jaundice
2. Abdominal pain and mass
3. Acholic stools
4. Signs and symptoms of cholangitis
D. Diagnosis
1. Conjugated hyperbilirubinemia
2. Ultrasound and CT of the abdomen
3. HIDA scan
4. ERCP in older patients, which may be helpful
E. Treatment: cyst excision with Roux-en-Y hepaticojejunostomy

VI. Lymphangiomas

A. Mostly retroperitoneal intraoperatively
B. Lymph-filled cyst
C. Symptoms and signs: pain and tenderness
D. Treatment: laparoscopic or open operation (partial or near-total removal)

VII. Urachal Remnants

A. Midline swelling of the lower abdomen, which can be found anywhere from urinary bladder to umbilicus, along the course of urachus
B. Clinical features
1. Abdominal mass
2. Discharge from the umbilicus
3. Urinary complaints
C. Diagnosis
1. Ultrasound of the abdomen and pelvis
2. Voiding cystourethrogram
D. Treatment: exploration of umbilical region and excision of urachus remnant with repair of urinary bladder, if required

 ONCOLOGY

Although leukemia and lymphoma represent the most common cancer diagnoses in children, their management is generally medical and beyond the scope of a surgical text. This section will therefore focus on the most common solid tumors of infancy and childhood, where general pediatric surgical therapy is a mainstay of treatment.

I. Neuroblastoma

A. A solid tumor arising from primitive neural crest cells
B. Epidemiology
1. Incidence: 1 in 7,500 to 10,000
2. Age of onset: More than 50% present within 2 years of birth.
3. Relative frequency: 10% of childhood tumors, which represents the most common extracranial solid tumor in children

C. Sites: Locations tend to be in the distribution of derivatives of neural crest cells.
   1. Adrenal gland (50%)
   2. Paraspinal (25%)
   3. Mediastinum (20%)
   4. Neck (5%)
   5. Pelvis (less than 5%) pelvic organ of Zuckerkandl
D. Etiology
   1. Associated with the N-myc oncogene
   2. Associated genetic abnormalities of deletions on the p arm of chromosome 1, and gain of DNA on the q arm of chromosome 17, both of which confer a worse prognosis
E. Clinical features
   1. Typically appears as highly cellular, uniform tumor with varying degrees of stroma within the tumor on microscopy
   2. Graded on the Shimada scale
      a. Favorable factors are tumor rich in stroma, young age, and a low mitosis/karyorrhexis index (MKI).
      b. Unfavorable factors are nodular pattern, greater age at diagnosis, poor differentiation, and high MKI.
      c. MKI assesses the number of mitoses and karyorrhexis per 5,000 cells in the tumor.
   3. Typically present as a cervical, abdominal, or pelvic solid mass
      a. Cervical neuroblastoma
         (1) Rarely obstruct the airway
         (2) Arise from the cervical sympathetic chain and result in a Horner syndrome on the involved side
         (3) Nodal involvement common, distant metastasis rare
      b. Abdominal neuroblastoma
         (1) Most common presentation
         (2) Fixed hard mass arising in the abdomen, crossing the midline, arising from the adrenal medulla or midline sympathetic chain
         (3) Nodal involvement along the aorta or in the mediastinum is common.
      c. Pelvic neuroblastoma
         (1) Often found by parent by palpation
         (2) May lead to obstructive symptoms in the bowel or ureter
         (3) May involve sacral nerves, mandating close physical examination of lower extremity motor function and anal sphincter tone
   4. Associated signs/symptoms
      a. Periorbital ecchymosis due to venous congestion/rupture with metastasis to the eyes
      b. Myoclonus due to antitumor antibody cross-reaction with Purkinje fibers in the cerebellum
      c. Secretory diarrhea syndrome due to secretion of vasoactive intestinal peptide
F. Diagnosis
   1. Imaging with contrasted CT or MRI will show tumor extent.
   2. Metaiodobenzylguanidine (MIBG) scan
   3. Serum and urinary marker
   4. Biopsy is the mainstay of diagnosis and staging.
G. Treatment
   1. Low-risk tumor can be treated with resection alone.
   2. High-risk tumor should be treated with resection and central venous access device placement for chemotherapy and radiation.

II. Nephroblastoma (Wilms Tumor)

A. General principles
   1. A tumor of primitive metanephric blastema cells

2. The most common pediatric renal tumor and the fifth most common pediatric cancer

B. Etiology
1. Sporadic form results from two allele loss in a specific tumor suppressor gene.
2. *WTI*, an oncogene located on chromosome 11 involved in development of Wilms tumor
3. Associated with other clinical syndromes
   a. Denys–Drash syndrome: Wilms tumor, pseudohermaphroditism, glomerulonephropathy
   b. WAGR syndrome: Wilms tumor, aniridia, genitourinary malformation, and mental retardation
   c. Beckwith–Wiedemann syndrome
   d. Hemihypertrophy

C. Clinical features
1. Typically presents with a palpable abdominal or flank mass, with or without abdominal pain
2. Other signs include hematuria, hypertension, and/or tumor necrosis with associated fever.

D. Diagnosis
1. Imaging
   a. Renal ultrasound is often the initial study obtained to assess renal mass and renal vascular involvement.
   b. CT of the chest, abdomen, and pelvis allows assessment of tumor, differentiation from neuroblastoma of the adrenal gland, assessment of the opposite kidney, and nodal or distant metastasis.
2. Staging, which requires surgical resection
   a. Stage 1: tumor confined to kidney and completely resected
   b. Stage 2: tumor completely excised, but with extension beyond renal capsule, or biopsy of confined tumor with local spillage
   c. Stage 3: tumor incompletely excised, positive lymph nodes, peritoneal implants, or intra-abdominal tumor spillage
   d. Stage 4: hematogenous or lymph node metastasis beyond the abdominal cavity
   e. Stage 5: simultaneous bilateral involvement, with each side staged 1 to 3 separately

E. Treatment
1. Surgical resection is required for treatment and staging.
2. Chemotherapy is required for all patients with Wilms tumor diagnosis and consists typically of doxorubicin, dactinomycin, and vincristine.
3. Radiation therapy is used for stage 3 to 5 disease.
4. If found to be unresectable by CT scanning, surgery can be delayed until after cytoreductive chemotherapy.

III. Hepatoblastoma

A. General principles
1. Hepatoblastoma is the most common liver malignancy in the pediatric population.
2. A relatively rare tumor, with an approximate incidence of 1 in 1,000,000 per year (more frequent in patients 6 months to 3 years of age)
3. Associated with Beckwith–Wiedemann syndrome and familial adenomatous polyposis

B. Pathology: Several histologic variants occur.
1. Epithelial
   a. Fetal (31%)
   b. Embryonal (19%)

    c. Macrotrabecular (3%)

    d. Anaplastic (3%)

  2. Mixed epithelial/mesenchymal (44%)

C. Diagnosis

  1. Most patients present with a palpable abdominal mass, with or without abdominal swelling, pain, irritability, GI disturbances, fever, pallor, and/or failure to thrive.

  2. Alpha-fetoprotein levels are significantly elevated with hepatoblastoma (greater than 90%).

  3. Imaging

    a. Abdominal X-ray may show hepatomegaly.

    b. CT reveals a heterogenous mass and is the imaging procedure of choice to assess metastasis, but it is less sensitive than MRI for primary diagnosis.

    c. MRI is the imaging procedure of choice.

  4. Staging requires resection.

    a. Stage 1: complete surgical resection

    b. Stage 2: microscopic positive margins without regional spread, confined to one lobe of the liver

    c. Stage 3: partially resected tumor, spillage of tumor at time of surgery, involving two lobes of the liver with positive lymph nodes

    d. Stage 4: distant metastasis

D. Treatment

  1. Typically, neoadjuvant chemotherapy with doxorubicin and cisplatin prior to surgical resection is used.

  2. Following cytoreduction, surgical resection with hepatic lobectomy is the procedure of choice, although in rare instances, a wedge resection may be used for small, peripherally located tumors.

  3. Liver transplantation (up to 6% of patients)

PHYSIOLOGIC CONSIDERATIONS IN PEDIATRIC SURGERY

It is often said that children are not just "little adults." There are important physiologic differences between children and adults that must be taken into account when caring for the pediatric surgical patient.

A. Fluid balance

  1. At birth, total body water is approximately 75% of total weight. This falls to 60% by age 1 year.

  2. Extracellular fluid volume is approximately 45% of total body weight at birth, and it falls to 20% by 1 year of age.

  3. Infants and children have a lower glomerular filtration rate and a reduced renal concentrating ability. Because of this, they tolerate dehydration poorly and cannot excrete salt or water loads as well as adults.

    a. Adequate urine output for an infant is 1 to 2 mL/kg/hr, as opposed to 0.5 mL/kg/hr for adults.

  4. Higher insensible losses due to higher body surface:weight ratio

  5. In general, fluid requirements follow the 4-2-1 rule: 4 mL/kg/hr for the first 10 kg, 2 mL/kg/hr for the second 10 kg, and 1 mL/kg/hr thereafter.

    a. In neonates, 70 mL/kg/24 hr in the first day of life and 100 mL/kg/24 hr thereafter.

B. Nutrition

  1. Infants have higher caloric requirements than adults or older children.

  2. Protein requirements are the highest during infancy.

  3. In infants and young children, TPN is indicated if nutrition is inadequate for 3 days or more, as opposed to 7 days in adults.

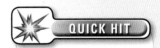

QUICK HIT

Gastric dilation is common in children (especially after trauma) and may result in vomiting, aspiration, and vagal bradycardia and hypotension. Treatment is gastric decompression.

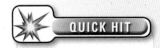

QUICK HIT

Intentional trauma is the most common cause of fatal injury in the first year of life and must be a consideration when injury patterns and mechanism are inconsistent.

C. Shock
  1. Hypovolemic and septic shock are most common.
  2. Shock response in infants is significantly different from older children and adults.
     a. Children and infants have much higher physiologic reserve and may tolerate much higher volume loss for longer periods of time before they become hypotensive.
     b. May become bradycardic in earlier stages of shock than older children and adults
     c. May not show hemodynamic compromise until shock becomes refractory
     d. Initial management includes fluid boluses in 20 mL/kg increments.
        1. If needed, blood is given in 10 mL/kg boluses.

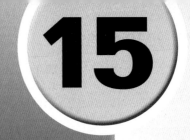

Orthopedic Surgery

Michelle Bramer, John Tidwell, and Stephanie Burkhardt

 TRAUMA/FRACTURES

I. General Principles

A. History and physical examination
1. A thorough history and physical are essential to make the diagnosis. Important aspects of the history include the mechanism of injury as well as the overall health status of the patient.
2. The injury must first be suspected in order to ensure proper imaging is obtained.
3. Always inspect and palpate the entire body to ensure injuries are not missed.
4. In trauma patients, always follow advanced trauma life support (ATLS) protocol.

B. Classification
1. Basis for classification: location
2. Fracture type: open or closed
3. Injury energy: high or low

C. Commonly used abbreviations for weight-bearing restrictions in orthopedic trauma patients (see Clinical Pearl 15-1).

D. Deep venous thromboses are a common sequela and complication of orthopedic injuries and surgical interventions. They are most commonly associated with pelvic trauma, lower extremity trauma, hip replacements, and knee replacements. Mobilization and mechanical prophylaxis should be encouraged in all orthopedic patients. For high-risk injuries and procedures, pharmacologic prophylaxis should also be considered.

II. Open Fractures

A. Introduction
1. Open fractures are usually caused by high-energy trauma.
2. The mechanism may be from the outside in, as in a penetrating trauma, or from the inside out, as in a bone spike that ruptures the skin.
3. Regardless of the mechanism, open fractures are a surgical urgency and require prompt diagnosis and treatment. Intravenous (IV) antibiotics, irrigation and debridement, and stabilization of the fracture are necessary.
4. Timely antibiotic administration is the most important factor to preventing infection.

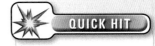

QUICK HIT

Timing of antibiotics administration is the most important factor to prevent infection with open fractures.

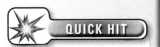

QUICK HIT

Diagnosis is made primarily by radiography. At least two radiographs of the bone/joint taken at right angles to each other are necessary to assess the fracture type. Always obtain a radiograph of the joint above and the joint below a known fracture/injury.

CLINICAL PEARL 15-1

Commonly Used Abbreviations for Weight-Bearing Restrictions

NWB	Non–weight bearing	LUE	Left upper extremity
TDWB	Touch-down weight bearing	LLE	Left lower extremity
PWB	Partial weight bearing	RUE	Right upper extremity
WBAT	Weight bearing as tolerated	RLE	Right lower extremity

B. History and physical
1. The mechanism of the injury as well as the timing of the injury and where it occurred are important parts of the history.
2. The history is usually consistent with a high-energy trauma such as a motor vehicle crash or fall from height. Open fractures in the elderly or those with osteoporotic bone may occur with a low-energy trauma.
3. The tetanus status of the patient should be obtained.
4. Important aspects of the physical examination include inspection of the entire involved extremity. In many cases, an obvious deformity is noted, but some open fractures may be subtle. Skin must be examined thoroughly and carefully on all injured extremities.
5. All abrasions and lacerations should be probed to see if they communicate with the fracture. Exposed bone should be placed back in the skin to prevent pressure necrosis.

C. Diagnosis
1. Two orthogonal radiographs, usually AP and lateral, should be obtained as soon as possible.
2. Radiographs of the joint above and the joint below the fracture should be obtained for complete evaluation of the injury.
3. In most cases, splints should be taken off to minimize the risk of inadequate films. If the patient has come from the scene and radiographs can be taken quickly, it is appropriate to provisionally splint the extremity with a pillow or other device and wait until after the radiographs have been taken to splint the patient.

D. Classification
1. There are three major types based on the mechanism of injury, degree of soft-tissue damage, configuration of the fracture, and the amount of contamination (see Clinical Pearl 15-2).
2. The most commonly used classification system is the Gustilo and Anderson system.

E. Treatment
1. Early treatment involves rapid IV antibiotics and tetanus prophylaxis, stabilization of the fracture and wound management, followed by aggressive rehabilitation.
2. Antibiotics are given based on the classification and the amount of contamination. They are typically given every 4 hours before surgery and then every 8 hours after surgery for a duration of 24 to 48 hours (see Clinical Pearl 15-3).
3. Surgical options vary, depending on the type of fracture and the area of the body.
   a. For types I, II, and some IIIA open fractures, definitive surgical stabilization can be carried out, usually in the form of intramedullary devices or plates and screws.
   b. For types IIIB and IIIC fractures, external fixation is usually required, with subsequent trips to the operating room for repeat irrigation and debridement before closure and definitive fixation.
   c. For types IIIB and IIIC fractures, plastic surgery is usually consulted for skin closure with flaps or grafts because the wounds require definitive closure 7 days from the time of injury to prevent secondary colonization of bacteria. Vascular surgery is consulted for repair as indicated by injury.

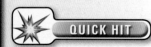

QUICK HIT

If a spine fracture is identified, always obtain imaging of the entire spine (cervical, thoracic, lumbar, sacral) because of the high incidence of associated fractures.

Orthopedic Surgery

CLINICAL PEARL 15-2

Classification of Fracture Type, Configuration and Degree of Contamination

Type I fractures	Skin opening ≤1 cm; soft tissue damage is usually minimal
Type II fractures	Skin opening >1cm; soft tissue damage is more extensive than type I fractures
Type III fractures	Extensive skin and soft tissue damage; three subgroups:

- IIIA – Sufficient soft tissue to provide adequate bone coverage
- IIIB – Require skin grafts or flaps to provide coverage
- IIIC – Involve vascular injury requiring repair

CLINICAL PEARL 15-3

Antibiotic Treatment of Open Fractures

Type I and II fractures	First-generation cephalosporin, typically cefazolin
Type III fractures	First-generation cephalosporin plus an aminoglycoside, usually gentamicin
Farmyard contamination, vascular compromise, extensive soft-tissue crush injuries	First-generation cephalosporin plus an aminoglycoside and add penicillin
Water injuries	First-generation cephalosporin plus an aminoglycoside and add fluoroquinolone (i.e., ciprofloxacin)

III. Fractures of the Distal Radius

A. Introduction

1. Fractures of the distal radius are very common. They include a wide spectrum of fractures, ranging from simple fractures requiring minimal treatment to complex fractures requiring open reduction and internal fixation (ORIF).

2. Fractures of the distal radius have a bimodal distribution, occurring commonly in children from 6 to 10 years of age and in adults from 60 to 69 years of age.

B. History and physical

1. Important aspects of the history include the age of the patient and his or her associated medical conditions, the mechanism of the injury as well as previous injuries to the wrist.

2. Important aspects of the physical examination include a thorough inspection of the skin and associated deformities as well as the neurovascular status of the involved extremity (see Clinical Pearl 15-4).

C. Imaging

1. Imaging of the upper extremity should include anteroposterior (AP) and lateral radiographs of the wrist as well as radiographs of the forearm and elbow.

2. Radiographic parameters in the normal wrist include the radial inclination (normally 23 degrees), the radial height (normally 12 mm), as well as the volar tilt (normally 11 degrees).

3. Radiographic signs in the fractured wrist include the level of the fracture (distance from the radiocarpal joint), loss of radial height, amount of dorsal comminution, extension of the fracture into the radiocarpal joint, and loss of volar tilt (resulting in dorsal tilt) (Fig. 15-1).

D. Classification

1. Numerous classification systems exist for fractures of the distal radius. For simplicity, and the ability to describe the injury to a coworker, an anatomic description as well as a description of the radiographic signs is most commonly used.

2. Eponymous descriptions are still widely used and include Colles, Smith, Chauffeur, and Barton fractures.

a. Colles fractures are transverse, extra-articular fractures of the distal radius. The distal fragment is displaced dorsally, resulting in the classic "dinner fork" deformity.

b. Smith fractures are reverse Colles fractures, in that the displacement of the distal fragment is volar (palmar).

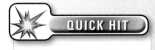

QUICK HIT

Most extra-articular distal radius fractures only require reduction and casting.

CLINICAL PEARL 15-4

Neuromuscular Assessment Clinical Pearls

Nerve	Motor	Muscle	Sensation
Radial	"Thumbs up" sign	Extensor pollicis longus	Radial aspect of the thumb
Median	"A-OK" sign	Flexor pollicis longus	Palmar surface of the index finger
Ulnar	Abduct the fingers	Dorsal interossei	Ulnar aspect of the small finger

Orthopedic Surgery

Distal radius fractures: external fixation and supplemental K-wires.

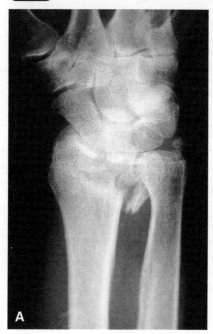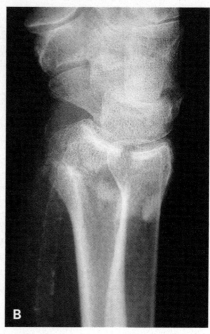

Anteroposterior view (**A**) and lateral view (**B**) of underlying unstable distal radius fracture.
(Reprinted with permission from Koval KJ, Zuckerman JD. *Atlas of Orthopaedic Surgery: A Multimedia Reference*. Philadelphia, PA: Lippincott Williams & Wilkins; 2004.)

    c. Chauffeur's fractures are intra-articular fractures of the radial styloid.

    d. Barton fractures are intra-articular fractures that result from a shearing force and are best seen in the lateral radiograph. Barton fractures are classified as either dorsal or volar, depending on which cortex the fracture extends into.

E. Treatment

  1. Treatment options are based on the fracture pattern and the stability of the fracture. Factors that influence operative treatment over nonoperative treatment based on the initial injury radiographs are age (older than 60 years), extension into the radiocarpal joint, loss of radial height (greater than 0.5 cm), amount of dorsal comminution, and loss of volar tilt (dorsal tilt greater than 20 degrees).

  2. Nonoperative distal radius fractures can be treated with closed reduction and casting in the emergency department.

    a. Options for anesthesia include reduction without anesthesia, oral/IV analgesia, hematoma block, Bier block, conscious sedation, and general anesthesia. Typically, a hematoma block using local anesthetic agents augmented with oral analgesia is used.

    b. Based on the stability of the reduction, patients can usually be maintained in a sugar tong splint with a three-point mold.

  3. Operative interventions vary depending on the experience of the surgeon. The two main methods include (1) ORIF (with a volar or dorsal plate) and (2) external fixation.

IV. Fractures of the Hip

A. Introduction

  1. It is estimated that the incidence of hip fractures (femoral neck and inter-trochanteric proximal femur fractures) is more than 300,000 per year in the United States alone. The risk of falling doubles between the ages of 65 and 85 years. Combined with the increased incidence of osteoporosis in this age group, the risk of sustaining an associated hip fracture increases hundredfold.

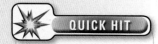

Hip fractures are usually secondary to osteoporosis. They can cause significant mortality within 1 year.

2. Fractures in elderly patients
    a. Significant low-energy injuries may result from osteoporosis or neoplasm.
    b. Although subtrochanteric, femoral shaft, and distal femoral fractures may occur in elderly patients due to low-energy trauma, usually high-energy trauma such as a fall from height or an automobile, motorcycle, or all-terrain vehicle crash is necessary.

B. History and physical
    1. Important aspects of the history include the patient's age, the mechanism of injury, current medications (including blood thinners), and associated medical comorbidities.
    2. Important aspects of the physical examination include a thorough neurovascular examination because some patients may sustain injuries to the sciatic nerve or develop compartment syndrome as a result of bleeding from the fracture site.

C. Imaging
    1. Most fractures of the proximal femur, including femoral head/neck fractures and intertrochanteric and subtrochanteric fractures, can be seen on an AP pelvis X-ray.
    2. Additional radiographs include full-length femur AP and lateral views. Occasionally, a computed tomography (CT) scan or magnetic resonance imaging (MRI) is necessary to evaluate for an occult fracture in an elderly patient with continued hip pain after a fall.

D. Classification
    1. Fractures of the femur are generally classified based on the anatomic location. The different locations are the femoral head, neck, intertrochanteric region, subtrochanteric region, shaft, and distal femur (Fig. 15-2).
    2. Femoral neck fractures are typically classified using the Garden classification.
        a. Type I: incomplete, valgus impacted
        b. Type II: complete, nondisplaced
        c. Type III: complete, partially displaced in varus alignment
        d. Type IV: completely displaced, with no contact between the fracture fragments
    3. Intertrochanteric femur fractures are more difficult to classify.
        a. Most systems classify the fracture patterns as stable or unstable, with special attention placed on reverse obliquity patterns.
        b. The stability of the fracture is generally based on the integrity of the posteromedial cortex (calcar femorale), which allows native bone to withstand compressive loads after reduction and fixation.

E. Treatment
    1. Treatment of hip fractures is based on the age of the patient, the patient's comorbidities, the quality of the patient's bone, and the pre-injury level of activity.
    2. Goals of treatment focus on improving the mobility of the patient and allowing immediate progressive weight bearing. Complications with remaining on bed rest include pneumonia, decubiti, urinary tract infections (UTIs), and deep vein thromboses (DVTs).
    3. For treatment purposes, fractures may be classified as Garden I/II and Garden III/IV.
        a. Stable (Garden I and II) fractures are usually treated with closed reduction and percutaneous pinning of the fracture. Usually, three screws are placed into the femoral head from the lesser trochanter.
        b. Unstable (Garden III and IV) fractures are usually treated with a unipolar hemiarthroplasty, a bipolar hemiarthroplasty, or a total hip arthroplasty with or without cement (Fig. 15-3).
    4. Intertrochanteric femur fractures can be fixed with a variety of implants, based on the surgeon's preference. Common implants include a compression hip screw with a side plate, cephalomedullary nails, and 95-degree angled blade plates.

Orthopedic Surgery

FIGURE 15-2 Intertrochanteric fracture with a close-up of femoral neck fracture.

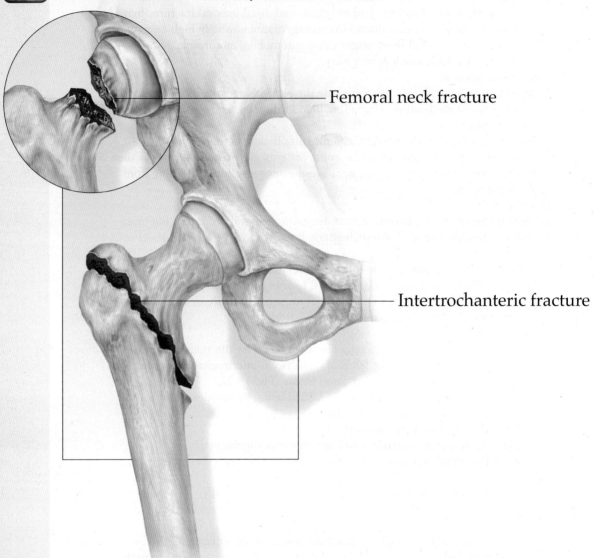

Femoral neck fracture

Intertrochanteric fracture

(Reprinted with permission from Anatomical Chart Company, Lower Extremity Disorders, 2008-10-21 0338, Diseases & Disorders, ACC Diseases and Disorders, ACC.)

FIGURE 15-3 Hemiarthroplasty of the femoral neck. Anteroposterior radiograph of the pelvis demonstrates a displaced, left femoral neck fracture.

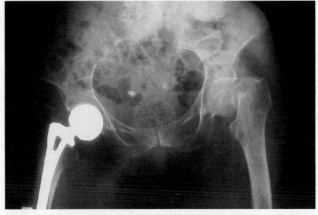

(Reprinted with permission from Koval KJ, Zuckerman JD. *Atlas of Orthopaedic Surgery: A Multimedia Reference*. Philadelphia, PA: Lippincott Williams & Wilkins; 2004.)

V. Sprains/Fractures of the Ankle

A. Introduction

1. The ankle is one of the most frequently injured areas of the body.

2. There is a continuum from sprains to fractures based on the mechanism of the injury and the amount of energy involved.

B. History and physical

1. Important aspects from the history are the energy and mechanism of the injury, previous injuries to the same area, and the associated medical comorbidities.

2. Important aspects of the physical examination are the condition of the skin, associated swelling or bruising, and a detailed examination of the nerves, arteries, and muscles that cross the ankle.

C. Imaging

1. The Ottawa ankle rules determine the appropriateness of obtaining ankle radiographs. These rules state that radiographs are indicated if there is pain in the malleolar zone of the ankle and one or more of the following is present:

a. Age older than 55 years

b. Bone tenderness at posterior edge of distal 6 cm

c. Tip of medial or lateral malleolus

d. The inability both to weight bear immediately after injury and walk four steps

2. Three views of the ankle are required to accurately assess fractures. Standard films include AP, lateral, and mortise views.

D. Classification

1. There are several ankle classification systems, including the AO-OTA and the Lauge–Hansen classifications. However, the most common practical classification system is based on a description of the fracture pattern involving the three malleoli of the ankle: lateral, medial, and posterior malleoli.

a. Fractures of the lateral malleolus are classified based on the level of the fracture via the Weber classification, with a Weber A fracture being below the level of the distal tibiofibular joint, a Weber B fracture being at the level of the joint, and a Weber C fracture being above the level of the joint (Fig. 15-4).

b. Fractures of the medial malleolus are usually described by the fracture pattern and the amount of displacement.

c. Fractures of the posterior malleolus are described based on the amount of joint space involvement and the amount of articular step-off.

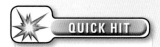

QUICK HIT

The Ottawa rules help guide indication for radiographs with ankle pain.

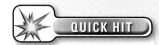

QUICK HIT

Ankle sprains are the most common musculoskeletal injury. The anterior talofibular ligament (ATFL) is the most commonly injured ligament in an inversion ankle sprain.

Orthopedic Surgery

FIGURE
15-4 Schematic diagram and case examples of the AO/OTA classification of ankle fractures.

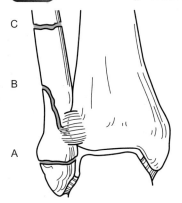

There are three types of ankle fractures in the AO/OTA classification: type A, type B, and type C. Each type is further subdivided into three groups: an anteroposterior radiograph of a type A distal fibula fracture in which the fracture line is completely below the level of the syndesmosis; a radiograph of a type B ankle fracture in which the fibula fracture begins anteriorly at the level of the distal tibiofibular syndesmosis; a mortise radiograph of a type C injury with disruption of the syndesmosis up to the level of the fibula fracture, which is completely above the distal syndesmotic ligament complex. There is a medial deltoid ligament injury.
(Reprinted with permission from Bucholz RW, Heckman JD, eds. *Rockwood & Green's Fractures in Adults*. 5th ed. Philadelphia, PA: Lippincott Williams & Wilkins; 2001.)

FIGURE
15-5 Bimalleolar ankle fractures: open reduction and internal fixation.

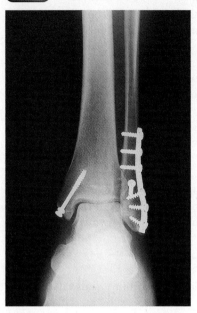

(Reprinted with permission from Koval KJ, Zuckerman JD, eds. *Atlas of Orthopaedic Surgery: A Multimedia Reference.* Philadelphia, PA: Lippincott Williams & Wilkins; 2004.)

    2. Fractures of more than one malleolus are called bimalleolar and trimalleolar ankle fractures, with descriptions of the fracture pattern of each malleolus involved.

E. Treatment

    1. Treatment of ankle sprains includes rest, ice, immobilization, elevation, and compression. It usually includes a period of nonweight bearing.

    2. Treatment of ankle fractures is based on restoration of the normal anatomy of the tibiotalar (ankle) joint.

    3. Isolated fractures of the lateral malleolus (Weber A or B) are usually treated nonoperatively. Small avulsion fractures of the tip of the lateral malleolus can be treated with an Aircast. Weber B fractures usually require a short leg walking cast.

    4. Isolated Weber C fractures are typically unstable and require ORIF.

    5. Isolated medial malleolus fractures may be treated nonoperatively if the fracture is nondisplaced. However, the treatment is a short leg cast with nonweight bearing for several months.

    6. Bimalleolar and bimalleolar equivalent fractures usually require ORIF with a plate and screw construct (Fig. 15-5).

    7. Trimalleolar ankle fractures typically require operative treatment. ORIF is most often the surgical procedure of choice.

VI. Shoulder Dislocations

A. Introduction

    1. Shoulder dislocations are common injuries, most often associated with high-energy injuries. They occur most commonly from motor vehicle crashes, falls from height, and athletic injuries.

    2. Most common joint in the body to dislocate

    3. The most common dislocation is anterior because of the bony and soft-tissue anatomy as well as the direction of the applied force.

B. History and physical

    1. History includes mechanism of injury, time of injury, age and activity level of patient, and medical comorbidities of the patient.

    2. Physical exam demonstrates pain in the shoulder as well as decreased mobility of the arm. Because of the proximity to the brachial plexus, a thorough and complete neurovascular exam must be performed.

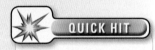

QUICK HIT

Axillary radiographs are required to make the diagnosis of shoulder dislocations.

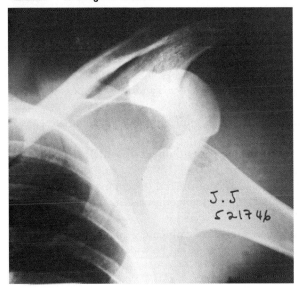

FIGURE 15-6 Subglenoid dislocation. Note that the humeral head is completely inferior to the glenoid fossa.

(Reprinted with permission from Bucholz RW, Heckman JD, eds. *Rockwood & Green's Fractures in Adults.* 5th ed. Philadelphia, PA: Lippincott Williams & Wilkins; 2001.)

  3. Special attention should be paid to axillary nerve function (sensation over lateral upper arm and motor function of the deltoid) because it is the most commonly injured nerve with a shoulder dislocation.
  4. Posterior dislocations are associated with seizures and electrocution.
 C. Imaging
  1. AP and axillary views of the shoulder are required to diagnose a dislocation. Because of the anatomy of the shoulder, an AP view may appear normal if the shoulder is dislocated directly anteriorly or posteriorly (Fig. 15-6).
  2. It may be difficult to obtain an axillary view secondary to pain, so assistance may be needed when obtaining this view.
 D. Classification
  1. Shoulder dislocations are classified based on the axillary view radiograph as either anterior or posterior.
 E. Treatment
  1. Mainstay of treatment is urgent closed reduction of the dislocation. There are many techniques for reducing a shoulder dislocation, including traction/countertraction, external rotation, and Stimson technique (prone technique with traction).
  2. Closed reductions routinely require pain control. This can include oral and IV analgesics, intra-articular injections of local anesthetics, conscious sedation, or even general anesthesia.
  3. Reduction must be confirmed by AP and axillary radiographs.
  4. Patient is placed into a sling for a short time period and then begins range-of-motion exercises and physical therapy to restore strength and motion.

VII. Compartment Syndrome
 A. Introduction
  1. Compartment syndrome is characterized by increased pressure in an enclosed space (fascial compartment) with the potential to cause irreversible damage to its contents, including nerves and blood vessels.
  2. It is an orthopedic emergency that necessitates prompt diagnosis and treatment.
  3. It is usually associated with a crush injury or a fracture of a long bone, most commonly in the forearm or lower leg.

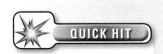

QUICK HIT

The key exam findings for compartment syndrome are pain out of proportion to injury and pain with passive stretch of that compartment.

B. History and physical
1. History usually includes a high-energy injury to a long bone or a crush injury to an extremity. Often associated with prolonged extrication from motor vehicles or enclosed spaces.
2. Physical exam findings include swelling, pain out of proportion to injury, and pain with passive stretch of the involved compartment (e.g., dorsiflexion of ankle causes pain in calf).
3. Late findings include pallor, paresthesias, paralysis, and pulselessness.
C. Diagnosis
1. The diagnosis of compartment syndrome is clinical in an awake and alert patient.
2. However, in an obtunded or intoxicated patient, direct measurement of the compartment pressures may be required.
3. Diagnosis of compartment syndrome is confirmed if the compartment pressure is within 30 mm Hg of the patient's diastolic blood pressure.
D. Treatment
1. Compartment syndrome is treated surgically with emergent fasciotomy. Skin, subcutaneous fat, and fascial layers must all be widely decompressed and left open.
2. If compartment syndrome is associated with a fracture, rigid stabilization of the bone is necessary.
3. After the initial insult has subsided, the wounds may be closed primarily or may require split-thickness skin grafting.

 PEDIATRIC ORTHOPEDICS

I. General Principles
A. History and physical
1. In all pediatric patients, it is important to obtain a birth and developmental history. Specifically, gestational age at birth, breech position in utero, age of crawling, age of walking, and family history of developmental delay or difficulties.
2. Remember that children are not just small adults from a musculoskeletal standpoint. They have significant changes with bony and soft-tissue growth throughout childhood. From a skeletal standpoint, pediatric patients have growth plates (physes) that can affect length and alignment of bones if injured.
B. Common pediatric orthopedic problems include developmental disorders, anatomic variants, genetic disorders, and trauma.

II. Developmental Dysplasia of the Hip (DDH)
A. Introduction
1. Abnormal development of the hip secondary to soft-tissue laxity and uterine positioning may present with frank hip dislocation.
2. Risk factors include breech position, female gender, family history, and first born. The left hip is most commonly affected because of intrauterine positioning.
3. Treatment and prognosis change significantly if the diagnosis is made after 6 weeks of age.
B. History and physical
1. A family and personal delivery history of breech position must be taken.
2. A physical exam is extremely important for detecting hips that may be affected. A focused exam of the hip should be performed on every newborn. Any test abnormalities below warrant a further workup:
   a. Ortolani maneuver: reduction of a dislocated hip with femur elevation and abduction ("hip clunk")
   b. Barlow maneuver: subluxation or dislocation of the affected hip with adduction and posteriorly directed force
   c. Galeazzi sign: clinical appearance of a shortened femur on the affected side
   d. Asymmetrical abduction of the affected hip when compared to contralateral side

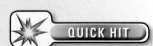

QUICK HIT

DDH risk factors: breech, firstborn, female, and family history.

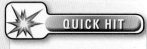

QUICK HIT

A hip clunk, not click, with Ortolani maneuver should raise suspicion for DDH.

FIGURE 15-7 Proper positioning of an infant in a Pavlik harness. The harness is composed of shoulder straps, stirrups, and a chest strap. It is placed on both legs, even if only one hip is dislocated.

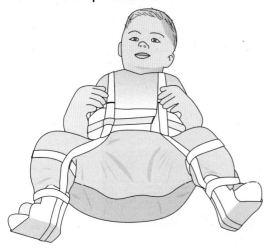

(Reprinted with permission from Klossner NJ, Hatfield NT. *Introductory Maternity & Pediatric Nursing.* 2nd ed. Philadelphia, PA: Lippincott Williams & Wilkins; 2009.)

C. Diagnosis
1. Physical exam should make a practitioner highly suspicious for DDH.
2. Diagnosis is confirmed via dynamic ultrasound demonstrating an unreduced or dislocated hip. Because the femoral head does not ossify until 4 to 6 months of age, plain radiographs may not be helpful during this time period.

D. Treatment
1. Treatment is focused on obtaining and maintaining a concentric hip reduction. The treatment course depends on the patient age at diagnosis.
   a. Zero to 6 weeks: Pavlik harness (Fig. 15-7)
   b. Six weeks to 1 year: A Pavlik harness is applied if hip is reducible; otherwise, closed or open reduction with possible soft-tissue releases followed by casting is performed.

III. Slipped Capital Femoral Epiphysis (SCFE)

A. Introduction
1. Pathology is displacement of proximal femoral epiphysis posteriorly and medially relative to metaphysis.
2. This is seen in children ages 10 to 15 years who are commonly obese, male, and African-American. Up to 25% of cases may be bilateral.
3. Younger patients (<10 years old) and bilateral cases are more commonly associated with an underlying endocrine abnormality (e.g., hypothyroidism, renal failure, growth hormone deficiencies).

B. History and physical
1. Most common complaint may be knee pain secondary to referred pain. All children with knee pain require a radiograph of the hip. Also, patients commonly present with limited rotation of the hip or a limp.
2. On physical exam, all patients have obligatory external rotation with flexion of the hip. They also commonly have limited hip rotation. Pain may be present in groin, thigh, or knee.

C. Diagnosis
1. AP pelvis and frog-leg lateral radiographs of bilateral hips will show displacement of the femoral head epiphysis through the physis. If concerned for bilateral slips, consider an endocrine workup (Fig. 15-8).
2. Radiographic findings may be subtle in early slips. Often, the only abnormality may be seen on the lateral view of the affected hip. It is helpful to compare the affected hip to the unaffected hip on the same image.

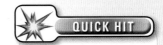

QUICK HIT

SCFE is common in obese adolescents with hip or knee pain. The femoral neck moves relative to the femoral epiphysis through the physis.

**FIGURE
15-8** Slipped capital femoral epiphysis.

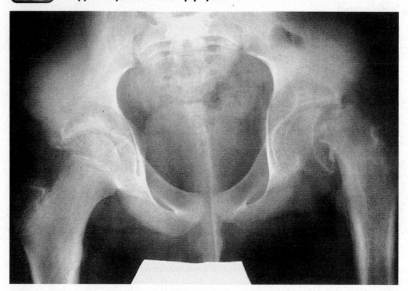

(Reprinted with permission from Swiontkowski MF, Stovitz SD, eds. *Manual of Orthopaedics*. 6th ed. Philadelphia, PA: Lippincott Williams & Wilkins; 2006.)

    3. Loder classification
       a. Stable: The patient is able to weight bear with or without crutches.
       b. Unstable: The patient is unable to weight bear secondary to pain.
  D. Treatment
    1. SCFE is treated with operative intervention.
    2. Usually, in situ percutaneous pinning of the femoral neck and head is preferred.

IV. Osgood-Schlatter Disease
  A. Introduction
    1. This is an overuse disease most common in males that usually presents in late childhood or early adolescence.
    2. This results from a partial avulsion of the anterior portion of the tibial tuberosity through the apophysis. The cause is recognized as a juvenile traction osteochondrosis of the tibial tuberosity due to stress from the knee extensor mechanism (patellar tendon).
  B. History and physical
    1. Patients often present with a history of knee pain that is worse with activity and often participate in sports. They may complain of a prominence or "bump" on the front of their knee.
    2. Physical exam demonstrates a tender prominence over the tibial tuberosity.
  C. Diagnosis
    1. Diagnosis is often made by history and physical alone. If pain is severe, may consider obtaining AP and lateral plain radiographs of the knee and tibia
    2. Lateral radiograph may show avulsion and fragmenting of the tibial tubercle.
  D. Treatment
    1. The disorder is usually self-limiting.
    2. Often, decreasing activity, resting, and taking anti-inflammatories helps the symptoms.
    3. Occasionally, the avulsion will not heal after the patient has finished growth. If painful, this area may be excised surgically.

V. Osteogenesis Imperfecta (OI)
  A. Introduction
    1. OI is a skeletal dysplasia caused by a defect in type I collagen that causes abnormal cross-linking of collagen and "brittle bones."

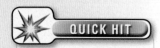

QUICK HIT

OI (genetic collagen disease) patients have blue sclerae and sustain multiple low-energy fractures.

2. Common clinical findings include bowing of long bones, multiple fractures, short stature, scoliosis, hearing loss, blue sclera, and tooth defects.

3. There are multiple types of OI, with different inheritance patterns.

B. History and physical

1. Family history is important to obtain because many of the types of this disorder have an inheritance pattern, usually autosomal dominant or autosomal recessive.

2. A history of multiple fractures in childhood, sometimes present at birth, is a hallmark. Fractures tend to cease at puberty.

3. Physical exam may show short stature, bowing of lower extremities, and scoliosis. Check the eyes for blue sclera and mouth for tooth defects.

C. Diagnosis

1. Diagnosis is made based on clinical presentation and physical exam findings. Often, family history is positive.

2. Radiographs may show history of multiple fractures. The bones tend to have thin cortices and be diffusely osteopenic.

3. A fracture of the olecranon process in pediatric patients is pathognomonic for OI.

D. Treatment

1. Treatment includes management of fractures, correcting scoliosis, and improving function.

2. Often, surgical procedures are required for fracture stabilization. These can become quite complicated secondary to the deformity of the long bones and the fact that they must continue to allow for growth of the child.

VI. Septic Arthritis

A. Introduction

1. Septic arthritis occurs in children, most often under 3 years of age. However, it can occur in any age. The hip is the commonly affected joint.

2. Most commonly caused by hematogenous spread; however, it may spread from a bone infection (osteomyelitis) when the metaphysis of the bone is intra-articular (hip, elbow, ankle, or shoulder).

3. Common organisms (by age of patient)

   a. <12 months → group B *Streptococcus, Staphylococcus aureus, Haemophilus influenzae*

   b. 6 months to 5 years → *Haemophilus influenza, Staphylococcus aureus*

   c. 5 to 12 years → *Staphylococcus aureus*

   d. 12 to 18 years → *Staphylococcus aureus, Neisseria gonorrhoeae*

B. History and physical

1. Patient will present with fever, pain, and limping or inability to bear weight on the affected limb. With young infants, pain with diaper changes or decreased movement of the affected limb may be the only clues present.

2. Common physical exam findings include fever, pain (especially with range of motion of the joint), limping, or decreased use of the affected limb.

C. Diagnosis

1. The Kocher criteria are helpful to evaluate patients to diagnose septic hip arthritis.

2. These criteria are (1) temperature >101.5° F, (2) white blood cell (WBC) count >12,000, (3) erythrocyte sedimentation rate (ESR) >40 mm/hr, and (4) inability of the patient to weight bear (see Clinical Pearl 15-5).

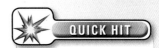

QUICK HIT

Use the Kocher criteria to correctly distinguish septic arthritis and transient synovitis of the hip.

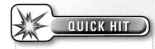

QUICK HIT

Staphylococcus aureus is most common bacteria for joint and bone infections.

CLINICAL PEARL 15-5

Kocher Criteria for Septic Arthritis

Number of Criteria Met	Chance That the Child Has Septic Arthritis
4/4	99%
3/4	93%
2/4	40%
1/4	3%

3. Ultrasound can be useful to help evaluate for the presence of a joint effusion. If present, aspiration should be performed to obtain a fluid sample for laboratory analysis. Joint fluid analysis findings consistent with septic arthritis are:
   a. WBC >50,000/mm^3
   b. Decreased glucose
   c. Increased protein
   d. Positive gram stain
D. Treatment
   1. Septic arthritis in children is a surgical emergency. Pus is chondrolytic and destroys cartilage.
   2. Emergent irrigation and debridement of the affected joint is performed in the operating room, followed by a course of IV antibiotics.

VII. Salter-Harris Fractures

A. Introduction
   1. Fractures in the long bones of children can injure the growth plate (physis) near the ends of the bones. If the fracture damages the growth plate, growth arrest can occur. This can lead to an angular deformity (if only a portion of the growth plate is damaged) or, in some cases, complete growth arrest. In the lower extremity, this leads to leg length discrepancies.
   2. Correctly identifying and classifying growth plate injuries allows for a detailed discussion with the patient and the family regarding expected prognosis and complications.
B. History and physical
   1. History and physical exam are usually consistent with a traumatic injury. Pain, deformity, and swelling are common with fractures. Remember to examine for open wounds.
C. Diagnosis
   1. Like in adult fractures, AP and lateral views of the involved area are required to diagnose the injury. Remember to image the entire bone as well as the joint above and the joint below.
   2. Classification of pediatric fractures is by the Salter-Harris classification (Fig. 15-9). It is based on the amount of the growth plate involved and location of other fracture lines:
      a. Type I: fracture through the physis
      b. Type II: fracture through the physis and the metaphysis, sparing the epiphysis
      c. Type III: fracture through physis and epiphysis, sparing the metaphysis
      d. Type IV: fracture through all three elements of the bone (physis, metaphysis, and epiphysis)
      e. Type V: compression fracture of the physis, resulting in a decrease in the perceived space between the epiphysis and metaphysis
D. Treatment
   1. Fractures that are nondisplaced are usually treated conservatively with casting. Displaced fractures that can be reduced may also be treated conservatively.

FIGURE

15-9 Salter-Harris classification of physical fractures.

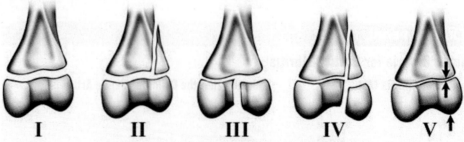

I II III IV V

(Reprinted with permission from Strickland JW, Graham TJ, eds. *Master Techniques in Orthopaedic Surgery: The Hand.* 2nd ed. Philadelphia, PA: Lippincott Williams & Wilkins; 2005.)

2. Fractures that involve the articular surface (types III and IV) require anatomic reduction via surgical intervention, specifically ORIF. Irreducible fractures also require ORIF.

VIII. Child Abuse (Nonaccidental Trauma)

A. Introduction

1. As a physician, it is state law to report suspected child abuse.
2. Fractures in children younger than 2 to 3 years of age should raise suspicion, especially lower extremity fractures in children not yet walking.

B. History and physical

1. A history of multiple visits to the emergency department should raise suspicion. Also, a story told by the caregiver that does not seem to fit the circumstances should raise red flags.
2. Exam findings can include multiple fractures at various stages of healing, multiple healing bruises, skin marks (hand prints), burns, malnutrition, and other signs of neglect.

C. Diagnosis

1. The most common locations of fractures in child abuse are humerus, tibia, and femur. For suspected cases, a skeletal survey can be useful to evaluate for multiple old and new fractures.
2. Common fracture patterns in child abuse are metaphyseal (corner) and spiral fractures. However, any fracture in children could be from abuse.

D. Treatment

1. Notification to child protective services is *mandatory* for any suspected cases of child abuse. If abuse is missed:
   a. One in three children will have further abuse.
   b. There is a 5% to 10% chance of death in these children.
2. Routine fracture care

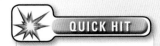

SPORTS MEDICINE

I. General Principles

A. History and physical

1. A thorough history and physical are essential to make the diagnosis. Important aspects of the history include the mechanism of injury as well as the overall health status of the patient.
2. These are often soft-tissue injuries. Most commonly, ligaments, cartilage, tendons, and muscle insertions are injured around joints. These joints must be examined for instability and resulting loss of range of motion.

II. Anterior Cruciate Ligament (ACL) Injuries

A. Introduction

1. The ACL prevents anterior translation of tibia with respect to femur. It is an intra-articular ligament of the knee.
2. These injuries are commonly associated with lateral meniscal tears (approximately 50%) and medial collateral ligament (MCL) tears.
3. ACL origin: lateral femoral condyle
4. ACL insertion: anterior tibia

B. History and physical

1. Mechanism of injury is a noncontact twisting injury to the knee (soccer and basketball players).
2. Patients state they felt a "pop" deep within knee and have immediate swelling and hemarthrosis (blood within joint).
3. Commonly, a significant knee effusion is present.
4. Lachman test is the most sensitive exam for ACL tear: With knee in 30 degrees of flexion and hamstrings relaxed, stabilize distal femur in one hand and translate the proximal tibia anterior with other hand. A positive test reveals no good endpoint and is asymmetric with contralateral extremity.

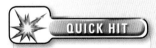

C. Diagnosis
1. This is a clinical diagnosis based on history and physical.
2. Radiographs may reveal Segond fracture, an avulsion fracture of lateral proximal tibia, which is pathognomonic of an ACL tear.
3. MRI is usually used to confirm the diagnosis. Primary utility of MRI is to preoperatively rule out additional pathology such as meniscal tears that may require surgical attention (Fig. 15-10).

D. Treatment
1. Clinic or ED disposition: Place patient in knee immobilizer in full extension. They can bear weight with brace but may require crutches. Orthopedic follow-up within 1 week. If high-energy mechanism or concern for knee dislocation, perform pulse exam and ankle–brachial index to rule out vascular injury.
2. Nonsurgical treatment (bracing and physical therapy) is reserved for low-demand patients or patients with little or no instability.
3. Surgical treatment is reserved for active patients with signs of instability. The ACL is reconstructed with either autograft (patient's patellar or hamstring tendons) or allograft (cadaver tendons). This procedure is generally performed arthroscopically.

FIGURE
15-10 Anterior cruciate ligament tear.

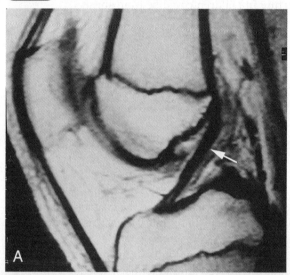
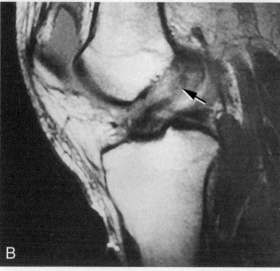

A. Proton density-weighted MRI, sagittal knee. Note the normal low signal intensity anterior cruciate ligament (ACL) in this pediatric patient (*arrow*). **B.** Proton density-weighted MRI, sagittal knee. Observe that the ACL has been avulsed from its proximal femoral attachment (*arrow*). Note the retraction of the ligament and surrounding hemorrhagic edema.

(Reprinted with permission from Yochum TR, Rowe LJ. *Yochum and Rowe's Essentials of Skeletal Radiology*. 3rd ed. Philadelphia, PA: Lippincott Williams & Wilkins; 2004.)

III. Posterior Cruciate Ligament (PCL) Injuries

A. Introduction

1. The PCL prevents posterior translation of the tibia with respect to the femur.
2. These injuries are often missed at first presentation.
3. PCL origin: medial femoral condyle
4. PCL insertion: posterior tibia

B. History and physical

1. Mechanism of injury is a posteriorly directed force to anterior proximal tibia with a flexed knee.
2. Physical exam acutely will be limited secondary pain and swelling.
3. Posterior drawer test: With the knee in 90 degrees of flexion and stabilizing patient's foot with body, place posteriorly directed force at proximal tibia. A positive test reveals no good endpoint and asymmetry with contralateral extremity.

C. Diagnosis

1. This is a clinical diagnosis based on history and physical exam.
2. Radiographs usually are negative.
3. MRI is used to confirm the diagnosis if planning surgery. The primary utility of MRI is to preoperatively rule out any additional pathology, such as meniscal tears, that may require surgical attention.

D. Treatment

1. Clinic or ED disposition: Place patient in knee immobilizer in full extension. They can bear weight with brace but may require crutches. Orthopedic follow-up within 1 week. If high-energy mechanism or concern for knee dislocation, perform pulse exam and ankle–brachial index to rule out vascular injury.
2. Nonsurgical treatment (bracing) is mainstay of treatment for isolated low- and medium-grade PCL tears. Surgical indications include complete tears and tears associated with other ligamentous injuries.
3. Surgical treatment is reserved for active patients with signs of instability. The PCL is reconstructed with either autograft (patient's tendons) or allograft (cadaver tendons). This procedure is generally performed arthroscopically.

IV. Meniscal Tears

A. Introduction

1. The menisci are C-shaped collagenous structures that function as shock absorbers and secondary joint stabilizers in the knee joint.
2. These are extremely common injuries.
3. Medial tears (usually degenerative) are more common than lateral tears (usually associated with acute ACL injury).

B. History and physical

1. There may be a history of major or minor traumatic events for acute injuries.
2. Degenerative tears tend to present with insidious onset of pain.
3. Pain is localized over the medial or lateral joint line that may be worse with twisting motions or with deep knee flexion (increased forces through meniscus in flexion).
4. These injuries may present with mechanical symptoms (locking or catching) of knee.
5. Joint line tenderness on palpation is almost always present.
6. McMurray test: While bringing the knee from extension to flexion and placing an external rotation and valgus force, a pop or click will be felt for medial meniscal tears. An internal rotation and varus force should be used for lateral meniscal tears. If this only reproduces pain, many surgeons generally still consider this a positive test.

C. Diagnosis

1. History and physical are significant for raising suspicion of a meniscus injury.
2. Radiographs usually are negative. They may be used to evaluate for arthritic changes of the knee, which are common with degenerative tears.
3. MRI: Linear signals extending through two surfaces of menisci indicate a tear. Although this is necessary to confirm diagnosis for suspected acute injuries, it is not as paramount for suspected degenerative tears in presence of arthritic changes of knee (Fig. 15-11).

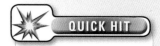

QUICK HIT

PCL tears are common with "dashboard injuries" when a flexed knee sustains a posteriorly directed force to proximal tibia.

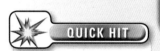

QUICK HIT

Meniscal tears present with history of a twisting knee injury and joint line tenderness. McMurray test is present for the patients.

Orthopedic Surgery

FIGURE 15-11 The knee, showing the lateral and medial meniscus (with the patella removed for clarity). Insert (lower left) shows meniscus tear.

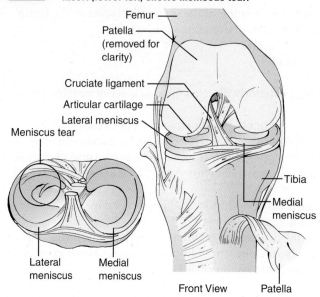

(Reprinted with permission from Porth CM, ed. *Pathophysiology: Concepts of Altered Health States.* 7th ed. Philadelphia, PA: Lippincott Williams & Wilkins; 2005.)

D. Treatment
1. Clinic or ED disposition: They can bear weight with brace but may require crutches. If acute, a knee brace may be used for pain control. Nonemergent orthopedic follow-up is acceptable. MRI should be ordered at the discretion of the orthopedist.
2. Symptomatic treatment consists of nonsteroidal anti-inflammatory drugs (NSAIDs), rest, and physical therapy for degenerative tears.
3. Surgical treatment is considered for acute tears in young, active patients who have failed nonsurgical treatment and have no or minimal signs of arthritic changes. Arthroscopic treatment consists of meniscal debridement or repair depending on patient characteristics and meniscal pathology.

V. Patellar Dislocation
A. Introduction
1. The patella is the largest sesamoid bone (intratendinous bone) in the body. It increases leverage and force transmission of the quadriceps for knee extension.
2. The patella dislocates (generally laterally) from the trochlear groove in the distal femur.
3. Medial patellofemoral ligament (MPFL): primary restraint to lateral dislocation
4. Associated with women, ligamentous laxity, and increased Q angle (angle between line from anterior superior iliac spine [ASIS] to central patella and line from central patella to tibial tubercle)
B. History and physical
1. Mechanism of injury is a noncontact twisting injury to the knee with the knee in extension.
2. Most dislocations will reduce with reflexive quadriceps contraction prior to examination.
3. Physical exam will be limited secondary pain and swelling.
4. A significant knee effusion is present, and tenderness to palpation medially (MPFL)
C. Diagnosis
1. This may be a clinical diagnosis based on history and physical, especially if the patella spontaneously reduced prior to presentation.

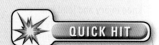

QUICK HIT

Patellar dislocations are common in females with increased Q angles and ligamentous laxity.

2. Radiographs may reveal associated lateral femoral condyle or medial patella facet fracture. Ensure patella is reduced in trochlear groove and rule out loose intra-articular bodies.

3. MRI: Not routinely ordered. Used only to confirm no loose bodies or fractures. Additionally, if considering surgical procedures, would be used to confirm MPFL tear and to plan reconstruction.

D. Treatment

1. Clinic or ED disposition: After appropriate pain control, reduce patella into trochlear groove and confirm radiographically. Place patient in knee immobilizer in full extension. They can bear weight with brace but may require crutches. Nonemergent orthopedic follow-up is acceptable.

2. Nonsurgical treatment (NSAIDs, temporary immobilization, and physical therapy) is appropriate for the majority of patients, especially acute first-time dislocators.

3. Surgery is indicated to remove intra-articular loose bodies, and fracture fixation may be warranted for associated fractures. MPFL autograft or allograft reconstructions or bony procedures could be indicated for chronic dislocators.

VI. Lateral Epicondylitis ("Tennis Elbow")

A. Introduction

1. Although seen with tennis players, this is an overuse injury associated with repetitive forearm pronation and supination with the elbow extended.

2. Most commonly associated with tendinosis and inflammation at origin of extensor carpi radialis brevis (ECRB) muscle on the lateral epicondyle of the distal humerus.

B. History and physical

1. Repetitive forearm rotational movement during athletics or work (tennis players and manual laborers) will cause pain over the lateral humeral epicondyle.

2. Tenderness to palpation is present at the origin of the extensor wad on the lateral humerus.

3. Pain is present with resisted wrist extension with the elbow extended.

C. Diagnosis

1. This is a clinical diagnosis based on history and physical exam.

2. Radiographs will be negative but may be used to rule out alternative pathology.

D. Treatment

1. Clinic or ED disposition: Common diagnosis that may be treated at first in primary care setting. Referral to orthopedics with continued symptoms or concern for alternate pathology.

2. Nonsurgical treatment consists of activity modification, NSAIDs, and potential physical therapy to strengthen extensor muscles. Modifications to activities can include a larger grip (racquet or hammer), lower racquet tension, and a higher flexibility racquet.

3. A tension strap worn around proximal forearm may alleviate symptoms and should be the first line of treatment. This is successful up to 95% of the time.

4. Steroid injections may be performed by an orthopedist for recalcitrant cases to decrease inflammation at the origin of the ECRB (maximum of three injections).

5. Surgical intervention consists of releasing the ECRB at the insertion on the lateral epicondyle and debriding the inflamed tissue. This is reserved for recalcitrant cases after 1 year of failed nonoperative treatment.

VII. Plantar Fasciitis

A. Introduction

1. The plantar fascia (PF) is a thin, longitudinal connective tissue layer supporting the arch of the foot that originates on the plantar calcaneus.

2. This disorder is also associated with Achilles tendonitis.

3. May develop from chronic repetitive overuse syndrome resulting from microtears in the PF

B. History and physical

1. The hallmark symptom is sharp, stabbing, plantar (bottom) surface heel pain with first steps, especially in the morning or after prolonged inactivity.

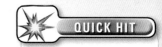

Pain with repetitive wrist extension such as tennis players is indicative of lateral epicondylitis. The pathology is in the ECRB muscle origin.

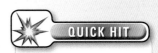

Painful heel pain that is worse with the first step in the morning is a classic finding for plantar fasciitis. Stretching is first-line treatment.

Orthopedic Surgery

2. Heel pain improves with movement but worsens by the end of the day.
3. Tenderness to palpation over the proximal plantar calcaneus is often present.

C. Diagnosis
1. This is a clinical diagnosis based on history and physical exam findings.
2. Radiographs may reveal heel spurs at PF or Achilles insertion.

D. Treatment
1. Clinic or ED disposition: Diagnosis and treatment can be performed by primary care physicians. Refer to orthopedics if suspect alternative diagnosis or for recalcitrant disease.
2. Mainstay of nonsurgical treatment is PF and Achilles specific stretching exercises to be performed five times daily. Symptom relief can take up to 6 months. Cushioned heel inserts can be prescribed for symptomatic control. NSAIDs may be prescribed for pain control.
3. Alternative treatments include corticosteroid injections, high-intensity ultrasound, and surgical release. These should be reserved for patients with symptoms lasting longer than 9 months under a supervised care program.

VIII. Achilles Tendonitis

A. Introduction
1. The Achilles tendon is constituted of the gastrocnemius and soleus tendons, whose function is as the primary plantar flexor of the ankle.
2. Chronic repetitive overuse syndrome of Achilles insertion into calcaneus can lead to tendonitis.
3. Middle-aged patients are most commonly affected.
4. Can be associated with plantar fasciitis

B. History and physical
1. The hallmark symptom is sharp, stabbing, posterior surface heel pain that worsens with increased activity and dorsiflexion of ankle.
2. Tenderness to palpation is present over the posterior calcaneus.
3. Thompson test: In prone position with knee flexed, squeeze proximal calf and evaluate for ankle plantar flexion. If asymmetric with contralateral side, consider Achilles tendon rupture.

C. Diagnosis
1. This is a clinical diagnosis based on history and physical exam.
2. Radiographs may reveal heel spurs at PF or Achilles insertion.

D. Treatment
1. Clinic or ED disposition: Diagnosis and treatment can be performed by primary care physicians. Refer to orthopedics if suspect alternative diagnosis or for recalcitrant disease. If acute onset of pain with a palpable gap in the tendon is present, consider Achilles tendon rupture with urgent orthopedic referral.
2. Mainstay of nonsurgical treatment is Achilles tendon–specific stretching exercises and strengthening exercises. A period of nonweight bearing in a short-leg walking cast or boot walker may be necessary to decrease inflammation. This disease can have a prolonged course. NSAIDs may be prescribed for pain control.
3. Surgical debridement of the Achilles tendon only considered for patients who fail nonsurgical treatment as described earlier for extended periods of time, who have concurrent abnormal calcaneal anatomy, or who have rupture of the Achilles tendon.

Hand

I. General Principles

A. Hand disorders include congenital deformities, acquired deformities, trauma, and nerve compression injuries.
B. History and physical
1. There are many complex biomechanics of the function of the bones, joints, and tendons of the hand. A detailed physical exam can help to determine which of the many anatomical structures may be causing pathology.

II. Ganglion Cyst of the Wrist

A. Introduction

1. A ganglion is a mucinous-filled cyst adjacent to a joint capsule or tendon sheath that contains clear and colorless fluid (70% on dorsal wrist, 30% on volar wrist).
2. These are more common in women than men.
3. They are the most common soft-tissue mass of the hand.

B. History and physical

1. This often presents as a slow-growing, painful mass about the wrist that may fluctuate in size and appearance.
2. These cysts are firm and well-circumscribed superficial masses, usually on the dorsum of the wrist.
3. Mass will transilluminate with a pen light.
4. Tenderness may be present over cysts with palpation.

C. Diagnosis

1. This is a clinical diagnosis based on history and physical exam.
2. Radiographs are nondiagnostic. Advanced imaging studies are not usually necessary.

D. Treatment

1. Clinic or ED disposition: Diagnosis and treatment can be performed by primary care physicians. Refer to orthopedics if suspect alternative diagnosis or for concern regarding other soft-tissue masses or tumors.
2. Many patients will resolve the cyst without intervention, so observation may be warranted depending on the scope of symptoms. Aspiration of dorsal cysts with placement of a compressive dressing and brief immobilization has a 50% recurrence rate but is diagnostic and avoids surgery in many patients. Avoid volar aspiration, given proximity of radial artery. NSAIDs may be prescribed for pain control.
3. Surgical excision of the cyst is indicated for recalcitrant, symptomatic dorsal cysts or symptomatic volar cysts. It is important to remove the complete stalk of the cysts from the joint for decreased recurrence rates.

III. Boxer's Fracture

A. Introduction

1. Boxer's fractures are defined as fractures of the fifth metacarpal neck.
2. These are common in younger males, often from closed-fist punching injuries.
3. Although usually a closed injury, they can be open fractures depending on impact.

B. History and physical

1. Mechanism of injury is trauma, likely an impact to a closed fist. If an open fracture is present, question what the patient struck during the trauma.
2. Tenderness to palpation is present over the ulnar border of the hand.
3. Perform a neurovascular exam on fingertip.
4. Evaluate for any open wounds, which may be concerning for open fracture. These are often termed "fight bites" because the fist commonly strikes an opponent's teeth.

C. Diagnosis

1. This is a radiographic diagnosis. Three radiographic views of the hand are preferred (Fig. 15-12).
2. The angulation of the fracture is measured on AP and lateral radiographs. Evaluate for additional fractures and fracture into the metacarpophalangeal (MCP) joint. Subcutaneous air indicates open injuries. Acceptable angulation for nonsurgical treatment is up to 60 degrees of angulation.

D. Treatment

1. Clinic or ED disposition: Manual reduction of fracture after local anesthetic injection is commonly performed in the emergency department. The patient is then placed into an ulnar gutter splint in intrinsic plus position (MCP flexed and interphalangeal joints extended). Patients should follow up with orthopedic surgeon within 1 week. Maintain splint or short-arm ulnar gutter cast until the fracture is healed at 4 to 6 weeks.

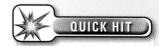

QUICK HIT

Superficial masses on dorsum of wrist that transilluminate usually represent ganglion cysts.

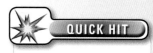

QUICK HIT

Boxer's fractures are fracture of the fifth metacarpal neck.

Orthopedic Surgery

FIGURE 15-12 Boxer's fracture.

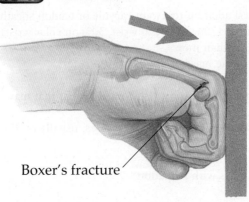

Boxer's fracture

(Reprinted with permission from Anatomical Chart Company, Upper Extremity Disorders, 2008-06-20 0431, ACC Anatomy 2, 5 MCC Emergency Medicine group.)

2. If an open fracture is present, the patient will need an urgent orthopedic surgical consultation along with tetanus and antibiotic administration.
3. Surgical intervention may be warranted for closed fractures if closed reduction, and percutaneous pinning (CRPP) may be required for patients with residual angulation greater than 60 degrees or if combined with other hand fractures or dislocations.

IV. Carpal Tunnel Syndrome (CTS)

A. Introduction
1. This is a compression neuropathy of the median nerve (most common compression neuropathy) within the carpal tunnel of the wrist.
2. Some believe it is caused by patients who perform repetitive activities of the wrist.
3. It is also associated with diabetes mellitus, pregnancy, and rheumatoid arthritis.
4. The carpal tunnel consists of nine wrist and finger flexors, as well as the median nerve.

B. History and physical
1. Patients describe numbness and tingling in radial three and a half fingers that is worse at night.
2. The carpal tunnel compression test, performed by compressing the carpal tunnel with examiner's fingers, is the most sensitive test. A positive test results in reproduction of symptoms within 30 seconds of administration of pressure.

C. Diagnosis
1. This is a clinical diagnosis based on history and physical exam. Radiographs are unnecessary and will be negative if CTS is the correct diagnosis.
2. Electromyography (EMG) and nerve conduction studies (NCS) may be used to ensure accurate diagnosis in difficult cases. They would show increased nerve latencies, nerve conduction velocities, and decreased motor strength.

D. Treatment
1. Clinic or ED disposition: Although most patients will be diagnosed by primary physicians, an elective orthopedic hand referral is appropriate.
2. Nonsurgical treatments include the use of wrist splints both during activity and at night to prevent extremes of motion (both flexion and extension), NSAIDs, and activity modification. Steroid injections into the carpal tunnel can be performed for both diagnostic and therapeutic reasons. If positive result with injection, prognosis is better for surgical procedures.
3. Open or endoscopic carpal tunnel release is commonly performed and is indicated for patients with refractory disease or who present with atrophy of their thenar eminence, a sign of long-standing disease.

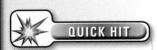

QUICK HIT

Carpal tunnel presents with numbness in radial three fingers that is worse at night.

Spine

I. General Principles

A. History and physical

1. A detailed history and neurologic exam is required for any patient presenting with a potential spine injury or disorder. This allows the practitioner to delineate which levels of the spine may be affected. This exam includes motor, sensory, and reflex exams.

2. Any detectable neurologic deficit requires urgent consultation with spine surgery.

II. Lumbar Spinal Stenosis

A. Introduction

1. Reduction in spinal canal volume causes spinal nerve root compression at the cauda equina (the spinal cord usually ends at level L1 to L2 in adults).

2. Most commonly caused by degenerative changes to bone, disc, or ligamentous anatomy of spine

3. A more acute presentation could be secondary to lumbar disc herniation.

B. History and physical

1. Low back, buttock, and leg pain (neurogenic claudication) will be present.

2. Symptoms worsen with lumbar extension (standing) and improve with lumbar flexion (sitting, leaning forward).

3. Neurogenic claudication symptoms slowly resolve with rest, whereas vascular claudication symptoms resolve more quickly with rest.

4. Symptoms are often bilateral but may be unilateral.

5. Perform vascular exam (ankle–brachial index) to rule out vascular claudication.

C. Diagnosis

1. Distinguish neurogenic claudication from vascular claudication based on history and physical exam.

2. AP/lateral lumbar spine radiographs will show degenerative changes of the spine, including disc space narrowing and osteophyte formation.

3. MRI should be ordered to assess extent and location of the stenosis. If MRI is unobtainable, then a CT myelogram may be a sufficient examination.

4. Diagnosis is based both on clinical and radiographic findings.

D. Treatment

1. Clinic or ED disposition: Rarely will patients present with cauda equina syndrome (acute spinal nerve root compression causing urinary retention, fecal incontinence, and saddle anesthesia). This would require emergent surgical consultation and MRI. Otherwise, patients may be referred to an orthopedic spine surgeon electively.

2. Nonsurgical treatments include anti-inflammatory medications, physical therapy for flexion/extension strengthening, weight loss, and activity modification.

3. Epidural steroid injections may be indicated for some patients at the spine surgeon's discretion with an opportunity to alleviate symptoms obviating surgical intervention. Lumbar bracing may help pain.

4. Surgical treatment is for patients who have failed conservative care. Indications are continued neurogenic claudication and/or cauda equina syndrome. Back pain is not an indication for surgical intervention. Surgery consists of decompression of appropriate spinal levels.

III. Lumbar Disc Herniation

A. Introduction

1. Disc herniations are acute or chronic tears in the disc annulus that can lead to extrusion of the nucleosis pulposus, causing impingement of lumbar spinal roots.

2. Most herniations are asymptomatic, and most asymptomatic herniations resolve without any treatment.

3. They are more common in males and occur most frequently between the ages of 30 and 50 years old.

4. Ninety-five percent of disc herniations are at L4/L5 and L5/S1 discs, with the latter being more common.

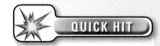

QUICK HIT

Buttock and leg pain that improves with flexion (grocery cart sign) is a symptom of lumbar stenosis.

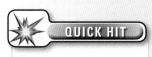

QUICK HIT

L4–L5 disc herniation usually affects the L5 nerve root, whereas L5–S1 disc herniations usually affect the S1 nerve root.

Orthopedic Surgery

FIGURE
15-13 Far lateral disc herniation: lumbar spine.

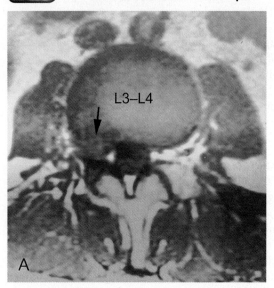
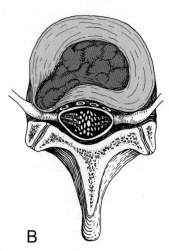

A. T1-weighted MRI, axial L3-L4. **B.** Diagram: L3-L4. Observe the far lateral disc herniation at L3-L4 (*arrow*). The normal epidural fat has been displaced by the disc material, obscuring the far lateral recess.
(Reprinted with permission from Yochum TR, Rowe LJ. *Yochum and Rowe's Essentials of Skeletal Radiology.* 3rd ed. Philadelphia, PA: Lippincott Williams & Wilkins; 2004.)

5. Paracentral disc herniation will affect traversing nerve root (nerve root from level below disc), whereas far lateral disc herniation will affect exiting nerve root (nerve from level above disc) as seen in Figure 15-13.
B. History and physical
1. Most commonly, these patients will present with sciatica (radicular extremity pain), but beware of cauda equina syndrome.
2. A full neurologic examination will be needed but deficits would be as seen in Clinical Pearl 15-6.
3. A straight-leg raise is positive with reproduction of radicular pain between 30 and 70 degrees of hip flexion with knee fully extended.
C. Diagnosis
1. Lumbar spine radiographs should be ordered to rule out other diagnoses and may show disc space narrowing or other degenerative changes.
2. MRI without gadolinium will confirm diagnosis and show anatomy.
3. The diagnosis is based both on clinical and radiographic findings.
D. Treatment
1. Clinic or ED disposition: Primary care physicians will diagnose and manage condition regularly. Nonemergent orthopedic referral for continued symptoms despite nonsurgical treatment. MRI to be ordered if concern for tumor, infection, high-energy trauma, cauda equina syndrome, or persistent symptoms.
2. Nonsurgical treatments are highly successful and include anti-inflammatory medications (NSAIDs or steroids), physical therapy for flexion/extension strengthening, lumbar stretching exercises, weight loss, and activity modification. Bed rest is not appropriate.

CLINICAL PEARL 15-6

Key Features of Neuromuscular Examination of the Lumbo-Sacral Spine

Nerve Root Level	Motor Deficit	Sensory Deficit	Reflex
L4	Ankle dorsiflexion (tibialis anterior)	Anterior knee, medial leg	Knee jerk
L5	Great toe extension (extensor hallucis longus)	Lateral leg, dorsum of foot	None
S1	Ankle plantar flexion (gastrocsoleus complex)	Posterior leg, lateral foot	Ankle jerk

3. Nerve root block with steroid injections may be used for refractory or severe cases for pain control. These can also be diagnostic and prognostic for surgical interventions.

4. Lumbar discectomy (remove the extruded disc from the spinal canal) would be considered for large herniations and patients with recalcitrant symptoms. These procedures are most helpful for radicular pain and may not alleviate the back pain component of symptoms.

IV. Compression Fracture

A. Introduction

1. These are vertebral body fractures that are the most common osteoporotic fracture in the elderly.

2. Osteoporosis is defined by a T-score < -2.5 on dual energy X-ray absorptiometry (DEXA) scan. The bone has normal architecture but has significantly decreased bone mass.

3. Many patients have pain but never present for evaluation.

4. The fractures are most common in lower thoracic and upper lumbar vertebral bodies.

5. With one fragility fracture, the risk of future fragility fractures (compression fracture, distal radius fracture, and femoral neck fracture) increases significantly over time.

B. History and physical

1. Patient may give history of very minor trauma such as twisting in chair or lifting small child.

2. Back pain and tenderness to palpation will be present at area of compression fracture.

3. Rarely will these present with any neurologic deficit.

4. Make sure to elicit personal and family history of cancer, constitutional symptoms, or infection.

C. Diagnosis

1. AP and lateral standing radiographs of entire spine should be ordered because other noncontiguous fractures are commonly identified (Fig. 15-14).

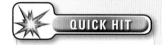

QUICK HIT

Compression fractures are commonly the first sign of osteoporosis.

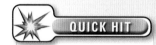

QUICK HIT

A DEXA T-score less than –2.5 represents osteoporosis.

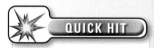

QUICK HIT

Cauda equina is severe compression of nerve roots causing bowel and bladder dysfunction and is a surgical emergency.

Orthopedic Surgery

FIGURE 15-14 Isolated compression fracture: thoracic spine.

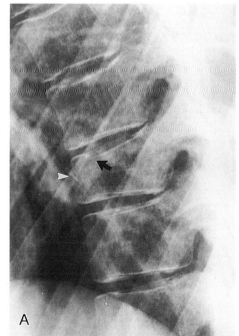
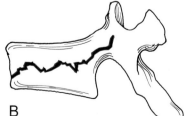
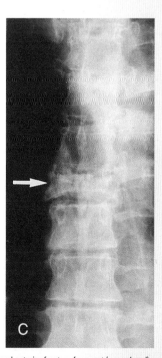

A. Lateral thoracic spine. Note the focal depression of the superior endplate (*arrow*) of the T10 vertebral body, with a displaced anterior fracture fragment (*arrowhead*). A characteristic trapezoidal vertebral shape has been formed owing to anterior compression of the superior vertebral endplate. **B.** Diagram. The usual precipitating force is an anterior compression injury focusing the compressive forces to the anterior aspect of the vertebral body. **C.** AP thoracic spine. Observe that the most notable features are a decrease in vertebral height, with approximation of the vertebral endplates, and associated lateral displacement of the vertebral body margins (*arrow*). (Panel A courtesy of Richard M. Nuzzi, DC, Denver, Colorado. Panel C courtesy of Lawrence P. Rosenbaum, MA, DC, MD, Linkoping, Sweden.)

2. Lab work to rule out infection or tumor may be necessary.
3. Although not commonly needed, MRI with gadolinium should be ordered for atypical fractures, such as fractures that include upper thoracic vertebrae, fractures not consistent with patient's age and mechanism of injury, or if there is concern for infection and/or tumor.

D. Treatment
1. Clinic or ED disposition: Although most patients will be diagnosed by primary physicians, an elective orthopedic spine referral is appropriate for most patients.
2. Nonsurgical treatments include anti-inflammatory medications, physical therapy strengthening and stretching once acute pain has decreased, and activity modification. Some patients may find bracing effective for pain control. With osteoporotic fractures, medical management of osteoporosis is indicated by either a primary care physician or rheumatologist.
3. Surgical treatment is indicated for patients who have failed a 6-week course of the nonsurgical treatments described earlier without symptom relief. Kyphoplasty, injection of cement into the vertebral body, may be performed at that time but is only indicated for pain relief because this procedure does not correct kyphotic deformity.

Neurosurgery

16

Stanley Zaslau and Charles Rosen

CONGENITAL MALFORMATIONS AND DISORDERS OF CEREBROSPINAL FLUID CIRCULATION

I. Hydrocephalus

A. General principles
1. May be congenital or acquired
2. Caused by an obstruction to the flow of cerebrospinal fluid (CSF). The most common causes are:
   a. Intraventricular hemorrhage in a premature infant
   b. Stenosis of the aqueduct
   c. Chiari malformation
3. The most common type of Chiari malformation is downward herniation of the fourth ventricle and the cerebellar tonsils.

B. Clinical features
1. Patients may present with bulging fontanelles, dilation of scalp veins, and increased head circumference.
2. Parinaud syndrome (altered upward gaze), nausea, vomiting, ataxia, lethargy, and irritability may result.

C. Diagnosis: Computed tomography (CT) scan or magnetic resonance imaging (MRI) confirms the diagnosis.

D. Treatment
1. Shunt placement to divert ventricular fluid is necessary.
2. The most commonly used shunt is a ventriculoperitoneal shunt.
3. Ventriculoatrial shunts may be considered in very small infants because of the smaller absorptive surface of their peritoneum.

II. Spinal Dysraphism

A. General principles
1. This is a defective fusion of the raphe, with associated physical defects on examination.
2. Findings may include hair tufts, nevus, lipoma, abnormal blood vessels, gluteal cleft, or dimples.
3. Examples include spina bifida, meningocele, and myelomeningocele.
   a. Spina bifida results from failure of fusion of the arches of the vertebrae.
   b. Meningocele is a saclike midline herniation of the dura.
   c. Myelomeningocele is herniation of the dura and neural elements.

B. Clinical features
1. Patients with spina bifida and meningocele can be asymptomatic.
2. Neurologic defects are common with myelomeningocele.

C. Diagnosis: Physical examination and CT or MRI confirm the diagnosis.

D. Treatment: Therapy for the associated congenital abnormalities may be required, such as for the cosmetic defects associated with each condition.

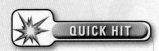

INTRACRANIAL BLEEDING

I. Epidural Hematoma

A. General principles
  1. This condition is seen in patients with head trauma with associated skull fracture.
  2. Fracture involves laceration of the middle meningeal artery, leading to laceration and expansile hematoma formation.
  3. Increased intracranial pressure produces brain compression and can lead to herniation.

B. Clinical features
  1. Loss of consciousness without obvious neurologic deficits may occur.
  2. Patient loses consciousness in a rapid and progressive fashion.
  3. Consciousness should be assessed with the Glasgow Coma Scale (GCS).
    a. Patients with severe injuries and a GCS of less than 8 require airway protection with endotracheal intubation.
    b. Immediate neurosurgical evaluation is compulsory.

C. Diagnosis: CT scan indicates the diagnosis.

D. Treatment
  1. Emergency decompression is performed for patients with problems in the following areas: airway control, altered and decreased level of consciousness, and a depressed skull fracture.
  2. Creation of a burr hole over the area of hematoma removes the blood clot and lowers the intracranial pressure.
  3. The dura is fixed to bone to prevent hematoma reaccumulation. The bleeding middle meningeal artery is ligated.

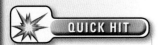

II. Subdural Hematoma

A. General principles
  1. Subdural hematoma is a low-flow, low-pressure cause of intracerebral bleeding.
  2. Bleeding is secondary to either spontaneous or traumatic bleeding of bridging veins that drain the superior sagittal sinus.
  3. Consider this diagnosis in an elderly patient with known cerebral atrophy and who is taking oral anticoagulants such as warfarin.

B. Clinical features
  1. Patients present with headache, drowsiness, and hemiparesis.
  2. Patients rarely have seizures or papilledema.

C. Diagnosis: CT scan confirms the diagnosis.

D. Treatment: Burr hole decompression is required in patients with a significant mass effect and neurologic deficits.

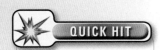

III. Subarachnoid Hemorrhage

A. General principles
  1. The most common cause is trauma. However, this hemorrhage may be secondary to arteriovenous malformation (AVM) or aneurysm.
  2. Blood fills the subarachnoid space instead of CSF.
  3. Development may be spontaneous.
  4. Fifteen percent of patients have multiple aneurysms.
  5. Fifteen percent of patients have no angiographic evidence of subarachnoid hemorrhage.

B. Clinical features
  1. Sudden onset of severe headache is characteristic. Nausea, vomiting, stiff neck, photophobia, and altered mental status can occur.
  2. Third nerve palsy results from aneurysm of the posterior communicating artery.
  3. Monocular visual field cuts result from aneurysm of the internal carotid-ophthalmic vessels.

C. Diagnosis
1. CT scan reveals the diagnosis in nearly 90% of cases.
2. If the CT scan is negative and does not reveal mass effect, lumbar puncture may establish the diagnosis.
D. Treatment: Therapy involves surgical clipping and resection of the aneurysmal defect.

IV. Arteriovenous Malformation

A. General principles
1. AVMs are congenitally abnormal connections between arteries and veins, without intervening small vessels to decrease pressure and flow.
2. This allows high flow and high pressure arterial blood to rupture the AVM.
3. AVMs are located in the brain parenchyma and can cause intracerebral hematoma.
B. Clinical features
1. Neurologic presentation depends on location of the AVM.
2. Aphasia and contralateral arm and/or leg hemiplegia can result from intracerebral hematoma.
3. Visual field defects can result from occipital hematomas.
C. Diagnosis
1. CT scan reveals an intracerebral hematoma.
2. Angiography may reveal smaller AVMs.
D. Treatment
1. Patients with elevated intracranial pressure and evidence of herniation require surgical evacuation of the hematoma.
2. Small AVMs diagnosed by angiography may be observed initially, but definitive removal is recommended.
3. Radiosurgical techniques may be feasible for AVMs smaller than 3 cm and in locations of the brain that are difficult to approach surgically.

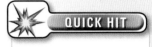

QUICK HIT

It is important to identify the level of spinal injury.

DISEASES OF THE SPINE: SPINAL CORD INJURY

I. General Principles

A. Spinal cord injuries may result from vertebral fracture, subluxation, or hyperextension of the cervical spine.
B. Penetrating injuries from gunshot or stab wounds can also result in these injuries.
C. Patients with head injury should be immobilized and placed on a backboard, with immobilization and stabilization of the cervical spine.
D. Next, a complete evaluation and radiologic assessment must be completed.

II. Clinical Features

A. Patients may have tenderness of the spine upon palpation.
B. Numbness, paresthesias, respiratory distress, and hypotension may be present and suggest possible spinal cord injury. Hypotension can occur with lesions above T5.
C. In complete lesions, loss of all motor and sensory function occurs below the lesion. This may include areflexia and autonomic paralysis.
D. Incomplete spinal cord lesions can present with ipsilateral motor paralysis, loss of position/vibration sensation, and contralateral loss of pain and temperature sensation below the level of injury. This is known as the Brown–Sequard syndrome.
E. With cord injury above C3, complete loss of respiratory function occurs. Spinal cord injury can lead to ileus and gastric distension.

III. Diagnosis

A. Hemodynamic stability must be achieved.
B. Patients with a cervical collar need complete imaging of the cervical spine.
C. Complete imaging studies include CT scans, MRI, and myelography.

Neurosurgery

IV. Treatment

A. The goal of treatment is correction of spinal alignment, protection of normal neural tissues, and achievement of spinal stability.

B. Cervical dislocation is corrected with closed or open reduction techniques.

C. Thoracic and lumbar are treated with immobilization. Surgery may be required at a later date.

BENIGN AND MALIGNANT CENTRAL NERVOUS SYSTEM TUMORS

I. Ependymoma

A. General principles

1. These well-circumscribed lesions occur near the ventricles.

2. They are spread via CSF pathways.

3. Median survival approaches 5 years.

B. Clinical features

1. Elevated intracranial pressure is characteristic.

2. Nausea, vomiting, and lethargy often occur.

C. Diagnosis: A CT scan or MRI reveals an irregularly enhancing lesion with well-defined borders near the ventricle.

D. Treatment

1. Aggressive surgical resection

2. Radiation therapy

II. Medulloblastoma

A. General principles

1. This malignant tumor of the fourth ventricle or vermis occurs due to a maturation arrest of neuroectodermal cells during development.

2. It is most common before age 20 years and more common in males.

3. The 10-year survival approaches 30% but can be improved with total mass resection and postoperative radiotherapy.

B. Clinical features

1. Cerebellar and brain stem dysfunction occur due to increased intracranial pressure.

2. Lesions are most common in the midline or lateral cerebellar hemisphere.

C. Diagnosis: CT scan or MRI reveals a nonhomogeneous mass that enhances with contrast and is located near or in the fourth ventricle.

D. Treatment

1. Surgical resection and radiotherapy

2. CSF seeding is possible.

3. Chemotherapy is used in young children, whereas radiotherapy is reserved for older individuals.

III. Astrocytoma

A. General principles

1. This slow-growing tumor has a peak incidence in the fourth decade of life.

2. Prognosis relates to a variety of factors, including patient age, neurologic status, and tumor histopathology.

3. Patients with low-grade astrocytomas have a median survival of 5 years, whereas those with anaplastic astrocytomas survive approximately 2 years. Survival is worst with glioblastoma, which has a 1-year median survival rate.

B. Clinical features: Patients may present with seizures, headaches, and focal neurologic defects.

C. Diagnosis: CT scan or MRI reveals an irregular, nonhomogeneous enhancing mass with a zone of edema surrounding the lesion.

D. Treatment

1. Aggressive and complete surgical resection

2. Radiotherapy

Neurosurgery

3. Possible boost radiation therapy to the tumor bed. Brachytherapy may also be considered.
4. Chemotherapy

IV. Meningioma

A. General principles
1. These lesions account for 15% of intracranial neoplasms.
2. They are near the dura with a well-circumscribed border.
3. They often contain calcium, which leads to edema and corresponding cerebral compression.
4. Prognosis relates to the location of the lesion as well as its size.
B. Clinical features: Headache, focal neurologic defects, and seizures may occur.
C. Diagnosis: CT scan and MRI may reveal a homogeneous, contrast-enhancing mass with a well-circumscribed border.
D. Treatment
1. Surgical excision
2. Radiation therapy
3. Chemotherapy for malignant lesions

V. Acoustic Neuroma

A. General principles
1. This lesion arises from the vestibular portion of cranial nerve VIII.
2. Prognosis relates to size of tumor and extent of resection.
B. Clinical features
1. Patients present with tinnitus, hearing loss, and balance disturbance.
2. Hearing loss is gradual. Ability to discriminate speech affected first.
3. Physical examination may reveal facial weakness and loss of corneal reflex.
4. Nystagmus and gait ataxia are seen with lesions that compress the cerebellum.
C. Diagnosis
1. CT and MRI reveal a mass in the internal auditory meatus.
2. Brain stem–evoked potentials and audiometric evaluation may reveal cranial nerve VIII defects.
D. Treatment
1. Surgical resection
2. Stereotactic radiosurgery

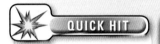

QUICK HIT

Patients with acoustic neuroma present with tinnitus, vertigo, and high-frequency sensorineural hearing loss.

VI. Metastatic Tumors

A. General principles
1. The most common sources include tumors of the lung, breast, kidney, prostate, and skin (malignant melanoma).
2. Twenty percent of cancer patients develop brain metastasis.
3. Patients with a single metastasis can survive at least 1 year.
B. Clinical features. Increased intracranial pressure, obstructive hydrocephalus, neurologic deficits, and spontaneous cerebral bleeding are seen.
C. Diagnosis
1. CT or MRI reveals a well-circumscribed, contrast-enhancing mass surrounded by cerebral edema.
2. Multiple cerebral lesions are common.
D. Treatment
1. Surgical resection should be considered for solitary lesions.
2. Whole-brain radiotherapy may be considered.
3. Corticosteroids may be used.

Neurosurgery

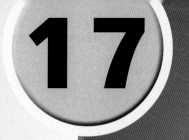

17

Urology

Chad Morley, Chad Hubsher, and Stanley Zaslau

 KIDNEY

I. Development

A. Three kidney systems are formed embryologically in cranial-to-caudal sequence: First is the vestigial pronephros in the fourth week of gestation, second is the mesonephros, and third is the metanephros in the fifth week of gestation, which is considered the definitive kidney (Table 17-1). Embryologic abnormalities of kidney formation are shown in Table 17-1.

B. Nephrons are formed from the metanephric mesoderm and consist of the glomeruli and the excretory tubules (i.e., the proximal convoluted tubule, the loop of Henle, and the distal convoluted tubule).

C. The collecting system of the permanent kidney arises from the ureteric bud, an outgrowth of the mesonephric duct.

D. The ureteric bud penetrates the metanephric tissue and then dilates to form the renal pelvis and splits into the calyces.

II. Anatomy

A. General principles
1. The kidneys are bean-shaped bilateral structures in the retroperitoneum.
2. They are encased in Gerota fascia.

B. Arterial supply
1. The arterial supply of the kidney is branched with four or more segmental vessels (five is most common). The renal arteries are found posterior to the renal veins.
2. The right renal artery leaves the aorta and then travels behind the inferior vena cava.

TABLE 17-1 Embryologic Abnormalities of Kidney Formation	
Embryologic Abnormality	**Description**
Pelvic kidney	As the kidneys ascend from the pelvis, they sometimes cannot pass through the umbilical arteries and remain in the pelvis.
Horseshoe kidney	While ascending from the pelvis, the kidneys sometimes get pushed together as they pass through the umbilical arteries and then they fuse at the lower poles. They usually get trapped at the lower lumbar vertebrae by the inferior mesenteric artery.
Renal agenesis	May be unilateral or bilateral. Bilateral agenesis is not compatible with life. It is termed Potter syndrome and is diagnosed by fetal oligohydramnios and absent kidneys on prenatal ultrasound. Renal agenesis is usually secondary to either a failure of the ureteric bud to form or an absence of the nephrogenic ridge.

3. The left renal artery is shorter than the right renal artery and originates directly from the aorta.
4. The segmental arteries come from the main renal artery.
   a. These then branch into lobar arteries as they course deeper into the renal parenchyma. These further branch into interlobar arteries, arcuate arteries, interlobular arteries, and afferent arterioles of the glomerulus.
   b. After entering the glomerulus, they branch into efferent arterioles and then filter into the vasa recta capillary system.
C. Venous supply
   1. The venous system begins at the capillaries of the nephron, which drain into progressively larger parts of the venous system. In order, these are the interlobular veins, arcuate veins, lobar veins, and the segmental veins.
   2. The right renal vein is short and enters the inferior vena cava directly.
   3. The left renal vein crosses anterior to the aorta. It receives three other veins prior to draining into the inferior vena cava. These include the lumbar vein, left gonadal vein, and left adrenal vein.

III. Physiology
A. The kidneys receive 20% of the resting cardiac output and filter the plasma to remove waste, toxins, and metabolites. The plasma is filtered by the renal tubules.
B. The Bowman capsule filters 20% of the plasma
C. The proximal convoluted tubules absorb 70% of the filtrate.
D. The loop of Henle receives the solute and concentrates the urine to a certain osmolality.
E. The renin-angiotensin system is an important regulator of blood pressure.
   1. Renin is an enzyme released from the juxtaglomerular apparatus in the kidney. It regulates blood pressure by responding to the changes in the pressure of the afferent arteriole.
   2. Renin acts on angiotensinogen to produce angiotensin I and then angiotensin II.
   3. Angiotensin II is a potent vasoconstrictor, and it also affects the release of aldosterone from the adrenal cortex.

IV. Diseases of the Kidney
A. Polycystic kidney disease
   1. Autosomal dominant polycystic kidney disease
      a. This disease is commonly called adult polycystic kidney disease.
      b. The incidence is about 1 in 1,000 people.
      c. It always occurs bilaterally and causes the kidneys to become massive in size and full of cysts. It accounts for 10% of chronic renal failure.
      d. Symptoms include hematuria, flank pain, hypertension, and proteinuria.
      e. Between 10% and 30% of patients have cerebral berry aneurysms.
   2. Autosomal recessive polycystic kidney disease
      a. This rare disorder of bilateral kidney disease presents in infants and young children.
      b. The kidneys are fairly smooth on the outside but are enlarged by multiple dilated collecting ducts.
      c. The liver is usually cystic as well and can cause hepatic fibrosis.
      d. Death is secondary to renal failure and congenital hepatic fibrosis.
B. Renal cell carcinoma (RCC) (Fig. 17-1)
   1. Three percent of all visceral cancers, and 85% of all renal cancers, are RCC.
   2. The male:female ratio is 2:1.
   3. Histologic patterns include clear cell (70%), chromophobe RCC (5%), and papillary RCC (15%).
   4. RCC usually occurs in patients in their 50s and 60s.
   5. An important risk factor is tobacco smoking.
   6. Ten percent of patients have the classic symptom triad, which includes hematuria, dull flank pain, and a palpable mass.

FIGURE 17-1 Abdomen axial CT.

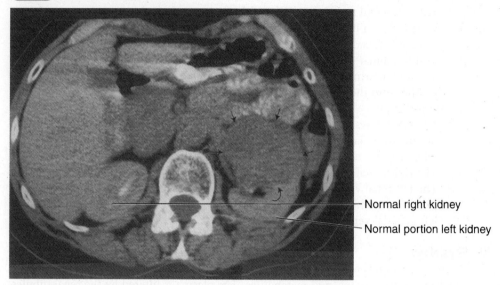

— Normal right kidney
— Normal portion left kidney

Left renal cell carcinoma (*straight arrows*). The mass lesion is solid, and its border with the normal kidney (*curved arrow*) is poorly defined. (Reprinted with permission from Erkonen WE, Smith WL, eds. *Radiology 101: The Basics and Fundamentals of Imaging.* 2nd ed. Baltimore, MD: Lippincott Williams & Wilkins; 2005.)

7. Diagnosis is made by computed tomography (CT) or magnetic resonance imaging (MRI).
   a. There is no role for percutaneous biopsy because of the high rate of false-negative results.
   b. Definitive diagnosis is made after surgical removal of the mass.
8. Treatment is surgical, and the standard of treatment is radical nephrectomy if the contralateral kidney is normal.
   a. Laparoscopic radical nephrectomy has shown to have similar survival in the literature and has less recovery time for the patient.
   b. Nephron-sparing partial nephrectomy is indicated in a solitary kidney, bilateral kidney tumors, and von Hippel–Lindau disease.
      (1) Relative indications for partial nephrectomy include a small tumor (4 cm or smaller) with a normal contralateral kidney.
      (2) Local recurrence is less than 10%.
      (3) There is a high incidence of urinary fistula, which is treated with conservative management including a ureteral stent and Foley catheter drainage.
      (4) RCC sometimes invades the inferior vena cava.
9. Chemotherapy for RCC has limited success. Two adjuvant therapies used are interleukin-2 and interferon.
10. Metastatic RCC may still be managed surgically if there are solitary metastasis or for purposes of cytoreduction. RCC is thought to metastasize via both the lymphatics and hematogenous spread.
11. Recurrence of RCC is rare for patients with stage T1 and T2 tumors. Five-year survival for patients with stage T3 tumors is about 40%.
12. Follow-up after surgical removal of RCC is performed at 6-month intervals and includes liver function testing, chest X-ray (CXR), urinalysis, and CT scan of the abdomen and pelvis.

V. Urinary Tract Calculi
A. Incidence is 20 in 10,000, and it is more common in males.
B. Types of kidney stones
   1. Calcium oxalate (60%)
   2. Calcium phosphate (10% to 20%)
   3. Struvite (10%): These stones form in the presence of urease-producing infectious organisms.

4. Uric acid (10%): These stones are radiolucent and cannot typically be seen on plain films, but they can be seen on CT scan.

5. Cystine (1%)

C. Kidney stones typically become lodged and cause obstruction at one of the following anatomic places:

1. Ureteropelvic junction

2. Mid to distal ureter at the location that the iliac vessel crosses the ureter

3. Ureterovesical junction

D. Clinical features

1. Flank pain is colicky in nature, with nausea and vomiting.

2. Hematuria may occur.

E. Diagnosis

1. CT scan without contrast is the most common test ordered in the emergency department for flank pain. This test also shows whether or not a stone causes obstruction and hydronephrosis (Fig. 17-2).

2. Ultrasound: This test is not optimal for calculi, but it will show whether or not there is hydronephrosis. Sometimes stones can be visualized as well.

3. X-rays of the kidneys, ureter, and bladder (plain X-ray of the abdomen and pelvis)

   a. Advantages: It is inexpensive and a good way to monitor the progression of a stone.

   b. Disadvantages: It does not show all stones (especially the radiolucent stones such as uric acid or cystine stones), and it does not typically show hydronephrosis.

4. Urinalysis: may reveal microscopic hematuria

5. Creatinine: reveals acute renal insufficiency from obstruction secondary to stones

F. Treatment

1. Medical management

   a. Patients may be given a trial of passage of the stone. Typically, stones less than 5 mm can be passed.

      (1) The patient is given pain medication and instructed to drink plenty of water and strain their urine.

      (2) Any stones passed should be kept and analyzed for their organic composition.

FIGURE 17-2 Urolithiasis.

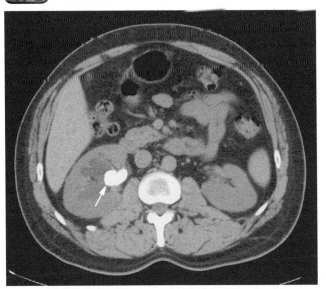

Computed tomographic scan of a patient with right renal collecting system calculus. The *arrow* points to a large staghorn calculus. (Reprinted with permission from Zaslau S, ed. *Blueprints Urology*. Baltimore, MD: Lippincott Williams & Wilkins; 2004.)

Urology

b. Patients who are frequent stone formers should have serum parathyroid hormone and calcium levels taken to evaluate for hyperparathyroidism. They should also have citrate levels and uric acid levels as well as a 24-hour urine study.

2. Surgical management

a. Extracorporeal shock wave lithotripsy (ESWL) is a method in which focused high-pressure shock waves are aimed at the stones with the use of fluoroscopy or ultrasound. The stones are then broken into smaller fragments, so that the patient can pass them.

(1) Complications of ESWL include transient hypertension, subcapsular renal hematoma, failure to completely break stones, urosepsis, and Steinstrasse syndrome. Steinstrasse syndrome is a large quantity of stone fragments, which may accumulate and block the ureter.

(2) Contraindications include inability to localize the stone secondary to the stone being radiopaque, pregnancy, and bleeding disorders.

b. Ureteroscopy is a method in which a small-caliber instrument called a ureteroscope is advanced into the ureter and into the kidney. The stone can then be retrieved with a basket or grasper and endoscopically removed from the urinary tract.

(1) If the stone is too large to safely remove manually, it may be broken into smaller fragments with a laser and then removed.

(2) Complications include damage to the ureter including perforation, strictures, avulsion, and sepsis.

c. Percutaneous nephrolithotripsy is a method for stone removal that is usually reserved for patients with a staghorn calculus, a significant stone burden, or any stones that the surgeon is unable to remove with the aforementioned methods.

(1) The patient has a nephrostomy access placed.

(2) Next, a scope is advanced into the renal pelvis and the stones are removed manually.

(3) If the stones are too large to remove manually, they may be broken up with laser fibers prior to removal.

d. Open surgery for stone retrieval has largely fallen out of favor, secondary to the invasive nature of this procedure. It is still performed occasionally for large complete staghorn calculi.

BLADDER

I. Development

A. The bladder is formed during the fourth to seventh weeks of development. It is formed by the division of the cloacae into an anal canal posteriorly and a urogenital sinus anteriorly. The largest portion of the urogenital sinus becomes the bladder.

B. The apex of the bladder is connected to the urachus during development. The urachus eventually becomes the median umbilical ligament.

II. Anatomy

A. General principles

1. The bladder sits atop of the prostate in the male. It is anterior to the vagina in the female.

2. Three layers of muscle make up the bladder: the inner longitudinal layer, the middle circular layer, and the outer longitudinal layer. The inner layer is covered by transitional epithelium.

3. The inside view of the bladder includes the lateral walls of the bladder, dome of the bladder, and the triangular base of the bladder, which is known as the trigone.

4. The ureteral orifices are the two holes by which the ureters are connected to the bladder. They enter the bladder on either side of the trigone at the base of the bladder.

B. Vascular blood supply of the bladder
  1. The arterial supply of the bladder is supplied by the inferior vesical and superior vesical artery. Both arteries are branches of the internal iliac artery.
  2. Venous drainage of the bladder terminates in the internal iliac veins.
C. Innervation of the bladder
  1. Sympathetic innervation of the bladder originates from T10 to L2 spinal nerves.
  2. Parasympathetic innervation of the bladder comes from S2 to S4 spinal nerves.

III. Transitional Cell Carcinoma

A. General principles
  1. Transitional cell carcinoma (TCC) comprises 90% of all bladder cancers.
  2. The tumors can be papillary, sessile, or ulcerative.
  3. TCC is newly diagnosed in about 53,000 people in the United States annually.
  4. TCC of the bladder is a slow-growing tumor. However, it is often recurrent. About 50% of low-grade cancers recur, and 80% to 90% of high-grade cancers recur.
  5. Factors that cause TCC include smoking, exposure to cyclophosphamide, or industrial exposure to arylamine.
B. Clinical features
  1. The most common presentation for TCC of the bladder is gross or microscopic hematuria. This is the presenting symptom in about 90% of patients with newly diagnosed TCC.
  2. Patients may also have irritative voiding symptoms, also known as lower urinary tract symptoms. These include urgency, frequency, and dysuria.
C. Diagnosis
  1. A voided urine specimen may be sent for cytology to screen for malignant cells.
  2. Imaging studies may find a suspicious bladder wall thickening or a large bladder mass. Imaging modalities include CT scan, ultrasound, and MRI.
  3. The standard for diagnosis of a bladder cancer is cystoscopy. Cystoscopy can be performed under local anesthesia. A flexible cystoscope or a rigid cystoscope may be used to enter the bladder. Masses are found by direct visualization.
D. Treatment
  1. Initial staging of the bladder cancer must be determined by transurethral resection of the bladder tumor (TURBT).
     a. This procedure is performed by inserting a resectoscope through the urethra and into the bladder.
     b. The tumor is then resected off of the bladder wall. Hemostasis is achieved with electrocautery.
     c. The tissue is then sent to pathology to diagnose the extent of invasion.
     d. Complications include bladder wall perforation.
  2. If the TCC is stage T1, management includes surveillance cystoscopy with TURBT for any recurrence. The patient should have surveillance cystoscopy every 3 months for 2 years, then every 6 months for 2 more years, and then every year thereafter.
  3. Bacillus Calmette–Guérin (BCG) therapy is performed by intravesical infusion of an attenuated strain of *Mycobacterium bovis*. This exerts an antitumor effect by an unknown mechanism. This is a very effective therapy for patients with carcinoma in situ to prevent recurrence.
  4. Other chemotherapeutic agents include mitomycin C (Thiotepa) and doxorubicin.
  5. Partial cystectomy is a procedure for removing the part of the bladder that is affected by the tumor. It is reserved for tumors that cannot be resected via TURBT secondary to bladder wall thinning at that region. An example would be a tumor inside of a bladder diverticulum.
  6. Radical cystectomy is the standard of care for muscle-invasive TCC of the bladder.
     a. This procedure includes removal of the prostate and seminal vesicles in men and removal of the uterus, cervix, and ovaries in women.
     b. A lymph node dissection is also performed at the time of cystectomy.

Urology

  c. The ureter drainage must be diverted. There are many methods of diversion; including continent diversions, as well as the more common noncontinent urostomies such as the ileal conduit. The ileal conduit is the most common choice for urinary diversion in the United States.

   (1) In this diversion, a piece of the ileum that is about 20 cm from the ileocecal valve is utilized to bring a urostomy to the skin.

   (2) The ureters are implanted to the ileal pouch and then drain the urine into an ostomy bag.

IV. Neurogenic Bladder

 A. General principles

  1. Neurogenic bladder is the loss of normal function of the bladder secondary to damage to part of the nervous system.

  2. Causes include any disease process that can damage the nerve fibers that innervate the bladder. These include traumatic spinal cord injury, spinal cord neoplasm, spina bifida, stroke, multiple sclerosis, cerebral palsy, Parkinson disease, and others.

 B. Clinical features: Symptoms include urinary incontinence, urinary retention, frequent urinary tract infections, pyelonephritis, urinary urgency, and urinary frequency.

 C. Diagnosis

  1. Tests should be performed to locate the neuroanatomic lesion. These tests include CT or MRI of brain, electroencephalography, and films of the spine.

  2. The standard test for diagnosis of neurogenic bladder is cystoscopy with complex urodynamics.

   a. The urodynamics procedure is performed by inserting a urethral catheter and placing electrodes on the perineum to assess the contractions of accessory muscles and the detrusor contraction, during filling as well as voiding.

   b. Urodynamics can detect detrusor hyperreflexia as well as sphincteric dysfunction.

 D. Treatment

  1. Behavioral therapy

   a. Clean intermittent catheterization is an excellent way of managing a patient with urinary retention and neurogenic bladder. Patients are instructed to void on their own and then to catheterize themselves to remove the post-void residual urine in their bladder.

   b. Scheduled voiding can be used for patients with urinary incontinence. This decreases the number of episodes of incontinence during the day.

  2. Medical management

   a. Anticholinergic therapy is used to decrease the bladder contractility and thus to decrease the amount of involuntary bladder contractions.

    (1) This treatment works by inhibiting the postganglionic parasympathetic receptors in the bladder smooth muscle.

    (2) The agents do have significant side effects for the patient, including dry mouth and constipation.

   b. Prophylactic antibiotics may be considered for patients with recurrent urinary tract infections.

  3. Surgical management

   a. Bladder augmentation is performed to increase the bladder size with accessory tissues.

   b. Paralytic agents such as botulinum toxin may be injected to relax the urethral sphincter.

V. Interstitial Cystitis

 A. General principles

  1. Interstitial cystitis (IC) is a constellation of symptoms including pelvic pain, urgency, frequency, dyspareunia, and severe dysuria.

  2. The female:male ratio is 8:1.

3. Findings at cystoscopy include glomerulations (submucosal hemorrhages) on the bladder mucosa. The patients also may have diffuse cystitis.

4. Patients with symptoms consistent with IC must be evaluated for urinary tract infection, cancer, or other urinary tract disorders prior to the diagnosis of IC.

5. The etiology of IC is not known. Many theories have been proposed. These include the presence of a fastidious infectious organism and that the condition results from an autoimmune disfunction. The current theory is that the condition results from a defect in the glycosaminoglycan layer of the bladder mucosa. This defect is proposed to leave the bladder mucosa permeable to small molecules such as potassium. These molecules are thought to irritate the bladder mucosa and cause bladder mast cells to secrete inflammatory mediators. Nerve stimulation and detrusor muscle depolarization also occur.

B. Diagnosis
1. IC is a diagnosis of exclusion. Urine cultures should be negative, and urine-voided cytology should be negative for malignant cells.

2. An upper urinary tract study is warranted to evaluate the possibility of upper urinary tract disease causing the symptoms. Such a study should consist of either an ultrasound of the kidneys or a CT scan of the abdomen and pelvis.

3. Cystoscopy should be performed to evaluate the bladder mucosa. Often, patients with IC have evidence of cystitis cystica (inflammation of the bladder) or glomerulations of the bladder mucosa.

C. Treatment
1. Medical management
a. Tricyclic antidepressants are frequently utilized to stabilize the mast cells and block histamine receptors. They also treat neuropathic pain.

b. Anticholinergic therapy may be used to treat the symptoms of urgency and frequency by inhibiting parasympathetic receptors.

c. Sodium pentosan polysulfate (Elmiron) is a heparin-like glycosaminoglycan. It is partially excreted in the urine.
(1) It is given orally and has been shown to have some effect on pelvic pain associated with IC.
(2) It takes 3 to 6 months for a patient to experience a significant response.

d. Intravesical dimethyl sulfoxide is a treatment administered into the bladder. It acts as an anti-inflammatory agent and also modulates the immune system.

2. Surgical management
a. There is no role for cystectomy in patients with IC.

b. Sacral neuromodulation is a surgical therapy that is gaining popularity for refractory cases of urgency/frequency.
(1) This is a procedure in which an electrode is inserted into the S3 sacral nerve foramen.
(2) A stimulator is connected to an implantable battery pack placed under the skin. The stimulator sends impulses that stimulate the S3 nerve root.
(3) It is thought that the electrical stimulation excites the pudendal nerves and then modulates a reflex to stabilize the bladder contractions. Preliminary results are promising.

c. Hydrodistention of the bladder is an effective method that provides temporary relief of symptoms of IC.
(1) During this procedure, the bladder is distended above its capacity under anesthesia.
(2) This provides temporary relief from frequency for up to 6 to 8 months.

VI. Urinary Incontinence
A. General principles
1. Urinary incontinence is the complaint of involuntary leakage of urine.
2. There are four major clinical types of urinary incontinence.
a. Urge incontinence: The etiology is presumed to be due to uninhibited bladder contraction, also called detrusor overactivity.

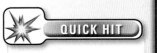

QUICK HIT

A classic finding on cystoscopy of an IC patient is a Hunner ulcer. This bladder ulceration can be found in IC patients with a particularly aggressive form of the disease.

Urology

    b. Stress incontinence: leakage that occurs with an increase in intra-abdominal pressure that overcomes the urinary sphincter closure pressure, in the absence of a bladder contraction

    c. Mixed incontinence: the combination of urge and stress incontinence; detrusor overactivity with impaired urethral sphincter function

    d. Continuous incontinence: continuous involuntary loss of urine. This is often due to a urinary fistula.

    e. Overflow incontinence (incomplete emptying): dribbling and/or continuous leakage associated with incomplete bladder emptying. Often due to impaired detrusor contractility and/or bladder outlet obstruction

B. Diagnosis

  1. A thorough history, physical examination, and urinalysis are necessary for the initial workup.

  2. Key components of the history include leakage frequency, volume, timing, and associated symptoms such as urgency, hesitancy, nocturia, straining, and incomplete emptying. Medications and precipitants, including caffeinated beverages, alcohol, physical activity, and laughing/coughing, should also be reviewed.

  3. A bladder diary, which incorporates patient recordings of the time and volume of all continent and incontinent voids, is a useful tool in elucidating the type of incontinence.

  4. Physical exam should include a genital exam in women to assess for vaginal mucosa atrophy, adequacy of pelvic support, and urethral hypermobility. In men, a digital rectal exam should be performed to evaluate the prostate. Furthermore, a generalized physical can help elucidate additional systemic etiologies causing urinary incontinence, such as neurologic disturbances or fluid overload.

  5. A urinalysis should be performed in all patients with an additional urine culture if an infection is suspected.

C. Clinical testing

  1. Stress test: This test is performed by asking the patient to stand, relax, and give a single cough or bear down while the patient has a full bladder.

  2. Postvoid residual volume: The patient is asked to void and the remaining volume of urine in the bladder is measured either by ultrasound or catheterization.

  3. Urodynamic testing: This is usually performed by a specialist and is considered the physiologic gold standard in evaluating urinary incontinence.

  4. Cystoscopy: Also performed by a specialist, this should be performed when surgery is considered, empiric therapy is unsuccessful, or the diagnosis is unclear.

D. Treatment

  1. Behavioral therapy

    a. Timed (scheduled) voiding: voiding by a routine schedule with a constant interval between voids. The goal is to empty the bladder before the incontinence occurs.

    b. Pelvic floor training: Previously known as Kegel or pelvic floor exercises, this is a regimen of repeated voluntary pelvic floor muscle contractions. This has been shown to improve stress, urge, and mixed incontinence and should be offered as first-line therapy.

    c. Fluid and dietary management: Avoid excessive fluid intake and bladder irritants, including caffeine, alcohol, spicy food, and acidic food.

    d. Weight loss in obese women can reduce urinary incontinence.

  2. Medical management

    a. Anticholinergics: can impair bladder contraction; however, may cause urinary retention and constipation. Examples: oxybutynin, tolterodine, fesoterodine, solifenacin.

    b. Alpha-agonists: can increase urethral sphincter tone; however, may cause urinary retention. Examples: nasal decongestants, imipramine.

    c. Alpha-antagonists: can decrease urethral sphincter tone. Examples include terazosin, doxazosin, tamsulosin, silodosin.

    d. Beta-3-agonists: can augment bladder relaxation at the level of the detrusor body. Examples include: mirabegron.

3. Surgical management
   a. Botulinum toxin: inhibits muscle contraction by blocking the release of acetylcholine at the neuromuscular junction. When injected into the bladder, it reduces urgency and urge incontinence by inhibiting detrusor overactivity.
   b. Sacral neuromodulation: modifies the voiding reflex by using direct electrical stimulation of the S3 nerve root. Indicated in patients who fail conservative treatment.
   c. Bladder augmentation: can increase bladder capacity and decrease detrusor overactivity. Involves either excising the overlying bladder detrusor muscle or suturing a detubularized segment of intestine to the bladder dome.
   d. Bulking agent injection therapy: A bulking agent is injected into the submucosa of proximal urethra and bladder neck via cystoscopy. This increases bladder outlet resistance and reduces stress incontinence.
   e. Urethral suspension (sling) procedure: Used in females, this increases urethral support and helps reduce stress incontinence.
   f. Artificial urinary sphincter: Used in males, this device is controlled by the patient and compresses the urethra until the patient releases the sphincter pressure so that voiding can occur.

 PROSTATE

I. Development
   A. The urogenital sinus develops from the cloaca at the 28th day of gestation.
   B. The prostate gland forms as an outgrowth of the urethra. The stimulus for this development is testosterone secreted from the testes and dihydrotestosterone (DHT).

II. Anatomy
   A. General principles
      1. The prostate is a bilobed firm glandular structure covered by a capsule.
         a. It is found between the bladder neck and the verumontanum, next to the external sphincter.
         b. It is bordered posteriorly by the rectum and thus is palpable in men on digital rectal examination (DRE).
      2. The zones of the prostate include the peripheral zone, the central zone, and the transition zone.
      3. The urethra runs through the center of the prostate.
      4. The prostate emits a molecule called prostate-specific antigen (PSA). The function of this molecule is to liquefy the seminal coagulum after ejaculation.
   B. Blood supply
      1. Arterial supply is from the prostatic artery, which originates from the inferior vesical artery, which comes from the internal iliac artery.
      2. Venous drainage is via the hypogastric veins.

III. Prostate Cancer
   A. General principles
      1. The incidence of adenocarcinoma of the prostate is about 180,000 new cases per year. It is one of the most common cancers among men.
      2. Prostate cancer is more likely to occur at the peripheral zone of the prostate.
      3. The cause of prostate cancer is unknown. It is more likely to occur in a patient who has a first-degree relative with prostate cancer, and it is more likely in African-Americans.
      4. Prostate tumors spread by direct extension into the seminal vesicles or by extracapsular extension via the periprostatic nerve routes. Lymphatic metastasis also occurs. Most distant metastasis occurs in the bones.

Urology

5. Prostate cancer is a slow-growing cancer. The patients who have low-grade disease and are treated for their disease have a less than 10% chance of cancer-related mortality in 10 years.

6. Gleason grading is a system of tumor grading that takes into account the glandular differentiation of the cancer. The scores range from 2 to 10, with the higher numbers representing increasingly more aggressive tumors.

B. Clinical features

1. Patients with prostate cancer often report no symptoms. They may have symptoms of urinary obstruction, hematuria, and bone pain if distant metastasis has occurred.

2. DRE may reveal a prostate nodule. Absence of a nodule does not exclude the presence of cancer, and presence of a nodule does not automatically mean that the patient has disease.

C. Diagnosis

1. PSA is the most useful laboratory test. The American Cancer Society recommends that serum PSA and yearly DRE be performed in men over the age of 50 years who have a life expectancy of greater than 10 years. The cutoff for an abnormal PSA is any value over 2.0 ng/mL. However, controversy exists as to whether this number is arbitrary or should be allowed to increase with age. Acid phosphatase is another serum marker.

2. Prostate needle biopsy is a transrectal, ultrasound-guided procedure to obtain prostatic tissue for pathologic diagnosis. Several cores are obtained from each lobe of the prostate as well as at the transitional zone. This procedure is often performed under local anesthesia in the office setting.

3. Bone scans are used to assess for distant bone metastasis.

4. CT and MRI are used to view the potential of local invasion and lymph node metastasis.

D. Treatment

1. Radical prostatectomy is the standard of therapy for a patient who is expected to survive greater than 10 years and has organ-confined disease.
   a. This surgical procedure is usually performed open via retropubic approach or using a robotics approach to assist in dissection.
   b. It is common practice to perform nerve-sparing procedures to help reduce the amount of postoperative erectile dysfunction (ED).
   c. Approximately 6% of patients also experience significant urinary incontinence from the procedure.

2. Brachytherapy is a less invasive therapy for organ-confined prostate disease. This procedure consists of ultrasound-guided placement of radioactive seeds into the prostate that emit radiation to destroy prostatic tissue.
   a. Results are better for prostate cancer with a lower Gleason score.
   b. Some side effects include urinary retention, urethritis, and irritative voiding symptoms.

3. External beam radiation therapy is the treatment preferred for T3 disease with extracapsular extension.
   a. Complications of this therapy include radiation cystitis, hematuria or hemorrhagic cystitis, and ED.
   b. The side effects are decreasing because techniques are improving to protect the bladder from stray radiation.

4. Bilateral orchiectomy is removal of the testicles. This procedure is performed for advanced prostate cancer to remove all androgens. Because prostate cancer is receptive to androgens, ablating the androgens causes about 40% of the tumors to regress. Side effects include hot flashes and loss of libido as well as ED.

5. Medical castration has the same principle as surgical castration, which is to remove all androgen activity. This is accomplished medically by administering luteinizing hormone–releasing hormone (LHRH) agonists. LHRH agonists cause an initial increase in testosterone followed by a decrease in the receptors.
   a. The medication is administered either monthly or every 3 to 4 months.
   b. Side effects are the same as those caused with surgical castration.

IV. Benign Prostatic Hyperplasia

A. General principles

1. Benign prostatic hyperplasia (BPH) is caused by benign growth in prostate tissue as men age. Up to 50% of men older than 50 years of age have BPH, but it is not usually clinically significant.

2. Causes of BPH are not fully understood. According to some theories, BPH is caused by increasing estrogen levels in men as they age.

3. BPH forms in the transitional zone of the prostate, which is the zone that encircles the urethra. This often causes obstructive voiding symptoms in patients who suffer from BPH.

B. Clinical features

1. Patients who have BPH often complain of a decreased urine stream, urinary hesitancy, frequency, urgency, and straining to void.

2. Patients can have episodes of urinary retention.

C. Diagnosis

1. Serum PSA may be slightly elevated in patients with BPH.

2. Imaging studies such as renal ultrasound are sufficient to evaluate the kidneys and ureters for hydronephrosis. Hydronephrosis is usually bilateral if caused by BPH.

3. Cystoscopy is the standard for evaluating a patient with obstructive voiding symptoms and possible BPH.

   a. Because the prostate can be visualized while advancing the cystoscope through the prostatic urethra, cystoscopy is an excellent way to visualize the size of the prostate and the amount of bladder outlet obstruction the prostate is causing.

   b. Other findings on cystoscopy include thickening of the bladder wall musculature, known as trabeculations, which is caused by a bladder that is constantly straining to achieve micturition.

4. Postvoid residual (PVR) is a useful study that can be performed by having the patient empty his or her bladder and then using an ultrasound bladder scanner to assess the amount of urine that remains after micturition. This value can also be obtained with a simple straight catheterization of the bladder. Patients with BPH often have a PVR greater than 50 to 100 mL.

5. Urodynamics is a useful study that can rule out other causes of voiding dysfunction for a patient with obstructive voiding symptoms and possible BPH. This also measures the flow rate during voiding, which is often markedly decreased in patients with BPH.

D. Treatment

1. Medical management

   a. Alpha blockers are often used to treat patients with BPH. These medications work on the alpha-1-adrenoreceptors found in the prostate and bladder. The blockade of alpha receptors causes a decrease in the amount of alpha-receptor-moderated muscle tone in the prostate and bladder. Examples include terazosin, doxazosin, tamsulosin, and alfluzasin.

      (1) Treatment with these medications results in improved urinary flow rate and symptom scores.

      (2) Side effects include hypotension, dizziness, and retrograde ejaculation.

   b. 5-Alpha reductase inhibitors such as finasteride and dutasteride are competitive selective inhibitors of 5-alpha reductase.

      (1) These agents decrease the amount of prostatic DHT, which then causes a decrease in the size of the prostate.

      (2) Side effects include loss of libido and ejaculatory dysfunction.

2. Surgical management

   a. The most common method of resection of BPH is transurethral resection of the prostate (TURP). This method uses electrocautery to remove excess prostatic tissue. This is performed using a resecting endoscope inserted through the penis.

      (1) Patients may have significant hematuria, ED, or even urinary incontinence after the procedure.

(2) Another risk is transurethral resection syndrome, caused by absorption of the hypotonic irrigating solution that is infused into the prostatic venous system during the procedure. This can cause hypervolemia and hyponatremia, which leads to confusion, visual disturbances, and cardiac arrhythmias.

b. Laser TURP is a relatively new variation of TURP. This uses the same principle as traditional TURP. However, a laser is used to resect the prostatic tissue as opposed to electrocautery. Advantages of this procedure are a decreased amount of hematuria after the procedure and a decreased risk of transurethral resection syndrome.

c. Open prostatectomy is used when the prostate is too large (over 100 grams) to remove transurethrally.

V. Prostatitis

A. General principles
1. Prostatitis can be broken down into three groups.
   a. The first group is less common and is called acute bacterial prostatitis. This type of prostatitis is caused by a severe urinary tract infection and causes significant pain as well as fevers and chills. A bacterial organism is cultured from the prostatic secretions of the urine.
   b. The second group is chronic bacterial prostatitis. This type of prostatitis causes symptoms such as chronic pelvic, perineal, or low back pain. Patients may also have pain after ejaculating or irritative voiding symptoms. Recurrent bacterial organisms can be cultured in the urine or prostatic secretions.
   c. The third group, the most common group, is called chronic nonbacterial prostatitis or chronic pelvic pain syndrome. The symptoms are the same as chronic bacterial prostatitis. However, no organisms can be cultured.

B. Diagnosis
1. Diagnosis of prostatitis is usually based on history.
2. Patients often experience reproduction of their pelvic pain upon DRE.
3. Attempt to culture an organism is made using either the voided urine specimen or by milking prostatic secretions and culturing the secretions.

C. Treatment
1. Treatment is via medical management. Patients are usually given 6 weeks of antibiotics as well as nonsteroidal anti-inflammatory drugs such as ibuprofen. Some patients require chronic prophylactic antibiotics.
2. Complications of prostatitis include prostatitic abscess. This can be diagnosed with transrectal ultrasound and can be drained by percutaneous drainage.

 PENIS

I. Development

A. The external genitalia in the male develops at 10 weeks of age.
B. The phallus elongates and pulls the urethral folds together until they form the urethral groove.
C. During the third month of gestation, the urethral folds close over the urethral plate to form the penile urethra.

II. Anatomy

A. General principles
1. Three tissue bodies comprise the penis. These include the paired erectile corpora cavernosa and the corpus spongiosum, which contains the urethra.
2. Sexual desire and parasympathetic stimulation causes erection by causing relaxation in the cavernosal arterial smooth muscles. Arterial engorgement of the corpora cavernosa prevents venous outflow from the corpora to cause erection.
B. Arterial supply to the penis comes from the internal pudendal artery. The deep artery of the penis runs through the center of the erectile body. Superficial blood supply is supplied by the external pudendal artery.
C. Venous drainage comes from the deep dorsal vein of the penis.

III. Priapism

A. General principles

1. Priapism is defined as a painful erection that lasts over 4 hours. This erection is not relieved by orgasm. This condition is a urologic emergency because it can damage the erectile tissue and cause impotence.

2. There are two types of priapism: high flow (nonischemic), and low flow (ischemic priapism).

   a. High-flow priapism can be idiopathic or as a result of trauma.

   b. Low-flow priapism can be idiopathic, can occur as a result of prescription or recreational drug abuse (especially cocaine), or can occur as a result of sickle cell disease or leukemia.

B. Diagnosis

1. History taking is important when evaluating a patient with priapism. This is to identify a cause for the problem, including drug abuse or past medical history.

2. Physical examination often reveals a firm penis with a flaccid glans. The penis is often very tender to palpation.

3. Laboratory values that must be obtained include a drug screen, a complete blood count (CBC), hemoglobin electrophoresis if sickle cell anemia is suspected, and a cavernosal blood gas.

   a. In high-flow priapism, the blood gas taken from the cavernosa is similar to that of the arterial blood gas (ABG) obtained peripherally.

   b. In low-flow priapism, the corporal blood gas usually reveals a pH of less than 7.25 and a PCO_2 of over 60.

4. Ultrasound of the cavernosa can be performed to determine if the priapism is high flow or low flow.

C. Treatment

1. Low-flow priapism

   a. The initial treatment includes corporal aspiration and irrigation.

   b. After aspiration and irrigation, corporal injection of alpha agonists should be performed.

      (1) The alpha agonists that should be injected include epinephrine and phenylephrine. The patient should be on a cardiac monitor while these medications are being injected.

      (2) If the penis does not reach detumescence, then the injection of epinephrine or phenylephrine may be repeated every 5 minutes up to three times.

   c. If the penis is still erect, then a distal cavernosal shunt (Winter shunt) may be performed.

   d. If the condition recurs, then a proximal cavernosal-spongiosal shunt may be performed.

2. High-flow priapism

   a. Treatment begins with a pelvic angiogram with embolization or observation. Embolization may be repeated if the penis is still erect.

   b. Failure of embolization can be treated with surgical management as discussed earlier.

IV. Peyronie Disease

A. General principles

1. Peyronie disease is defined as an idiopathic curvature of the penis that is acquired, and it commonly presents in men age 40 years and over.

2. It is caused by scarring or fibrosis of the tunica albuginea and causes a fibrous plaque. Causes of the disease are thought to be secondary to microtrauma to the penis.

3. The incidence is less than about 2% of the male population and is more common in Caucasian men.

4. The disease has been associated with patients who also have Dupuytren contracture of the hands.

Urology

B. Diagnosis
1. Patients with Peyronie disease often complain of curved, painful erections, and a palpable plaque on the shaft of the penis.
2. Physical examination usually reveals a palpable fibrous plaque.
3. Ultrasound is not necessary but may be utilized when the examination findings are not impressive enough to make the diagnosis.

C. Treatment
1. Medical management
   a. Potassium para-aminobenzoate to reduce pain and improve curvature
   b. Vitamin E supplements
   c. Nonsteroidal anti-inflammatory agents
   d. Calcium-channel blockers
2. Surgical management: Surgery, including plaque excision with graft to the excised portion of tunica albuginea, is the most effective treatment for refractory cases of Peyronie disease that cause impotence or severe deformity.

V. Erectile Dysfunction

A. General principles
1. It is estimated that up to 25 million American men suffer from ED.
2. There are many causes of ED. Its origins may be vasculogenic, psychogenic, neurogenic, endocrine, or iatrogenic.
   a. Vasculogenic causes include diabetes mellitus, atherosclerosis, thromboembolic disease, or smoking.
   b. Psychogenic causes include anxiety, depression, and post-traumatic stress disorders.
   c. Neurogenic causes include diabetic neuropathy and any disease that causes lesions in either the peripheral or central nervous system (e.g., multiple sclerosis, spinal cord injury).
   d. Endocrine causes include any disease that causes primary or secondary hypogonadism (e.g., Prader-Willi syndrome, Kallmann syndrome).
   e. Iatrogenic causes include drugs such as alcohol and selective serotonin reuptake inhibitors.

B. Diagnosis
1. A careful history should be taken to attempt to determine the cause of the ED.
2. Physical examination should be performed to assess the neurologic, vascular, and genitourinary systems.
3. Laboratory values necessary to evaluate a patient for ED include prolactin level, testosterone level, fasting blood sugar, and even cholesterol studies.
4. Nocturnal penile tumescence testing measures the ability of a patient to achieve erection while sleeping. The normal number of erections is four or more per night.

C. Treatment
1. Medical management
   a. Phosphodiesterase inhibitors include sildenafil, vardenafil, and tadalafil.
      (1) These agents work by inhibiting the enzyme phosphodiesterase to achieve elevated levels of cyclic guanosine monophosphate (GMP). Cyclic GMP then causes an increase in nitric oxide, which in turn causes engorgement of the corpora cavernosa.
      (2) Side effects include headache, visual disturbance, flushing, and hypotension. These drugs may not be used in patients taking nitrates secondary to risk of hypotension.
   b. Intracavernosal injection therapy is with prostaglandin E1, an injectable agent that the patient must inject into the corpora cavernosa prior to intercourse. It is very effective. However, side effects include burning and pain, as well as corporal fibrosis.

Urology

c. Vacuum erection devices are mechanical treatments that involve using a pump to create a pressure gradient that causes filling of the cavernosa.

d. If a patient has low testosterone, topical testosterone cream may assist with increasing the patient's libido.

2. Surgical management

a. Surgical management is reserved for refractory cases. This treatment involves placement of a penile prosthesis. There are several types of penile prostheses, including mechanical, inflatable, and malleable devices.

(1) Malleable rods are paired implants that are placed into the corpora cavernosa. The patient has a constant semirigid penis.

(2) Inflatable devices are placed and allow the patient to pump the penis to the erect state prior to intercourse.

b. Complications of penile prosthesis include infection, erosion, and device malfunction requiring revision.

VI. Penile Cancer

A. General principles

1. The incidence is about 1 in 100,000.

2. Risk factors include uncircumcised phallus, balanitis, Bowen disease, poor hygiene, and human papillomavirus.

3. The 5-year survival rate is 65% to 80% for patients without palpable adenopathy and 20% to 50% for patients with palpable adenopathy.

4. The most common pathologic type of penile cancer is squamous cell carcinoma.

B. Diagnosis

1. Diagnosis is by physical examination of the penis and foreskin, which reveals an abnormal skin lesion.

2. Biopsy is necessary for pathologic diagnosis.

3. CT scan or MRI is needed to assess lymph node involvement.

C. Treatment

1. If lesion is confined to prepuce, circumcision is indicated.

2. Tumors of the glans or penile shaft should be resected surgically, with partial or total penectomy (removal of penis) with at least a 2-cm margin.

3. Patients with palpable inguinal lymphadenopathy require inguinal lymph node dissection.

URETHRA

I. Development and Anatomy

A. Development: The urethral folds close over the urethral plate to form the penile urethra during the third month of gestation.

B. Anatomy

1. General principles

a. The male urethra is divided into four parts, which include (from proximal to distal): the prostatic urethra, the membranous urethra, the bulbar urethra, and the penile urethra.

b. The type of epithelium in the urethra changes from transitional epithelium to squamous epithelium at the distal portion.

2. Blood supply: The urethra obtains arterial blood supply from the internal pudendal artery, and its venous drainage goes to the internal pudendal vein.

II. Hypospadias

A. General principles

1. Hypospadias is a congenital malformation in which the urethral meatus opens onto the ventral side of the penis. This results from incomplete fusion of the urethral folds in utero.

2. Incidence is 1 in 300 live male births.

3. There are five classifications of hypospadias:
  a. Coronal, in which the meatus is at the coronal sulcus
  b. Glandular, in which the meatus is on the proximal glans penis
  c. Meatal opening on the penile shaft
  d. Scrotal hypospadias, in which the meatus is at the base of the penis at the scrotal level
  e. Penoscrotal hypospadias, in which the meatus opens onto the perineum
4. Significance
  a. Hypospadias does not usually cause any problems for an infant.
  b. It becomes problematic as the child ages and is unable to urinate with a straight stream.
  c. Associated with chordee (curvature of the penis), which can make intercourse difficult once the patient becomes mature.
B. Diagnosis: based on physical examination findings of the previously described classification of hypospadias
C. Treatment
  1. Surgical correction is the only treatment for hypospadias.
  2. Hypospadias can be surgically corrected after 4 months of age but should be done prior to the child entering school. The child should not be circumcised prior to surgical correction of hypospadias.
  3. There are many different methods of surgical correction. The repair usually involves straightening the penis by removing the chordee and urethral reconstruction using a graft that usually comes from the excess foreskin.
  4. Complications of hypospadias repair include urethrocutaneous fistula in up to 30% of patients. This is repaired surgically.

 SCROTUM

I. Development and Anatomy
A. Development: The male bilateral scrotal swellings fuse at the scrotal septum during development.
B. Anatomy
  1. General principles
    a. The scrotum houses the testicles and epididymis.
    b. The scrotal sac consists of skin, dartos muscle, external spermatic fascia, cremasteric muscle, internal spermatic fascia, and tunica vaginalis.
  2. Blood supply
    a. The anterior scrotum derives its blood supply from the external pudendal artery.
    b. The posterior scrotum derives its blood supply from the cremasteric and testicular arteries.

II. Hydrocele
A. General principles
  1. Hydroceles are a collection of fluid between the parietal and visceral layers of the tunica vaginalis.
    a. In infants, they are caused by a patent processus vaginalis that allows peritoneal fluid to enter the scrotum.
    b. In adults, they are thought to be from a secretory imbalance in the tunica vaginalis.
  2. Hydroceles present as a scrotal swelling that transilluminates.
    a. In infants, they are usually painless.
    b. In adults, they can become large enough to cause discomfort or pain.
B. Diagnosis
  1. Hydroceles present as a scrotal swelling that transilluminates to light on physical examination.
  2. Ultrasound of the scrotum can be performed to confirm the diagnosis.

C. Treatment
1. In infants, hydroceles can be monitored until 1 year of age. This is unlike inguinal hernias, which should be fixed as soon as possible; secondary to a risk of incarceration of the hernia sac. Many hydroceles spontaneously resolve by 1 year of age.
2. In infants older than 1 year of age with continued hydrocele, surgical management is indicated. Hydrocelectomy is performed to ligate the patent processus vaginalis.
3. In adults, surgical management is indicated only if the hydrocele is large enough to bother the patient's daily life or if the hydrocele is painful.

III. Fournier Gangrene
A. General principles
1. Fournier gangrene was first described by a French physician named Fournier in the late 1800s.
2. This condition is defined by a necrotizing fasciitis of the scrotum that travels up the lower abdomen. This is a urologic emergency with mortality rates up to 50%.
3. Symptoms include a painful, erythematous scrotum that rapidly progresses within hours and can travel up the abdomen. Crepitans of the erythematous region can be palpated if the offending organism is a gas-forming bacteria.
4. Risk factors include obesity, diabetes, history of perineal fistula or urethral stricture, and trauma to the pelvic region.
5. Many microorganisms can be responsible for this condition, including *Staphylococcus, Streptococcus, Enterobacteriaceae–Bacteroides,* and *Clostridium.*
B. Diagnosis
1. Diagnosis is made by physical examination. The physician must have a high index of suspicion.
2. Laboratory values needed include CBC and serum electrolytes. If the patient is septic, he or she must be resuscitated appropriately.
3. Wound cultures and blood cultures are needed to determine the microorganism responsible.
C. Treatment
1. Medical management includes broad-spectrum intravenous antibiotics as soon as possible. Once wound and blood cultures have been obtained, antibiotic therapy can be tailored for the offending organism.
2. Surgical management includes wide excision of the involved devascularized region with debridement of the tissue. The patient may require multiple debridements after the initial procedure. Urinary diversion, such as a suprapubic tube, may be necessary.

 SPERMATIC CORD

I. Development and Anatomy
A. Development: The testes descend into the scrotum during development and pass through the abdominal wall at the level of the internal inguinal ring. Each testicle is attached to the spermatic cord which contains blood vessels, nerves, lymphatics, and the vas deferens.
B. Anatomy
1. General principles: The spermatic cord is covered with internal spermatic fasciae, cremasteric fasciae, and external spermatic fasciae.
2. Blood supply and other contents of spermatic cord
   a. The arterial contents of the spermatic cord include the testicular artery, the cremasteric artery, and the artery to the vas deferens.
   b. The testicular veins form the pampiniform plexus.
   c. Lumbar lymphatics are found in the spermatic cord.
   d. The nerves in the spermatic cord include the genital branch of the genitofemoral nerve and branches of the hypogastric plexus. The ilioinguinal nerve is found at the floor of the inguinal canal.

Urology

II. Varicocele

A. General principles

1. A varicocele is a dilated varicosity of the internal spermatic vein that produces a fullness surrounding the spermatic cord.
2. It may be slightly tender and is more common on the left side.
3. The incidence is 10% to 20% of males.
4. Varicoceles are more prevalent in patients who have male factor infertility. The mechanism is not fully understood, but it is theorized that the increased blood supply from the dilated veins increases the temperature in the scrotum and impedes sperm maturation.

B. Diagnosis: Diagnosis is made by physical examination but may be confirmed with a scrotal ultrasound.

C. Treatment

1. Treatment is necessary if the patient is having fertility problems, experiences chronic pain of the testicle, or has an atrophic growth pattern (in adolescents).
2. Surgical management is performed by varicocele ligation from a retroperitoneal, inguinal, or subinguinal approach.
3. Newer methods of treatment include angiographic interventional radiology techniques to coil or sclerose the varicocele.
4. Most patients have a 70% rate of improvement of semen quality. Fertility improves about 6 months after varicocelectomy.

 TESTIS

I. Development and Anatomy

A. Development: The sex cords migrate along into the genital ridge at the sixth week. They differentiate into the testes by the seventh week.

B. Anatomy

1. General principles
   a. The testes are bilateral male reproductive organs that lie within the scrotal sac. The testis is the site of sperm production and maturation. An epididymis attaches to the dorsum of each testis. The epididymis terminates into the vas deferens, which carries the sperm to the ejaculatory duct and into the urethra.
   b. The inside of the testis is compartmentalized into lobules. Each lobule contains Sertoli cells to assist with spermatogenesis. Seminiferous tubules are interspersed in the testis.
   c. The testes are about 4 to 5 cm in length. They are suspended in the scrotum by the spermatic cord. Each testis is covered by the tunica vaginalis.

2. Blood supply
   a. The arterial supply of the testis is from the internal spermatic arteries, which arise below the renal arteries. Additional arterial anastomoses include the cremasteric arteries and the arteries of the vas.
   b. The venous drainage of the testis is from the pampiniform plexus and spermatic veins. The right spermatic vein enters renal vein.

II. Cryptorchidism

A. General principles

1. The incidence of undescended testis is about 1% of live male births. It is unlikely that the testicles will descend in an infant over 3 months of age.
2. Locations of the undescended testis include intra-abdominal, suprapubic, superficial inguinal, femoral, and perineal.
3. Men with a history of cryptorchidism are predisposed to infertility, although early surgical repair of cryptorchidism increases the chances of future paternity.
4. Testicular malignancy is up to 35 times more likely in a patient with a history of cryptorchidism.

B. Diagnosis
1. The diagnosis of cryptorchidism is by physical examination. Sometimes the testis can be milked into the scrotum. If the testis remains in the scrotum after traction is released, no surgical intervention is indicated.
2. If the undescended testis is not palpable, CT scan may be indicated to find the location of the testis.
C. Treatment: Surgical management, in the form of orchidopexy, is indicated for patients over 6 months of age and must be completed by 2 years of age. Newer data suggest that fertility increases with earlier orchidopexy. The surgical procedure is performed via an inguinal incision.

III. Orchitis

A. General principles: Symptoms of acute orchitis usually include fever and testicular pain. The involved testis is swollen and tender.
B. Etiology
1. There are several causes of orchitis, including viral, bacterial, traumatic, chemical, fungal, parasitic, and idiopathic.
2. Mumps orchitis is caused by the mumps virus. This usually occurs about 6 days after the onset of parotid involvement. It often causes infertility.
C. Treatment
1. Medical management is the appropriate therapy and thus varies greatly based on the cause of the orchitis.
   a. Treatments include antibiotics, antifungals, and antiparasitic agents.
   b. Supportive care includes treatment of pain, scrotal support, and icing the scrotum.
2. Surgical management may include aspiration of an inflammatory hydrocele and may give some relief from pain. Abscess of the testicle is rare, but when it occurs, it requires debridement or removal of the testicle (orchiectomy).

IV. Testicular Cancer

A. General principles
1. The incidence is 4.5 per 100,000 people.
2. Cryptorchidism is a risk factor.
3. Most testicular cancers (95%) are germ cell tumors. These can be broken down into seminomatous and nonseminomatous germ cell tumors.
4. The types of testicular tumors are as follows:
   a. Classic seminoma (comprises 30% of all germ cell testicular tumors)
   b. Spermatocytic tumor
   c. Anaplastic seminoma
   d. Embryonal carcinoma
   e. Teratomas
   f. Choriocarcinoma
   g. Yolk sac tumor (the most common nonseminomatous germ cell tumor in children)
   h. Stromal tumors, which make up the minority of tumors and are classified as nongerminal tumors
5. Symptoms include a painless enlarging mass in the testicle.
B. Diagnosis
1. Physical examination reveals a palpable mass.
2. Ultrasound is an excellent imaging method for evaluating testicular neoplasm.
3. CT scan or MRI of chest, abdomen, and pelvis should be considered for evaluation of metastatic spread.
4. Serum tumor markers include beta-human chorionic gonadotropin, alphafetoprotein, and lactate dehydrogenase. Elevations in these tumor markers are much more likely in nonseminomatous germ cell tumors.
C. Treatment
1. Radical inguinal orchiectomy should be performed for all types of testicular cancer. Scrotal orchiectomy is discouraged because of the risk of nodal metastasis.

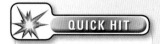

Orchidopexy increases the fertility rate among patients with cryptorchidism, but it does not decrease the incidence of testicular cancer.

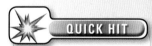

The standard of care in the United States for stage I seminoma is orchiectomy with radiation therapy.

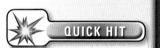

All nonseminomatous germ cell tumors should be managed with orchiectomy and RPLND because these tumors are more likely to undergo lymphatic spread.

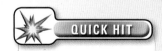

Left-sided testicular cancer usually metastasizes to the para-aortic nodes. Right-sided testicular cancer usually metastasizes to the interaortocaval nodes. The right-sided cancers can cross over to the para-aortic nodes, but left-sided testicular cancers cannot cross to the right.

Urology

2. Retroperitoneal lymph node dissection (RPLND) is indicated for all nonsemi-nomatous germ cell tumors because of the likelihood of nodal metastasis. Nonseminomatous germ cell tumors with bulky retroperitoneal lymphadenop-athy can also benefit from platinum-based chemotherapy prior to RPLND.

3. Radiation therapy is utilized for neoadjuvant therapy for almost all stage 1 seminoma patients. This is performed because there is a 15% rate of relapse of the tumor in the lymphatics.

4. Chemotherapy is effective for recurrent seminoma and is an excellent salvage therapy.

5. Testicular cancer is one of the most curable forms of cancer because most his-tiologic subtypes are sensitive to adjuvant therapy, such as radiation and che-motherapy.

V. Testicular Torsion

A. General principles

1. Testicular torsion occurs when the testis rotates upon itself in the scrotum. When this occurs, venous outflow is obstructed, and edema causes subsequent arterial compromise and necrosis of the testicle. Symptoms include an acutely painful, swollen testis.

2. This condition is a surgical emergency! Prognosis is good if the patient under-goes surgery within 4 to 6 hours.

3. The most common presenting age is 12 to 18 years.

4. There are two types of testicular torsion:

    a. Extravaginal torsion is more common in infants because the gubernaculum is free to rotate in the scrotum.

    b. Intravaginal torsion is more common in adolescents. This condition is thought to occur because of a short mesenteric attachment from the cord onto the testis and epididymis. This allows the testis to prolapse onto its side and rotate like a "bell in a clapper" (bell clapper deformity).

5. The appendix testis is a remnant of the müllerian duct. Torsion of the appen-dix testis can occur and may cause a gradual onset of testicular pain. Physical examination can reveal a blue dot that is visible through the scrotal wall.

B. Diagnosis

1. Diagnosis is made by physical examination.

2. Ultrasound is the gold standard for imaging a patient with acute scrotal pain. The ultrasound reveals vascular compromise.

C. Treatment: Testicular torsion is a surgical emergency, and the patient should be taken immediately to the operating room to attempt detorsion, testicular sal-vage, and orchiopexy. Sometimes the testicle can even be manually "de-torsed" by rotating the testicle as though opening a book (i.e., turning the left testicle counterclockwise and the right testicle clockwise).

Otolaryngology

Jordan Cain and Jason McChesney

 ## COMMON OTOLARYNGOLOGIC CONDITIONS

I. **Acute Sinusitis**
   A. General principles
      1. Infection of the paranasal sinuses for less than 4 weeks (4 to 12 weeks = sub-acute; >12 weeks = chronic)
      2. Most commonly results from a viral upper respiratory infection (URI)
      3. Minimal mucosal inflammation can obstruct the drainage of the sinuses, leading to bacterial infection of retained sinus secretions, typically during the second week of the URI.
      4. The most common bacterial pathogens are *Streptococcus pneumoniae, Haemophilus influenzae,* and *Moraxella catarrhalis.*
      5. Other common predisposing factors for bacterial infection include allergies, anatomic obstruction of the nose, odontogenic infection, intranasal drug abuse, immunodeficiency, and impaired mucociliary clearance (e.g., cystic fibrosis).
      6. Acute invasive fungal sinusitis may occur in immunocompromised patients or those with poorly controlled diabetes and is a medical emergency.
         a. Most common fungal organisms are *Mucor, Rhizopus,* and *Aspergillus.*
   B. Clinical features
      1. Nasal congestion
      2. Postnasal drip and purulent nasal drainage
      3. Facial pain or pressure that is worse when bending forward, maxillary tooth pain
      4. Headache
      5. Hyposmia/anosmia
   C. Diagnosis (see Clinical Pearl 18-1)
      1. Endoscopic evaluation: Visualize purulent drainage as well as septal deviation, nasal polyps, and other obstructing features that may cause blockage of sinus drainage.

CLINICAL PEARL 18-1

Criteria for the Diagnosis of Sinusitis*

Major Criteria
- Purulent anterior nasal discharge
- Purulent posterior nasal discharge
- Nasal congestion or obstruction
- Facial congestion or fullness
- Hyposmia or anosmia
- Fever (acute sinusitis only)

Minor Criteria
- Headache
- Ear pain, pressure, or fullness
- Halitosis
- Dental pain
- Fever (subacute or chronic sinusitis)
- Fatigue

*Diagnosis of sinusitis made in the presence of at least two major criteria or one major and two or more minor criteria.

2. Imaging: indicated in chronic/recurrent sinusitis or complicated cases of acute sinusitis
   a. Computed tomography (CT) scan: method of choice; can assess bony structures as well as evaluate for air–fluid levels and mucosal thickening
   b. Magnetic resonance imaging (MRI): does not image bone as well as CT but is good for differentiating soft-tissue masses from retained mucus, particularly when extra-sinus involvement is suspected
3. Laboratory studies: HIV and immunoglobulin serologies are useful in refractory cases of sinusitis if there is any evidence of an immunocompromised state.

D. Treatment
   1. Medical management
      a. Prevention
         (1) Nasal saline and/or nasal steroids
         (2) Allergy management (oral and/or nasal antihistamines, environmental control, immunotherapy)
         (3) Oxymetazoline spray: causes vasoconstriction of nasal mucosa; can cause rebound swelling. Therefore, short use (less than 3 days) is recommended.
      b. Antibiotics
         (1) Cornerstone of treatment of acute sinusitis
         (2) First-line: amoxicillin (or trimethoprim-sulfamethoxazole if the patient has a penicillin allergy) for 10 to 14 days
         (3) Second-line: amoxicillin/clavulanic acid or fluoroquinolones
   2. Surgical management
      a. Considered an option after failure of 4 to 6 weeks of maximum medical therapy, or for complicated acute infections
         (1) Complications: orbital infection, meningitis, intracranial abscess, cavernous sinus thrombosis, invasive fungal infection (see Clinical Pearl 18-2)
      b. Functional endoscopic sinus surgery aims to open the natural sinus ostia while preserving as much of the sinus mucosa as possible.
      c. Surgery does not treat the underlying inflammatory causes of sinusitis, and patients with chronic sinusitis must be managed medically following surgery in order to prevent recurrence.

QUICK HIT

Complications such as orbital infection, meningitis, intracranial abscess, and cavernous sinus thrombosis can result from an episode of acute sinusitis.

Otolaryngology

CLINICAL PEARL 18-2

Chandler Classification of Orbital Complications of Sinusitis

Group 1	Preseptal cellulitis	Inflammatory edema of the eyelids anterior to the orbital septum
Group 2	Orbital cellulitis	Diffuse edema of the orbital contents due to inflammation and bacterial infection, without abscess
Group 3	Subperiosteal abscess	Abscess formation between the orbital periosteum and the bony orbital wall; may cause proptosis with the globe displaced away from the abscess, decreased ocular mobility, and/or decreased visual acuity
Group 4	Orbital abscess	Discrete abscess within the orbit; often associated with severe, symmetric proptosis; complete ophthalmoplegia results, and permanent loss of vision may occur
Group 5	Cavernous sinus thrombosis	Progression of phlebitis into the cavernous sinus and to the opposite side, with resultant bilateral symptoms; may lead to meningitis and/or sepsis

II. Bacterial Pharyngitis

A. General principles

1. Pharyngitis: inflammation of the pharynx (most commonly the oropharynx), which has many etiologies: bacterial or viral infection, carcinoma, reflux disease, allergy, postnasal drip, environmental exposures

2. Bacterial pharyngitis accounts for 5% to 10% of cases of pharyngitis and commonly affects the palatine tonsils, uvula, soft palate, and posterior pharyngeal wall.

B. Clinical features

1. Sore throat, odynophagia, fever, chills, malaise, headache, neck stiffness, and anorexia

2. Cervical adenopathy, pharyngeal erythema and edema, gray-white tonsillar exudates, and petechiae on the soft palate

3. Cough is typically absent.

4. Pharyngitis can lead to peritonsillar or retropharyngeal abscess, rheumatic fever, scarlet fever, and poststreptococcal glomerulonephritis.

C. Diagnosis

1. History and physical examination (Centor criteria): fever, tender anterior cervical adenopathy, tonsillar exudates, absent cough

2. Rapid antigen test (70% to 90% sensitivity, 90% to 100% specific)

3. Antistreptolysin titers are not helpful in diagnosis of acute pharyngitis.

D. Treatment

1. Medical management with a 10-day course of antibiotics

   a. Penicillins (penicillin V, amoxicillin)

   b. Macrolides (azithromycin, clarithromycin, erythromycin) for penicillin-allergic patients

   c. Cephalosporins may be used in instances of recurrent infection refractory to the previously mentioned therapies.

2. Surgical management: Tonsillectomy is appropriate for those patients with recurrent bacterial pharyngitis, whose episodes do not decrease with appropriate antibiotic therapy.

III. Epiglottitis

A. General principles

1. In children, median age for occurrence is 6 to 12 years old.

2. Most common pathogen associated with this disease is *Haemophilus influenzae* B (HIB).

3. Incidence has decreased 90% since the introduction of the HIB vaccine.

B. Clinical features

1. Abrupt onset (within hours) and rapid progression of fever, as well as "the 3 Ds": <u>d</u>ysphagia, <u>d</u>rooling, and <u>d</u>istress caused by sore throat with severe odynophagia

2. Children with this condition are often sitting up in the "tripod" or "sniffing" position—trunk leaning forward with the neck hyperextended and chin thrust forward—and may be reluctant to lie down.

3. Biphasic stridor is a late sign.

C. Diagnosis

1. Lateral neck X-ray: "thumbprint sign" (thickened epiglottis). Can confirm the diagnosis but is often unnecessary. Best for use in children in which epiglottitis is a possibility, but another diagnosis is more likely.

2. Direct visualization should be performed in a setting in which the airway could be secured immediately if necessary (e.g., in the intensive care unit or operating room, with anesthesia nearby for intubation).

D. Treatment

1. Surgical management: Airway maintenance is the first priority. If the patient develops respiratory arrest during examination in operating room, endotracheal intubation or tracheotomy may be needed to maintain the airway.

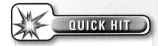

QUICK HIT

Fever, malaise, headache, and sore throat are present, but cough is classically absent in group A beta-hemolytic streptococcal (GABHS) pharyngitis.

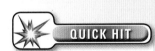

QUICK HIT

In a pediatric patient with suspected epiglottitis, examination of the pharynx should be performed only in a controlled setting, by an otolaryngologist with an anesthesiologist on hand.

Otolaryngology

2. Medical management
   a. Antibiotics: third-generation cephalosporin (ceftriaxone/cefotaxime) *and* an antistaphylococcal agent active against methicillin-resistant *Staphylococcus aureus* (MRSA) (clindamycin/vancomycin)
   b. Corticosteroids

IV. Laryngeal Trauma

A. Blunt injury
   1. Most common causes include motor vehicle accidents, all-terrain vehicle accidents, assaults, strangulation, and "clothesline" injuries.
   2. The larynx is an essential component of the airway, so trauma to this structure is life-threatening.
B. Penetrating injury
   1. Most common causes include stabbings and gunshot wounds.
   2. Mass and velocity determine damage to neck.
   3. Often associated with damage to surrounding structures in the neck
C. Intubation injury
   1. Both the act of intubation and the removal of an endotracheal tube with the cuff inflated can cause arytenoid dislocation.
   2. Prolonged intubation can cause glottic edema, ulceration, and pressure necrosis of the larynx/trachea. This can lead to granulation tissue with subsequent fibrosis and subglottic/tracheal stenosis in the healing process.
D. Clinical features
   1. Hoarseness, anterior neck pain, dysphagia, odynophagia, and dyspnea
   2. Hemoptysis, stridor, and crepitus over laryngeal cartilage
   3. Damage to surrounding structures (esophagus, vessels): hematemesis, subcutaneous emphysema, expanding hematoma, and bruit
E. Diagnosis
   1. Flexible laryngoscopy: Check for vocal cord movement and symmetry of the arytenoids. Can also evaluate for granulation tissue or stenosis, suggesting intubation trauma.
   2. Plain films of the neck may show air around the trachea or chest that may compromise the airway.
   3. CT scan: best radiographic tool to evaluate for laryngeal injury, especially when physical examination is normal
F. Treatment
   1. Airway, breathing, and circulation (ABC)
      a. Secure the airway.
      b. Immobilize the cervical spine.
      c. Stabilize the patient hemodynamically while controlling any bleeding.
      d. Auscultate the chest because low neck injuries may involve intrathoracic structures as well.
   2. Medical management: can be used on those patients with a stable airway
      a. Humidified air
      b. Elevate the head of the bed.
      c. Voice rest
      d. Antibiotics, if there are any defects in the laryngeal mucosa
      e. Serial laryngoscopic examinations
      f. Steroids
   3. Surgical management
      a. Blunt neck trauma
         (1) Lacerations of the laryngeal mucosa, vocal fold immobility, exposed cartilage, and comminuted laryngeal fractures necessitate surgical correction.
         (2) Early intervention has been shown to have favorable long-term outcome, compared to delayed treatment.
      b. Penetrating neck trauma: All unstable patients (those with massive hemorrhage, expanding hematoma, hemodynamic instability, hemothorax/hemomediastinum, or hypovolemic shock) require immediate exploration.

If stable, the need for surgical intervention depends on the zone of involvement.

(1) Zone I: sternal notch to cricoid cartilage

    (a) Surgical approach to structures made difficult by nearby bony structures

    (b) Obtain angiography and esophageal studies to assess for injuries and determine need for surgical intervention.

(2) Zone II: cricoid cartilage to angle of mandible

    (a) Most frequently involved region

    (b) Often explored without imaging, unless damage to another neck zone is suspected. A select group of patients may be managed with close observation if there are no signs of significant injury to the major vessels or aerodigestive tract.

(3) Zone III: angle of mandible to skull base

    (a) Also difficult to approach surgically due to bony protection

    (b) Angiography is usually performed to assess need for surgery.

    (c) Serial intraoral examination should be performed to assess for development of any parapharyngeal hematomas.

CONGENITAL CONDITIONS

I. Branchial Cleft Cysts

A. General principles

1. Caused by failure of branchial clefts to obliterate during the fetal period
2. Comprise approximately one-third of all congenital neck masses
3. Most are second branchial cleft cysts (found just inferior to the angle of the mandible and anterior to the border of sternocleidomastoid muscle).

B. Clinical features

1. Nontender, fluctuant mass
2. Can enlarge when they become inflamed and form an abscess
3. Typically diagnosed in children or young adults but may present at any age

C. Diagnosis

1. Ultrasound: helps differentiate between cystic and solid masses. Least invasive and does not expose patient to radiation.
2. CT: helps evaluate proximity and relationship to surrounding structures. Allows more complete evaluation of the mass and should be obtained preoperatively if surgical intervention is planned.
3. MRI: indicated for masses that may require further delineation of soft-tissue characteristics (e.g., infiltrative lesions, concern for perineural spread). High cost and need for extensive patient cooperation make this less than ideal for an initial study.

D. Treatment

1. Medical management: antibiotics to treat infection
2. Surgical management: Complete excision of the cyst is the only definitive treatment.

    a. Incision and drainage is avoided if possible (makes excision more difficult).

    b. Aspiration can be beneficial in preoperative decompression of the mass.

II. Infantile Hemangioma

A. General principles

1. Most common tumor of infancy, with a 4% to 10% prevalence at 1 year of age
2. Rapid postnatal growth (most rapid during the first 5 months, with some growth lasting up until 12 months), followed by slow regression (beginning around 12 months, with 50% completely involuted by age 5 years and 90% involuted by age 9 years)
3. Most commonly appear during first 6 weeks of life but are often not seen in the newborn nursery. A subset of congenital hemangiomas is present at birth and does not demonstrate rapid postnatal growth.

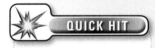

QUICK HIT

Branchial cleft cysts often present in late childhood or early adulthood, when the cysts become infected after a URI.

Otolaryngology

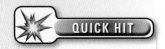

B. Clinical features
1. Superficial presentation most common
   a. Bright red nodule, papule, or plaque, which is well-circumscribed. Often referred to as "strawberry" or "capillary" hemangioma.
2. Deep/subcutaneous presentation less common
   a. Raised, skin-colored nodule with a bluish hue $+/-$ central telangiectatic patch. Often referred to as "cavernous" hemangioma.
3. Combined hemangiomas consist of both superficial and deep components.
4. Common complications include ulceration, bleeding, and infection.
5. May also create visual defects if they involve periorbital structures (most commonly the upper medial eyelid)
6. Subglottic hemangioma may lead to airway obstruction with hoarseness, stridor, and eventual respiratory failure.
7. Visceral hemangiomas: include hepatic hemangiomas, which can create large vessel shunts leading to hepatomegaly and heart failure (high-output type)

C. Diagnosis
1. Can typically be made on the basis of history and physical examination alone
2. Imaging techniques (ultrasound, CT, or MRI) may be helpful in assessing the extent of the lesion and infiltration into surrounding structures.

D. Treatment
1. Medical management
   a. Watchful waiting
   b. Propranolol may be used for lesions with the potential to impair function or cause disfigurement.
   c. Corticosteroids are useful in lesions associated with high-output heart failure. Oral steroids are preferred to intravenous. Intralesional may also be used, with a more rapid response typically noted in the first 2 weeks of treatment.
   d. Interferon or vincristine may be considered if a lesion is refractory to corticosteroid treatment.
2. Surgical management
   a. Involves removal of residual tissue after involution of lesion
   b. Performed via pulsed dye laser or open surgical resection if clinical symptoms such as visual defects, stridor, or congestive heart failure (CHF) are present

III. Thyroglossal Duct Cyst

A. General principles
1. Comprises approximately one-third of congenital neck masses
2. Usually found midline over the hyoid bone
3. Can be found anywhere between the foramen cecum and thyroid gland
4. Up to 65% contain thyroid tissue.

B. Clinical features
1. Usually asymptomatic
2. May cause mild dysphagia
3. Infection may occur, leading to enlargement of the cyst, localized pain, and significant dyspnea and/or dysphagia.

C. Diagnosis
1. History and physical examination
2. Ultrasound is useful to demonstrate the cystic nature of the lesion but provides little information regarding relationship to surrounding structures (e.g., hyoid bone).
3. CT scan can confirm the diagnosis and help evaluate size, extent, and location with regards to surrounding structures.
4. Radionucleotide uptake scan can identify the presence of ectopic thyroid tissue.
5. Fine-needle aspiration (FNA) is often performed to confirm the diagnosis and rule out alternative diagnoses.
6. Thyroid function tests should be evaluated preoperatively.

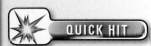

Otolaryngology

D. Treatment
  1. Medical management: Treat infection with antibiotics.
  2. Surgical management: Sistrunk operation (thyroglossal duct cyst excision)
     a. Small cuff of tissue (including center portion of hyoid bone) is excised.
     b. A small percentage of cysts contain thyroid carcinoma; therefore, they must all undergo histologic examination.

IV. Lymphatic Malformations

A. General principles
  1. Vascular malformation that results from sequestered lymphatic vessels that do not connect to the lymphatic system
  2. Can occur anywhere on the body, although head and neck regions are most commonly affected (80%)
  3. May be present at birth

B. Clinical features
  1. Often present as deep mass lesions with normal-appearing overlying skin
  2. Tend to grow in size slowly as the patient grows and rarely involute spontaneously
  3. May enlarge rapidly with hemorrhage into the lesion or due to inflammation in conjunction with a URI
  4. Microcystic
     a. Usually suprahyoid and often involve mucosal surfaces such as the oral cavity with associated vesicular lesions
     b. Tend to invade local tissues
     c. Usually present at birth
  5. Macrocystic
     a. Usually involve the infrahyoid portions of the neck
     b. Less likely to infiltrate into local tissues
     c. Lesions are typically soft and compressible.

C. Diagnosis
  1. History and physical examination
  2. MRI is the preferred imaging modality.
     a. Hyperintense on T2-weighted images, with low intensity on T1-weighted images
     b. Macrocystic lesions tend to show sharp demarcations of the cystic areas on imaging, whereas microcystic lesions are isodense and poorly defined.

D. Treatment
  1. Medical management
     a. Sclerotherapy with intralesional injection of ethanol, sodium tetradecyl sulfate, doxycycline, tetracycline, cyclophosphamide, bleomycin, or OK-432. This stimulates fibrosis and shrinking of the lesion.
     b. OK-432 is an inactivated strain of *Streptococcus pyogenes,* which is currently undergoing clinical trials in the United States with very encouraging results in macrocystic lesions.
  2. Surgical management
     a. Manage airway complications with tracheostomy if necessary.
     b. Surgical resection offers the best chance at complete cure if the complete resection is achieved, but this is often difficult to accomplish, and recurrence rates are high. However, surgery is often more effective than sclerotherapy in the treatment of microcystic lesions.
     c. Laser surgery is often an acceptable option in more superficial lesions.

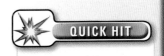

QUICK HIT

Recurrence of lymphatic malformations after surgery is very common, especially if all disease is not removed.

OTITIS

I. Otitis Externa

A. General principles
  1. Inflammatory/infectious process in the external auditory canal (EAC)
  2. Most common pathogens
     a. *Pseudomonas aeruginosa* (approximately 40%)
     b. *Staphylococcus aureus* (approximately 10%)

Otolaryngology

c. *Staphylococcus epidermidis* (approximately 10%)
d. Fungi
3. Risk factors (cause breakdown of the skin-cerumen barrier)
a. Heat
b. Humidity/moisture
c. Trauma to the skin of the EAC
d. Occlusion of the EAC (hearing aids, ear plugs)
e. Prior radiation therapy
4. Malignant otitis externa
a. Osteomyelitis involving the skull base, most frequently found in elderly and diabetic patients as a complication of otitis externa
b. *Pseudomonas* is the most common pathogen implicated.
B. Clinical features
1. Otalgia, otorrhea, pruritus, and tenderness to palpation/manipulation of the pinna
2. Possible hearing loss, depending on the amount of edema of the EAC
3. Adjacent lymphadenopathy and cellulitis of the EAC and/or pinna
C. Diagnosis: history and physical examination
D. Treatment
1. Medical management
a. Cleaning of the EAC with removal of purulent debris
b. Topical therapy
(1) Antibiotic drops: ofloxacin, ciprofloxacin, polymyxin B, neomycin, gentamicin, or tobramycin
(2) Steroids: help decrease edema and pain
c. Analgesics: nonsteroidal anti-inflammatory agents, opioids, steroids
2. Surgical management: Patients with malignant otitis externa often need to be taken to the operating room for debridement of the affected temporal bone.

II. Acute Otitis Media

A. General principles
1. Inflammation of the middle ear cavity, most commonly due to bacterial infection, which is usually preceded by viral URI
2. Generally due to dysfunction of the eustachian tube
3. Incidence peaks around 6 to 18 months of age, with a smaller peak around 5 to 6 years of age (upon entering school).
4. Most common bacteria
a. *Streptococcus pneumoniae* (40%)
b. *Haemophilus influenzae* (20% to 30%)
c. *Moraxella catarrhalis* (10% to 20%)
5. Risk factors are largely environmental and include:
a. Tobacco smoke exposure
b. Daycare exposure
c. Lack of breastfeeding
d. Seasonal variations of respiratory infections
B. Clinical features
1. Fever
2. Irritability in infants who pull at their ears
3. Earache in older children
4. Hearing loss (conductive)
C. Diagnosis
1. Pneumatic otoscopy is the accepted standard.
a. Thickened, dull, hyperemic tympanic membrane with decreased mobility
2. Laboratory results: leukocytosis, bacteremia
3. Ear discharge can be cultured in cases in which first-line treatment fails.

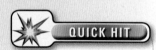

QUICK HIT

In an elderly patient with diabetes, granulation tissue in the EAC is indicative of malignant otitis externa, which is osteomyelitis of the temporal bone.

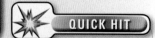

QUICK HIT

A patient with otitis media diagnosed 2 days ago who suddenly experiences the abrupt relief of otalgia most likely has perforated his or her tympanic membrane.

Otolaryngology

D. Treatment
  1. Medical management
     a. Antibiotics
        (1) Current guidelines recommend that all children age 6 months and younger should be treated with antibiotics if otitis media is suspected. In children older than 6 months, antibiotic treatment should be initiated for those patients in which the diagnosis is certain or the symptoms are severe (moderate to severe otalgia or fever ≥39°C). If the diagnosis is uncertain and symptoms are not severe, observation with close follow-up is preferred.
        (2) Amoxicillin is first-line therapy, but resistance is developing. There may be a need to add clavulanic acid to antibiotic therapy (Augmentin).
        (3) For patients with penicillin allergy, acceptable alternatives include second- or third-generation cephalosporins (cefdinir, cefuroxime) or macrolides (azithromycin, clarithromycin).
     b. Analgesics and antipyretics
  2. Surgical management: Myringotomy with ventilation tubes is usually reserved for cases refractory to medical therapy (recurrent or chronic otitis media) or where a complication has occurred.

 FRACTURES

I. Temporal Bone Fractures
  A. General principles
     1. Twenty percent of all skull fractures
     2. Males 21 years of age and under are at high risk for temporal bone fractures due to more frequent involvement in at-risk activities.
     3. Most common cause is motor vehicle accidents (30%), followed by assaults, falls, and motorcycle collisions.
     4. Blunt trauma to the lateral skull often results in a temporal bone fracture.
     5. Two common types of temporal bone fractures are longitudinal (70% to 90%) and transverse (10% to 30%), although many fractures may be a combination of these or oblique, and the more important factor is whether or not the fracture involves the otic capsule.
  B. Clinical features
     1. Battle sign: postauricular ecchymosis, resulting from bleeding from the postauricular artery or mastoid emissary vein
     2. Raccoon eyes: periorbital ecchymosis, often associated with a temporal bone fracture
     3. Other findings may include cerebrospinal fluid (CSF) leak, otorrhea, hemotympanum, facial nerve paralysis, and conductive hearing loss on the side of the fracture.
  C. Diagnosis
     1. CT scan of head and facial bones
     2. Tuning fork test: Weber test results in sound localizing to the side of the fracture.
     3. Audiometry: can be performed a few weeks after the injury if ear symptoms persist
  D. Treatment
     1. Medical management
        a. Can observe fracture if nondisplaced or asymptomatic
        b. Onset of facial nerve paralysis can be delayed up to 2 weeks after the injury and will most commonly resolve spontaneously.
        c. A course of systemic corticosteroids may be used to treat patients with delayed-onset facial paralysis, although there is no definitive evidence that this will affect the patient's outcome.

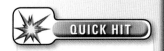

Blunt trauma to the lateral head that presents with unilateral hearing loss and unilateral facial nerve palsy should make one think of a temporal bone fracture.

Otolaryngology

2. Surgical management
  a. CSF leak that is persistent after a week should be surgically repaired.
  b. Tympanic perforation that persists should be surgically repaired with a tympanoplasty.
  c. Immediate-onset, complete facial nerve paralysis with inability to stimulate the nerve within the first week postinjury may require facial nerve decompression.

II. Midface Fractures

A. Le Fort I fractures
  1. General principles
    a. Transverse fractures of the maxilla above the maxillary tooth roots, which separate the palate from the midface
    b. Involves the pterygoid plates
  2. Clinical features
    a. Patients may present with malocclusion.
    b. Patients also may have an open bite deformity.
    c. In the most severe cases, patients can be found to have airway compromise.
  3. Diagnosis
    a. Clinical findings (stable midface but mobile palate on physical examination)
    b. CT scan of the facial bones
  4. Treatment
    a. The patient needs to be surgically managed by first being placed into class I occlusion. This is accomplished by aligning the mesiobuccal cusp of the maxillary first molar with the buccal groove of the first mandibular molar, followed by maxillomandibular fixation.
    b. The fracture should then be reduced and plated with titanium miniplates.
    c. If the patient has a relatively nondisplaced fracture, it can be managed solely with maxillomandibular fixation for 4 to 6 weeks.

B. Le Fort II fractures
  1. General principles
    a. Pyramidal fracture lines extending usually bilaterally from the nasal root through the medial orbit to the orbital floor and through the anterolateral maxillary wall anteriorly, as well as through the lower pterygoid plate posteriorly.
  2. Clinical features
    a. Mobility of the palate and upper midface, including the nasal unit. Often associated with other fractures and morbidities.
    b. CSF leak may be present due to fracture of the cribriform plate of the ethmoid bone.
  3. Diagnosis
    a. Physical examination findings
    b. CT scan of the facial bones
  4. Treatment
    a. Usually requires surgical intervention
    b. Patients should be placed into class I occlusion via maxillomandibular fixation, followed by plating of the fracture sites with titanium miniplates.

C. Le Fort III fractures
  1. General principles
    a. Usually occur with high-energy trauma
    b. Result in complete midface mobility (craniofacial dissociation) and are rare
    c. Involve the pterygoid plates, the frontonasal maxillary buttress, and the frontozygomatic buttress
  2. Clinical features
    a. Severe midface mobility
    b. CSF leak often present
  3. Diagnosis
    a. Physical examination findings
    b. CT scan of facial bones

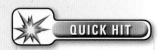

QUICK HIT

Patients with facial trauma who present with a mobile palate but with a stable midface should be evaluated for Le Fort I fractures.

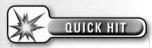

QUICK HIT

A patient who presents with a recent high-velocity trauma and has midface mobility on physical examination should be imaged and evaluated for Le Fort fractures.

Otolaryngology

4. Treatment
   a. Tracheotomy should be performed before fracture repair to secure a definitive airway.
   b. Patients should be placed into maxillomandibular fixation and often require multiple surgical approaches to stabilize the facial bones.

III. Mandible Fractures

A. General principles
   1. Occur in multiple types of traumas
   2. Patients often present several days after the injury due to the fact that they were under the influence of alcohol or illicit drugs at the time of injury.
   3. Fractures are classified based on location as favorable when natural muscle forces tend to pull the fragments together or unfavorable when natural muscle forces tend to displace the fracture sites (see Clinical Pearl 18-3).

B. Clinical features
   1. Pain with opening the mouth or chewing
   2. Malocclusion
   3. Numbness in the V3 distribution of the trigeminal nerve
   4. Fractures of the body, symphysis, and angle are often mobile on physical examination.
   5. Condylar fractures are often difficult to detect on physical examination.

C. Diagnosis
   1. Plain X-ray of the face or CT scan of the facial bones
   2. Panorex series can often be beneficial because they can differentiate a condylar fracture from an angle fracture.

D. Treatment
   1. Patients with nondisplaced fractures often need minimal intervention and may sometimes be managed with a soft diet alone for several weeks.
   2. Patients with displaced fractures often need to be placed into maxillomandibular fixation. This approach requires the patient to have immobilization of the jaw for 4 to 6 weeks.
   3. Open reduction and fixation using titanium miniplates is often performed, and some surgeons will allow the patient to resume mastication almost immediately after surgery.
   4. The type of repair system often depends on the surgeon, and in some instances, both approaches are used to achieve fixation of the fracture.
   5. Patients typically require prophylactic antibiotics postoperatively due to the contaminated nature of the fracture site.

IV. Sinus Fractures

A. General principles
   1. Motor vehicle accidents are the most common cause of sinus fractures.
   2. Patients are often under the influence of alcohol.

B. Clinical features
   1. Patients with sinus fractures often sustain loss of consciousness as the result of the trauma.
   2. Patients with sinus fractures can present with facial numbness, crepitus, and step-offs on palpation.

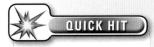

QUICK HIT

A patient with a history of trauma who presents with pain with mastication and numbness in the distribution of V3 should be evaluated for a mandible fracture.

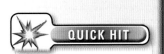

QUICK HIT

Patients with a history of trauma who present with bony step-offs on physical examination should be evaluated thoroughly for sinus fractures.

Otolaryngology

CLINICAL PEARL 18-3

Unfavorable Mandible Fractures

Horizontally unfavorable	Almost all fractures of the angle; superior and medial displacement of the proximal segment occurs due to the action of the masseter, medial pterygoid, and temporalis muscles
Vertically unfavorable	Fractures of the angle in which the proximal segment is displaced medial by the pterygoid muscles; also, fractures of the body that are distracted by the action of the mylohyoid and suprahyoid muscle group

C. Diagnosis
1. CT scans of the head and facial bones are the gold standard for making the diagnosis of facial fractures.
2. The CT scan of the facial bones should include axial, sagittal, and coronal series, with thin cuts to allow for accurate visualization of fracture sites.
3. Imaging should be correlated with physical examination findings to make the diagnosis.

D. Treatment
1. Patients with displaced sinus fractures may require surgical intervention to restore the normal contour of the face.
2. Fractures involving both the anterior and posterior tables of the frontal sinus may require surgical intervention to prevent development of intracranial complications.

NEOPLASMS

I. **Acoustic Neuroma**
A. General principles
1. Also referred to as vestibular schwannoma
2. Nerve sheath tumor of the eighth cranial nerve
3. Originate in the medial internal auditory canal or lateral cerebellopontine angle
4. These tumors are benign in nature and slow-growing, but they may interfere with the anatomy in this region via compressive mass effect and cause symptoms.

B. Clinical features
1. These patients often present with hearing loss, which can be progressive and is unilateral in most cases.
2. A large subset of patients with these tumors also present with tinnitus and disequilibrium.
3. Patients may also present with facial numbness and numbness in the distribution of the sensory component of the facial nerve. They may also experience effects on the motor component of the facial nerve.

C. Diagnosis
1. MRI with gadolinium contrast along with clinical correlation of symptoms is considered the gold standard in securing this diagnosis.
2. CT scan with contrast can be used in situations where MRI is not readily accessible. It is not as sensitive in diagnosing these tumors.
3. A standard auditory evaluation using pure-tone audiometry, speech discrimination score, and acoustic reflex should be used to evaluate patients who present with unilateral hearing loss, unilateral tinnitus, or disequilibrium.

D. Treatment
1. Treatment options include surgical resection, radiation therapy, or observation.
2. Due to the benign, slow-growing nature of these tumors, many patients can be managed conservatively with observation and at least yearly follow-up imaging and audiometry, particularly in the instance of a small tumor in an elderly or otherwise poor surgical candidate.
3. If the growth rate is more than 2.5 mm per year or patient experiences significant worsening of symptoms, intervention via either surgery or radiation therapy should be considered.
4. Radiation therapy approaches include conventional fractionated radiation therapy, stereotactic radiotherapy, stereotactic radiosurgery, and proton beam therapy.
5. Radiation therapy is sometimes elected in patients with relatively well-preserved hearing with the goal of preventing permanent hearing loss and/or facial nerve dysfunction.

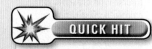

QUICK HIT

An adult patient presenting with asymmetric hearing sensorineural hearing loss should make one suspicious of a possible acoustic neuroma.

Otolaryngology

II. Glomus Tumor

A. General principles

1. Also referred to as paragangliomas
2. The most common of these is a carotid body tumor (60%). There are also two glomus tumors in the temporal bone: the glomus tympanicum, which arises in the middle ear, and glomus jugulare, which arises in the jugular foramen.
3. Females are affected more commonly than males (6:1).

B. Clinical features

1. Patients with a paraganglioma in the temporal bone may present with pulsatile tinnitus and hearing loss.
2. Physical examination of the tympanic membrane often reveals a reddish-blue mass behind the tympanic membrane, due to the highly vascular nature of the tumor. This will often blanch with positive pressure applied via pneumatic otoscopy (Brown sign).
3. Some paragangliomas secrete catecholamines and may be associated with sympathetic symptoms such as tachycardia, palpitations, flushing, diarrhea, headaches, or poorly controlled hypertension.
4. Extensive glomus tumors, particularly those that arise in the jugular foramen, may be associated with multiple ipsilateral cranial nerve palsies.

C. Diagnosis

1. High-resolution CT of the skull base is typically the initial study used to evaluate these tumors.
2. MRI of the skull base may be useful to further delineate a tumor's association with surrounding soft-tissue structures.
3. Magnetic resonance angiography can also be useful to evaluate for intraluminal involvement of the carotid artery or occlusion of the jugular vein and/or sigmoid sinus.

D. Treatment

1. Complete surgical removal of these tumors using a microsurgical technique is recommended.
2. Alternatives to surgical intervention—particularly for recurrent or residual tumors—include external beam radiation therapy or stereotactic radiosurgery in order to halt tumor growth and stabilize neurologic symptoms.

III. Juvenile Nasopharyngeal Angiofibroma

A. General principles

1. Occur primarily in young males
2. Highly vascular tumors, which arise near the junction of the posterior nasal cavity and lateral nasopharynx

B. Clinical features

1. Nasal obstruction
2. Recurrent epistaxis
3. Nasal drainage, serous otitis media, and resultant conductive hearing loss may also be present.

C. Diagnosis

1. Endoscopic examination of the nasal cavities and nasopharynx
2. CT scan with contrast is the preferred initial imaging modality, in order to evaluate the surrounding bony structure as well as the vascularity of the tumor.
3. MRI is useful in complement with the CT scan to delineate any intraorbital or intracranial extension of the mass.

D. Treatment

1. Surgical resection
2. Radiation and chemotherapy may be considered for the treatment of poor surgical candidates, recurrent disease, or significant intracranial extension that cannot be treated surgically.

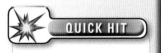

QUICK HIT

A young male with nasal obstruction and severe, recurrent epistaxis should make one think of juvenile nasopharyngeal angiofibroma.

Otolaryngology

IV. Recurrent Respiratory Papillomatosis

A. General principles
   1. Most common benign laryngeal tumor in children, usually diagnosed between 2 and 3 years of age
   2. Caused most commonly by human papillomavirus (HPV) strains 6 and 11
B. Clinical features
   1. Hoarseness
   2. Abnormal cry
   3. Advanced disease may be associated with dyspnea, stridor, and respiratory distress.
C. Diagnosis: microlaryngoscopy with biopsy of the lesion to establish a definitive diagnosis
D. Treatment
   1. Microlaryngeal surgery with debulking of the lesions via CO_2 laser is the most common treatment modality.
   2. Patients often require multiple procedures up to the age of puberty, when the disease tends to regress.
   3. Tracheotomy should be avoided if possible due to the possibility of extralaryngeal spread of the disease.

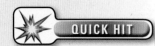

> **QUICK HIT**
>
> A young child with stridor and dyspnea, who otherwise does not appear to be clinically ill, should make one think of recurrent respiratory papillomatosis.

SQUAMOUS CELL CARCINOMA

I. Squamous Cell Carcinoma of the Oral Cavity

A. General principles
   1. The oral cavity contains the lips, anterior two-thirds of the tongue, buccal mucosa, hard palate, floor of the mouth, alveolar ridges, and retromolar trigone.
   2. More predominant in males
   3. Tobacco and alcohol use are synergistic in the development of squamous cell carcinoma (SCC).
   4. Betel nut quid use is carcinogenic and is considered a risk factor for oral cavity cancer in India and Southeast Asia.
B. Clinical features
   1. Patients typically present with nonhealing ulcers or lesions in the oral cavity.
   2. Patients may also present with unilateral otalgia, trismus, bleeding, or dysphagia.
   3. Leukoplakia and erythroplakia are considered premalignant lesions and should be monitored closely for malignant transformation.
C. Diagnosis
   1. It is important to perform a thorough head and neck examination in any patient with a suspicious lesion of the mouth.
   2. CT and/or MRI of the head and neck are appropriate to establish the extent of the lesion as well as to evaluate for lymph node metastasis.
   3. Biopsy of the lesion is also needed to establish a histologic diagnosis.
   4. Panendoscopy including direct laryngoscopy, esophagoscopy, and bronchoscopy is generally performed to evaluate the extent of the lesion and to search for any synchronous lesions.
D. Treatment
   1. Primary resection of the tumor using a surgical technique is typically the first choice.
   2. Radiation therapy can be used postoperatively or in patients with tumors that are difficult to manage surgically.

II. Squamous Cell Carcinoma of the Oropharynx

A. General principles
   1. The oropharynx consists of the posterior third of the tongue, tonsillar fossa, soft palate, and the posterior pharyngeal wall.
   2. The chances of occurrence increase with the consumption of alcohol and tobacco.

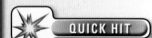

> **QUICK HIT**
>
> A male patient who presents with a long history of tobacco use and has a nonhealing oral ulcer should be considered at high risk for an oral cavity SCC.

Otolaryngology

B. Clinical features
1. Signs of symptoms include sore throat, dysphagia, odynophagia, and bleeding.
2. These tumors are often silent and difficult to detect in the early stages of the disease.
3. Patients can also present with unilateral otalgia, which is referred pain from the oropharynx.

C. Diagnosis
1. It is important to perform a thorough head and neck examination on any patient with a suspicious lesion of the mouth.
2. Panendoscopy including direct laryngoscopy, esophagoscopy, and bronchoscopy is generally performed to evaluate the extent of the lesion and to search for any synchronous lesions.
3. Biopsy of the lesion is also needed to establish a histologic diagnosis.
4. CT and/or MRI of the head and neck should be done to evaluate the extent of tumor involvement and lymph node disease.
5. Positron emission tomography (PET) scans may be ordered as part of the workup for patients with advanced disease to evaluate for metastatic disease.

D. Treatment
1. Chemotherapy combined with radiation therapy is typically the treatment of choice for SCC of the oropharynx
2. Surgical resection is generally reserved for patients who fail chemoradiation.

III. Squamous Cell Carcinoma of the Nasopharynx

A. General principles
1. More common in Chinese Americans
2. Associated with Epstein–Barr virus, sawdust inhalation, and smoke inhalation
3. Smoking increases the risk of disease.

B. Clinical features
1. Cervical adenopathy or neck mass
2. Unilateral otitis media with effusion with associated hearing loss
3. Nasal obstruction
4. Epistaxis

C. Diagnosis
1. Nasopharyngoscopy
2. Biopsy of the lesion with endoscopic guidance
3. CT and/or MRI to evaluate for involvement of tumor

D. Treatment
1. Patients with nasopharyngeal carcinoma usually undergo radiation therapy.
2. This is the treatment of choice because it is difficult to obtain surgical margins in the nasopharynx.

IV. Squamous Cell Carcinoma of the Larynx

A. General principles
1. The vast majority of patients with laryngeal cancer have an extensive history of alcohol and tobacco use.
2. Gastroesophageal reflux disease is controversial risk factor.
3. HPV infection is a risk factor for all head and neck SCC, including the larynx.
4. Laryngeal cancers are divided into supraglottic, glottic, and subglottic.

B. Clinical features
1. Signs and symptoms include dysphonia, sore throat, dysphagia, ear pain, dyspnea, stridor, and hemoptysis.
2. Physical examination should include a complete head and neck exam, including a thorough neck examination, to evaluate for any lymph node disease.
3. Flexible laryngoscopy is typically performed in clinic to evaluate the extent of laryngeal involvement, vocal cord mobility, and airway patency.

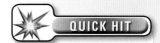

QUICK HIT

A patient who presents to the clinic with unilateral ear pain and unilateral tonsillar hypertrophy should make one think of oropharyngeal carcinoma.

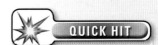

QUICK HIT

An adult patient who presents with unilateral serous otitis media and nasal obstruction should make one suspicious of a nasopharyngeal carcinoma.

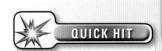

QUICK HIT

A patient with a long history of smoking and alcohol consumption who presents to clinic with a neck mass, hoarseness, and weight loss should make one think of laryngeal SCC.

Otolaryngology

C. Diagnosis
1. CT and/or MRI of the head and neck should be done to evaluate the extent of tumor involvement and lymph node disease.
2. Panendoscopy including direct laryngoscopy is typically performed in the operating room to evaluate the extent of tumor involvement for surgical planning. Biopsies are also performed at this time for histologic diagnosis.
3. PET scans are typically ordered as part of the workup for patients with advanced laryngeal cancer to evaluate for metastatic disease.
D. Treatment
1. Medical management: Radiation and chemotherapy are alternatives to surgery.
2. Surgical management
   a. Tracheotomy may need to be performed prior to definite surgical treatment for large lesions causing airway obstruction.
   b. Microlaryngoscopy with endoscopic excision can be done for some small T1 lesions.
   c. Partial laryngectomy
      (1) Involves removing the affected portions of the larynx while leaving enough of the unaffected larynx to maintain adequate speech and swallowing
      (2) Options include hemilaryngectomy, supraglottic laryngectomy, supracricoid laryngectomy, and near-total laryngectomy.
      (3) Patient typically must have good preoperative lung function.
   d. Total laryngectomy
      (1) Involves removing the entire larynx including the hyoid bone and cricoid cartilage
      (2) It is usually reserved for patients with extensive disease.
      (3) Patients have a permanent tracheal stoma after this procedure.

19

Cardiothoracic Surgery

Mary Carolyn C. Vinson and Kevin J. Tveter

Cardiothoracic surgery is a broad field that includes acquired and congenital disease. It also comprises treatment for some of the leading causes of death: coronary artery disease (CAD) and lung cancer. This chapter discusses diagnostic testing, cardiac disease, pulmonary disease, and mediastinal and chest wall diseases.

 ## DIAGNOSTIC TESTS

I. **Imaging Studies**
   A. Computed tomography (CT) shows anatomic localization and spread of disease process and can evaluate lymphadenopathy, cavitations, and additional pathology.
   B. Positron emission tomography (PET) uses 2-[18F]-fluoro-2-deoxy-D-glucose (FDG-18), detects areas of increased metabolic activity, and is combined with CT to increase detection of malignancy and determine the extent of spread of cancers.
      1. Sensitivity for the detection of lung cancer is approximately 95%.
      2. Some benign processes, including several types of infectious lesions, can simulate cancer with this test; biopsy is required to confirm the diagnosis.
   C. Echocardiography (ECHO) is an ultrasound examination of the heart and major vessels. It may be performed through a transthoracic or transesophageal approach. ECHO allows more accurate evaluation of valve morphology.
      1. Measures left ventricular ejection fraction (LVEF) accesses
      2. LVEF is most commonly used measure of overall cardiac function.
      3. Ejection fraction is simply the proportion of blood that is expelled from the ventricle with each heartbeat.
      4. Example: If the left ventricle (LV) ejects 60% of its blood volume with each beat, the LVEF is 0.6. (A normal LVEF is 0.5 or greater.)
   D. Multiple gated acquisition (MUGA) scan: useful noninvasive tool for assessing the function of the heart, uses red blood cells tagged with technetium 99; useful in patient selection for high-risk cardiac surgery and for following cardiac function in patients receiving chemotherapeutic agents that are cardiotoxic
      1. Advantages of MUGA scan over other techniques (e.g., ECHO)
      2. Measuring the LVEF, highly accurate and highly reproducible
   E. Electrocardiogram (EKG) may reveal rhythm disturbance, chamber enlargement, or evidence of recent and old infarcts.
   F. Chest X-ray (CXR) is readily available and may be useful in detecting a primary tumor and demonstrating its size and location.
      1. Not sensitive in detecting lymph node involvement
      2. May show a pleural effusion, destruction of ribs or vertebrae, and elevation of hemi-diaphragm (phrenic nerve injury/involvement)

II. Other Studies

A. Pulmonary function testing (PFT) and arterial blood gases (ABGs) are helpful in determining a patient's ability to tolerate cardiac procedures and suitability for pulmonary resections.

B. Bronchoscopy is the diagnostic or therapeutic evaluation for the airway from trachea to segmental bronchi. It may also be used to clear secretions, remove foreign objects, drain infections, and/or as biopsy or culture.

C. Mediastinoscopy is the introduction of a lighted instrument through a small incision above the suprasternal notch and behind the sternum to evaluate mediastinal structures.

1. Common procedure used for the diagnosis of thoracic disease and the staging of lung cancer and to obtain tissue for pathologic diagnosis of mediastinal lymphadenopathy

2. Of lymph nodes greater than 1 cm

3. Can only evaluate anterior mediastinum

4. Is the gold standard for mediastinal staging with an 89% sensitivity and 100% specificity for nonsmall cell lung cancer

5. Complications include hemorrhage, pneumothorax, and nerve injury (recurrent laryngeal).

D. Endobronchial ultrasound (EBUS)-guided fine-needle aspiration biopsy of mediastinal nodes

1. Less invasive alternative for histologic sampling of the mediastinal nodes

2. Requires a specialized bronchoscope

3. Widely adopted and may replace mediastinoscopy in the future

E. Cardiac catheterization (CATH) allows invasive angiography to visualize cardiac anatomy. Percutaneous transluminal coronary angioplasty (PTCA) allows angioplasty and stenting of some coronary obstructive lesions.

1. CATH is useful to determine the transvalvular gradient and to evaluate LVEF from the left ventriculogram.

2. Right-sided heart catheterization is also used to calculate the aortic valve area (AVA) based on the Gorlin equation, as described earlier. CATH also may provide information about the presence or absence of other valve lesions.

CARDIAC DISEASE

I. Valve Disease

1. General principles: Cardiac function is largely dependent on proper valve function. The aortic and mitral valves are anatomically related to the conduction system.

2. Diagnosis is based on detailed history and physical and supplemented by CXR, EKG, ECHO, and CATH.

3. Physical examination findings in cardiac valve disease are presented in Table 19-1.

TABLE 19-1 Physical Examination Findings in Cardiac Valve Disease

Valve Pathology	Physical Finding
Aortic stenosis	Decreased pulse pressure Midsystolic murmur heard best at the base and radiating to the carotid arteries
Aortic insufficiency	Increased pulse pressure Diastolic murmur loudest at the left sternal border
Mitral regurgitation	Holosystolic murmur, widely split S_2 Hyperdynamic circulation
Mitral stenosis	Decreased opening snap and S_2 Pulmonary congestion may lead to rales
Tricuspid regurgitation	Pansystolic murmur and venous congestion

A. Aortic stenosis (AS)
1. Epidemiology: Calcified bicuspid aortic valve represents the most common form of congenital AS.
   a. Bicuspid aortic valves are present in approximately 2% of the general population.
   b. Gradual calcification of the bicuspid aortic valve results in significant stenosis most often in the fifth and sixth decades of life, earlier in unicommissural than in bicuspid valves and earlier in men than in women.
   c. Age-related degenerative calcific AS is currently the most common cause of AS in adults and the most frequent reason for aortic valve replacement (AVR).
   d. Most common cause of AS is degenerative calcification of the aortic valve.
      (1) Previously considered to be the result of years of mechanical stress on an otherwise normal valve
      (2) Evolving concept: Degenerative process leads to proliferative and inflammatory changes, with lipid accumulation, upregulation of angiotensin-converting enzyme (ACE) activity, and infiltration of macrophages and T lymphocytes.
   e. Rheumatic AS represents the least common form of AS in the adult population.
   f. Rheumatic AS, rarely an isolated disease, usually occurs with mitral valve stenosis.
2. Early stage of rheumatic AS is characterized by edema, lymphocytic infiltration, and revascularization of the leaflets, whereas the later stages are characterized by thickening, commissural fusion, and scarred leaflet edges.
3. Clinical features: angina pectoris, syncope, and ultimately heart failure
4. Physiologic compensation
   a. Adaptations include increased left ventricular mass, decrease in ventricular compliance, increase in end-diastolic pressure, and pulmonary congestion. Diastolic dysfunction may lead to congestive heart failure (CHF) in 15% to 40% of cases.
   b. Early relief of obstruction may reverse ventricular adaptations.
5. Diagnosis
   a. Signs/symptoms
      (1) Systolic ejection crescendo-decrescendo murmur that radiates to the neck and is often accompanied by a thrill
      (2) Regurgitant systolic murmur represents rupture of the mitral chordae tendineae.
      (3) Classic pulsus parvus, or small pulse, is a sign of severe AS or decompensated AS; occurs when stroke volume and systolic and pulse pressures fall.
      (4) Wide pulse pressure: Severity is measured with noninvasive testing.
   b. CATH is generally performed prior to surgical valve replacement.
      (1) CAD may be present in up to 25% of patients with AS who do not have angina.
      (2) CATH performed in most patients to assess coronary anatomy and evaluate need for combined AVR and myocardial revascularization
   c. Exercise testing is contraindicated in symptomatic patients.
6. Treatment
   a. No medical therapy is proven.
   b. Diuretics and digitalis may improve the symptoms of CHF.
   c. ACE inhibitors are relatively contraindicated in patients with AS.
   d. Afterload reduction therapy is contraindicated in patients with AS because it can reduce coronary perfusion pressure.
7. Indications for surgical AVR
   a. Replacement of the valve should be considered in patients who have symptoms secondary to the AS.
   b. Symptomatic patients with uncorrected AS have a 25% 1-year mortality and a 50% 2-year mortality.
   c. Balloon aortic valvotomy for acquired AS is useful only for palliation for symptomatic patients who are not operative candidates: Complications are as high as 10%.

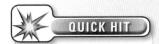

QUICK HIT

Acute aortic insufficiency can develop due to trauma, aortic dissection, or endocarditis. In this setting, there is no time for the LV to adapt, leading to rapid decrease in cardiac output and eventual cardiovascular collapse.

Cardiothoracic Surgery

    d. Percutaneous AVR represents a new, less invasive approach to the treatment of AS: This has been applied successfully in high-risk patients with severe symptomatic AS who are not candidates for conventional surgery.

    e. AVR in asymptomatic patients is currently controversial: Asymptomatic patients, with mild or moderate AS, should be followed with serial echocardiographic evaluation.

B. Aortic insufficiency/regurgitation: poor leaflet co-optation

  1. Etiology

    a. Diastolic reflux of blood from the aorta into the LV owing to failure of co-aptation of the valve leaflets during diastole

    b. Insufficiency results from an intrinsic leaflet abnormality or distortion of the aortic root.

    c. Causes include:

      (1) Infective endocarditis, rheumatic fever, annuloaortic ectasia, Marfan syndrome, aortic dissection, collagen vascular disease, syphilis, and calcific disease. Calcific aortic disease and myxomatous proliferation of aortic valve tissue all prevent the valve cusps from closing properly.

      (2) More recently, anorectic medications, such as fenfluramine and phentermine, have been found to cause aortic valve distortion from accelerated degeneration of valve leaflets.

    d. Most commonly, aortic valvular insufficiency is seen in combination with AS, often seen in aortic disease, rheumatic valvular disease, or myxomatous degenerative disease.

  2. Clinical features

    a. Signs/symptoms: widened pulse pressure from augmentation of total CO, leading to distention of the peripheral arterial system followed by a quick collapse from regurgitant flow

    b. Leads to many classic physical findings

      (1) "Water-hammer" pulse (Corrigan pulse)

      (2) Head bobbing with each heartbeat (de Musset sign)

      (3) Capillary pulsations at the lips and fingers (Quincke pulses)

    c. Other findings are associated with CHF if present (e.g., rales, S_3).

    d. Death may be due to pulmonary edema, ventricular arrhythmia, electromechanical dissociation, and circulatory collapse.

  3. Physiologic compensation

    a. Effect of aortic insufficiency is to decrease the effective stroke volume (SV)

    b. Leads to increased ventricular mass (left ventricular hypertrophy)

    c. May remain asymptomatic and well compensated until late in course

    d. Increases myocardial oxygen consumption

    e. Compensated chronic aortic insufficiency may be well tolerated.

  4. Diagnosis

    a. Signs and symptoms are all that are needed to make diagnosis.

    b. If diagnosis is unclear or need to quantify the severity of disease, diagnostic tests can help, including an EKG, ECHO, CATH, and MRI.

    c. ECHO is the most useful diagnostic modality in both the initial diagnosis and continued monitoring of patients with aortic regurgitation (AR).

    d. Exercise tolerance testing ensures patients are not unconsciously self-limiting activity in response to symptoms and will unmask left ventricular dysfunction.

  5. Treatment

    a. AVR is currently *not* recommended for patients who are asymptomatic, even with severe chronic AR.

    b. Asymptomatic or minimally symptomatic patients should be followed yearly for deterioration of ejection fraction (EF).

    c. Goal is valve replacement before irreversible damage to the LV occurs.

d. Operative criteria may include ventricular decompensation, increased LVEF diameter greater than 55 mm, EF less than 55% at rest, and increased left ventricular end-diastolic volume.

C. Mitral stenosis (MS)

1. Epidemiology and etiology
   a. Isolated MS is almost exclusively the result of rheumatic heart disease, affecting women more than men. It is now rare.
   b. Etiologic agent for acute rheumatic fever is group A beta-hemolytic streptococcus RF only occurs in about 3% of untreated group A strep. Table 19-2 describes the Jones Criteria for the diagnosis of rheumatic heart disease.
   c. Nonrheumatic causes: mitral annular and/or leaflet calcification, congenital mitral valve deformities, malignant carcinoid syndrome, neoplasm, left atrium (LA)thrombus, endocarditic vegetations, previous commissurotomy, or an implanted prosthetic

2. Clinical features
   a. MS is a continuous and progressive lesion.
   b. There is a long latency before onset of symptoms.
   c. Association of pregnancy and clinical onset of symptoms of MS is common.
   d. Once symptoms begin, the 10-year life expectancy is 0% to 15%.
   e. Atrial fibrillation occurs in 30% to 40% of patients with MS.

3. Signs/symptoms: eventually develop and are associated primarily with pulmonary venous congestion or low cardiac output (e.g., dyspnea on exertion, orthopnea, or paroxysmal nocturnal dyspnea and fatigue)
   a. Dyspnea often is precipitated by events that elevate LA pressure, such as physical or emotional stress or atrial fibrillation.
   b. Systemic thromboembolism, occurring in approximately 20% of patients, may be the first symptom of MS.
   c. Patients may be thin and frail (cardiac cachexia), indicative of long-standing low CO, CHF, and inanition.
   d. Peripheral arterial pulse generally is normal.
   e. Heart size usually normal, normal apical impulse on chest palpation
   f. Auscultatory findings include a presystolic murmur, a loud S_1, an opening snap, and an apical diastolic rumble.

4. Diagnosis
   a. EKG is not accurate and in many cases may be completely normal.
   b. ECHO is the chief diagnostic tool for assessing severity of MS.

5. Treatment
   a. For the asymptomatic patient in sinus rhythm with mild MS, treatment is directed.
   b. For mild symptoms or evidence of pulmonary hypertension, mechanical relief such as balloon valvotomy is indicated.
   c. Balloon valvotomy may be performed if no cuspal or annular calcification, subvalvular chordal fusion and distortion, atrial fibrillation, or clot exists.

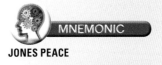

MNEMONIC

JONES PEACE

TABLE 19-2 JONES Criteria for Diagnosis of Rheumatic Heart Disease	
Major Criteria	**Minor Criteria**
J: Joints (polyarthritis, hot swollen joints)	P: Previous rheumatic fever
O: Heart (carditis, valve damage)	E: EKG with PR prolongation
E: Erythema nodosum (painless rash)	A: Arthralgias
S: Sydenham chorea (flinching movement disorder)	C: CRP and ESR elevated
	E: Elevated temperature

CRP, C-reactive protein; EKG, electrocardiogram; ESR, erythrocyte sedimentation rate.

d. Other options are open commissurotomy, mitral valve reconstruction, or replacement.

e. In those patients with established atrial fibrillation, surgical interventions may be combined with Cox maze (ablative) procedure to ensure postoperative sinus rhythm.

D. Mitral regurgitation/mitral valve prolapse

1. Etiology
   a. This valvular disease is the most common valvular heart disease, affecting 2% to 6% of the population.
   b. Both acquired (*fibroelastic deficiency* in older patients) and congenital or heritable, with excess spongy, weak fibroelastic connective tissue constituting the leaflets and chordae tendineae
      (1) Dysfunctional or uncoordinated interaction valvular ventricular complex (VVC)
      (2) VVC: mitral annulus and leaflets, chordae tendineae, papillary muscles, LA, and LV
   c. Common causes
      (1) Myxomatous degeneration of the mitral valve, also known as floppy mitral valve or mitral valve prolapse
      (2) Other causes: collagen vascular disease, infective endocarditis, rheumatic fever, ischemic disease, or nonischemic cardiomyopathy
      (3) Although incidence is decreasing in United States, rheumatic fever remains a common cause of mitral regurgitation around the world.
         (a) Barlow syndrome
            i. Large amounts of excessive leaflet tissue and marked annular dilatation are coupled with extensive hooding and billowing of both leaflets.
            ii. Most common cause of mitral regurgitation in patients undergoing surgical evaluation in the United States.
      (4) Mitral regurgitation with normal leaflet motion can result from annular dilatation, often secondary to LV dilatation (e.g., patients with dilated cardiomyopathy or ischemic cardiomyopathy).
   d. Mitral valve prolapse appears to be more widespread in women.

2. Clinical features
   a. Subtle signs of heart failure, usually manifest as declining stamina and fatigue: may be the presenting complaint in 25% to 40% of symptomatic patients with mitral valve prolapse (MVP)
   b. The syndrome of MVP includes palpitations, chest pain, syncope, and dyspnea.
   c. In younger patients, the initial clinical sign is a midsystolic click, which later evolves into a click followed by a late systolic murmur.
   d. Only 5% to 10% of patients progress to severe mitral regurgitation, and the majority remain relatively asymptomatic.

3. Physiologic compensation
   a. Mitral regurgitation allows unloading of the LV into the LA during systole.
   b. The LV compensates by increasing ejection volume (increased EF).
   c. Eventually, the LV is not able to compensate, leading to eccentric cardiac hypertrophy and CHF.
   d. Because chronic mitral regurgitation is associated with LA enlargement and only mild elevations in LA pressure, increases in pulmonary vascular resistance usually do not develop.
   e. Intervention should be before left ventricular decompensation occurs.

4. Diagnosis
   a. EKG: are not particularly useful; atrial fibrillation is a late finding.
   b. ECHO: allows assessment of mitral regurgitation as well as left ventricular function
   c. CATH before surgery to evaluate for concomitant CAD

5. Treatment
   a. Asymptomatic MVP patients should be evaluated every 3 to 5 years clinically and by ECHO.
   b. Yearly ECHO is indicated for patients with mild mitral regurgitation and no symptoms or cardiac enlargement.
   c. EF should not fall below the normal range before referral for intervention.
   d. Successful mitral valve repair or replacement usually is associated with clinical improvement, augmented forward stroke volume with lower total stroke volume, smaller LV end-diastolic volume, and regression of LV hypertrophy.
   e. Mitral valve repair results in better late outcome, lower operative mortality, better preservation of LV function, and less need for anticoagulation.
   f. During mitral valve replacement, attempt should be made to preserve chordal structures and connections to avoid reduction in mitral regurgitation function.
   g. Surgical repair is indicated only for significant mitral regurgitation, changes in LV dimensions, or for flail leaflet due to chordal rupture.

E. Tricuspid regurgitation
   1. Etiology
      a. The most common cause of tricuspid regurgitation is secondary to mitral valve disease.
      b. Tricuspid regurgitation is usually due to right ventricular dilation, with secondary distortion of the tricuspid valve.
      c. Severe tricuspid regurgitation has poor prognosis, due to underlying right ventricular dysfunction.
      d. Eisenmenger syndrome and primary pulmonary hypertension lead to the same pathophysiology of progressive right ventricular dilatation, tricuspid annular enlargement, and valvular incompetence.
   2. Diagnosis
      a. Signs/symptoms
         (1) Fatigue and weakness related to a reduction in cardiac output.
         (2) Right-sided heart failure leads to ascites, congestive hepatosplenomegaly, pulsatile liver, pleural effusions, and peripheral edema.
         (3) In the late stages, patients are wasted with cachexia, cyanosis, and jaundice.
         (4) Atrial fibrillation is common.
         (5) Auscultatory findings: S_3 increases with inspiration and decreases with Valsalva maneuver; parasternal pansystolic murmur increasing with inspiration
      b. CXR: cardiomegaly, increased right atrial and ventricular size, a prominent azygous vein, possible pleural effusion, and upward diaphragmatic displacement owing to ascites
      c. ECHO best test for degree of regurgitation, structural abnormalities of the valve, pulmonary artery pressures (PAPs), and right ventricular function

II. Endocarditis

A. Epidemiology
   1. Predisposing factors for infective endocarditis are cardiac abnormalities that disrupt the endocardium and presence of bloodborne microorganisms that colonize these abnormal surfaces.
   2. It is associated with rheumatic heart disease (24%), congenital abnormality (23%), hypertrophic cardiomyopathy, and MVP.
   3. Congenitally bicuspid aortic valve is the most common predisposing lesion for endocarditis of the aortic valve.
   4. It affects left-side valves more than the right side.
   5. Mortality occurs in 10% to 15% of patients.
B. Endocarditis may be precipitated by any cause of transient bacteremia; dental procedures can produce transient bacteremia; streptococcal infections are often associated.

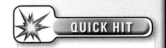

QUICK HIT

There is a very high rate of thromboembolic complication with mechanical prostheses in the tricuspid position despite adequate anticoagulation.

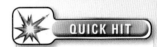

QUICK HIT

The now-discontinued anorectic (diet) drugs fenfluramine and phentermine are associated with left- and right-sided valve regurgitation, secondary to valve fibrosis. Prevalence is related to the duration of therapy. Patients who had this treatment should undergo annual cardiovascular physical and ECHO examination.

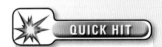

QUICK HIT

Endocarditis associated with intravenous drug use is often right-sided, and *Staphylococcus aureus* is often the responsible organism.

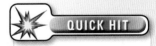

QUICK HIT

Postoperative endocarditis is associated with *Staphylococcus epidermidis* infection.

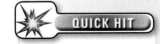

QUICK HIT

Perivalvular abscess is associated with *S. aureus* infection and may occur in 20% of cases of endocarditis.

Cardiothoracic Surgery

C. Causes of endocarditis are *S. aureus* and alpha-hemolytic streptococcal infections (*Streptococcus viridans*); *S. aureus* is associated with higher morbidity and more virulent course.

D. Endocarditis due to gram-negative bacteria is uncommon, but it is often resistant to antibiotic therapy and may cause serious complications; *Haemophilus*, *Actinobacillus*, *Cardiobacterium*, *Eikenella*, and *Kingella* (the HACEK group) are grouped together due to their characteristic fastidiousness.

E. Fungal endocarditis is rare but extremely serious; *Candida albicans* and *Aspergillus fumigatus* are most common cause.

F. Infection of a diseased valve tends to have a subacute, indolent course, whereas infection of a normal valve can present with a fulminant course.

G. Culture-negative endocarditis may occur with prior antibiotic treatment, fungal infections, and noninfective endocarditis as seen in systemic lupus erythematosus, otherwise called Libman–Sacks endocarditis.

1. Depending on virulence of microorganism, normal aortic valves can also be affected; intravenous drug users are particularly susceptible to infective endocarditis, which often occurs in structurally normal heart valves.

2. Patients with prosthetic heart valves have a constant risk of developing infective endocarditis.

3. Prosthetic valve endocarditis occurs in 1% to 2% of prosthetic valves.
   a. Accounts for 15% to 30% of endocarditis
   b. Early prosthetic valve endocarditis is caused by contamination of the valve at the time of implantation by perioperative bacteremia.
   c. Most common: *Staphylococcus epidermidis*, *S. aureus*, and *Enterococcus faecalis*

4. The incidence of nosocomial endocarditis is increasing because more patients undergo invasive procedures. Most often caused by *Staphylococcus aureus* or other staphylococci.

5. Infective endocarditis in hemodialysis patients is rare and is associated with high mortality.

H. Clinical features

1. Classified into acute and subacute
   a. Acute endocarditis caused by virulent microorganism (e.g., *S. aureus*): Clinical course is acute, often fulminating, and antibiotics alone seldom cure the infection.
   b. Subacute endocarditis is caused by less virulent microorganisms (e.g., *Streptococcus viridans*).
      (1) Clinical course is subtle, low-grade fever and malaise, and antibiotics alone cure most cases.
      (2) Splenomegaly is common.

I. Signs and symptoms of endocarditis are presented in Table 19-3.

J. Diagnosis

1. Diagnostic studies include ECHO and serial blood cultures.

2. Transesophageal ECHO is better than transthoracic ECHO at detecting vegetations as small as 1 or 2 mm in size. It is more reliable in native than in prosthetic valve endocarditis.

3. The Duke criteria are used to establish diagnosis of infective endocarditis.

TABLE 19-3 Signs Associated with Endocarditis

Sign	Manifestation
Roth spots	Retinal spots
Osler nodes	Raised, painful nodes on soles and palms
Janeway lesions	Flat, painless lesions on soles and palms
Splinter hemorrhages	Hemorrhages on fingernails

K. Treatment
1. Appropriate antibiotic is the most important aspect of the management of patients with infective endocarditis. Surveillance blood cultures are performed in 48 hours to monitor the efficacy of antibiotic therapy.
2. Anticoagulation is not effective in preventing embolization of vegetations and is associated with an increased risk of neurologic complications.
L. Early surgical treatment should be considered in patients with:
1. Signs of CHF, acute valve dysfunction, paravalvular abscess or cardiac fistulas, recurrent systemic embolization
2. When aortic valve vegetations are present
3. Persistent sepsis despite adequate antibiotic therapy for more than 4 to 5 days
4. Prosthetic valve endocarditis, particularly in patients with mechanical valves
5. Acute endocarditis of the aortic valve due to *S. aureus*
6. Reinfection after surgery is 1% to 13%.
M. Complications
1. Postoperative complications are common after surgery for active infective endocarditis.
2. Septic patients may have severe coagulopathy and may bleed excessively after cardiopulmonary bypass.
3. Fungal vegetations may produce stenosis due to their bulk.

III. Types of Valves
A. Mechanical valves
1. Mechanical valves have good long-term durability, but there is a risk of thromboembolism and bleeding secondary to anticoagulation.
2. The most common valve-related morbidity is secondary to anticoagulation (1% to 3% of patients per year).
B. Bioprosthetic or tissue valves
1. Types of tissue valves include porcine and pericardial valves, allograft for aortic or mitral valves, and autograft of pulmonic valve into the aortic position (also called the Ross procedure).
2. All tissue valves have low risk of thromboembolism and do not require anticoagulation after 3 months.
3. These degenerate over time; they have about a 40% failure at 10 years.

IV. Cardiac Indications for Anticoagulation
A. Mechanical prosthesis
B. Intracardiac thrombus
C. Atrial fibrillation with or without previous embolism or cardiomyopathy
D. Anticoagulation is not indicated for infective endocarditis, aortic valve disease, or mitral valve prolapse or disease.

V. Acquired Heart Disease
A. Coronary anatomy
1. The left and right coronary arteries are the first branches of the aorta originating just above the aortic valve, most commonly in the sinuses of Valsalva.
2. The left coronary divides into the left anterior descending (LAD) artery and the left circumflex artery. The branches of the LAD artery are the septals and diagonal coronary arteries.
3. The branches of the circumflex are the obtuse marginal arteries.
4. The right coronary artery arises more anteriorly, and after supplying the sinus node, it divides on the inferior surface of the heart into the posterior descending and posterolateral arteries.
5. The posterior descending artery (PDA) may arise from the left circumflex coronary artery in about 10% of people, in which case it is called a left dominant system. This is important because the PDA supplies the atrioventricular node and its occlusion can result in heart block.

QUICK HIT

Valve selection is dependent both on size and patient factors. Bioprosthetic valves are indicated for patients over 65 years, those patients in whom anticoagulation is contraindicated or unwilling to take warfarin, and those with a life expectancy less than 10 years. Mechanical valves are for younger patients who tolerate lifelong anticoagulation.

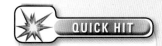

QUICK HIT

The majority of coronary blood flow occurs during diastole.

VI. Ischemic Heart Disease

A. Etiology and epidemiology

1. Atherosclerotic plaques are composed of smooth muscle, collagen, lipids, elastin, and other matrix components.
2. Disruption in the plaque surface results in thrombogenic ulcerations.
3. Risk factors include age, genetic predisposition, male gender, hypertension, diabetes, hyperlipidemia, and smoking.
4. This disease is more likely to be underdiagnosed or undertreated in women, and therefore results more often in death and disability.

B. Pathophysiology

1. Atherosclerotic disease directly compromises coronary blood flow, resulting in an imbalance of blood supply and myocardial demand.
2. Atherosclerotic disease results in decreased ventricular compliance, decreased myocardial contractility, and potential myocardial necrosis and scarring.

C. Clinical features

1. Continuum of three interrelated ischemic clinical syndromes: angina pectoris, myocardial infarction (MI), and ischemic cardiomyopathy
2. May be asymptomatic
3. Ischemic cardiomyopathy is an atypical presentation, resulting from loss of ventricular function due to myocardial scarring. This is also seen in patients with multiple MIs resulting in heart failure due to loss of ventricular muscle.

D. Signs and symptoms

1. Angina pectoris typically presents as substernal chest pain lasting 5 to 10 minutes.
2. Angina may be described as stable, unstable (new-onset or increasing frequency), or occurring at rest.

E. Diagnosis

1. History is vital.
2. EKG may be normal. Abnormal findings include ST-segment changes and T-wave changes.
3. Exercise stress testing and radionucleotide scans assist in evaluation and in delineating areas of ischemia and infarction.

F. Treatment

1. Medical management
   a. Prevention and risk factor reduction is the mainstay of treatment.
   b. Among the pharmacologic agents used to treat are beta-blockers, aspirin, ACE inhibitors, and statins.
   c. Nitrates are prescribed for symptom management.
2. Cardiac angiography (catheterization)
   a. CATH is an invasive evaluation of coronary vascular anatomy.
   b. Diagnostic and therapeutic: angiography assessment, as well as potential intervention with angioplasty and stent placement, to alleviate myocardial injury
   c. Intervention is indicated for patients with intractable symptoms and proximal lesions that put a large amount of myocardium at risk.
   d. Percutaneous intervention is usually not indicated for lesions in the left main coronary artery, if target vessel is less than 2 mm, and if multiple obstructions are present within the same vessel.
3. The advent of newer high-resolution CT angiograms may alter the invasive study of CAD.

G. Surgical management: coronary artery bypass graft (CABG).

1. Indications for CABG include: Surgical treatment may be indicated in left main disease, triple-vessel disease, double-vessel disease including the LAD artery, unstable angina, post-MI angina, symptoms uncontrolled with medical therapy and lifestyle, coronary artery rupture, dissection or thrombosis with PTCA, and CAD in patients with diabetes.

II. Procedure

1. The diseased artery is bypassed, thereby reestablishing blood flow beyond the area of stenosis.

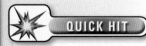

QUICK HIT

Cardiac disease must be included in the diagnosis of any presenting complaint from the jaw to umbilicus. Patients with diabetes are at greater risk for silent MI. Women more often have atypical symptoms.

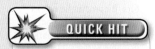

QUICK HIT

All patients with known CAD should take aspirin and lipid-lowering agents in the absence of contraindication.

2. The internal mammary artery is used most commonly. Radial arteries or greater saphenous veins are also used when additional grafts are needed. Nearly all (95%) of internal mammary arteries and 50% to 60% of vein grafts are patent at 10 years.
3. Cardiopulmonary bypass and cardioplegia are used to stop the heart and achieve a quiet, bloodless field. The surgery can also be performed on a beating heart, otherwise called the off-pump bypass grafting.

VII. Complications

A. Postoperative complications include MI, arrhythmias, tamponade, infection, hemorrhage, graft thrombosis, sternal dehiscence, stroke, and postpericardiotomy syndrome.
B. Operative mortality is greatly dependent on ventricular function.
C. The mortality rate for CABG is 1% to 3%.
D. Reoperative CABG has a higher mortality rate (5% to 8%).
E. The 5-year survival rate is 90%, and 10-year survival rate is 80%.

VIII. Extracorporeal Circulation

A. Extracorporeal circulation is artificial pumping and oxygenation, allowing removal of blood from the superior and inferior vena cava and returning it to the aorta, allowing cardiac arrest during procedures.
B. It provides constant pulsatile or nonpulsatile flow.
C. It requires anticoagulation with heparin and is reversed with protamine.
D. Heparin rebound is the phenomenon of increased anticoagulation after bypass as heparin returns to circulation from peripheral tissues.
E. Atrial fibrillation may occur in one-third of patients after bypass.
F. Complications of extracorporeal circulation are presented in Table 19-4.

IX. Cardiac Tumors

A. Epidemiology
   1. The most common cardiac tumors are secondary tumors from lung (men) or breast (women).
   2. Primary tumors are rare, and 80% are benign.
B. Pathology: Types of cardiac tumors include:
   1. Myxoma
      a. Most common tumor of the heart, more common in women, usually in adulthood
      b. Majority (75%) are found in the LA.
      c. May present with thromboembolic events and/or constitutional symptoms
   2. Rhabdomyoma: usually found in children and mortality is 80% at 1 year (often multiple)
C. Clinical features: embolic, unexplained murmur, CHF, or dysrhythmia
D. Diagnosis: Tumors are usually diagnosed when ECHO is performed for other indications.
E. Treatment: excision; if resection is not possible, then relief of obstruction may give good long-term results

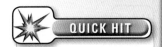

QUICK HIT

Dressler syndrome is pericarditis after MI. Postpericardiotomy syndrome is pericarditis after cardiac surgery. Both are treated with NSAIDs and sometimes steroids.

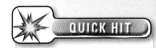

QUICK HIT

Closure of the pericardium after open-heart surgery facilitates reentry into the sternum but increases risk of tamponade.

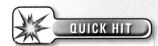

QUICK HIT

The most common tumor in all groups is metastasis from a remote organ.

TABLE 19-4 **Complications of Extracorporeal Circulation**
Trauma to blood elements resulting in hemolysis and platelet destruction
Pancreatitis due to low flow
Heparin rebound
Stroke
Failure to wean from bypass
Systemic inflammatory response syndrome (SIRS)

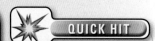

Diaphragmatic paralysis can be a complication of pericardial disease.

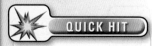

Beck acute cardiac compression triad: (1) falling arterial pressure, (2) rising venous pressure, and (3) a small, quiet heart.

X. Pericardium

A. Anatomy
   1. The serous and fibrous pericardium together composes the parietal pericardium.
   2. The visceral pericardium (epicardium) covers the heart and great vessels.
   3. Phrenic nerves lie in the parietal pericardium.
   4. Superiorly, it merges with the adventitia of the great vessels.
   5. Inferiorly, it attaches to the central tendon of the diaphragm.
   6. Normally contains 15 to 50 mL of straw-colored serous fluid

B. Physiology
   1. Structural functions include mechanical protection and anchoring, prevention of acute cardiac distention, and serving as an infection barrier.
   2. Chemical functions include absorption. Mechanoreceptors govern blood pressure and heart rate, and the pericardial fluid has fibrinolytic properties.

C. Acute pericarditis
   1. Produces a typical serofibrinous exudate on the pericardium that may or may not produce an effusion
   2. Typical presentation for acute pericarditis is pleuritic chest pain relieved by leaning forward.
   3. A pericardial friction rub is common on examination.
   4. EKG findings include diffuse ST elevations in all leads except V1 and aVF along with diffuse PR depressions.
   5. Infectious pericarditis
      a. Viral pericarditis: caused by coxsackievirus B (most common), echovirus, adenovirus, influenza virus, mumps, varicella, Epstein-Barr virus, or hepatitis B virus. Treatment is supportive with nonsteroidal anti-inflammatory drugs (NSAIDs) +/− colchicine.
      b. Bacterial pericarditis: most commonly due to streptococcal, pneumococcal, or staphylococcal organisms. Treated with antibiotics and supportive care.
      c. Tuberculosis (TB) pericarditis: results in an exudative pericardial inflammation in the setting of an active TB infection. Management is mainly medical with triple-drug therapy.
      d. Fungal pericarditis: treated medically with antifungals and NSAIDs

D. Neoplastic pericarditis
   1. Rarely due to primary tumors, commonly from metastatic disease or contiguous spread
   2. Most common tumors include breast, lung, and lymphoma.
   3. Neoplastic effusions are drained for palliation only with repeated drainage and/or sclerosing agents such as doxycycline.

E. Dressler syndrome
   1. Can occur about 2 weeks following an acute MI when a diffuse pericarditis ensues
   2. Indicates a worse prognosis for an acute MI
   3. Does not generally cause effusions that require drainage and is treated supportively with NSAIDs with/without colchicine

F. Metabolic causes
   1. Uremic pericarditis usually resolves within 2 weeks of aggressive dialysis.
   2. May result in bloody effusions and lead to tamponade
   3. Drainage is reserved for large, symptomatic, or refractory effusions.

G. Other causes
   1. Rheumatoid arthritis and TB exposure may also result in acute pericarditis, but they are generally more commonly associated with constrictive pericarditis.

XI. Constrictive Pericarditis

A. The heart is contained by a thickened, fibrotic pericardium.
B. The pericardial space may be obliterated or effusion-filled.
C. Can develop as a late sequela of acute pericarditis
D. Most common etiology in Western countries is idiopathic, followed by prior cardiac surgery and mediastinal irritation.

E. Most common cause in developing world is TB.

F. Clinical features
1. Low cardiac output (fatigue, hypotension, tachycardia) and/or elevated venous pressures (hepatomegaly, edema, ascites, shortness of breath on exertion)
2. Kussmaul sign is an increase in jugular venous distention with inspiration.
3. Pericardial knock is a loud third heart sound produced by rapid diastolic ventricular filling.
4. Some patients (25%) have atrial fibrillation or flutter.
5. A pericardial calcification is pathognomonic.

G. Treatment
1. Surgical stripping via median sternotomy or left anterolateral thoracotomy
2. Pericardium is resected anteriorly from phrenic nerve to phrenic nerve and down to the diaphragmatic reflection.

XII. Cardiac Tamponade

A. Etiology
1. Cardiac tamponade is a hemodynamically significant cardiac compression due to accumulating pericardial contents.
2. Acute accumulation of 100 to 200 mL may produce tamponade.
    a. Causes: trauma, open heart surgery, uremia, complex pericarditis
3. Chronic effusion may allow accumulation of liters before tamponade occurs.
4. Tamponade usually occurs when pericardial pressures rise to 20 to 30 mm Hg.

B. Clinical features
1. Diagnosis in a postoperative patient: drop in cardiac index, elevated filling pressures, hypotension, narrowed pulse pressure, and oliguria
2. Classic findings of Beck triad: distended neck veins, muffled heart sounds, hypotension
3. Clinical findings include dyspnea and tachycardia.
4. Pulsus paradoxus is usually present with a fall in systolic blood pressure of 10 mm Hg during inspiration.

C. Diagnosis is confirmed through the use of ECHO; cardiac manometry may reveal equalization of ventricular pressures.

D. Treatment
1. Needle pericardiocentesis or surgical drainage (pericardial window); the approach to the pericardium can be subxiphoid, thoracotomy, or sternotomy.

XIII. Pericardiocentesis

A. A long, large-gauge needle with a sheath is inserted just to the left of the xiphoid process and aiming at a 45-degree angle for the left shoulder. The needle is slowly advanced until fluid is aspirated.

B. ECHO or fluoroscopy is mandatory for guidance in the absence of an emergency.

C. Pericardiocentesis is useful for diagnosis of the etiology of effusion or treatment of tamponade.

D. Pericardial biopsy and surgical drainage; open surgical drainage may be necessary for bloody, purulent, or recurrent effusions.

XIV. Pericardectomy

A. Usually for constrictive pericarditis, chronic malignant effusion, and/or unresponsive effusions

B. Care must be taken to preserve both phrenic nerves.

XV. Pediatric Cardiac Disease

A. General principles
1. Congenital heart disease occurs in 3 in 1,000 live births.
2. Etiology is usually unknown. However, rubella infection in the first trimester is associated with congenital heart disease, and Down syndrome is associated with endocardial cushion defects.
3. Most common congenital heart defects are listed in Table 19-5.

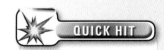

QUICK HIT

Children with congenital heart disease may present with poor feeding, fatigability, poor exercise tolerance, and frequent pulmonary infections.

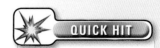

QUICK HIT

Cyanotic heart disease is caused by the five Ts: tetralogy of Fallot, truncus arteriosus, total anomalous pulmonary venous return, tricuspid atresia, and transposition of the great vessels.

TABLE **19-5** Congenital Heart Defects by Type	
Cyanotic: R-to-L Shunt (The Five Ts)	**Cyanotic: L-to-R Shunt (The Ds)**
Tetralogy of Fallot	Ventral septal defect
Transposition of great vessels	Atrial septal defect
Tricuspid atresia	Patent ductus arterious
Truncus arteriosus (persistent)	Congenital aortic stenosis
Total anomalous pulmonary arteries	

XVI. Acyanotic Defects: Left-to-Right Shunts (The Ds)

A. Atrial septal defect (ASD)
   1. Patent foramen ovale
      (1) Results from failure of fusion of the septum secundum and septum primum
      (2) Present in 27% of the population at autopsy and does not cause significant shunting. It may allow for paradoxical embolization.
      a. Secundum ASD
      (1) Prior to birth, a patent ostium secundum allows shunting of blood from the inferior vena cava to the LA. The increase in left atrial pressure at birth closes this pathway.
      b. Normal cardiac septation occurs between the third and sixth weeks of development.
      c. ASD is third most common congenital heart defect, occurring in 1 of 1,000 live births, and it accounts for 10% of congenital defects.
      d. More common in premature infants
B. Signs and symptoms
   1. Adult population: Eisenmenger syndrome
   2. Neonatal population
      a. CHF
      b. Pulmonary overcirculation
      c. Systemic hypoperfusion
         (1) Fixed splitting of S2 and a systolic ejection murmur at the left sternal border
         (2) CXR cardiomegaly
         (3) EKG right axis deviation with incomplete right-bundle-branch block
         (4) ECHO confirms diagnosis and defines anatomy.
C. Treatment
   1. Intervention is recommended for all patients with symptomatic ASDs and all asymptomatic patients with significant ASDs due to long-term complications.
   2. Repair usually occurs prior to school age.
   3. Transcatheter repair is possible for small to moderate secundum ASDs and for patent foramen ovale.
   4. Surgical repair may be primary closure of the defect or with Dacron, Gore-Tex, or pericardial patch.

XVII. Ventricular Septal Defect (VSD)

A. General
   1. VSDs are the most common congenital heart anomaly, with 4 per 1,000 live births.
   2. VSDs represent 40% of congenital anomalies.
   3. Some VSDs (30%) close spontaneously.
   4. VSDs are classified based on location into perimembranous (80%) versus inlet, outlet, and trabecular.

TABLE 19-6 Signs and Symptoms of Ventricular Septal Defect		
Tachypnea	**Hepatomegaly**	**Poor Feeding**
Failure to thrive	Holosystolic murmur (louder with small defects)	Increased vascular markings on chest X-ray
Electrocardiographic right ventricular hypertrophy	Echocardiography confirms diagnosis	Cardiac catheterization used in older children and adults in who elevated pulmonary vascular resistance is suspected

B. Physiologic compensation
   1. Increases pulmonary blood flow due to left-to-right shunting during systole, increasing volume load on the left heart. The right side of the heart is pressure loaded.
   2. After birth, the shunt volume is low because pulmonary vascular resistance is high. As pulmonary vascular resistance falls, the volume will increase.
   3. Patients may be asymptomatic at birth but become symptomatic at several weeks of age.
   4. Most VSDs are restrictive and tend to close spontaneously by 1 year.
   5. Large VSDs are not restrictive, and CHF symptoms develop by 2 months.
   6. Pulmonary vascular disease usually develops by 2 years of life.
   7. There is a small risk of endocarditis.
C. Clinical features: Table 19-6 presents the signs and symptoms of VSDs.
D. Treatment
   1. Severe, symptomatic VSDs should be repaired early.
   2. If symptoms may be moderated with medical therapy, then surgical intervention can be delayed until school age to allow for possible spontaneous closure.
   3. Repair with patch: Care is taken not to interrupt the conduction system.

XVIII. Congenital Aortic Stenosis
   1. Left ventricular outflow obstruction
   2. AS represents 4% of congenital heart disease.
   3. Twenty percent occur in conjunction with other cardiac defects, most commonly coarctation of the aorta, but also with patent ductus arteriosus, VSD, and MS.
   4. The male:female ratio is 4:1.
   5. At birth, critical AS is an emergency managed with intubation, inotropic support, and prostaglandins to maintain patent ductus arteriosus patency.
   6. Physiologic compensation: Severe AS is well compensated during development by increasing right ventricular output via a patent ductus.
A. Treatment
   1. Urgent intervention may be required.
   2. Treatment includes percutaneous balloon valvuloplasty, surgical valvotomy, or AVR.

XIX. Patent Ductus Arteriosus
A. In utero, prostaglandins E1 and E2, and hypoxia keep the ductus open.
B. In normal-term infants, the pulmonary circulation causes increased oxygen levels with breakdown prostaglandins, resulting in duct closure in the first days of life.
C. Failure of closure may be asymptomatic, although a small number develop heart failure and pulmonary vascular disease.
D. Clinical features and diagnosis
   1. Patients may present with signs and symptoms of CHF.
   2. Continuous machinery murmur is detected.
   3. Widened pulse pressure and bounding peripheral pulses are observed.

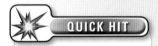

QUICK HIT

Eisenmenger syndrome is irreversible pulmonary hypertension and cyanosis that develops when the ventricular shunt becomes right to left. The only treatment is a heart–lung transplant.

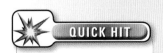

QUICK HIT

Prostaglandins act to maintain patency of the ductus. Indomethacin inhibits prostaglandins to promote closure of the ductus.

E. Treatment
   1. Indomethacin is a prostaglandin inhibitor used to close the duct in preterm infants with simple symptomatic patent ductus.
   2. Coil closure in the catheterization laboratory using a percutaneous approach
F. Surgical treatment is ligation of the ductus, and it is indicated if patency persists after 2 to 3 years or if it causes symptoms of heart failure earlier.

XX. Cyanotic Heart Defects in Right-to-Left Shunts (The Five Ts)
A. Tetralogy of Fallot
   1. Tetralogy of Fallot is the most common congenital, cyanotic heart condition.
      a. Mnemonic "PROVe"
      b. Pulmonary stenosis
      c. Right ventricular hypertrophy
      d. Overriding aorta
      e. VSD
B. Resistance to right ventricular outflow exceeds systemic resistance, resulting in a right-to-left shunt with cyanosis and desaturation.
C. Clinical features
   1. Cyanosis in 30% of children at birth and in 30% at 1 year
   2. Presenting signs include cyanosis and dyspnea on exertion.
   3. Squatting temporarily alleviates symptoms (Tet spells): increasing systemic vascular resistance and increasing pulmonary flow
   4. Cerebrovascular accidents and brain sepsis may be life-threatening events.
   5. Cardiac failure is rare.
D. Diagnosis
   1. Evaluation reveals cyanosis, clubbing, polycythemia, and systolic murmur.
   2. A boot-shaped heart is revealed on CXR, due to right ventricular enlargement.
   3. CATH can determine the level of obstruction and anatomy of pulmonary and coronary arteries.
E. Treatment
   1. Correction timing is controversial: early primary repair versus Blalock shunting and complete repair later
   2. Most agree on complete repair by age 2 years.
   3. Treatment is palliative, and systemic to pulmonary shunt may be performed prior to correction.
   4. Risk depends on age and degree of cyanosis.
   5. Dramatic improvement occurs after correction.

XXI. Transposition of the Great Arteries
A. Two separate and parallel circuits result from the aorta arising from the right ventricle and the pulmonary artery arising from the LV.
B. An anomalous communication is required for survival, such as an ASD, patent ductus arteriosus, or VSD.
C. Diagnosis is based on ABG, CXR, and ECHO. An enlarged, egg-shaped heart is seen on CXR.
D. Treatment involves septostomy to improve mixing followed by definitive correction.

XXII. Obstructive Congenital Anomalies
A. Coarctation of the aorta
   1. Severe narrowing of the aorta usually adjacent to the ductus arteriosus
   2. Occurs in males twice as often as in females
B. A majority (60%) are associated with intracardiac defects.
C. Clinical features
   1. May be asymptomatic for a variable length of time
   2. Presenting symptoms and signs: CHF, headaches, dizziness, and lower-extremity weakness
D. Diagnosis
   1. Upper extremity hypertension with absent or diminished lower extremity pulses and asystolic murmur are found.
   2. CXR in older individuals may show rib notching due to indentation by collateral circulation via intercostal arteries.

3. ECHO and CATH further define anatomy and evaluate for associated cardiac defects.

E. Treatment

1. Surgical correction is indicated, although it may be delayed in asymptomatic patients.
2. Correction may involve resection with end-to-end anastomosis, placement of a prosthetic graft, or use of subclavian artery used to enlarge the area of coarctation.
3. Hypertension may persist postoperatively.
4. Spinal cord ischemia and mesenteric ischemia are rare postoperative complications.

XXIII. Pulmonary Disease

A. Spontaneous pneumothorax

1. General principles
   a. This occurs with rupture of a subpleural bleb, allowing lung collapse.
   b. Incidence: usually occurs in young adults 18 to 24 years old
   c. Clinical features: Presenting symptoms include chest pain and shortness of breath.
2. Diagnosis: Physical examination and CXR are the basis of diagnosis
3. Treatment
   a. Initial treatment is chest tube drainage.
   b. Surgical videothoracoscopy with chemical and/or mechanical pleurodesis is indicated for recurrent or persistent pneumothorax. Any bullae present are resected at the same time.
   c. Tension pneumothorax is a clinical diagnosis based on tracheal deviation and absence of breath sounds, and it is a life-threatening emergency.

XXIV. Disorders of the Pleura and Pleural Space

A. Empyema/abscess: Pus in the pleural space usually is secondary to pulmonary infection.

B. Forms in three stages

1. Acute phase: approximately 7 days, serous pleural fluid collection
2. Transitional phase: from day 7 to 21, characterized by fibropurulent fluid collecting in dependent areas
3. Chronic phase: after 21 days, organization of fluid collection with abscess formation

C. Treatment

1. Early-course treatment may involve aspiration, antibiotics, and sometimes fibrinolytic therapy.
2. Late-course treatment requires continuous drainage or surgical debridement and decortication.

XXV. Mesothelioma

A. Mesothelioma is a pleural tumor usually related to asbestos exposure.

B. Malignant mesothelioma usually presents with malignant pleural effusion.

C. The condition is usually fatal.

D. Surgery has a limited role and is usually palliative.

XXVI. Lung Lesion: Solitary Pulmonary Nodule

A. Pulmonary nodule is a neoformation of unknown origin that appears at CXR as a well-defined opacity of 1 to 3 cm in diameter, surrounded by normal pulmonary parenchyma and not associated to atelectasis or adenopathy.

B. General principles

1. A small minority (5% to 10%) are malignant.
2. Risk factors for malignancy include size greater than 1 cm, indistinct margins, documented growth, and increasing age.
3. Half of lesions are malignant in smokers older than 50 years of age.

C. Diagnosis

1. If found incidentally, old films are reviewed. If the lesion is stable over 2 years, no further evaluation is needed.

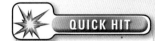

QUICK HIT

Ebstein anomaly is a congenital anomaly associated with lithium during pregnancy. The tricuspid valve is placed low in the right ventricle, decreasing the size of the ventricle. The result is tricuspid regurgitation and decreased right-sided output.

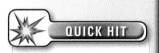

QUICK HIT

The right mainstem bronchus is more often intubated when an endotracheal tube is advanced too far due to the less oblique angle of the left main bronchus.

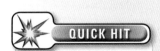

QUICK HIT

If a patient is younger than 40 years of age, then two-thirds of nodules are benign.

TABLE 19-7 Key Features of Pulmonary Cancer

Squamous Cell	Adenocarcinoma	Small (Oat) Cell	Large Cell
Usually centrally located	Usually peripheral	Centrally located	Usually peripheral
Slow growing, late metastasis	Rapid growth with hematogenous and nodal metastasis	Highly malignant	Highly malignant
Associated with smoking	Associated with lung scarring	Strong association with smoking	
May be associated with Pancoast tumor			
		Neuroendocrine tumor	
		Usually unresectable	
		Treatment: chemotherapy and radiation	

2. Additional testing may include tuberculin skin testing, sputum cultures, chest CT, PET scan, CT-guided biopsy, and excisional biopsy.
3. Differential diagnosis includes infection, granulomatous disease, benign neoplasm, and malignancy.

D. Treatment
1. Lesions can be followed without a tissue diagnosis if they are stable over 2 years or if popcorn calcifications (indicative of hamartoma) are present.
2. If a pulmonary nodule is present in the setting of hypertrophic osteoarthropathy, there is a 75% chance of carcinoma.

XXVII. Cancer

A. General principles (Table 19-7)
1. Lung cancer is the leading cause of cancer-related deaths and the second cause of overall mortality.
2. Majority of patients present with distant disease.
3. Resection is the mainstay of treatment; however, only about 20% of cancers are resectable at presentation (stage I to IIIa).
4. Risk decreases to that of never smokers after 10 years.

B. Clinical features and diagnosis
1. Presenting signs and symptoms may include cough, hemoptysis, hoarseness, weight loss, fatigue, and recurrent infections.
2. CXR is not an effective screening tool because lesions are not visible on the X-ray until they reach 1 cm. At that size, most neoplasms have metastasized.
3. Treatment: Lung cancer treatment can be divided into small and nonsmall cell tumors.

XXVIII. Nonsmall Cell Lung Cancer

A. Staging
1. Stage I: any tumor size without extension to chest wall, mediastinum, pericardium, or diaphragm, with no nodes or metastasis, and at least 2 cm from the carina
   a. Treatment is surgical resection.
   b. The 5-year survival is 65%.
2. Stage II: a stage I tumor with positive ipsilateral hilar or peribronchial nodes and no distant metastasis
   a. Treatment is surgical resection.
   b. The 5-year survival is 45%.

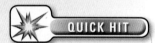

QUICK HIT

Pancoast tumor is a tumor at the apex of the lung that may involve the brachial plexus, sympathetic ganglia, and vertebral body, leading to pain, upper extremity weakness, and Horner syndrome.

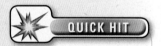

QUICK HIT

Horner syndrome is miosis, ptosis, and ipsilateral decreased sweating due to involvement of cervical sympathetic chain.

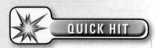

QUICK HIT

Hypertrophic pulmonary osteoarthropathy (proliferation of long bones and in the bones of the hand) is seen in 10% of patients with lung cancer.

3. Stage IIIa: any tumor size with local spread, not involving the heart, aorta, pulmonary artery, trachea, or esophagus, or with positive subcarinal or mediastinal nodes and no distant metastasis
   a. Treatment is surgical resection and chemotherapy with or without radiation.
   b. The 5-year survival is 30%.
4. Stage IIIb: nodal involvement beyond that listed previously, with mediastinal extension and no distant metastasis
   a. Treatment is chemotherapy and radiation.
   b. The 5-year survival is less than 10%.
5. Stage IV: any tumor with distant metastasis
   a. Treatment is chemotherapy.
   b. The 5-year survival is 0%.
B. Contraindications to surgical resection of lung cancer
   1. Superior vena cava (SVC) syndrome
   2. Supraclavicular or scalene node metastasis
   3. Carinal involvement
   4. Small-cell tumor
   5. Poor pulmonary function (forced expiratory volume in 1 second [FEV_1] less than 1)
   6. Metastatic disease

XXIX. Reoperative Evaluation
A. Risk assessment prior to resection includes cardiac evaluation, PFT, and room air ABG.
   1. An individual with a preoperative FEV_1 greater than 2 can tolerate pneumonectomy.
   2. An individual who can climb five flights of stairs can likely tolerate pneumonectomy, but one who cannot climb one flight is unlikely to tolerate a pulmonary resection.

XXX. Surgical Resection of Pulmonary Metastases
A. Pulmonary metastasis is a common presentation and may be the only site of metastasis.
B. Resection of metastatic lesions may be part of a treatment protocol.

XXXI. Benign Tumors of the Lung
A. Hamartoma is the most common benign lung tumor.
B. This presents as a solitary lung nodule.

XXXII. Carcinoid Syndrome
A. An amine precursor uptake and decarboxylation tumor of the bronchus is slow growing but may be malignant.
B. It may present with bronchial obstruction or stenosis.
C. Biopsy has to be undertaken with care because significant hemorrhage is possible.
D. Carcinoid syndrome is rare with pulmonary carcinoid. This syndrome consists of episodic flushing, abdominal cramps, diarrhea, and right-sided heart valve damage.
E. Most bronchial adenomas have malignant potential. Other bronchial adenomas include mucoepidermoid carcinoma, mucous gland adenoma, and adenoid cystic carcinoma.

XXXIII. Paraneoplastic and Other Cancer-Related Syndromes
A. These syndromes are associated with cancers with symptoms in distant parts of the body from the tumor. The cause may be endocrine activity of tumor cells or may be unknown.
B. Manifestations of paraneoplastic syndromes include Cushing syndrome of inappropriate secretion of antidiuretic hormone (SIADH), hypercalcemia, Eaton–Lambert syndrome, cerebellar ataxia, hypertrophic osteoarthropathy, acanthosis nigricans, and thrombophlebitis.
C. Small-cell carcinoma can cause Lambert–Eaton syndrome, Cushing syndrome, or SIADH.

D. Hypercalcemia can result from parathyroid hormone production by a squamous cell tumor.

E. SVC syndrome results from compression of the SVC with impaired drainage. Patients present with edema and plethora of the head and neck, as well as central nervous system symptoms.

XXXIV. Pulmonary Sequestration

A. Abnormal lung tissue with separate blood supply and no communication with tracheobronchial airway

B. Benign, may be asymptomatic, with possible recurrent infections

C. Classified as interlobar (contained within visceral pleura) or extralobar (outside normal lung with separate pleural covering)

D. Treatment is resection if indicated.

XXXV. Mediastinum

A. Anterior mediastinal anatomy includes the thymus, extrapericardial aorta and its branches, great veins, and lymphatic tissue.

B. Anterior mediastinal masses
   1. Thymoma, teratoma, thyroid disease, and lymphoma
      a. Usually occurs in adolescents
      b. The vast majority (80%) are benign.
      c. Derived from branchial cleft pouch
      d. Contain all tissue types
      e. Treatment is surgical excision.

XXXVI. Lymphoma

A. Half of patients with lymphoma have mediastinal involvement; only 5% have isolated mediastinal disease.

B. Present with cough, chest pain, fever, and weight loss

C. Diagnosis with imaging and lymph node biopsy

D. Treatment is nonsurgical.

XXXVII. Germ Cell

A. Very rare mediastinal tumors present with vagus involvement.

B. Treatment is resection.

XXXVIII. Middle Mediastinal Anatomy Includes the Heart, Intrapericardial Great Vessels, Pericardium, and Trachea.

A. Middle mediastinal masses
   1. Pericardial cysts
   2. Bronchogenic cysts
   3. Lymphoma
   4. Ascending aortic aneurysms

B. Posterior mediastinal anatomy includes the esophagus, vagus nerves, thoracic duct, sympathetic chain, and the azygous vein system.
   1. Posterior mediastinal masses: neurogenic tumors

XXXIX. Treatment for Mediastinal Masses

A. Needle aspiration of suspected cysts

B. Resection either via minimally invasive techniques or sternotomy/thoracotomy

XL. Chest Wall

A. Thoracic outlet syndrome
   1. This compromised subclavian vessel flow is caused by a cervical rib or muscular hypertrophy.
   2. Presentation is unilateral upper extremity claudication.

B. Treatment is surgical removal of obstruction (rib resection).

 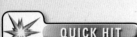

QUICK HIT

The differential diagnosis of a mediastinal mass is based on anatomic location. The most common primary anterior mass in adults is a thymoma. The most common primary anterior mass in children is a teratoma.

QUICK HIT

Differentiate thoracic outlet syndrome from subclavian steal syndrome by history. Subclavian steal presents with central nervous system symptoms, although both have unilateral upper extremity claudication.

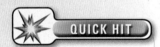

QUICK HIT

Fibrous dysplasia occurs posteriorly and laterally, chondromas occur anteriorly, and osteochondromas can occur anywhere.

QUICK HIT

The majority (60%–90%) of primary chest wall tumors are malignant. Chondrosarcoma is the most common, usually occurring in individuals 10–40 years of age.

XLI. Chest Wall Tumors

A. Benign tumors
1. Fibrous dysplasia of the rib may occur as part of McCune–Albright syndrome.
2. Tumors are slow growing.
3. Chondroma is the most common benign tumor.
4. Osteochondroma is also a common benign tumor.

B. Malignant tumors: fibrosarcoma, chondrosarcoma, osteogenic sarcoma, myeloma, and Ewing sarcoma
1. Treatment is wide excision with reconstruction of the chest wall.

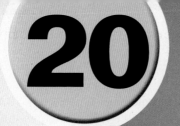

20

Transplantation

Glenn Warden and Brenner Dixon

 IMMUNOBIOLOGY

I. Terminology

A. Types of grafts

1. Autograft (isograft): transplantation of tissue from an individual to itself, usually a different site (e.g., split-thickness skin graft, parathyroid tissue, bone from iliac crest, autotransfusion of blood). An autograft requires no immunosuppression (Fig. 20-1A).
2. Allograft: transplantation of tissue between genetically nonidentical individuals of the same species (e.g., solid organ transplants, allogeneic bone marrow transplants, cornea, blood transfusions). Allografts require

FIGURE
 Types of grafts.

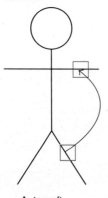
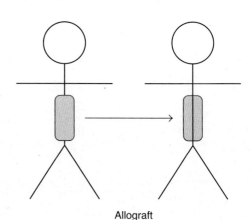

Autograft

A

Allograft

B

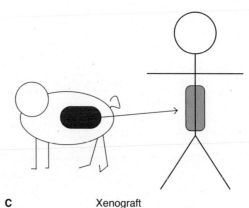

C   Xenograft

A. Autograft. **B.** Allograft. **C.** Xenograft.

immunosuppression to prevent rejection of the transplanted donor tissue by the recipient's intact immune system (Fig. 20-1B).

3. Xenograft: transplantation of tissue between members of different species (Fig. 20-1C)

B. B cells
  1. These lymphocytes arise and partially mature in bone marrow.
  2. They respond by directly binding antigen (Ag) to immunoglobulin (Ig) on the surface of the cell. Thus, activated B cells proliferate (clonal selection) to terminally differentiate into antibody (Ab)-producing plasma cells.
      a. Antibodies are glycoproteins secreted by plasma cells.
      b. Antibodies are constructed from two light polypeptide chains and two heavy polypeptide chains.
          (1) There are two isotypes of light chains: κ (kappa) and λ (lambda).
          (2) There are five isotypes of heavy chains: μ, (mu), γ (gamma), ε (epsilon), α (alpha), and δ (delta), responsible for the five isotypes of circulating antibody: IgM, IgG, IgE, IgA, and IgD.

C. T cells
  1. These lymphocytes arise in the bone marrow and mature in the thymus.
  2. They are responsible for cell-mediated immunity as well as facilitating B-cell response.
  3. They are broadly classified as CD4+ or CD8+. CD is the abbreviation for cluster determinant.
      a. CD4+ T cells have been termed helper cells, or helper T cells (T_H), in that their function is crucial in promoting both B- as well as T-effector function.
      b. Helper (CD4+) T lymphocytes are further classified as Th1 and Th2, depending upon the profile of cytokines they produce in response to antigen stimulation.
          (1) Th_1 cells produce interleukin-2 (IL-2) and interferon-gamma (IFN-γ) to stimulate macrophages and cytotoxic T cells.
          (2) Th_2 cells produce IL-4, IL-5, and IL-10 to increase production of immunoglobulin.
      c. CD8+ T cells effect the T-cell response. This frequently involves direct cytotoxicity, and effector T cells have also been termed cytotoxic T cells (T_c).

D. Major histocompatibility complex
  1. T cells normally recognize (nonself) antigen only in the context of self major histocompatibility complex (MHC). Antigen is bound to the MHC molecule on antigen-presenting cells (APCs). This limitation on antigen recognition is referred to as MHC restriction.
  2. MHC is a cluster of genes, found in all mammalian species, that allows an individual to differentiate self from nonself.
  3. This restriction of the T-cell recognition occurs during development and maturation in the thymus. At this stage, T cells that would react to self-antigens and T cells that do not recognize self MHC as such are eliminated or inactivated (T-cell selection).
  4. Three genetic loci of the human MHC (HLA) are described—class I, class II, and class III. These loci code for class I, class II, and class III antigens.
      a. Class I and II region genes code for several highly polymorphic cell surface proteins (HLA antigens).
          (1) Class I is additionally subdivided into HLA-A, HLA-B, and HLA-C. Class I antigens are present on all nucleated cells.
          (2) Class II region genes code for HLA-DR, HLA-DQ, and HLA-DP. Class II antigens are present on B cells, dendritic cells (DCs), macrophages, and activated T cells.
      b. Class III region genes code for some proteins of the complement system.
      c. Some other cell types (e.g., endothelial cells) may be induced to express class II antigen by cytokines (e.g., IFN-γ).

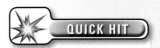

QUICK HIT

The human MHC is termed the human leukocyte antigen (HLA) complex. It is coded on the short arm of chromosome 6.

Transplantation

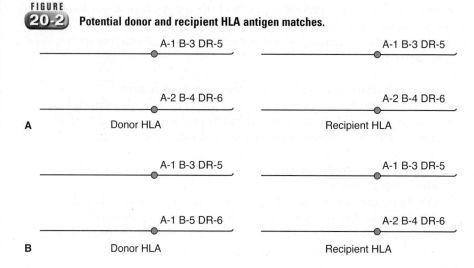

FIGURE 20-2 Potential donor and recipient HLA antigen matches.

5. HLA-A, HLA-B, and HLA-DR have been termed major histocompatibility antigens. These have been most closely associated with the host's immune response (rejection) to transplanted allogeneic tissue.
   a. Because each individual has two #6 chromosomes (one maternal and one paternal), there are potentially six distinct major HLA antigens expressed on cells.
   b. If donor tissue and the recipient have the same HLA-A, HLA-B, and HLA-DR, this is referred to as a "six-antigen match" (Fig. 20-2A). An individual may be homozygous for any of these antigens (e.g., A-1) (see Fig. 20-2B).
6. Although in the previous example, donor and recipient HLA are not identical, the donor is a "zero-antigen mismatch" with the recipient because the donor has no HLA antigens that mismatch with the recipient.
7. APCs process and present nonself antigen to T cells in the context of MHC. APCs include macrophages (Mϕ), DCs, activated T_H, and B cells.

II. Rejection

A. Transplant rejection is the host response (antibody-mediated, cell-mediated, or both) directed against nonself alloantigens (transplanted tissue) (Table 20-1).
B. Hyperacute rejection
   1. This type of rejection is mediated by preformed (already present at the time of transplant) antibodies against donor antigen (HLA antigen). These antibodies may be IgG against HLA antigen and/or IgM against an ABO mismatch. Hyperacute rejection is also controlled by activation of the complement

TABLE 20-1	Type of Rejections		
	Hyperacute Rejection	**Acute Rejection**	**Chronic Rejection**
Time course	Immediate	Days	Weeks to years
Rejection conferred by	Preformed Ab	T-cell-dependent immunity	T-cell-dependent immunity
Rejection mediated by	HLA-Ab ABO, DP, DQ, DR	Cell-mediated immunity	Cell-mediated immunity
"Buzz" words	Graft thrombosis (rapid)	Lymphocytic infiltrate Vasculitis	Loss of structure Graft fibrosis Atherosclerosis
Treatment	Pretransplant crossmatch Immediate retransplant	Alter regimen for immunosuppression Burst steroids	Minimize acute rejection May require retransplantation

TABLE 20-2 Renal Recipient versus Renal Donor Blood Type	
Donor	**Recipient**
O	O, A, B, AB
A	A, AB
B	B, AB
AB	AB

system, which causes acute vascular injury, and activation of the coagulation cascade. Rapid and irreversible graft loss is due to ischemia from thrombosis.

2. Hyperacute rejection occurs within minutes to hours after organ reperfusion.
3. There are no effective treatments for hyperacute rejection. The clinical strategy is to avoid hyperacute rejection.
   a. Pretransplant crossmatches are performed to detect preformed anti-HLA antibodies. The rules regarding compatibility are generally the same as those for blood transfusion (Table 20-2).
   b. Hyperacute rejection is prevented by careful matching of ABO blood groups and by screening for preformed anti-HLA antibodies with the pretransplant crossmatch.
   c. Blood group A may clinically present as Al or A2. A2 individuals are clinically blood group A but express significantly less A antigen. A2 organs have been successfully transplanted into blood group O and B recipients with low titers of anti-A antibody.
4. In the absence of meticulous preparation and manipulation of the immune response, transplantation across blood group compatibilities will fail with hyperacute rejection due to preformed antibodies.
5. Experimental protocols to remove circulating antibody (plasmapheresis) and antibody-producing cells (splenectomy and/or treatment with rituximab [anti-CD20]) have had some success in permitting transplantation across blood groups.

C. Accelerated acute rejection
1. This type of rejection is also antibody mediated but does not present clinically until 2 to 5 days after transplantation. This type of rejection is due to an anamnestic response from prior exposure (sensitization). Sensitization may result from previous blood transfusions, transplants, or pregnancy
2. Accelerated acute rejection has been successfully treated with plasmapheresis to remove antibody and intravenous (IV) IgG, anti-lymphocyte antibodies, or rituximab to manipulate further antibody production.

D. Acute rejection
1. Most acute rejections are cell mediated. Cell-mediated acute rejections are generally easier to reverse than antibody-mediated acute rejections.
2. This type of rejection occurs days to months following transplantation.
3. Acute rejection may present with fever, chills, arthralgias, and systemic toxicity (consistent with tumor necrosis factor alpha [TNF-α] and/or IL-1).
4. With current immunosuppression protocols, acute rejection often lacks these clinical features and presents as allograft dysfunction.
5. The diagnosis of rejection is most definitively established by allograft biopsy. The Banff classification scheme is frequently used to describe and grade the severity of acute rejection on renal allograft biopsy specimens.

E. Chronic rejection
1. This insidious process is the leading cause of late allograft loss.
2. Chronic rejection likely encompasses both immunologic as well as nonimmunologic (drug toxicity, infection, metabolic and biochemical alterations) factors.
3. Chronic rejection may present differently in different transplanted organs.
4. A Banff classification scheme can be used to grade the histopathology of chronic rejection in renal allografts.

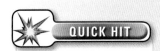

QUICK HIT

Chronic rejection comprises both immunologic as well as nonimmunologic factors.

Transplantation

III. Immunosuppression

A. Current clinically applicable immunosuppression is nonspecific. Ideal immunosuppression would specifically suppress only those cellular subsets of the immune system that are genetically programmed to respond to donor antigen.

B. Except in the case of transplantation between monozygotic twins, allografts between individuals will elicit an immune response. Immunosuppressive drugs are administered to suppress the immune response.

1. Although high-dose immunosuppressive therapy might eliminate rejection, it would be associated with an intolerable and unacceptable degree of morbidity and mortality.

2. Giving no immunosuppressive therapy would be associated with no drug-related toxicity but would lead to allograft loss from rejection.

C. Current immunosuppression protocols are designed to achieve acceptable allograft survival rates with minimal toxicities and side effects. The therapeutic window between lack of efficacy and toxicity/side effects is very narrow for most immunosuppressive medications.

D. Immunosuppressive agents are divided into two groups—agents used for induction therapy immediately after transplantation and drugs used for maintenance therapy.

E. Five basic categories of immunosuppressive agents are used in organ transplantation: corticosteroids, calcineurin inhibitors, antiproliferative agents, monoclonal antilymphocyte antibodies, and polyclonal antilymphocyte antibodies. Each type works to block a particular step of rejection.

1. Corticosteroids

a. A corticosteroid is a glucocorticoid-based medication that works principally to block T cell and APC-derived cytokine and cytokine-receptor expression. The major elements blocked are IL-1 and IL-6. Secondary effects of corticosteroids include the blocking of IL-2, INF-γ, and TNF-α. These elements, notably IL-1, are essential for lymphocyte-APC communication—a decrease in production effectively obstructs an APC's capacity to activate allograft-specific lymphocytes. As a result, threat of acute rejection is reduced. Corticosteroids have a hydrophobic structure that allows them to easily diffuse into cells and bind to specific cytoplasmic receptors. The resulting complexes progress to the nucleus, where they are able to inhibit the transcription of the genes of the cytokines named earlier.

b. Corticosteroids are also able to inhibit cytokine production in macrophages. This subsequently inhibits the macrophage phagocytosis and chemotaxis properties. Corticosteroids are also potent nonspecific anti-inflammatory agents—administration of corticosteroids results in an acute reduction of circulating lymphocytes and monocytes.

c. **Side effects** observed with corticosteroid use include hypertension, hyperlipidemia, osteoporosis, weight gain, a cushingoid appearance, opportunistic infection, glaucoma, ulcer formation, and hyperglycemia (usually progressing to steroid diabetes).

d. Corticosteroids can be used to prevent as well as to treat acute rejection. Oral as well as IV routes are commonly used.

e. A high dose of IV methylprednisolone is usually given immediately before and during the transplantation procedure. Methylprednisolone or prednisone is often continued postoperatively for several days at high doses and is then tapered to a maintenance dose. Dose and taper schedule varies with the organ transplanted.

f. Maintenance doses consist of orally administered prednisone and are normally 5 to 10 mg/day.

2. Calcineurin inhibitors

a. The mechanisms of calcineurin inhibitors converge at the inhibition of the calcineurin. This inhibition ultimately inhibits the production and secretion of **IL-2**. The interaction between **IL-2** and the **IL-2 receptor** is crucial in the activation and differentiation of B and T cells. Therefore, halting the rejection process at this step is highly effective at combating rejection.

b. Cyclosporine is a small fungal cyclic peptide that is used to prevent allograft rejection. Cyclosporine works by binding a protein found in the cytosol: cyclophilin. This complex inhibits calcineurin. The rest of the mechanism is outlined previously. Cyclosporine is a highly effective immunosuppressant. In fact, cyclosporine is generally hailed as the cornerstone of immunosuppression. The clinical introduction of cyclosporine significantly increased graft survival and significantly reduced the occurrence of acute rejection in patients.

c. **Side effects** observed with cyclosporine use include nephrotoxicity (improves when drug is discontinued), hypertension, tremor, coronary artery disease (dose related and reversible), hirsutism, gingival hyperplasia, opportunistic infections, malignancies, hyperuricemia, hepatoxicity, and hypertrichosis.

d. Cyclosporine is available in form of emulsions and microemulsions. Maintenance doses consist of orally administered cyclosporine, normally 5 to 10 mg/kg/day given in two doses. This is usually taken along with an antiproliferative agent and prednisone as part of an immunosuppression regimen. IV solutions also exist, with only a third of the oral dose required for this form.

e. Tacrolimus is a macrolide antibiotic that works in a mechanism similar to that of cyclosporine to prevent allograft rejection. Tacrolimus binds the cytosolic protein FKPB-121. This complex inhibits calcineurin in a manner parallel to cyclosporine.

f. **Side effects** observed with tacrolimus use include nephrotoxicity (improves when drug is discontinued), hypertension, hyperkalemia, hypomagnesemia, alopecia, hyperglycemia, opportunistic infections, and malignancies.

g. Tacrolimus is available in oral pills. A maintenance dose is usually 0.15 to 0.3 mg/kg/day given in two doses. There is also an IV form available, dosing of which is usually 0.03 mg/kg intravenously for 24 hours.

3. Antiproliferative agents

a. Antiproliferative agents are used in maintenance immunosuppression and treatment of rejection. Antiproliferative agents are drugs that work to block the proliferative phase of acute cellular rejection. They are an integral part of most immunosuppression regimens.

b. Azathioprine is rapidly hydrolyzed in the blood to 6-mercaptopurine. In this form (a purine analog and antimetabolite), it incorporates into the DNA, inhibiting nucleotide synthesis by causing feedback inhibition in the early stages of purine metabolism. This ultimately prevents mitosis and proliferation of rapidly dividing cells, such as activated B and T lymphocytes. Through this action, azathioprine is able to block most T cell functions and inhibit primary antibody synthesis. Azathioprine has little effect on established immune responses and is therefore effective only in the prevention (not treatment) of acute rejection.

c. Side effects observed with azathioprine use include: bone marrow depletion/suppression thrombocytopenia, anemia pancreatitis, hepatoxicity, neoplasia.

d. Azathioprine is normally taken orally, at a rate of 1 to 2 mg/kg/day. An IV form is also available. Azathioprine is used as part of a triple immunosuppression regimen, along with prednisone and a calcineurin inhibitor.

e. Mycophenolate mofetil (MMF) is absorbed and rapidly hydrolyzed in the blood to its active form: mycophenolic acid (MPA). MPA inhibits the key enzyme in the de novo pathway of purine biosynthesis, IMPDH1. Rapidly dividing cells, such as activated lymphocytes, depend on the **de novo pathway** for the production of purines necessary for RNA and DNA synthesis. In this way, activated lymphocytes are selectively inhibited because they are not allowed to proliferate once activated.

f. **Side effects** observed with MMF use include: leucopenia, thrombocytopenia, nausea opportunistic infection, malignancies, gastrointestinal (GI) upsets.

g. MMF is normally taken orally, 1 to 1.5 g twice daily. An IV form is also available.

h. Sirolimus is a highly potent macrolide antibiotic that has a chemical structure similar to tacrolimus. Sirolimus binds to the same protein as tacrolimus: FKBP-12. Instead of inhibiting calcineurin as tacrolimus does, this complex inhibits mTOR. This inhibition prevents the progression of T cells from the G1 to the S phase of the cell cycle by blocking signaling downstream of the **IL-2 receptor**. It therefore is able to block **delayed-type hypersensitivity (DTH)** immune reactions, **cytotoxic T lymphocyte (CTL)** activity, and humoral responses directed against a transplanted organ. Because cyclosporine and sirolimus have different mechanisms, the clinical combination of the two in an immunosuppression regimen results in effects that are synergistic.

i. **Side effects** observed with sirolimus use include leucopenia, thrombocytopenia, hypercholesterolemia, and hypertriglyceridemia. Sirolimus is taken orally at a recommended rate of 2 to 5 mg once a day.

4. Monoclonal antibodies

a. Monoclonal antibodies are used in early rejection prophylaxis and treatment of rejection. Monoclonal antibodies are antigen-specific immunosuppressants that will reduce immune response to alloantigens of the graft while preserving the response to alloantigens to unrelated antigens. These agents are specific to blocking T-cell activation, resulting in rapid depletion of T cells from the circulation by binding of antibody-coated T cells to Fc receptors on phagocytic cells. The most recently U.S. Food and Drug Administration (FDA)-approved monoclonal antibodies are the IL-2 receptor antagonists genetically engineered to possess both human and murine antibody sequences. The chimerization of these antibodies is an attempt to decrease the immunogenicity of the agent. Other monoclonal antibody–based drugs are still in clinical trials for FDA approval.

b. Muromonab-CD3 is the first type of murine monoclonal antibody directed against the epsilon chain of the CD3 molecule (an integral part of the T-cell receptor complex) and modulates the receptor and inactivates T-cell function, blocking both naive T cells and CTLs. This results in rapid depletion of T cells from circulation and cytokine release. This antibody is used to treat acute rejection and steroid-resistant rejection. Several severe adverse effects as a result of muromonab-CD3 are thought to be a product of the cytokine release inherent in the mechanism of the agent's efficacy.

c. Side effects observed with muromonab-CD3 use include acute clinical syndrome (cytokine release syndrome) after first few doses, aseptic meningitis, opportunistic infections, lymphoma (without cyclosporine, no lymphoma), malignancies, hypersensitivity reactions, human antimouse antibodies (HAMA) reaction

d. The recommended dose for muromonab-CD3 is 5 mg IV push once a day for 7 to 14 days.

e. IL-2-receptor antagonist (basiliximab): Basiliximab (Simulect) is a chimeric (70% human and 30% murine) monoclonal antibody used in the prevention of acute organ rejection. This monoclonal antibody has a specificity and high affinity for the a subunit of the IL-2 receptor (IL-2Ra, also known as CD25 or Tac) preventing IL-2 from binding to the receptor on the surface of activated T cells. By acting as an IL-2Ra antagonist, basiliximab inhibits IL-2-mediated activation and proliferation of T cells, the critical step in the cascade of cellular immune response of allograft rejection. Therefore, basiliximab has a long half-life of approximately 7 to 12 days and saturates the IL-2 receptor for up to 59 days. Due to its high percentage of humanization in its antibody sequences, the occurrence and acuteness of adverse effects is significantly lower when used with standard immunotherapy.

f. Side effects observed with IN-2 receptor antagonist use include GI disorders.

g. The prescribed dose of basiliximab is 20 mg IV 2 hours prior to transplant and 20 mg 4 days after transplant surgery. This immunosuppressant is given as part of the immunotherapeutic regimen.

Transplantation

h. Daclizumab is a similar agent as basiliximab but is a more humanized IgG monoclonal antibody (90% human and 10% murine). It also binds to and inhibits the a-subunit of IL-2 receptor. Daclizumab has a half-life of about 20 days and saturates the IL-2 receptor for up to 120 days (twice as long as basiliximab).

i. Side effects observed with IN-2 receptor antagonist use include GI disorders; it does not appear to increase the incidence of opportunistic infections or malignancies.

j. Daclizumab is given as a part of the immunosuppressant therapy in place. The first dose is 1 mg/kg IV given around the surgery and then every 14 days for four more doses.

5. Polyclonal antibodies

Polyclonal antibodies are directed against lymphocyte antigens, but instead of the single-specificity of the monoclonal antibodies, these anti-lymphocyte antibodies are directed against multiple epitopes. The agents are used in induction therapy and can be given to avoid the nephrotoxic effects of calcineurin inhibitors and to postpone or avert refection of the allograft.

Early rejection prophylaxis, treatment of rejection: Drawbacks from using these polyclonal antibodies include unpredictability, variable efficacy, and adverse reactions (increased risk of infections, lymphoproliferative disease due to over-immunosuppression—this is not specific).

a. Antithymocyte globulin is a polyclonal antibody derived from either horses (Atgam) or rabbits (Thymoglobulin). The agents contain antibodies specific for many common T-cell antigens including CD2, CD3, CD4, CD8, CD11a, and CD18. The antithymocyte globulin binds lymphocytes that display the surface antigens previously listed. This effectively depletes T-cell concentration in the body through complement-dependent cytolysis and cell-mediated opsonization (define in rejection portion or glossary) following with T-cell clearance from the circulation by the reticuloendothelial system (RES).

b. Side effects observed with antithymocyte globulin use include leukopenia serum sickness (cross-reactivity with other tissue antigens), adverse effects on the ability of the patient to make antibodies against foreign protein, thrombocytopenia, pruritus, fever, arthralgias, opportunistic infections, and malignancies.

c. Antithymocyte globulin can be a part of the induction therapy or acute rejection treatment. The recommended dose of Atgam is 10 to 20 mg/kg/day administered daily through an IV for up to 14 days. The recommended dose of Thymoglobulin is 1.5mg/kg administered daily through an IV for 7 to 14 days.

IV. Infection

A. General principles

1. Immunosuppressed patients are susceptible to familiar bacterial infections (e.g., pneumonia, wound infection, line infection, urine infection) as well as unusual infections (e.g., viral, fungal, protozoal, and atypical bacteria and mycobacteria). The time after transplant is an important factor in determining the etiology of an infection.

2. Immunosuppressed patients frequently present with subdued clinical (and laboratory) signs and symptoms of infection. As a consequence, immunosuppressed patients may present later in the course of an infection.

3. The key to successful management of infections in immunosuppressed patients is a high level of clinical suspicion and an aggressive approach to diagnosis and treatment.

4. Reduction of immunosuppression may be a necessary part of successful management of infection.

a. The overall degree (intensity) of immunosuppression correlates with the risk and severity of infection.

b. As the risk of certain ("unusual") infections is well known, drug prophylaxis protocols are used to reduce the risk of these infections.

B. Types of infections
  1. Cytomegalovirus (CMV)
     a. This member of the herpes family of viruses is a ubiquitous virus with many different serotypes. It can infect any cell type.
     b. In a nonimmunosuppressed individual, CMV usually occurs as a mild and self-limiting infection. An elevated anti-CMV IgG indicates previous CMV infection. The viral genome can persist without symptoms, for life.
     c. The CMV can be transferred with any solid organ transplant. CMV infection in transplant recipients has been associated with increased risk of rejection, increased risk of additional infections, and increased risk of malignancy (post-transplant lymphoproliferative disorder [PTLD]).
     d. In an immunosuppressed individual, CMV may occur as a primary or secondary infection.
        (1) A primary CMV infection occurs in a naive, seronegative individual upon exposure to the CMV.
        (2) A secondary infection occurs in a seropositive individual. A secondary infection may represent reactivation from a latent virus or exposure to a new serotype.
     e. CMV disease denotes a more symptomatic infection (fever, "viral syndrome," leukopenia). Invasive CMV disease may cause serious pneumonitis, hepatitis, encephalitis, and GI invasion with bleeding and/or perforation.
     f. CMV disease and invasive CMV is treated with ganciclovir or valganciclovir. CMV strains resistant to ganciclovir may be treated with foscarnet. Foscarnet has a significant renal toxicity.
     g. Effective prophylaxis can reduce incidence and severity of CMV disease. Prophylaxis is provided by ganciclovir, valganciclovir, acyclovir, or CMV immune globulin.
  2. Epstein–Barr virus (EBV)
     a. This member of the herpes family of viruses most frequently infects B lymphocytes. It is the most common causative agent of mononucleosis. Elevated IgG against EBV viral capsid antigen and/or EBV nuclear antigen indicates previous infection. The EBV genome may persist in lymphocytes.
     b. Because all transplantable solid organs contain some donor lymphocytes, EBV may be transmitted by transplantation. EBV has been clearly associated with the development of PTLD (see following text), especially in EBV-naive recipients.
     c. Primary and secondary EBV infections may occur (as with CMV), but the severity is generally less.
     d. Prophylaxis used for CMV (e.g., acyclovir, ganciclovir) may have some ameliorating effect on EBV.
  3. Varicella zoster virus (VZV)
     a. This is a member of the herpes family of viruses. It is the etiologic agent of chickenpox. The virus persists for life in the dorsal root ganglia.
     b. Reactivation of the VZV is responsible for clinical shingles (herpes zoster). Varicella zoster disease in immunosuppressed patients is due to reactivation. Disseminated disease is rare and usually occurs in previously serologically naive patients who are infected by the usual respiratory route.
     c. Prophylaxis (like that for CMV) appears to be effective in that the incidence of clinical VZV disease is low during such prophylaxis.
  4. Other
     a. Parvovirus B19 is the etiologic agent of fifth disease. In immunosuppressed individuals, parvovirus B19 can cause a profound and refractory anemia. The anemia may respond to IV IgG.
     b. BK virus is a polyomavirus. In renal transplant patients, BK virus infection may present as progressive allograft dysfunction, mimicking acute rejection. It can be differentiated on biopsy and polymerase chain reaction. There are no specific, good therapies, and treatment usually is reduction of immunosuppression.

c. *Pneumocystis carinii* is the etiologic agent of pneumocystis pneumonia. Previously classified as a protozoan, *P. carinii* is now classified as a fungus.

    (1) Treatment of pneumocystis pneumonia is with IV trimethoprim-sulfamethoxazole or IV pentamidine. The pentamidine is associated with a high incidence of side effects, including potentially severe pancreatitis.

    (2) Effective prophylaxis is achieved with trimethoprim-sulfamethoxazole, dapsone, or inhaled pentamidine.

d. Fungal infections have increased incidence and severity in immunosuppressed patients.

    (1) Risk factors include indwelling catheters, diabetes, use of high-dose steroids, intensity of immunosuppression, and use of broad-spectrum antibiotics.

    (2) Invasive fungal infections may be treated with fluconazole, itraconazole, or amphotericin B.

    (3) *Candida* infection, especially in the early post-transplant period, is most common. Effective prophylaxis against oral or esophageal candidiasis is provided by nystatin or clotrimazole.

V. Malignancy

A. There is an increased incidence and aggressiveness/virulence of certain tumors in immunosuppressed individuals.

  1. This now appears to be more due to suppression of natural defenses than to direct oncogenic properties of individual immunosuppressive medications.

  2. The incidence of these tumors is related to the intensity and duration of immunosuppression.

B. Malignant tumors that may metastasize to the transplanted organ in a donor harboring a malignancy may be transferred to the recipient of that organ.

  1. Such tumors may exhibit aggressive behavior in the immunosuppressed host.

  2. Potential organ donors with cancer are excluded (consideration may be given to prospective donors with nonmelanoma skin cancer and primary central nervous system [CNS] tumors).

C. Because immunosuppression may alter the innate defense against malignant cells, it is usually recommended that an individual not be transplanted/immunosuppressed until 2 to 5 years after curative therapy for cancer in a prospective transplant recipient.

D. Squamous cell carcinoma of the skin demonstrates the greatest increased incidence of these cancers. Prophylaxis against ultraviolet exposure (sunscreen, clothing), and appropriate dosing of immunosuppression are helpful preventive options

E. Lymphoma has an increased incidence in immunosuppressed individuals. These are usually (greater than 90%) non-Hodgkin B-cell lymphomas.

F. PTLD has been ascribed to EBV infection of B cells.

  1. In immunocompetent patients, an EBV infection causes a polyclonal proliferation of B cells. This proliferation may not be controlled in immunosuppressed individuals, leading, through mutation, to an independent monoclonal expansion (lymphoma). Extranodal involvement (CNS, liver, kidney, intestines) is much more common than with lymphomas in immunocompetent individuals.

  2. These lymphomas are much less responsive to standard chemotherapy and radiation treatments, which may increase the level of immunosuppression and worsen the prognosis.

  3. These lymphomas may respond to aggressive reduction or cessation of immunosuppression. In some cases, antiviral (oligoclonal) therapy has been reported to be beneficial.

G. There is a moderate increased incidence of Kaposi sarcoma (herpes virus 8) and cervical cancer (human papilloma virus).

H. There is no increased incidence of common solid tumors such as colon, breast, and lung cancer.

ORGAN SUPPLY AND DEMAND

I. Organ Allocation

A. There is a large discrepancy between the demand (number of patients awaiting transplantation) and the supply (number of actual organ donors and transplantable organs). For deceased donor organs, there is also a discrepancy between the location of the donor and the potential recipient who, according to current algorithms, might best use these transplantable organs.

B. The national Organ Procurement and Transplant Network (OPTN) was established in 1984 through the National Organ Transplant Act, passed by the Congress of the United States. The intent of the act is to ensure that scarce transplantable organs are distributed equitably, safely, and efficiently.

C. The federal contract to administer the OPTN has been awarded to the United Network for Organ Sharing (UNOS), which has its headquarters in Richmond, Virginia.

   1. All organ transplant centers, organ procurement organizations (OPOs), and tissue typing laboratories must meet and maintain standards set by UNOS to maintain membership in the network and access to deceased donor organs.

   2. UNOS maintains the national "waiting list" of patients awaiting a transplant.

      a. Each time a deceased donor organ becomes available for transplantation anywhere in the nation, this computerized database is searched, and transplant candidates are ranked according to predetermined parameters.

      b. It is important to note that the "list" is not merely a static ordinal rank of waiting time. The results of a match run are determined by multiple factors, of which waiting time is only one factor and not the most important factor for any organ.

D. The Scientific Registry of Transplant Recipients (SRTR) is responsible for maintaining a very extensive database on all listed patients awaiting transplantation and follow-up on all transplanted patients. SRTR data are easily accessible at http://www.ustransplant.org, and this website is a useful source of information for patients and health care providers.

E. Another useful resource is the United States Renal Data System (USRDS) (http://usrds.org), which maintains an extensive database on all patients who have enrolled in the End-Stage Renal Disease Program.

F. There is a different allocation algorithm for different deceased donor organs. These algorithms take in consideration multiple factors related to the recipient, donor, and logistics.

   1. Recipient factors include severity of illness for liver transplantation, loss of access for dialysis for renal transplantation, age (pediatric recipients receive a slight increased preference), and the likelihood of receiving a transplant (e.g., panel reactive antibody [PRA] for patients awaiting renal transplants).

   2. Donor factors include donor age, past medical history, social history, donor stability, and biopsy results of donor organs.

   3. Logistics primarily considers the distance (time of transport) between donor and recipient hospitals.

G. OPOs identify potential deceased organ donors. The 57 nonprofit OPOs provide service to all 50 states and Puerto Rico.

   1. OPOs facilitate and coordinate organ recovery, preservation, and transport. Law requires that all deaths are reported to the OPO.

   2. OPOs are also charged with education of health care providers and the lay public regarding organ donation.

II. Donor Organs from Diseased Individuals

A. Organ donation: Organs for transplantation may be recovered from individuals who meet the criteria for brain death or from individuals who have massive and irreversible brain damage and for whom an independent decision to withdraw life support has been made (nonheart-beating donor [NHBD], or donation after cardiac death).

   1. The basic legal framework for defining brain death is described in the Uniform Determination of Death Act (1980), which has been adopted by all states.

In this act, brain death is defined as the "irreversible cessation of all functions of the entire brain, including the brainstem."

2. Detailed specifics for clinical brain death (e.g., length of time for apnea), and requirements for confirmatory testing (e.g., electroencephalogram, cerebral blood flow studies) are the prerogative of individual hospitals.

3. The standards to determine brain death are rigorous to exclude any conceivable potentially reversible factors (e.g., hypothermia, alcohol, drugs, severe metabolic abnormalities).

4. The criteria for brain death include:
   a. A known and irreversible brain injury
   b. Coma on a ventilator
   c. Absent brain stem reflexes (e.g., pupillary, corneal, gag, vestibuloocular, oculocephalic)
   d. Apnea off a ventilator
   e. Absence of exclusionary criteria

5. Some hospitals require confirmatory tests (brain blood flow tests, electroencephalogram), although these have not been listed as mandatory in formal criteria.

6. NHBDs are comatose individuals with severe, irreversible damage, who do not meet all the formal criteria (usually, some remnant of brain stem activity) for brain death and for whom an independent decision has been made to withdraw life support. Organ recovery is performed after there is cessation of cardiac function in the donor.

7. Recoverable solid organs for transplantation include the heart, lung, liver, pancreas (whole organ, or islets of Langerhans), kidney, and intestine. Donors may also donate tissue, including bone, tendons, heart valves, and corneas.

8. The criteria for what is considered an acceptable organ for transplant have expanded as the number of people awaiting transplant has increased. The clinical need of an individual patient is taken into account when deciding on the suitability of a given organ offer.

9. Contraindications to organ donation include malignancy, HIV, systemic infection, hepatitis B surface antigen positivity, hepatitis C antibody (many centers use organs from hepatitis C+ donors for hepatitis C+ recipients).

B. Organ preservation: Because the tolerance of transplantable organs to normothermic ischemia is measured in minutes, effective steps must be taken to protect against cell damage and cell death.

1. Normothermic cellular metabolism in the absence of oxygen and the metabolic substrates supplied by an intact circulation leads to cell damage and death. The products of anaerobic cellular metabolism play a major role in reperfusion injury (e.g., oxygen-free radicals) upon the reestablishment of normothermic circulation to the transplanted organ.

2. The strategy of organ preservation is to minimize cellular metabolism.

3. Hypothermia (less than 5°C) is a cornerstone of all organ preservation. Oxygen consumption is reduced by 95% at 5°C. Freezing, with intracellular ice-crystal formation, must be avoided.
   a. Hypothermia does not totally stop metabolic processes, and the end products of metabolism accumulate over time. This is a major factor in the tolerable length of time between organ recovery and transplantation.
   b. Energy-independent cell functions are less affected by hypothermia (e.g., passive diffusion of extracellular sodium across thecal membrane). Organ preservation solutions approximate the intracellular environment with a high potassium and low sodium concentrations.
   c. Cellular swelling is a natural consequence of hypothermic storage due to passive diffusion of water into the higher oncotic pressure of the cell. Impermeable oncotic agents (e.g., hetastarch, mannitol, raffinose) are included to prevent cell swelling.

4. Accumulation of lactic acid from low-level anaerobic metabolism leads to a progressively lower pH within the stored organ. Phosphates are the usual buffer for organ preservation solutions.

5. Several commercial organ preservation solutions with different components and concentrations have been approved for clinical use, including Collins, ViaSpan (University of Wisconsin Solution), and Custodiol (HTK).

6. Optimal organ preservation begins with careful clinical management of the deceased donor, with special attention to hemodynamic and metabolic parameters. Hypotension is common, and many donors have diabetes insipidus and marked hypernatremia. Severe hypernatremia in the donor has been associated with allograft dysfunction (especially liver allografts).

C. Organ recovery

1. The operative approach is directed toward minimizing warm ischemia time as well as surgical injury to the recovered organs.

2. Proximal and distal control of the aorta for cold perfusion is carried out early in the operation. Access to the vena cava is required to vent blood and flush solution.

3. In a stable donor, time may be expended to do a preliminary dissection, mobilizing individual organs and looking for anatomic variants (e.g., replaced right and/or left hepatic arteries). However, many transplant programs prefer to use a rapid technique of en bloc excision after cold perfusion with dissection and separation on the back table.

TRANSPLANTATION OF SPECIFIC ORGANS

I. Kidney

A. Indications

1. End-stage renal disease with a glomerular filtration rate (GFR) less than 20 mL/min^{-1} or maintenance hemodialysis are prerequisites for a deceased donor transplant.

2. Preemptive renal transplant (GFR greater than 20 mL/min, or patient not yet on dialysis) may be performed using living donors.

3. Conditions that are some of the more common causes of renal failure leading to renal transplantation, such as diabetic nephropathy, hypertensive nephropathy, glomerulonephritides, polycystic kidney disease, chronic pyelonephritis, obstructive uropathy, or congenital abnormalities

B. Contraindications

1. Chronic, untreated infection: HIV, hepatitis B, and hepatitis C are no longer absolute contraindications to transplantation, but they must be approached with a meticulous plan for long-term management.

2. A recent malignancy (except small nonmelanoma skin cancer and, at some centers, carcinoma in situ) or metastatic cancer: A 2- to 5-year disease-free interval following curative treatment of a malignant tumor is required at most centers.

3. Severe comorbid conditions that make the risk of surgery and/or chronic immunosuppression prohibitive.

4. A history of recurrent noncompliance is a warning sign for inability to comply with the complicated postoperative management requirements.

C. Preoperative evaluation

1. A complete history and physical examination may identify many significant, but correctable, potential problems for transplantation. Evaluation of the lower urinary tract is often indicated based on history (e.g., recurrent infections, diabetes mellitus [neurogenic bladder]). Anuric patients have no voiding symptoms.

2. Bilateral native nephrectomy is indicated for chronic infection, severe proteinuria, suspicion of cancer in the native kidneys, or massively enlarged kidneys from polycystic kidney disease with pain, infection, or bleeding. Bilateral native nephrectomy for refractory hypertension has been reported to be helpful in some cases.

3. The patient has HLA typing and screening for preformed anti-HLA antibodies (PRAs) prior to being placed on the UNOS waiting list.

D. Operation
1. The kidney is transplanted into the heterotopic location of the iliac fossa. The renal artery and vein are anastomosed to the respective iliac artery and vein.
2. Following reperfusion, the ureter is anastomosed to the urinary bladder. An antireflux maneuver (Litch technique [currently favored] or Politano-Lead [better] technique) is performed. The ipsilateral native ureter may be used.

E. Immediate postoperative care
1. Most aspects of management are the same as they would be for any general surgical patient. Attention to fluid and electrolyte management is particularly important. Hypovolemia (which can occur rapidly with a brisk diuresis) must be avoided.
2. Special attention must be paid to frequent monitoring of urine output. Approximately 20% of deceased donor renal transplants have delayed graft function with anuria or oliguria.
    a. Because serious and graft-threatening technical complications (e.g., thrombosis, urine leak) may present with low urine output, this must be a diagnosis of exclusion, and causes of low urine output must be diligently sought and treated.
    b. Causes of low urine output include hypovolemia and hypotension, an occluded Foley catheter, arterial or venous thrombosis, hydronephrosis or urine leak, and antibody-mediated rejection.

F. Surgical complications
1. Urine leak may occur in as many as 10% of cases and is most frequently caused by the poor blood supply to the distal transplant ureter. Urine leak may be diagnosed by biochemical analysis of fluid from the wound or nuclear scan.
    a. Urine leaks in the very early post-transplant period should be treated by surgical revision of the anastomosis.
    b. Urine leaks in the later post-transplant period should be evaluated with cystoscopy/retrograde or percutaneous nephrostogram because such leaks are frequently associated with ureteral stenosis.
2. Lymphoceles are collections of lymph from divided lymphatic vessels along the iliac vessels. Lymphoceles have been reported to occur in as many as 20% of patients.
    a. Many of these collections are small and have no clinical impact. These require no intervention.
    b. Large lymphoceles may cause allograft dysfunction (by compression or hydronephrosis), pain, or deep venous thrombosis (compression of iliac vein). Percutaneous drainage, sometimes combined with sclerotherapy of the cavity, may be adequate treatment. Lymphoceles may recur, and they are treated with internal drainage between lymphocele cavity and the peritoneal cavity (fenestration). Fenestration may be accomplished by either open or laparoscopic approach.

G. Recurrent disease: Many of the diseases that cause end-stage renal disease in the native kidneys may recur in the transplanted kidney (Table 20-3). Recurrent disease does not always lead to allograft loss from recurrent disease.

TABLE 20-3 Renal Diseases and Their Risk of Recurrence	
Renal Disease	**Risk of Recurrence (%)**
Oxalosis	75–100
Membranoproliferative glomerulonephritis (MPGN) type 2	80–100
Hemolytic uremic syndrome (HUS)	40–50
IgA nephritis	40–60
Focal segmental glomerulosclerosis (FSGS)	40–50
Membranoproliferative glomerulonephritis (MPGN) type 1	30–50
Diabetic nephropathy	75–100

TABLE 20-4 Kidney Donor Status and Survival		
Status of Donor	**1-Year Survival**	**5-Year Survival**
Living donor kidney transplant	95%	80%
Deceased donor kidney transplant	90%	65%

H. Long-term outcomes
  1. Current graft survival (dialysis independence) is shown in Table 20-4.
  2. There are no randomized prospective trials comparing chronic dialysis to transplantation.
  3. There are several "intent to treat" studies comparing outcomes of patients on dialysis awaiting transplant and those actually transplanted. After the increased mortality associated with the operation itself, and early higher dose immunosuppression, the survival of transplanted patients is superior to dialysis after 8 months.

II. **Pancreas**
  A. Indications
    1. The majority of pancreas transplants are performed in patients with type I diabetes mellitus. Diabetes mellitus affects nearly 14 million Americans, and it is the sixth leading cause of death (National Center for Health Statistics). It is a leading cause of blindness and renal failure.
    2. Pancreas transplantation is most frequently performed in combination with a kidney transplant (simultaneous pancreas-kidney [SPK] transplant). The pancreas may also be transplanted into nonrenal failure diabetics (pancreas transplant alone [PTA]), or into diabetics with a previous renal transplant (pancreas after kidney [PAK] transplant).
  B. Contraindications
    1. Contraindications for pancreas transplantation are essentially the same as those for kidney transplantation.
    2. Because the incidence of atherosclerotic disease is so high in patients with diabetes, especially in patients with renal failure, an aggressive investigation of coronary and peripheral vascular disease should be performed.
  C. Operation
    1. The pancreas is transplanted with the adjacent duodenum, with which it shares a blood supply. The spleen is separated from the tail of the pancreas prior to transplantation.
    2. There have been multiple techniques of implantation of the pancreas graft. The two main considerations are the location of the vascular anastomoses and the technique of managing exocrine drainage.
    3. The venous (portal) drainage is still most frequently into the systemic circulation (iliac vein or inferior vena cava [IVC]). Several centers advocate drainage directly into the portal venous system (superior mesenteric vein or splenic vein). There is good clinical evidence that portal drainage is associated with a lower incidence of rejection.
    4. Enteric drainage may be either into small bowel (Roux-en-Y or side-to-side anastomosis) or into the urinary bladder.
    5. Bladder drainage is associated with metabolic acidosis, due to obligatory loss of the high pH pancreatic secretions, dehydration, "reflux pancreatitis," cystitis, and bleeding. Monitoring of urinary amylase excretion may aid in the diagnosis of rejection, and the pancreas graft can be biopsied cystoscopically.
    6. A functioning pancreas allograft rapidly establishes euglycemia, and "rebound hypoglycemia" is rare.

D. Long-term outcomes
   1. The potential of normalized glucose control (as reflected by a normal hemo-globin [Hgb] A1C) to prevent the severity and progression of the complications of diabetes has been well demonstrated by the Diabetes Control and Complications Trial (DCCT) (see *New England Journal of Medicine.* 1993; 329[14]).
   2. Successful pancreas transplantation can establish euglycemia and a normalized Hgb A1C. Current data suggest that successful pancreas transplantation can improve peripheral neuropathy and stabilize or even reduce diabetic retinopathy. There is no evidence that successful pancreas transplantation reverses macrovascular disease.

E. Islet transplantation
   1. The whole pancreas transplanted to correct diabetes mellitus contains less than 2% of its mass, the insulin-producing islets of Langerhans. Experimental studies demonstrating that isolated islet transplantation can correct diabetes were published by Lacy and Ballinger more than 30 years ago. Clinical attempts to use islet transplantation had low success rates of marginal durability. The Edmonton Protocol (*New England Journal of Medicine.* 2000;343[3]) is a new immunosuppression protocol that uses daclizumab, tacrolimus, and sirolimus and is steroid-free. Seven consecutive patients were insulin independent, with median follow-up of 1 year.
   2. Islets of Langerhans can be isolated from the pancreas using a combination of mechanical and enzymatic techniques. The isolated islets are injected into a branch of the portal vein in the liver. Islets from two to three donor pancreases are usually needed to achieve sufficient islet mass to correct diabetes.

III. Liver

A. General principles
   1. Indications for liver transplantation include acute hepatic failure and chronic liver failure.
   2. Before the advent of surgery, the 1-year mortality for patients with decompensated liver failure reached more than 50%. Since transplantation has been available, the survival reaches 85% at 1 year and 70% at 5 years.

B. Transplantation for acute liver failure
   1. Acute liver failure is defined as acute decompensation of hepatic function, with the time from onset of jaundice to encephalopathy in less than 8 weeks.
   2. The most common reasons for fulminant liver failure in the United States are acetaminophen (Tylenol) overdose (20%), followed by non-A or non-E hepatitis (also called cryptogenic liver failure) (15%), and drugs (12%).
   3. Presentation and accurate diagnosis begins with a thorough history and physical examination.
      a. Most patients are encephalopathic on presentation, and history can be obtained from the family.
      b. Identify findings of depression and medication overdose.
      c. Additionally, patients may have anorexia and malaise.
      d. Symptoms are suggestive of a viral syndrome.
   4. Prompt treatment includes admission to the intensive care unit with appropriate resuscitation.
      a. Follow liver function tests and chemistries closely.
      b. Initiate lactulose therapy early when patient is encephalopathic.
      c. Treat acetaminophen overdose with N-acetyl cysteine.
      d. Early referral to transplant center is critical for successful outcomes.
   5. King's College and Clichy criteria identify the degree of disease and the appropriate candidates that would benefit from transplantation in a patient with acute hepatic failure.
   6. Research interest: Some centers use artificial liver support systems to bridge a patient to liver transplantation. These are temporary measures.

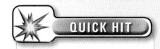

QUICK HIT

Treatment of encephalopathy is critical to prevent the devastating consequence of cerebral edema and herniation. Increased intracerebral pressures and cerebral edema are contraindications for transplantation.

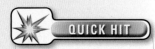

QUICK HIT

Identify the main porto-systemic shunts via the esophageal veins (causing esophageal varices), short gastric veins (causing gastric varices), umbilical vein (causing caput medusae), and rectal veins (causing hemorrhoids).

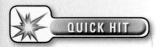

QUICK HIT

The degree of liver dysfunction is determined by the Child–Turcotte–Pugh classification. This scoring system takes into account the degree of ascites, hepatic encephalopathy, serum bilirubin, prothrombin time, and albumin.

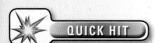

QUICK HIT

Priority on the waiting list is determined by the Model for End-Stage Liver Disease (MELD) score. This involves a complex mathematical equation that places patients with greatest metabolic disturbance higher on the list.

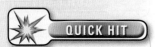

QUICK HIT

With liver transplantation, the donor organ is placed in the same area as the previous diseased liver, and therefore, such a placement is termed orthotopic transplantation. With kidney and pancreas transplantation, the donor organ is placed in the pelvis, and therefore, it is termed heterotopic transplantation.

C. Transplantation for chronic liver failure
  1. In the United States, common reasons for transplantation in a patient with chronic liver failure include alcohol-induced cirrhosis and the myriad of viral hepatitides. Other causes of liver failure include primary sclerosing cholangitis, primary biliary cirrhosis, hepatocellular carcinoma, biliary atresia, metabolic disorders such as hemochromatosis, Wilson disease, and enzymatic deficiencies in the urea cycle.
  2. The pathophysiology of chronic liver failure involves two basic concepts: portal hypertension and hepatocyte damage. The increased portal venous blood flow through the liver results in blood flow via the physiologic portosystemic shunts as a compensatory mechanism to increased portal blood flow. Hepatocyte damage results from insult at a cellular level by the virus or other toxins.
  3. Selection for liver transplantation involves identification of contraindications (HIV, advanced age, disseminated cancer), degree of liver disease, availability of psychosocial support group (to assist in postoperative care), and financial ability (postoperative care requires strict adherence to immunosuppressive regimens that may be expensive).
D. Surgical techniques
  1. Surgery can be especially difficult in a patient who is coagulopathic and has evidence of portal hypertension.
  2. The native liver is mobilized by releasing the attachments from the diaphragm. The portal triad, which includes the bile duct, portal vein, and the hepatic artery, are skeletonized in preparation of the donor organ. The suprahepatic IVC is mobilized. Following this, these structures are clamped and transected, releasing the liver from the bed.
  3. The donor organ is prepared in a similar way, followed by end-to-end anastomosis of the suprahepatic and infrahepatic IVC. The portal vein, hepatic artery, and finally the bile duct anastomosis are completed in that order.
  4. Occasionally, a split liver transplant may be performed in a child, wherein an adult liver cannot be accommodated into the abdomen.
E. Postoperative complications
  1. Bleeding: usually occurs when coagulopathy is not adequately addressed
  2. Primary nonfunction of the liver: This disastrous situation occurs when the liver is unable to function after transplantation. This condition warrants urgent retransplantation.
  3. Reperfusion injury: This scenario is common when the ischemic time on the organ is prolonged. The treatment is primarily supportive.
  4. Vascular complications: Following the hepatic arterial anastomosis, the artery may thrombose, leading to elevations of the transaminases, abscess formation, and biliary tract strictures. This usually results from a technical error.
    a. Acute portal hypertension after transplant should alert the physician to this complication.
    b. Treatment may be angiography with lytic therapy and stenting. Rarely portal vein thrombosis may occur.
  5. Biliary tract stricture: Strictures in the tract occur primarily due to ischemia of the tract. These can be treated with endoscopic retrograde cholangiopancreatography and stent placement.
  6. Rejection: Early rejection can occur if immunosuppressive therapy is not initiated early. The patient may be asymptomatic or may have a rise in the transaminases and bilirubin.
    a. The presence of inflammatory cells and lymphocyte-mediated bile duct injury as seen in the biopsy can be diagnostic. The diagnosis is confirmed by biopsy.
    b. This condition warrants the administration of immunoglobulin or high-dose steroids.
  7. Infection: Most commonly, CMV infection may result. One must always maintain a very low threshold for infection in a post-transplant patient. Workup includes blood, urine, and stool cultures for bacteria, fungi, and viruses.

8. Recurrence of native disease: Patients who are transplanted for hepatitis B and hepatitis C are prone to infecting the donor organ. Primary sclerosing cholangitis, biliary cirrhosis, hemochromatosis, and autoimmune hepatitis may occur in the donor organ.

9. PTLD: As mentioned earlier in the chapter, post-transplant patients may be susceptible to this malignancy.

F. Outcome: Since the advent of transplantation, approximately 10,000 liver transplants have been performed. This population has a 1-year patient survival rate of 90%, and a 5-year patient survival rate of 75%. More importantly, these patients have a dramatic improvement in their quality of life.

IV. Small Bowel

A. The importance of bowel transplantation has been recognized for decades, and yet the first successful transplant was not performed until 1988, in Germany. Very few centers in the United States currently undertake the daunting task of intestinal transplant.

B. Indications for this operation involve cases of short gut (less than 50 cm), intestinal disorders, or malabsorption syndromes. These include Crohn disease, trauma with multiple bowel resections, necrotizing enterocolitis, gastroschisis, and intestinal atresia. It is important to understand that there is no specific disease entity that warrants intestinal transplant.

C. The procedure involves the removal of the donor bowel, maintaining the superior mesenteric artery (SMA) and celiac axis. The transplant is conducted by anastomosis of the SMA to the aorta, with venous drainage into the IVC or the portal vein. The maximal ischemia time for bowel is about 6 hours.

D. Complications are failure of graft, infection, and rejection.

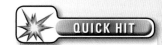
QUICK HIT

Patients who are offered this operation are usually dependent on total parenteral nutrition for life.

Transplantation

Questions

MOCK SHELF EXAMINATION #1

Time Limit: 2 hours 10 minutes

Number of Questions: 100

*Directions: Each of the numbered items or incomplete statements in this section is followed by answers or by completions of the statement. Select the **one** lettered answer or completion that is **best** in each case.*

1. A 29-year-old woman complains of left lower quadrant pain, cramps, and bloody diarrhea. She has been symptomatic for 1 year. She has a 20-lb weight loss. Her primary care physician diagnosed her with irritable bowel syndrome. Physical examination reveals minimal left lower quadrant tenderness. Stool cultures are negative for ova and parasites. What is the most appropriate next step in the management of this patient?
   A. Abdominal X-rays
   B. Repeat stool culture for ova and parasites
   C. Proctoscopy
   D. Small-bowel contrast study
   E. Reassurance

2. A 71-year-old woman in good health complains of anal pain, mucus discharge, and anal incontinence. Physical examination reveals protrusion of the full thickness of the rectum. What is the most appropriate treatment for this patient?
   A. Antibiotics
   B. Low anterior resection with rectopexy
   C. Rectal fixation to sacrum with mesh
   D. Left hemicolectomy with colostomy
   E. Reassurance

3. A 38-year-old man is brought to the emergency department complaining of anorectal pain and drainage of pus and blood. Physical examination reveals swelling and fluctuance in the left anorectal area approximately 2 cm from the anal verge. His white blood cell count is 14,000/mm³. What is the most appropriate treatment for this patient?
   A. Lateral internal sphincterotomy
   B. Stool softeners and sitz baths
   C. Oral antibiotics
   D. Incision and drainage
   E. Rubber band ligation

4. A 47-year-old man with multiple medical problems and recurrent cholecystitis is being considered for laparoscopic cholecystectomy. Physical examination reveals an obese man with right upper quadrant tenderness to palpation. Which of the following is the most significant potential contraindication to this procedure for this patient?
   A. Generalized peritonitis
   B. History of smoking
   C. Hypercholesterolemia
   D. Portal hypertension
   E. Prior history of wound infections

5. A 47-year-old woman with recurrent bouts of acute cholecystitis is hospitalized on the medicine service. Physical examination reveals right upper quadrant pain to palpation. Ultrasound reveals evidence of pericholecystic fluid and gallstones. Which of the following laboratory studies is most likely to be abnormal in this patient?
   A. AST
   B. Amylase
   C. Bilirubin
   D. Lipase
   E. Placental alkaline phosphatase

6. During a routine visit for high blood pressure, a 35-year-old man tells the physician his mother was recently diagnosed with lung cancer. Due to the patient's smoking history, he inquires about screening for lung cancer. He denies any respiratory symptoms. Which of the following is currently recommended as a screening tool for lung cancer?
   A. Computed tomography
   B. Chest X-ray
   C. No tool is recommended for screening.
   D. Serum antidiuretic hormone
   E. Sputum cytology

7. A 55-year-old man with a history of coronary artery disease including three-vessel disease undergoes bypass surgery. Following surgery, which of the following medications has been shown to reduce mortality and risk of ischemic complications and is routinely used after coronary bypass surgery?
   A. Aspirin
   B. Calcium-channel blocker
   C. Clopidogrel + aspirin
   D. Nitrates
   E. Simvastatin

8. A 6-week-old boy presents to the ambulatory care clinic with increasing stridor, wheezing, and occasional respiratory distress. His mother reports that he has been feeding well without vomiting or choking. His birth history is unremarkable with good Apgar scores. There is a family history of asthma. On exam, there is both inspiratory and expiratory stridor and subcostal retractions. A chest X-ray reveals an anterior indentation of the trachea, and an esophagram shows bilateral compression of the esophagus that is maintained during peristalsis. Which of the following is the most likely diagnosis?
   A. Asthma
   B. Infection
   C. Pneumothorax
   D. Tracheoesophageal fistula
   E. Vascular ring

9. A 50-year-old man presents to his physician with an "achy" pain in his right chest aggravated by movement. He also describes the pain being worse at night. On exam, the chest wall appears normal but is tender to palpation over the anterior sixth rib. An MRI of the chest shows a 6-cm mass projecting inward from the chest wall with irregular borders and bony invasion. A biopsy is performed and sent to pathology. Histologically, the tumor is composed of numerous spindle cells with moderate atypia and occasional mitotic figures. The cells do not stain with S100. Which of the following is the most likely diagnosis?
   A. Chondroma
   B. Fibrous dysplasia
   C. Malignant schwannoma
   D. Multiple myeloma
   E. Soft-tissue sarcoma

10. A 35-year-old man presents to the emergency department following a car accident where he sustained chest trauma. On examination and workup, the patient is suspected of having a hemothorax, and a chest tube will be required. Which of the following describes the best location for placement of the tube?

A. Anterior axillary line just below the fourth rib

B. Anterior axillary line just below the 12th rib

C. Midaxillary line just above the fifth rib

D. Midaxillary line just above the eighth rib

E. Midclavicular line just below the ninth rib

11. You are seeing a 52-year-old woman for routine screening. She has no complaints. Her past medical history includes hypertension, type 2 diabetes mellitus, and chronic renal insufficiency. Her surgical history includes open cholecystectomy 20 years prior and laparoscopic appendectomy 7 years prior. Vitals are normal. Physical exam is normal other than a right subcostal Kocher scar and three small laparoscopic incisions, which appear healed. Which statement listed below best defines McBurney point?

A. Two-thirds distance from the left anterior superior iliac spine to the umbilicus

B. Two-thirds distance from the right anterior superior iliac spine to the umbilicus

C. Two thirds distance from the umbilicus to the left anterior superior iliac spine

D. Two-thirds distance from the umbilicus to the right anterior superior iliac spine

12. A 44-year-old woman presents with epigastric pain of sudden onset. She describes it being in a similar location to the gnawing sensation she experiences with meals but worse and "faster." Her current medications include omeprazole, loratadine, and a multivitamin, and she reports a history of *Helicobacter pylori* infection. Physical exam reveals maximal abdominal tenderness in the epigastrium with involuntary guarding. Which action represents the best next step in management?

A. Colonoscopy

B. Computed tomography of the abdomen

C. Esophagogastroduodenoscopy

D. Upright abdominal X-ray

13. A 49-year-old man presents to the emergency department for abdominal pain. He describes worsening crampy pain in his left lower abdomen of 8-hour duration. He had been nauseous with diarrhea for 24 hours. He has a past medical history of hypertension, peptic ulcer disease status post–*Helicobacter pylori* eradication, and history of renal lithiasis. His medications include hydrochlorothiazide, rabeprazole, and over-the-counter MiraLAX. He has never had a colonoscopy. His last renal calculus episode was 19 years prior. Physical exam reveals a febrile, tachycardic male with abdominal tenderness and guarding over his left lower quadrant. Which of the following is the best means of diagnosis?

A. Colonoscopy

B. Computed tomography of the abdomen and pelvis

C. Esophagogastroduodenoscopy

D. No further diagnostics are necessary given this clinical diagnosis.

E. Magnetic resonance imaging

14. A 16-year-old boy presents to the emergency department with right lower quadrant pain. He first noted the onset of pain 10 days prior while doing homework, which worsened over 1 day. He experienced a warm sensation with relief of his pain 2 days after onset. His pain subsided for some time but began to recur 2 days prior to presenting. He noted fever and chills, nausea, and vomiting. Exam reveals a tachycardic, febrile young man in no acute distress. Abdominal exam reveals right lower quadrant tenderness with guarding. CT reveals appendiceal rupture with a walled-off abscess. Which of the following is the ideal treatment given the findings in this patient?

A. Conservative management

B. Interval appendectomy

C. Laparoscopic appendectomy

D. Open appendectomy

15. A 16-year-old boy with unremarkable general and surgical histories is brought to the emergency department by his parents for right-sided abdominal pain. He reports that the pain started 2 hours prior while doing sit-up drills with his cross-country team. He became nauseous and vomited after being picked up by his parents. He reported alleviation of pain sitting upright in the car. Vital signs are normal and stable. Exam reveals a young male in acute distress, with a diffusely tender abdomen without guarding or rebound. His CBC was normal as well. Which of the following is the best first step in attaining a diagnosis?

A. Complete physical examination

B. Computed tomography of the abdomen

C. Magnetic resonance imaging

D. Scrotal ultrasound

E. Upright KUB film

16. An 8-year-old girl with severe pectus excavatum is brought to the clinic by her parents to be evaluated for possible surgical correction. What is a benefit of the Nuss procedure over traditional costal cartilage resection in children?

A. The Nuss procedure avoids impairment in chest wall growth.

B. The Nuss procedure carries less chance of damage to thoracic organs.

C. The Nuss procedure carries significantly lower risk of infection.

D. The Nuss procedure carries significantly lower risk of pneumothorax.

E. The Nuss procedure carries significantly lower risk of recurrence of pectus excavatum.

17. A 3-year-old girl is brought in for evaluation of a neck mass. On physical exam, the child is found to have a soft, compressible mass about 2 cm × 2 cm in size but with poorly defined borders. The mass is located just posterior to the middle of the body of her left sternomastoid muscle. What is the likely cause of this mass?

A. Congenital malformation of lymphatic vessels

B. Failure of obliteration of the thyroglossal duct

C. Failure of resorption of the branchial clefts

D. Lymphoma

E. Torticollis

18. A 6-month-old boy is brought to the clinic for evaluation of a red lesion on his forehead. The mother of the child is concerned because the lesion has been rapidly increasing in size and the infant's maternal grandmother died of melanoma in her 60s. On physical exam, a red, raised lesion about 1 cm × 3 cm with irregular borders can be seen about 3 cm superior to his left eyebrow. What is the best treatment option for this child?

A. Do nothing

B. Embolization

C. Excision with wide margins

D. Laser photocoagulation

E. Systemic corticosteroid therapy

19. A 2-year-old boy is found to have hypertension during a checkup. The child was brought to the clinic because of recurrent fevers. He is in the 10th percentile for weight. A careful abdominal exam reveals a mass. Which of the following is the most likely condition in this child?
    A. Ewing sarcoma
    B. Nephroblastoma
    C. Neuroblastoma
    D. Rhabdomyosarcoma
    E. Teratoma

20. A 3½-year-old boy is brought to the clinic by his father because the father reports feeling "a bump in his belly" while tickling him 2 days ago. The father denies fevers, and he has been otherwise growing normally. He is in the 60th percentile for weight. A hard, golf ball–sized lump can be palpated in his right upper quadrant. Which of the following additional signs may also be seen in this patient?
    A. Aniridia
    B. Clubbed feet
    C. Cryptorchidism
    D. Imperforate anus (has been reported but rare, no known association)
    E. Webbed digits

21. A 39-year-old internist is playing football with his friends when he "rolls" his ankle. He says that he was jumping to catch the ball and came down on his toes with his ankle slightly plantar flexed. He present to the emergency department for evaluation. On exam, his lateral ankle appears swollen and erythematous with prominent bruising. There is no point tenderness, but a positive anterior drawer test of the ankle is done. The anterior drawer test is used to evaluate the stability of which of the following ligaments?
    A. Anterior talofibular ligament
    B. Calcaneofibular ligament
    C. Deep deltoid ligament
    D. Posterior talofibular ligament
    E. Talonavicular ligament

22. A 63-year-old man presents to his primary care physician with back pain, intermittent fevers, and anemia. He says his back pain started approximately 8 months ago and has not been getting better despite treatment with NSAIDs. Radiographs of the spine show a lytic lesion in his thoracic vertebrae. A biopsy of the lesion shows sheets of plasma cells. Which of the following is likely found on laboratory workup of this patient?
    A. Hypocalcemia
    B. Increased monoclonal heavy chain immunoglobulin in urine
    C. Increased monoclonal light chain immunoglobulin in urine
    D. Normal erythrocyte sedimentation rate
    E. Normal serum creatinine

23. An 18-year-old woman presents to the emergency department after being injured in a motor vehicle accident. She was driving the vehicle home from a party when she slid off the road and hit a tree at high speed. She says that during the crash she believes her knee hit the dashboard. She appears anxious and is complaining of right knee pain. On exam, she has an easily identifiable posterior dislocation of her right knee. The skin distal to the injury is warm, and pulses are palpable. Which of the following is the next best step in management?
    A. Administer an anxiolytic.
    B. Administer NSAIDs.
    C. Immediate knee reduction
    D. Perform ankle–brachial or arterial indices.
    E. Plain radiography

24. A previously well 4-year-old boy measuring in the 75th percentile for height and 55th percentile for weight is brought to the physician complaining of right leg and knee pain for the last month. His mother says he has been limping around as well. The mother reports no fever, morning stiffness, or history of trauma. His vital signs are within normal limits. On exam, his right knee is nontender to palpation and has a normal range of motion. Examination of his right hip reveals limited range of motion with hip flexion, abduction, and internal rotation. There is no observable trauma, erythema, or tenderness of the hip joint. Which of the following is the most likely diagnosis?

   A. Legg-Calve-Perthes disease

   B. Osteomyelitis of the hip

   C. Rheumatoid arthritis

   D. Septic arthritis of the knee

   E. Slipped capital femoral epiphysis

25. A 61-year-old man returns for a follow-up appointment for medial knee joint pain and "clicking." Other than mild arthritis, his past medical history is unremarkable. He has already tried nonsteroidal anti-inflammatory medications and physical therapy for his knee pain, and at his last appointment, he received an intra-articular steroid injection and reports no improvement of his symptoms. An MRI of his knee joint shows a medial meniscus tear and chondrosis of the underlying bone. Which of the following is the next best treatment?

   A. Arthroscopic partial meniscectomy

   B. Continued NSAID use and observation

   C. Intra-articular viscosupplementation

   D. Observation alone

   E. Total knee replacement

26. A 67-year-old woman undergoes upper endoscopy secondary to chronic dyspepsia, epigastric pain, weight loss, and melena. Endoscopic exploration reveals multiple small ulcerative erosions, one larger than the remainder. You biopsy all ulcers and obtain a CLO test. The subsequent pathology report indicates chronic gastritis and the presence of *Helicobacter pylori*. The largest lesion appears as a "dense infiltrate of lymphocytes in the lamina propria with reactive B-cell follicles," and immunohistochemical staining is positive for CD19 and CD20. Which of the following is the most appropriate management for this patient?

   A. PET scan to determine extent of disease

   B. Radiation therapy

   C. Repeat endoscopic biopsy based on improper collection site

   D. Surgical resection of underlying malignancy

   E. Treatment of underlying infectious process

27. A 35-year-old male bariatric patient who underwent Roux-en-Y gastric bypass 9 weeks prior presents for follow-up. Today, he has a new complaint of sweating, light-headedness, and chills with every meal. He seems disturbed when he informs you that during the last occurrence, he fainted while rushing to the bathroom to vomit. Which of the following is the most likely diagnosis?

   A. Anastomotic ulceration with subsequent leakage

   B. Conversion disorder

   C. Dumping syndrome

   D. Partial small bowel obstruction

28. A 54-year-old overweight man with a history of hypertension, obstructive sleep apnea, and type 2 diabetes mellitus presents with chronic complaints of reflux, belching, and excessive salivation with meals. His current medications include metformin, hydrochlorothiazide, and a multivitamin. He underwent laparoscopic cholecystectomy at 48 years old. He has no smoking history and drinks four to five beers on weekends. Which pharmacologic action is the mechanism of action for the most appropriate therapy for this patient?

A. Decreased production of prostaglandins via inhibition of COX-1 and COX-2 enzymes

B. Formation of a viscous gel along the gastric lining for protection against ulceration

C. Histaminergic antagonist that decreases volume and concentration of gastric acid

D. Irreversible blocking of the H^+/K^+-ATPase exchange pump at the gastric parietal cell

E. Synthetic prostaglandin analogue that decreases acid secretion and increases bicarbonate secretion

29. A 45-year-old man presents to his primary care physician for his annual follow-up. He has a past medical history of GERD, hypertension, and hypercholesterolemia. He underwent an indirect hernia repair 14 years prior. He brings with him outpatient laboratory results obtained earlier this week, pertinent for a hemoglobin of 9.7 but otherwise normal. His stool guaiac test obtained today is positive. Review of systems reveals the onset of dark tarry stools 6 months prior. Assuming that an upper GI bleed is the cause, which is the most common cause of a GI bleed in a 45-year-old man?

A. Gastric adenocarcinoma

B. GERD

C. Epistaxis

D. Low-dose daily aspirin

E. Peptic ulcer disease

30. A 61-year-old obese woman is referred to the clinic for refractory GERD. Her symptoms include dysphagia, heartburn, and nausea and have been consistent for 4 years. She has tried a host of over-the-counter and prescription medications without relief. She reports a pertinent family history of gastric adenocarcinoma, and you therefore recommend an upper endoscopy screening, during which you note several polypoid lesions throughout the gastric mucosa. Pathology results from your thorough biopsies indicate hyperplastic polyps. Which of the following is true regarding hyperplastic polyps of the stomach?

A. Rates of concurrent adenocarcinoma are as high as 20%.

B. They are commonly associated with familial polyposis syndromes.

C. Resolution occurs with successful eradication of *H. pylori*.

D. They are associated with a large artery that erodes the mucosa and causes massive hematemesis and hypovolemia.

E. Nitrate consumption is a risk factor for their development.

31. An 8 year-old boy is referred to the ambulatory care clinic with long-standing worsening headache over 1 year, dizziness, and a recent onset of frequent falling episodes. A CT obtained by an outside neurologist showed an enhancing mass located immediately adjacent to the fourth ventricle. Which of the following is the most appropriate first treatment option?

A. Chemotherapy

B. Palliative chemoradiation

C. Radiotherapy

D. Surgical resection

32. A 2-hour-old female neonate is examined in the nursery following delivery. She and her mother had been followed with serial ultrasounds for a maternal history of neural tube defects. Physical exam of this infant reveals an abnormal tuft of skin at the sacral area overlying herniated meninges and neural tissue. Which of the following is the most likely diagnosis?

A. Anencephaly

B. Arnold-Chiari deformity

C. Myelomeningocele

D. Spina bifida occulta

33. On your pediatrics rotation, you enter the room of a pleasant 3-year-old girl on a well-child visit. Her immunizations are up to date, and her mother reports that she has been healthy and has demonstrated normal milestones. You briefly review her growth charts, which appear normal also. Her physical exam is normal. Funduscopy reveals no papilledema. She has a right-sided eye droop, and her left pupil appears dilated relative to the right. Which of the following is the most likely diagnosis?

  A. Horner syndrome

  B. Left-sided acoustic neuroma

  C. Medulloblastoma

  D. Prolactinoma

  E. Right-sided facial nerve palsy

34. A 64-year-old woman presents to your clinic extremely anxious. Her brother has recently passed away due to autosomal dominant polycystic kidney disease (ADPKD), similar to her father and paternal grandmother. She is extremely concerned that she will suffer a similar fate. She has a benign medical history and a normal abdominal exam. Labs reveal a normal serum creatinine and urea. Urinalysis reveals no gross or microscopic hematuria. Renal ultrasound reveals normal-appearing, noncystic kidneys. Had she had been diagnosed with ADPKD, which of the following neurosurgical episodes is most likely to be seen in this patient?

  A. Epidural hemorrhage

  B. Subdural hemorrhage

  C. Subarachnoid hemorrhage

  D. Intraventricular hemorrhage

35. A 76-year-old woman is brought to the emergency department from her assisted-living residence due to altered mental status. She has multiple chronic medical morbidities. Her nursing staff noticed confusion 1 day prior to admission, and somnolence starting 8 hours prior. Vitals include a temperature of 39°C, heart rate of 110 bpm, and blood pressure of 105/80 mm Hg. Physical exam reveals a supine elderly woman not responsive to verbal commands but moaning and withdrawing in response to nuchal flexion. A spinal MRI obtained by emergency room physicians demonstrates an epidural fluid collection surrounded by inflammation with some enhancement. What is the most common cause of this patient's condition?

  A. Local spread of infection from an epidural procedure

  B. Lumbar disk herniation

  C. Hematogenous spread of infection

  D. Malignant process of the spinal canal

  E. Meningococcal vaccination reaction

36. A 61-year-old woman presents to the emergency department with acute abdominal pain and general malaise. She has been experiencing fevers with shaking chills for the past 12 hours, in addition to her constant abdominal pain. Her vitals are temperature 38.9°C, heart rate 113 bpm, blood pressure 105/60 mm Hg, and respiratory rate 19 breaths/min. On exam, she appears anxious. Her eyes are sunken, and her mucous membranes appear dry. Her abdomen is distended, guarded, and tender to palpation in the upper abdomen. Her labs show an elevated WBC count, as well as a lactic acid of 2.4 mmol/L. She is sent off for a CT scan, which shows air in the gallbladder. What is the best next management step?

  A. Laparoscopic cholecystectomy

  B. Percutaneous cholecystostomy

  C. Intravenous fluid bolus

  D. Broad-spectrum antibiotics

  E. Endoscopic retrograde cholangiopancreatography

37. A 47-year-old man presents to the emergency department with new-onset somnolence. He was previously healthy but over the last few days became progressively fatigued. He developed upper abdominal "cramping" over this time, which has been worsening in severity. His wife said he had a temperature of 101.2°F before she brought him in. His temperature is 38.7°C, heart rate 104 bpm, and blood pressure 103/53 mm Hg. On exam, he appears somnolent and jaundiced. His abdomen is guarded and nondistended. He grimaces when his upper abdomen is palpated, especially on the right side. His CBC shows a WBC count of 15.2 g and a HCT of 41%. A CMP is obtained, showing a total bilirubin of 8.2 mg/dL and alkaline phosphatase of 350 U/L. What is the best treatment for this condition?

A. Intravenous fluids and intravenous antibiotics alone

B. Intravenous fluids, intravenous antibiotics, and laparoscopic cholecystectomy

C. Intravenous fluids, intravenous antibiotics, and open cholecystectomy

D. Intravenous fluids, intravenous antibiotics, and endoscopic retrograde cholangiopancreatography

E. Intravenous fluids and endoscopic retrograde cholangiopancreatography

38. A 41-year-old man presents to his primary care physician with recent weight loss. He has lost 10 lb in the last 2 months, which he finds strange as "my bowels haven't flared up in 4 years." He also complains of some pruritus, which has come on rather insidiously. On review of systems, he declines any fevers, pain, shortness of breath, nausea, vomiting, or diarrhea. But he does recall that he has been feeling "tired lately." He is afebrile, and his vital signs are stable. On physical exam, he appears healthy and in no distress. He does not appear jaundiced, but there is some mild scleral icterus. The rest of his physical exam is unremarkable. Blood tests are ordered, which reveal an unremarkable CBC. But his CMP does show an elevated alkaline phosphatase and a total bilirubin of 4.7 mg/dL. Based on his history of inflammatory bowel disease, the primary care physician sends the patient to get a magnetic resonance cholangiopancreatography (MRCP) to evaluate him for possible primary sclerosing cholangitis (PSC). What anatomic finding on MRCP is characteristic of PSC?

A. Bile duct has alternating areas of dilation and stricture, appearing beaded.

B. Proximal bile duct is dilated, and distal bile duct is narrow.

C. Dilation of common bile duct and pancreatic duct (double duct sign)

D. Dilated common bile duct with filling defects within the duct

E. Ectasia of pancreatic duct branches

39. A 64-year-old woman presents to her family physician with chronic upper abdominal pain. She is not sure when it started but gradually she has noticed the pain more over the past 2 weeks. In addition, she has lost 20 lb unintentionally in the last 3 months. On exam, she is found to have a palpable abdominal mass in the right upper quadrant. Her labs are unremarkable. An abdominal CT scan shows a mass in the gallbladder, and she is diagnosed with a gallbladder tumor. Further imaging is performed, which does not show any distant metastases. An open cholecystectomy is performed, and the gallbladder is sent for frozen section. The results show gallbladder adenocarcinoma, with tumor invasion into the perimuscular fibrous tissue. What is the next step in treatment?

A. No further treatment required.

B. Biopsy of the sentinel lymph node (Calot node)

C. Extended resection of adjacent liver tissue with a 2-cm margin with lymphadenectomy

D. Extended resection of adjacent liver tissue with a 1-cm margin only

E. Extended resection of adjacent liver tissue with a 1-cm margin with lymphadenectomy

40. A 57-year-old woman presents to the emergency department with jaundice. She was previously healthy but over the last months became progressively jaundiced. She developed upper abdominal "cramping" over the past 2 weeks, which has been worsening in severity. She took her temperature at home today and found it to be 102°F. Her temperature in the emergency department is 38.9°C, heart rate 91 bpm, and blood pressure 123/73 mm Hg. On exam, she appears anxious. Her abdomen is soft and nondistended, but she is tender and guards when her upper abdomen is palpated, especially on the right side. Her CBC shows a WBC count of 10.2 g and a hematocrit of 41%. A CMP is obtained, showing a total bilirubin of 6.2 mg/dL and alkaline phosphatase of 290 U/L. What is the initial diagnostic test of choice?

A. Abdominal CT scan

B. Endoscopic retrograde cholangiopancreatography

C. Magnetic resonance cholangiopancreatography

D. Hepatobiliary iminodiacetic acid scan

E. Right upper quadrant ultrasound

41. A 62-year-old woman undergoes mammography to investigate a mass discovered on breast exam in the upper outer quadrant of her left breast. She has a variety of questions, including further workup and possible treatment options. Which of the following patients with breast cancer would be the best candidate for hormonal therapy?

A. A 34-year-old whose mother, maternal grandmother, and aunt all developed breast cancer

B. A 57-year-old man with no family history of breast cancer

C. A 58-year-old woman with an ER/PR positive tumor

D. A woman with *BRCA-1* mutation

E. A woman with *BRCA-2* mutation

42. A 68-year-old man complains of a lump that has been growing larger over the past few months. Which of the following features, if found, would suggest benign disease such as gynecomastia rather than cancer?

A. Fixation of mass to chest wall

B. Pain on palpation

C. Ulceration

D. Unilateral lesion

E. All of the above suggest cancer.

43. A 15-year-old young man complains of bilateral, tender breast enlargement first noticed 5 months ago. He is originally concerned that he may be developing breast cancer but is reassured by explanations that gynecomastia is much more likely. Which of the following would be the best treatment if he indeed has gynecomastia?

A. Chemotherapy

B. Duct drainage with fine-needle aspiration

C. Hormone therapy

D. Simple mastectomy

E. No intervention is necessary.

44. A 68-year-old woman who underwent a right modified radical mastectomy 10 years previously for breast cancer presents with a hard mass on her right anterior chest. On physical exam, a 0.8 cm × 0.6 cm lump is found in the midclavicular line at the level of the third rib of her right chest. The lump is firmly adherent to her chest wall. Which of the following would be the best next course of action?

A. Chemotherapy

B. Hormone therapy trial

C. Radiation therapy

D. Surgical removal of the lump and right pectoralis major muscle

E. No intervention is necessary.

45. A lump is discovered in the lower outer quadrant of a 47-year-old woman during a routine clinical exam. Mammography followed by fine-needle aspiration (FNA) confirms malignancy. Which of the following is the best prognostic indicator for this patient?

A. Axillary node status

B. Cellular appearance on FNA

C. Findings on mammography

D. Percentage of weight change in past 3 months

E. Tumor size

46. A 35-year-old black man has a small benign mole removed from his upper ear lobe. Six months later, he presents with a large, rubbery hypertrophic mass of tissue that appears to be invading the surrounding tissue. Biopsy shows wide bands and bundles of collagen in an unordered arrangement with brightly eosinophilic and glassy-appearing fibers. The edge of the tissue appears "tongue-like" and is pushing underneath the epidermis. There are horizontally arranged fibrous bands in the upper reticular dermis. Which of the following is the most likely diagnosis?

A. Basal cell carcinoma

B. Chronic folliculitis

C. Dermatofibroma

D. Hypertrophic scar

E. Keloid scar

47. A 35-year-old man presents to the emergency department following contact with a high-tension electrical power line while trying to fix his satellite dish. On exam, there is an entrance wound visible on the patient's right hand and an exit wound visible on his right upper arm. The patient is stabilized in the emergency room and scheduled for surgical debridement. Which of the following medications may this patient require to avoid renal failure?

A. Aluminum chloride

B. Dopamine

C. Epinephrine

D. Mannitol

E. Oxacillin

48. A 25-year-old woman comes to the physician because she is concerned about one of her "freckles" on her shoulder. She says that she has many freckles but that this one in particular has changed over the last several months with increased size and color changes. On exam, there are multiple small, pigmented lesions over her torso. On her left shoulder there is a larger, 1.8 cm in diameter, pigmented lesion that is asymmetrically shaped and has irregular borders. Which of the following is the next best step in management?

A. Application of 5FU

B. Excisional biopsy

C. Observation

D. Punch biopsy

E. Shave biopsy

49. A 50-year-old man who enjoys surfing presents with a lesion over the left forehead. The patient reports that it has been growing slowly over the last several years. On exam, there is a raised and waxy 1.3-cm skin mass over the left forehead. There is no lymphadenopathy, and the remainder of the exam is unremarkable. Which of the following is the most likely diagnosis?

A. Basal cell carcinoma

B. Congenital melanocytic nevus

C. Melanoma

D. Sarcoma

E. Squamous cell carcinoma

50. A 67-year-old retired businessman presents to the physician with a painful "nodule" on his lower lip that has not gone away despite home care with naturopathic remedies. He has a long history of smoking and reports that he enjoys golfing and drinking alcohol. On exam, there is a 0.7 cm × 0.5 cm lesion with central ulceration on his outer lower lip. Which of the following is the next best step in management?

A. Punch biopsy

B. Application of topical 5-fluorouracil

C. Shave biopsy

D. Observation

E. Topical antibiotics

51. A 32-year-old woman complains of frequent bruising. She reports that this bruising has been worsening over the last several months. Her physical exam is remarkable for several large areas of ecchymosis. After an exhaustive workup, the patient is diagnosed with immune thrombocytopenic purpura (ITP) and started on corticosteroids, intravenous immunoglobulin, and rituximab for 4 weeks. After several months of therapy with these medications and several others, her platelets fail to respond. Which of the following is the next best treatment for this patient?

A. Aspirin

B. Cyclophosphamide

C. Platelet transfusion

D. Rho(D) immunoglobulin

E. Surgery

52. A 30-year-old man with a history of intravenous drug use and endocarditis presents with fever and worsening abdominal pain. The patient localizes the pain to the upper left quadrant. On physical exam, there is mild splenomegaly and tenderness with guarding on the upper left abdomen. There is also mild dullness to percussion on the left lung base. A chest radiograph shows a left pleural effusion and elevated left hemidiaphragm. A CT scan shows several low-density, nonenhancing, and multiloculated lesions located within the spleen. Blood cultures grow multiple organisms. What is the best treatment option for this patient?

A. Broad-spectrum antibiotics and percutaneous drainage

B. CT-guided diagnostic percutaneous aspiration

C. Intravenous support and broad-spectrum antibiotics

D. Splenectomy and broad-spectrum antibiotics

E. Splenic artery embolization

53. A 55-year-old man with a long history of alcoholism presents with poor sleep, decreased appetite, loss of interest in hobbies, poor concentration, and lack of pleasure in activities he normally enjoys for the last 3 months. He reports that 6 weeks ago, he saw a psychiatrist who diagnosed him with clinical depression, and he was started on a selective serotonin reuptake inhibitor. On today's visit, he reports no improvement with his symptoms despite strict adherence to his medication regimen. He also complains of a new remitting and recurring painful swelling over the veins in his arms and legs. The patient's physical exam reveals a 10-lb weight loss since his last visit, along with mildly yellow skin. Which of the following is the most likely diagnosis?

A. Clinical depression

B. Hypothyroidism

C. Paget disease

D. Pancreatic cancer

E. Substance-induced depression

54. A 50-year-old obese man presents with painless jaundice and unexplained weight loss. His social history is remarkable for chronic alcoholism and a 40-pack year smoking history. His other medical problems include diabetes mellitus. He has a family history of multiple endocrine neoplasia type 1. Which of the following is not a risk factor for pancreatic cancer?

A. Alcohol

B. Diabetes mellitus

C. Multiple endocrine neoplasia type 1

D. Obesity

E. Smoking

55. A 70-year-old homeless man with a history of chronic alcoholism presents with severe pain in his upper belly that started several hours prior. He characterizes the pain as "10/10," with a "stabbing" quality and radiation to the back. His serum lipase and amylase are greatly elevated. Which of the following physical exam findings are associated with severe necrotizing pancreatitis?

A. Chronic papulovesicular eruptions on the extensor surfaces

B. Edema and bruising in the subcutaneous tissue around the umbilicus

C. Enlarged nodule in the left supraclavicular fossa

D. Palpable nodule bulging into the umbilicus

E. Visible swollen venous vessels that resolve and appear around the body

56. A 62-year-old man undergoes a triple coronary artery bypass graft. In order to monitor his cardiac output, a pulmonary artery catheter is inserted. The PCWP on the catheter reads 10 mm Hg. With which value does this measurement most closely correlate?

A. Inferior vena cava pressure

B. Left atrial pressure

C. Right atrial pressure

D. Right ventricular pressure during diastole

E. Right ventricular pressure during systole

57. A 74-year-old woman undergoes a partial nephrectomy for a tumor suspicious for renal cell carcinoma. During the night, the nurse calls to say that her heart rate is 112 bpm and blood pressure is 88/40 mm Hg and in distress. On physical examination, you find normal heart sounds; normal breath sounds; cold, clammy skin; and distended neck veins. From which type of shock is she most likely suffering?

A. Cardiogenic

B. Hypovolemic

C. Neurogenic

D. Obstructive

E. Septic

58. A 33-year-old morbidly obese man presents with 8 hours of worsening fever and chills following 5 days of a red, swollen, left lower extremity. He had tripped and cut his knee on a brick staircase outside his home and has not yet seen a doctor. Past medical history is significant for poorly controlled type 2 diabetes. His blood pressure is 86/42 mm Hg, and his pulse is 122 bpm. His skin is warm and flushed. From which type of shock is he most likely suffering?

A. Cardiogenic

B. Hypovolemic

C. Neurogenic

D. Obstructive

E. Septic

59. A 65-year-old, 60-kg woman undergoes a hemicolectomy for diverticulitis. Postoperatively, she exhibits poor respiratory drive and must remain intubated. Crackles are heard bilaterally. An arterial blood gas shows pH is 7.41, $PaCO_2$ is 41 mm Hg, PaO_2 is 110 mm Hg, and bicarbonate is 24 mEq/L. Current ventilator settings are 14 breaths/min, tidal volume 500 mL, PEEP is 5 mm Hg, and FiO_2 is 0.5. Which ventilator setting should be increased?

A. Breathing rate

B. FiO_2

C. PEEP

D. Tidal volume

E. No changes are necessary.

60. A 48-year-old morbidly obese man undergoes a penectomy for intractable cellulitis. His weight was decreased by 23 kg, and he is placed on a low-calorie diabetic diet. What is the best way to measure adequate protein intake in this patient?

A. Calculate protein content of food.

B. Daily weights

C. Hemoglobin level

D. Prealbumin level

E. Urinary urea nitrogen level

61. A 30-year-old woman presents with nausea, vomiting, chronic diarrhea, and frequent abdominal pain following meals. She reports she has been to many physicians in the past but has not yet been successful in controlling her symptoms. Laboratory studies show positive antiendomysial antibodies. Which of the following disease processes would be unlikely to be associated with this patient's condition?

A. Anemia

B. Increased risk of miscarriage

C. Lymphoma of small intestine

D. Sarcoma of the small intestine

E. Subfertility

62. A 24-year-old man presents with an 8-month history of diarrhea, malaise, recurrent abdominal pain, and occasional fevers. On physical exam, there is tenderness to palpation of the lower quadrants of the abdomen without rebound or guarding. Oral ulcers are noted on the physical exam. An upper gastrointestinal series shows a stenotic segment of small bowel in the ileum. Laboratory studies show:
Hemoglobin: 12.1 g/dL
Leukocytes: 13,000/mm^3
Albumin: 2.5 g/dL
C-reactive protein: elevated

The patient undergoes surgery with resection of the involved segment of small bowel. Which of the following is the most likely diagnosis?

A. Adenocarcinoma of the small intestine

B. Celiac disease

C. Crohn disease

D. Gastritis

E. Ulcerative colitis

63. A 45-year-old man presents with a 3-month history of epigastric pain. He describes the pain as dull, achy, and intermittent and states that it occasionally wakes him up at night. The pain does not radiate and has not changed in character since the onset. He admits that the pain is exacerbated by coffee intake but reports that eating seems to temporarily help the pain. He denies weight loss, vomiting, fever, chills, or gross blood in his stools. He does not drink alcohol or smoke. On physical exam, there is mild epigastric tenderness with palpation. There is no rebound or guarding. Which of the following is the most likely diagnosis?

   A. Crohn disease
   B. Duodenal ulcer
   C. Esophageal spasm
   D. Gastric ulcer
   E. Pancreatitis

64. A 3-day-old infant that was initially feeding well after birth presents with bilious vomiting, abdominal distention, and irritability. On exam, the patient has a palpable right upper quadrant mass and the abdomen appears distended. A barium enema reveals an acute tapering of bowel with a "bird beak" appearance and proximal dilation of small bowel. The infant is diagnosed with a midgut volvulus and emergently taken to the operating room. During the operation, it is noted that there is a 2-cm segment of dusky small bowel. The volvulus is repaired and blood flow restored to the area. Unfortunately, the viability of the bowel segment cannot be determined intraoperatively. Which of the following is the next best step in management?

   A. Close the patient and closely monitor for signs of peritonitis.
   B. Close the patient and provide nasogastric suction, antibiotics, and continued intravenous support.
   C. Close the patient, provide support, and repeat examination of the bowel in 12 to 36 hours.
   D. Remove the entire small bowel.
   E. Remove the portion of small bowel.

65. A 35-year-old woman with a recent diagnosis of valvular heart disease complains of flushing, vague abdominal pain, and watery diarrhea. A carcinoid tumor is suspected. Which of the following is the best initial test for diagnosis?

   A. 24-hour urine test for 5-HIAA
   B. Abdominal ultrasound
   C. Computed tomography imaging of the head
   D. Measurement of serum niacin levels
   E. Radionucleotide scan with octreotide

66. A 52-year-old man presents to his primary care physician for an annual physical examination. He has a new complaint of profound watery diarrhea, which started 2 months ago. He denies any blood or mucus in the stool. He also complains of skin flushing during bouts of diarrhea, which he never had before. On review of systems, he denies fevers and weight loss; he has some nausea with no vomiting and with no abdominal pain. A thorough physical exam shows no abdominal tenderness. A rectal exam is performed, which yields a normal prostate and nontender rectum. His stool is negative for occult blood. What is the most likely diagnosis?

   A. Carcinoid tumor
   B. Tropical sprue
   C. Bacterial gastroenteritis
   D. VIPoma
   E. Surreptitious laxative abuse

67. A 48-year-old woman presents to her physician with a new rash on her buttocks. She also complains of losing 20 lb over the past 3 months and feeling "a little off." On examination, the rash appears as an area of erythematous blisters on her lower buttocks down into her perineal region, along with some swelling of the area. Her blood tests show an elevated blood glucose level of 1,040 mg/dL as well as a hemoglobin of 8.4 g/dL. Your first concern is that her symptoms may be caused by a neoplasm. What is the origin of this neoplasm?

   A. Pancreatic alpha cell
   B. Zona fasciculata
   C. Pancreatic acini
   D. Adrenal medulla
   E. Pancreatic delta cell

68. A 62-year-old man presents with a chief complaint of a 4-month history of intermittent diarrhea and light-headedness. On further questioning, he reveals the symptoms are episodic in nature. He also complains of skin flushing and occasional "asthma attacks" during these episodes. On review of systems, he has a 15-lb weight loss, even though he has been "eating more than ever." His physical exam shows no abnormalities. On his laboratory results, he is found to have an albumin of 2.5 mg/dL and an INR of 1.8. His 24-hour urine is negative for VMA and is positive for the presence of 5-HIAA. In this condition, which amino acid is in highest demand?

   A. Alanine
   B. Tyrosine
   C. Tryptophan
   D. Threonine
   E. Histidine

69. A 57-year-old woman presents to the emergency department with acute abdominal pain and distension. She has vomited two times since she arrived and has not had a bowel movement in 2 days, which she says is "way behind schedule." She is diagnosed with a small bowel obstruction and is scheduled for surgery. In the operating room, the surgeon identifies a large duodenal tumor, which he sends to pathology for an intraoperative frozen section. The tumor is identified as a carcinoid tumor. What is the surgical treatment of choice for carcinoid tumor?

   A. Local excision only
   B. Pancreaticoduodenectomy
   C. Segmental intestinal resection
   D. Wide excision of bowel and mesentery
   E. Local excision and mesenteric lymph node dissection

70. A 62-year-old man presents to his primary care physician with a chief complaint, "I get all flushed and have trouble breathing sometimes." Upon further questioning, he describes a 2-month history of episodic wheezing and skin flushing. He also complains of diarrhea, which did not improve even though he tried to increase his dietary fiber. His physical exam is normal, as are his CBC and BMP. On further workup, he has a 24-hour urine study that is negative for VMA but is positive for the presence of 5-HIAA. What is the best medical treatment for his condition?

   A. Labetalol
   B. Phenoxybenzamine and atenolol
   C. Diphenhydramine
   D. Diphenhydramine and atenolol
   E. Octreotide

71. A 55-year-old obese and multiparous woman presents with urinary incontinence that is "quite stressful." She says that she has to wear pads to avoid embarrassment. She admits that she leaks a small amount of urine each time she coughs, sneezes, and laughs. She denies frequency, urgency, or dysuria. A genitourinary exam reveals a hypermobile urethra and urine loss with cough. After a thorough workup, the patient is diagnosed with pure stress incontinence. Which of the following initial treatment is most appropriate for this patient?

A. Intermittent catheterization and diet modification

B. Oxybutynin

C. Pelvic floor exercise, weight loss, and bladder training

D. Sacral nerve stimulation and anticholinergic medication

E. Vaginal sling

72. A 31-year-old man presents with a painless right testicular mass. He reports that it has been growing over the last several months. On exam, there is small but palpable, hard, nonmobile mass on the inferior right testicle. His serum placental alkaline phosphatase is increased. The tumor is excised and sent for pathologic examination. Gross examination of the tissue reveals a yellow, uniform, and well-circumscribed bulging mass. Histologic examination reveals sheets of uniform large cells with abundant cytoplasm and minimal mitotic figures. Which of the following is the most likely diagnosis?

A. Gonadoblastoma

B. Leydig tumor

C. Seminoma

D. Sertoli cell tumor

E. Teratoma

73. A 26-year-old man presents to the emergency department with severe right scrotal pain. The pain started when he was playing basketball an hour earlier and has been progressing since. He admits that he was recently on a business trip where he had a new sexual partner. His temperature is 102.5°F, blood pressure 130/85 mm Hg, pulse 100 bpm, and respirations 20 breaths/min. On exam, his left testicle appears swollen and erythematous. It is also tender to palpation. Urinalysis reveals increased leukocytes. Which of the following is the next best step in management?

A. Ceftriaxone

B. Observation

C. Scrotal biopsy

D. Testicular ultrasound

E. Urine culture

74. A 23-year-old man presents with fever and testicular pain that has been progressing over the last several days. His temperature is 38.1°C, blood pressure 120/80 mm Hg, pulse 89 bpm, and respirations 18 breaths/min. On exam, his right testicle appears swollen and is tender to palpation. He is subsequently diagnosed with viral orchitis. Which of the following is the best management for this patient?

A. Bed rest, hot/cold packs, and scrotal elevation

B. Ceftriaxone

C. Doxycycline

D. Acyclovir

E. Ganciclovir

75. A newborn infant presents for checkup after a nurse noticed an abnormal-appearing penis on the newborn exam. He was found to have a short phallus with the urethral meatus located on the dorsal penile shaft. Which of the following medical conditions is associated with the same embryologic defect?

A. Bladder exstrophy

B. Cryptorchidism

C. Ectopic scrotum

D. Hypospadias

E. Penile agenesis

76. A 60-year-old woman presents with progressive swelling in her thigh. Her vitals are stable, and she does not have any other symptoms. After a thorough physical exam and workup, a femoral hernia is diagnosed. An elective repair of the femoral hernia is scheduled. During surgery, which of the following is the most likely space in which a femoral hernia will be identified?

A. Between the femoral artery and vein

B. Between the femoral nerve and artery

C. Between the femoral vein and lymphatics

D. Rectovesical pouch

E. Retropubic space

77. A 75-year-old man with a history of advanced prostate cancer and dysfunctional bladder undergoes a cystoprostatectomy and cutaneous conduit diversion. Following the surgery, the patient develops a parastomal hernia. Which of the following surgical methods greatly reduces parastomal hernia occurrence?

A. Generous size of the stomal incision

B. Placing stoma lateral to the rectus sheath

C. Tension suturing

D. Utilizing large bowel

E. Utilizing small bowel

78. A 47-year-old man with cirrhosis secondary to chronic and ongoing alcoholism presents with worsening abdominal distention and a new umbilical hernia. His temperature is 36.9°C, blood pressure 146/85 mm Hg, pulse 70 bpm, and respirations 18 breaths/min. On physical exam, there is an enlarged firm and nodular liver. A shifting fluid wave can be percussed within the abdomen. A large umbilical hernia is apparent with skin ulceration and necrosis over the hernia and around the umbilicus. Which of the following is the next best step in management?

A. Intravenous hydration, broad-spectrum antibiotics, and observation

B. Emergent liver transplantation

C. Primary umbilical hernia repair

D. Umbilical hernia repair with peritovenous shunt

E. Reassurance

79. A 52-year-old woman presents to the emergency room with colicky abdominal pain and a left lower quadrant bulge that is difficult to reduce. She reports not having a bowel movement for the last several days. After a thorough workup involving CT imaging of her abdomen, she is diagnosed with a Spigelian hernia. Which of the following describes the path of a Spigelian hernia?

A. Between the internal oblique and transversus abdominis muscle, anterior to the external oblique aponeurosis

B. Between the internal oblique and transversus abdominis muscle, posterior to the external oblique aponeurosis

C. Medial to the inferior epigastric vessels

D. Lateral to the inferior epigastric vessels

E. Through the obturator canal

80. Which of the following structures separate the boundaries of a direct and indirect inguinal hernia?

A. Cooper ligament

B. Inferior epigastric vessels

C. Inguinal ligament

D. Rectus abdominis muscle

E. Superficial epigastric artery

81. A 25-year-old man is shot in the chest during an altercation on the freeway after he failed to use his turn signal. He arrives complaining of moderate shortness of breath. His blood pressure is 115/70 mm Hg, pulse 103 bpm, and respirations are 20 breaths/min. On exam, there is a single bullet hole in the outer left chest with an exit wound just lateral to the scapula. There are no breath sounds on the left lung base, and the left chest base is dull to percussion. A chest X-ray shows obliteration of the costophrenic angle on the left side. A chest tube is placed, which immediately drains 200 mL of blood. Although the patient's vitals remain stable, another 50 mL of blood is recovered over the next hour. Which of the following is the next best step in management?

A. Close observation and continued drainage

B. CT scan of the chest

C. Emergent bedside thoracotomy

D. Exploratory thoracotomy in the operating room

E. Ventilation perfusion scan

82. A 32-year-old man is involved in a head-on high-speed automobile collision. He is unconscious immediately after the accident but briefly regains consciousness during the ambulance ride to a large trauma center. On arrival to the emergency department, he is now comatose. He is intubated and started on intravenous hydration. Examination shows a fixed and dilated right pupil. Which of the following is the next best step in management?

A. Administer mannitol

B. CT scan of the head

C. Induce hypoventilation

D. MRI imaging

E. Neurosurgical consultation and emergent craniotomy

83. A 23-year-old college student is stabbed in the neck during an argument with a roommate. He arrives in the emergency department complaining of difficulty speaking and coughing up blood. He appears confused. His blood pressure is 130/75 mm Hg, pulse 107 bpm, and respirations 19 breaths/min. Examination of his neck shows a penetrating wound just superior and left of the cricoid cartilage with the knife still in place. Over the course of the trauma exam in the triage bed, a lump forms next to the wound that seems to be pulsating and expanding. An airway is immediately secured and large-bore intravenous lines established. Blood has already been sent to the laboratory for cross and type. Which of the following is the next best step in management?

A. Admission and observation in critical care area

B. Angiography

C. Direct laryngoscopy

D. Immediate removal of the knife with applied pressure

E. Immediate surgical exploration of the neck

84. A 35-year-old transient man with a history of alcohol abuse is trying to jump from a moving train when his backpack is caught on the door. He falls out of the train and has an uncontrolled landing where he says that he hit his head. The patient arrives in the emergency department fully immobilized on a long board with a semi-rigid collar in place. He is complaining of leg pain but denies pain in his back or neck. His breathing is clear and his oxygen saturation is 99% of 1 L of oxygen. His blood pressure is 115/75 mm Hg, pulse 80 bpm, and respirations 15 breaths/min. His pupils are round and reactive to light and accommodation, and there is mild bruising over his left temple. His right leg is mildly tender at the knee joint. Which of the following is a contraindication to clearing the cervical spine and removing the collar without additional imaging?

A. Bruising over the temple

B. History of alcohol abuse

C. Impaired motor function of his right knee

D. Normal sensation and reflexes

E. Presence of posterior midline tenderness

85. A 32-year-old woman is brought to the emergency department after being stabbed by her husband in the left abdomen. She complains of abdominal pain localized to the knife injury. On exam, there is a defect in the left abdominal wall with several protruding loops of small bowel. Her airway is clear, and she is not complaining of difficulty breathing. Her blood pressure is 135/85 mm Hg, pulse 95 bpm, and respirations 14 breaths/min. Which of the following interventions is the next best step in management?

A. Abdominal ultrasound

B. CT scan of the abdomen

C. Diagnostic peritoneal lavage

D. Immediate laparotomy

E. Reduce the bowel back into the abdomen and close the defect.

86. A 29-year-old woman with a history of Crohn disease complains of increasing symptoms over the last few months, including bloating, diarrhea, and abdominal pain relieved by defecation. She also complains of increased fatigue and a decreased energy level. She has no family history of colon cancer. She denies smoking and eats a balanced diet rich in fruits and vegetables. She denies fevers, chills, and gross blood in her stools. Her temperature is 37.1°C, blood pressure 125/82 mm Hg, pulse 65 bpm, and respirations 15 breaths/min. Physical examination is remarkable for mild right lower quadrant tenderness with deep palpation. A fecal occult blood test is negative. Laboratory studies show:
Hemoglobin: 8.5 g/dL
Hematocrit: 27%
MCV: 90 fL
MCHC: 35%
Platelets: 230,000/mm^3
Leukocyte count: 6,500/mm^3
Serum ferritin: 280 ng/mL

Which of the following is most likely to be found with additional studies?

A. Decreased total iron-binding capacity and decreased serum iron

B. Decreased total iron-binding capacity and increased serum iron

C. Howell-Jolly bodies on a peripheral blood smear

D. Increased total iron-binding capacity and decreased serum iron

E. Large red blood cells on a peripheral blood smear

87. A 30-year-old woman complains of abdominal cramping and discomfort during her periods. She also admits to fatigue, malaise, and heavy, irregular menstrual periods over the past year. She has no other medical problems. She denies taking any medications or supplements and uses condoms for birth control. Her vital signs are within normal limits. Her physical examination is remarkable for mild conjunctival pallor. Which of the following is the most likely diagnosis?

A. Anemia of chronic disease

B. Folate deficiency

C. Iron deficiency

D. Vitamin B$_6$ deficiency

E. Vitamin B$_{12}$ deficiency

88. A 63-year-old woman presents to her primary care physician with increasing tiredness and dyspnea. She has also lost 7 kg of weight over the last year. Five years earlier, she had been found anemic and was treated with oral iron supplements. She says she eats a well-balanced diet and admits to drinking two glasses of wine on the weekends. Her past surgical history is remarkable for an appendectomy at age 15 years. On physical examination, she has marked pallor and several areas of depigmentation on her lower legs. Her laboratory values show a hemoglobin of 7.5 g/dL and an MCV of 112 fL. Her liver enzymes are normal. A fecal occult blood test is negative, and a colonoscopy 3 years prior showed no abnormalities. Which of the following is the most likely cause of this patient's symptoms?

  A. Adenocarcinoma of the colon

  B. Alcohol consumption

  C. Anti-intrinsic factor antibodies

  D. Lack of dietary folate

  E. Lack of dietary vitamin B_{12}

89. A 31-year-old man with a past medical history of mild anemia presents to the ambulatory care clinic with 5 months of dysphagia, anorexia, and episodes of brown urine. He denies fatigue, shortness of breath, easy bruising or bleeding, or other symptoms. He does not take any medications. His vitals are within normal limits. Physical exam is remarkable for mild scleral icterus and pallor. There is no hepatosplenomegaly, but mild right upper quadrant abdominal pain is present with palpation. A urinalysis shows 4+ hemoglobin, hemosiderin, and no red blood cells present. Additional laboratory studies show:

Hemoglobin: 8.1 g/dL

Hematocrit: 31.9%

MCV: 95 fL

Reticulocytes: 4.6%

Platelet count: 42,000/mm^3

Leukocytes: 3,800/mm^3

Blood urea nitrogen: 35 mg/dL

Serum creatinine: 2.1 mg/dL

Serum total bilirubin: 3.4 mg/dL

Direct bilirubin: 0.4 mg/dL

Haptoglobin: decreased

Which of the following is the most likely diagnosis?

  A. Autoimmune hemolytic anemia

  B. Chronic myelogenous leukemia

  C. Glucose-6-phosphate dehydrogenase deficiency

  D. Immune thrombocytopenic purpura

  E. Paroxysmal nocturnal hemoglobinuria

90. A 78-year-old Vietnam veteran is rushed to the emergency department after tripping onto a sharp stick while "chasing some kids that trespassed on my land." On exam, there is a large penetrating wound to his upper abdomen, so he is brought to the operating room for surgical repair. He is stable until postoperative day 3, when he develops fever, disorientation, and oozing from his intravenous sites. His surgical incision is clean, dry, and intact. A Jackson-Pratt drain shows minimal output of serosanguineous fluid. Laboratory studies show a platelet count of 43,000/mm^3 and increased fibrin split products. Which of the following is the most likely diagnosis?

  A. Disseminated intravascular coagulation

  B. Hemolytic uremic syndrome

  C. Immune thrombocytopenic purpura

  D. Rebleeding at operative site

  E. Thrombotic thrombocytopenic purpura

91. A 78-year-old woman presents to her family physician complaining of dysuria. She has no prior medical or surgical history. Physical examination is performed. The physician asks the patient to perform the Valsalva maneuver. Upon doing this, the cervix descends to protrude into the vagina. What is the most likely cause?

  A. Age-related laxity of the broad and round ovarian ligaments
  B. Endometrial hyperplasia
  C. Fecal impaction of the sigmoid colon
  D. Nulliparity
  E. Tear in the urogenital diaphragm

92. A 3-year-old boy is diagnosed with a malignant germ cell tumor, which is later determined to be the most common testicular tumor of infancy and early childhood. Which of the following hormones will be elevated in this tumor?

  A. Alpha-fetoprotein (AFP)
  B. Follicle-stimulating hormone (FSH)
  C. Human chorionic gonadotropin (hCG)
  D. Luteinizing hormone (LH)
  E. Thyroid-stimulating hormone (TSH)

93. A 70-year-old woman presents to her family physician complaining of a constant bloody vaginal discharge, which she has had for 3 months. Physical examination reveals a mass on the posterior wall of the vaginal fornix. A biopsy of the mass is obtained, and the pathology report suggests potentially metastatic squamous cell carcinoma of the vagina. Considering the location of the lesion, to which lymph nodes are the malignant cells most likely to metastasize first?

  A. Deep inguinal
  B. External iliac
  C. Internal iliac
  D. Superficial inguinal
  E. Superficial internal pudendal

94. Which of the following poses the greatest risk of malignancy in an otherwise healthy 30-year-old woman?

  A. Adenomyosis
  B. Immature teratoma
  C. Infection with HPV type II
  D. Leiomyoma
  E. Mature teratoma

95. A 39-year-old woman undergoes bilateral mastectomy after a diagnosis of infiltrating ductal carcinoma. Her mother, aunt, and three other relatives have had similar procedures performed, also in attempts to treat infiltrating ductal carcinoma in one or both breasts. Which of the following is the most likely etiology of the cancer in this woman?

  A. A decrease in the expression of the c-erb allele
  B. A mutant p53 allele
  C. A mutant Rb allele
  D. Expansion of a CCG trinucleotide repeat
  E. Loss of a specific enzyme in the excision repair system

96. A 28-year-old woman presents to her primary care physician complaining of abdominal bloating coincident with her menses. Her physician notes a nodular texture of the uterus on bimanual examination, and ultrasound shows several asymmetric masses within and radiating from the uterine corpus on the left. Serum pregnancy test results are negative. What is the most likely explanation for this finding?

A. Adenomyosis

B. Endometrial hyperplasia

C. Endometriosis

D. Leiomyoma

E. Molar pregnancy

97. A 34-year-old G3P3003 presents to the pediatrician with her 3-year-old child. The mother is concerned that her son's testicles have yet to descend. Physical examination reveals bilateral undescended testicles, an empty scrotum, and a severely underdeveloped penis. An ultrasound of the abdomen reveals bilateral ovaries and the absence of testicles. What is the most likely cause of this condition?

A. Inadequate production of androgenic hormones by the adrenal gland

B. Inhibition of the enzymes needed for 21-hydroxylation

C. A lack of receptors for dihydrotestosterone on peripheral tissues

D. A karyotype of XO

E. Point mutations in the SRY gene

98. A 57-year-old man with a history of cellulitis of the right foot has been on intravenous antibiotics for 4 weeks. He now complains of left lower quadrant pain and watery diarrhea. Physical examination reveals moderate left lower quadrant pain to palpation. Peritoneal signs are absent. Stool cultures are positive for overgrowth of *Clostridium difficile*. What is the most likely cause of this condition?

A. Antibiotic therapy

B. Botulinum toxin food poisoning

C. Compromised immune system

D. Gastric ulcer

E. Mechanical obstruction of the left colon

99. A 46-year-old man with hepatitis and cirrhosis due to chronic alcoholism dies of overwhelming pneumococcal sepsis (with *Streptococcus pyogenes*) despite treatment with intravenous antibiotics and intensive therapy in the hospital's intensive care unit. Which of the following bacterial enzymes may explain the process of invasiveness in this patient?

A. C5a peptidase

B. Dehydrogenase

C. Elastase

D. Telomerase

E. Urokinase

100. A 54-year-old woman with a history of left-sided breast cancer has been in remission for 5 years following paclitaxel therapy coupled with surgical resection. She has now noticed a new lump in her left breast close to where the original tumor was excised. A biopsy reveals recurring cancer. After talking with her physician, she decides to undergo more chemotherapy. Her physician prescribes a drug that inhibits DNA topoisomerase. Which chemotherapy agent inhibits topoisomerase?

A. Cisplatin

B. Docetaxel

C. Erlotinib

D. Irinotecan

E. Vincristine

Answers

1. **Answer:** **C.** *General Surgery/Colon, Rectum, Anus/Ulcerative Colitis.* This patient likely has ulcerative colitis on the basis of her chronic history of left lower quadrant abdominal pain, bloody diarrhea, and weight loss. On the basis of this information, her diagnosis of irritable bowel syndrome should be questioned. Proctoscopy is a valuable test for diagnosis of ulcerative colitis, which should be suspected in this patient. It may reveal mucosal inflammation above the level of the dentate line. Biopsies can be taken to confirm the diagnosis.

   A. Abdominal X-rays may reveal distension but will not reveal the typical findings of friable mucosa typical of ulcerative colitis.

   B. Cultures of stool for ova and parasites will be negative in this patient.

   D. Small-bowel contrast study would be useful in a patient with Crohn disease and reveal ileocolonic disease with strictures and impaired transit through these areas.

   E. Reassurance is not an appropriate treatment option for this patient with inflammatory bowel disease.

2. **Answer:** **B.** *General Surgery/Colon, Rectum, Anus/Rectal Prolapse.* This patient has rectal prolapse. She is in good health. Her most appropriate treatment should be low anterior resection with rectopexy. This is an efficacious approach to this patient given her age and good overall health.

   A. Antibiotics would be useful in the setting of infection such as proctitis.

   C. An alternative choice may be rectal fixation to sacrum with mesh. However, this procedure can be associated with difficulty in stool elimination.

   D. There is no indication to perform a hemicolectomy with colostomy in this patient. There is no underlying neoplastic disease. Colostomy is not indicated in this patient.

   E. Reassurance may be considered for small rectal prolapse in the asymptomatic patient or the patient with multiple medical problems who is a poor surgical candidate.

3. **Answer:** **D.** *General Surgery/Colon, Rectum, Anus/Anorectal Abscess.* This patient has an anorectal abscess. The treatment of choice is incision and drainage and should be performed immediately. Presenting features include pain and fever. Depending on the location of the abscess, a swollen mass may be felt. In general, intrasphincteric abscesses do not present with overt perianal swelling.

   A. Lateral sphincterotomy is a treatment for anal fissure.

   B. Stool softeners are indicated for patients with hemorrhoids.

   C. Oral antibiotics may relieve swelling and pain, but only incision and drainage will allow for evacuation of the abscess.

   E. Rubber band ligation is a treatment for hemorrhoids.

4. **Answer:** **A.** *General Surgery/Colon, Rectum, Anus/Contraindications to Laparoscopy.* Relative contraindications to laparoscopic cholecystectomy include coagulopathy, cirrhosis, portal hypertension, and generalized peritonitis. In addition, pregnancy, adhesions from prior surgery, and severe cardiopulmonary disease may complicate laparoscopic cholecystectomy.

   B. History of smoking, unless complicated by severe COPD, would not present significant risk for laparoscopy.

   C. Hypercholesterolemia is not a contraindication to laparoscopy.

   D. Portal hypertension, not systemic hypertension, represents a relative contraindication to laparoscopy.

   E. Prior history of wound infections would not be a contraindication to laparoscopy; however, this patient may be at somewhat higher risk of port site infections.

5. **Answer:** **C.** *General Surgery/Colon, Rectum, Anus/Abnormal Laboratory Values in Acute Cholecystitis.* Serum bilirubin is elevated in approximately 50% of patients with acute cholecystitis. This is the most likely laboratory finding to be abnormal in patients with acute cholecystitis. However, this laboratory is seldom ordered as a single test; thus, the other parameters in this question are also important to know about.

   A. Serum AST is elevated in nearly 40% of patients.

   B. Amylase is elevated in nearly 15% of patients.

   D. Lipase is not elevated in patients with acute cholecystitis.

   E. Serum alkaline phosphatase is elevated in 25% of patients.

6. Answer: C. *Cardiothoracic Surgery/Epidemiology/Guidelines for Lung Cancer Screening.* Currently, the clinical practice guidelines issued by the American College of Physicians as well as the U.S. Preventative Services Task Force recommend against screening asymptomatic individuals for lung cancer.

A. Although recent studies have suggested computed tomography as an effective screening tool in high-risk individuals, it is not currently recommended for screening use in asymptomatic patients.

B. Chest X-ray has not been shown to be an effective screening tool for lung cancer.

D. Although serum antidiuretic hormone may be elevated in some small cell lung cancers, it is not a useful screening tool.

E. Sputum cytology has been shown to be an ineffective screening tool for lung cancer.

7. Answer: A. *Cardiothoracic Surgery/Pharmacology/CABG.* Aspirin has been shown to reduce the risk of death and ischemic complications in numerous studies. Additionally, it is considered safe and does not increase the risk of bleeding complications.

B. Although short-term use of calcium-channel blockers may be useful in patients with radial artery grafts, there is little evidence to support the routine use of calcium-channel blockers after CABG to reduce patient mortality and ischemic complications.

C. The addition of clopidogrel to aspirin as dual therapy after CABG is controversial. Some research has suggested a benefit, whereas other studies have shown no difference in mortality between patients receiving aspirin alone and combination therapy.

D. There is little evidence to support significant mortality benefits with nitrates after CABG surgery.

E. Although statins have been shown in some studies to reduce progression of atherosclerosis and decrease the occurrence of graft occlusion, they do not show the same mortality benefits as aspirin.

8. Answer: E. *Cardiothoracic Surgery/Pathology/Vascular Rings.* This patient is presenting with signs, symptoms, and imaging findings suggesting the presence of a vascular ring. Vascular rings are a set of rare congenital anomalies that occur during the development of the aortic arch and great vessels that may compress the trachea and/or esophagus. Symptoms of respiratory distress may occur. The barium esophagram is the most important imaging study to order and is diagnostic in the vast majority of cases. If symptomatic, patients may need surgery to correct the problem with the type depending on the specific vascular anomaly.

A. It would be highly unusual for asthma to present this early in life. Furthermore, the imaging studies are not consistent with a diagnosis of asthma.

B. This patient does not have symptoms consistent with infection.

C. Although respiratory distress is a symptom of pneumothorax, the other findings are not consistent with this diagnosis.

D. If this patient had a tracheoesophageal fistula, he would more likely present with excessive salivation as a newborn and associated choking, vomiting, or distress associated with feeding.

9. Answer: E. *Cardiothoracic Surgery/Pathology/Soft-Tissue Sarcomas.* This patient's tumor description is that of a malignant soft-tissue sarcoma. These tumors are relatively uncommon and may occur in the chest wall. They often present as a painless lump but may cause symptoms if invading into the bone or compressing nerves. There are numerous subtypes of soft-tissue sarcomas that appear histologically similar. The stage of the tumor depends on the size and histologic grade. Surgical resection is the most common form of treatment.

A. Chondromas are benign neoplasms of cartilage that may occasionally occur on the chest wall. They are composed of mature cartilage and would not have this histologic appearance.

B. Fibrous dysplasia is a benign condition characterized by abnormal bone growth and may occasionally occur on the chest wall. Treatment options include medication to strengthen bones and pain management. Surgery does generally not have a role in treatment.

C. Although malignant schwannomas (derived from neural tissue) may appear histologically similar to soft-tissue sarcomas, they are usually S100 positive.

D. Multiple myeloma is a malignancy of plasma cells that may result in bone pain that often involves the spine or ribs. Lytic lesions may be seen on imaging. A bone marrow biopsy may show increased percentage of plasma cells. Surgery is generally not indicated.

10. Answer: C. *Cardiothoracic Surgery/Pathology/Chest Tube Placement.* Proper chest tube placement is important skill because vital structures must be avoided. Complications from improper technique may easily be avoided with an understanding of important anatomical landmarks. A chest tube should be placed in the mid or anterior axillary line behind the pectoralis major muscle to avoid extensive muscle dissection. Placing the tube above the fifth rib or the level of the nipple is important because the diaphragm elevates to this level during inspiration. The incision should be placed along the upper border of the rib to avoid damaging the neurovascular bundles that travel along the bottom of each rib.

A. This chest tube placement would compromise the neurovascular bundle that runs below the fourth rib.

B. This chest tube placement would be much too low and would endanger the neurovascular bundle that runs below the rib.

D. This tube placement would be too low.

E. This chest tube would be too anterior, too low, and would endanger the neurovascular bundle.

11. **Answer: D.** *Surgery/Acute Abdomen/Abdominal Anatomy/McBurney point.* This question is testing basic abdominal anatomy, specifically that of McBurney point, the location commonly overlying the inflamed appendix in acute appendicitis. McBurney point lies between the umbilicus and the right anterior superior iliac spine (ASIS), specifically two-thirds distance toward the ASIS. A McBurney incision is located here (at the point of maximal tenderness) perpendicular to this line.

   A. This statement does not accurately describe McBurney point because this point overlies the appendix, which is located on the right.

   B. While closely describing McBurney point, the problem with this statement is that the point lies closer to the ASIS than the umbilicus. This statement is describing the point being closer to the umbilicus.

   C. This statement does not accurately describe McBurney point because this point overlies the appendix, which is located on the right.

12. **Answer: D.** *Surgery/Acute Abdomen/Epigastric Pain/PUD as a Cause for Acute Abdomen.* This patient's history of *H. pylori* makes peptic ulcer disease very likely, which should raise concern for perforation of a preexisting ulcer. This is further supported with the sudden onset of abdominal pain in the epigastrium. An upright abdominal X-ray in the setting of perforation can be very specific if it reveals subdiaphragmatic air. As an inexpensive diagnostic approach, it is the best first step.

   A. Colonoscopy is incorrect. The patient's history, symptoms, and exam indicate that the pathology involved is the upper gastrointestinal tract. A colonoscopy, therefore, would contribute little to this diagnosis.

   B. Computed tomography would be the next best step if the abdominal film appears normal. A CT study would provide more specifics about the perforation including size, severity, and location. In a stable patient, it could be useful in addition to an abdominal film for preoperative intraabdominal details.

   C. In the setting of a perforation (as in peptic ulcer perforation) and diverticulitis (when microperforations exist or can occur easily), endoscopy is contraindicated. This would therefore be not an ideal management step, although it is addressing the relevant organ.

13. **Answer: B.** *Surgery/Acute Abdomen/Diverticulitis/Role of CT in Diverticulitis.* Given the symptoms and physical exam findings, this patient is most likely suffering from acute diverticulitis. Although he is lacking a previous diagnosis of diverticulosis, we are also told he has never had a colonoscopy. His MiraLAX use suggests constipation, a condition that may predispose to diverticulosis (or may have been a symptom of the disease itself). CT is the diagnostic gold standard for acute diverticulitis based on sensitivity and specificity. CT studies reveals colonic stranding, thickening of bowel, and other involved processes (e.g., abscess, phlegmon, fistulae).

   A. Colonoscopy is relatively contraindicated in diverticulitis. There is a significant risk of bowel perforation through an affected diverticula. This patient is already showing signs of perforation based on peritoneal signs.

   C. Despite having a history of peptic ulcer disease, perforation of a peptic ulcer is a less likely diagnosis given the location of this patient's pain. Furthermore, patients with peritoneal signs due to an ulcer perforation would proceed to exploratory laparotomy, not esophagogastroduodenoscopy (EGD), which is contraindicated.

   D. The diagnosis is not certain. Although this would deviate from the classic, typical presentation of renal calculus disease (involving renal or ureteral colic on the patient's left side), it is still a possibility given this patient's history. Further workup is required.

   E. Magnetic resonance imaging (MRI) would contribute little to this clinical picture. The patient has a fairly classic presentation and physical exam findings for diverticulitis. Given that renal calculus disease is included in the differential based on his history, CT first would be more appropriate to determine which is the cause.

14. **Answer: B.** *Surgery/Acute Abdomen/Appendiceal Abscess/Interval Appendectomy for Appendiceal Abscess.* Select cases of acute appendicitis are prone to rupture; rupture predisposes to abscess formation and possible sepsis. In cases where the abscess is effectively walled off, it is established that interval appendectomy (appendectomy 8 to 12 weeks after allowing the abscess to "cool off") is the gold standard in the pediatric population. Variations on this standard treatment include whether or not to administer antibiotics and whether or not to begin with percutaneous drainage.

   A. Conservative management is partially correct, in that interval appendectomy involves 8 to 12 weeks of conservative management prior to removal of the appendix. This answer is incorrect because it does not mention the appendectomy that occurs later; therefore, B is a better answer.

   C. Laparoscopic appendectomy would be ideal in an uncomplicated case of acute appendicitis. A walled-off abscess is more so an indication for interval appendectomy.

   D. Open appendectomy would be an option for acute appendicitis. In the pediatric population, however, laparoscopic would be the preferred approach. A walled-off abscess, however, is more of an indication for interval appendectomy.

15. **Answer:** A. *Surgery/Acute Abdomen/Referred Abdominal Pain/Acute Scrotum as a Cause for Acute Abdomen*. This question is modeled after a published case report of a case of testicular torsion that presented with abdominal pain only. Although this clinical picture is atypical for this scenario, it is irrelevant because further workup for this patient (and any patient) should start with a complete, head-to-toe physical examination. Remember to include testicular torsion as a differential for abdominal pain and to always complete the history and physical prior to other diagnostics.

   B. CT is a reasonable choice given the symptom of abdominal pain. Although this would not provide the diagnosis of testicular torsion, it would rule out other diagnoses for right-sided abdominal pain such as appendicitis.

   C. MRI is incorrect. This would take place well after a complete history and physical examination. Additionally, CT would take precedence.

   D. A scrotal ultrasound would be recommended for this patient because this is describing a case of testicular torsion. However, scrotal ultrasound would take place after a complete physical exam, including a urogenital exam.

   E. A KUB film, or "kidneys, ureters, bladder" X-ray, is similar to an abdominal X-ray (AXR) and useful in beginning a workup for a patient with suspected renal or ureteral stones. Although it is urologic in nature, it has no bearing in testicular torsion and would not occur before a complete physical exam.

16. **Answer:** A. *Pediatric Surgery/Chest Wall Deformities/Pectus Excavatum*. The traditional operation involves resection of the affected costal cartilage, a wedge osteotomy to enable anterior elevation of the sternum, and placement of hardware to maintain the new configuration for a few months while healing occurs. In the Nuss procedure, a semicircular bar is thoracoscopically inserted under the sternum and ribs to hold the sternum in a neutral position and is left in place for 2 years to allow remodeling of the chest wall. Both procedures carry similar risks of infection, recurrence, pneumothorax, and other damage to thoracic organs, but the Nuss procedure does not impair growth of the chest wall, whereas this is a common complication of the traditional operation.

   B. Both procedures carry similar risks of infection, recurrence, pneumothorax, and other damage to thoracic organs. Thoracic organs can be damaged during thoracoscopic insertion of the bar during a Nuss procedure.

   C. Both procedures carry similar risks of infection, recurrence, pneumothorax, and other damage to thoracic organs.

   D. Both procedures carry similar risks of infection, recurrence, pneumothorax, and other damage to thoracic organs.

   E. Both procedures carry similar risks of infection, recurrence, pneumothorax, and other damage to thoracic organs.

17. **Answer:** A. *Pediatric Surgery/Neck Masses/Cystic Hygroma*. Neck masses can be grouped according to their location: midline or lateral. Midline neck masses include thyroglossal duct cysts or ectopic thyroid gland tissue. Lateral neck masses include cystic hygromas, branchial cleft cysts, lymphadenopathy, and torticollis. This child's mass most closely fits the description of a cystic hygroma. Cystic hygromas are congenital malformation of lymphatic vessels. They have poorly defined borders and are soft and compressible.

   B. Thyroglossal duct cysts are the result of the failure of thyroglossal duct obliteration. Furthermore, a thyroglossal duct cyst is a midline lesion.

   C. A branchial cleft cyst is a lateral neck lesion. It results when the branchial clefts that arise during embryogenesis on the sides of the neck fail to regress completely. They have well-defined borders and are found along the anterior border of the sternomastoid muscle or possibly near the ear.

   D. Lymphoma invasion of a cervical node produces a hard, fixed lateral neck lesion. The borders may be poorly defined, but the mass would not be easily compressible.

   E. Torticollis refers to a fibrosis and shortening of the sternomastoid muscle. The fibrotic region may present as a mass found in line with the sternomastoid muscle and accompanied by the head being twisted toward the contralateral side.

18. **Answer:** A. *Pediatric Surgery/Vascular Tumors/Capillary Hemangiomas*. This presentation is most consistent with a capillary hemangioma. These vascular tumors most often appear within the first few weeks of life and rapidly increase in size for about a year, after which they begin to spontaneously regress. Most of these hemangiomas, including the one in this question stem, should be left alone because they will most likely regress and pose no threat to the child's health. Indications for intervention include lesions that threaten to interfere with the eyes or airway or lesions so large they cause thrombocytopenia, congestive heart failure, or significant facial distortion. All of the responses represent possible appropriate interventions, but this patient's lesion does not currently require treatment of any kind.

   B. Embolization by interventional radiology may be an appropriate option in another scenario. This patient's lesion is currently not threatening the infant's health and should not be treated at this time.

   C. Excision of the hemangioma may be an appropriate option in another scenario. This patient's lesion is currently not threatening the infant's health and should not be treated at this time.

   D. Laser photocoagulation may be a good option in another scenario. This patient's lesion is currently not threatening the infant's health and should not be treated at this time.

   E. Systemic corticosteroid therapy may be a good option in another scenario. This patient's lesion is currently not threatening the infant's health and should not be treated at this time.

19. Answer: C. *Pediatric Surgery/Tumors/Neuroblastoma.* Neuroblastomas are the most common extracranial solid tumors of children. These tumors arise from neural crest cells. Most are found in the abdomen, usually in the adrenal medulla. An abdominal mass can often be felt. Systemic symptoms, such as the fevers, hypertension, and failure to thrive, seen in this patient, are common. Urine will have elevated levels of catecholamines and their breakdown products. Treatment may involve surgery, chemotherapy, and radiation because most children have metastases by the time of presentation.

- **A.** Ewing sarcoma is a tumor of the bone. It is most commonly found in the limbs, pelvis, or ribs and would not present as an abdominal mass. Furthermore, hypertension is associated with neuroblastoma but not Ewing sarcoma.
- **B.** Nephroblastoma, or Wilms tumor, generally presents as a painless, asymptomatic abdominal mass. Nephroblastoma may cause hypertension and other symptoms, but this occurs much more commonly with neuroblastomas. Neuroblastomas are more common in general than nephroblastomas.
- **D.** Rhabdomyosarcomas are generally asymptomatic tumors of skeletal muscle and are classified into two subgroups: embryonal (found younger children in the head, neck, and genitourinary tract) and alveolar (found in older children in the trunk and extremities). Neuroblastomas are more common than rhabdomyosarcomas.
- **E.** Teratomas are tumors made up of cells from more than one of the germ layers. In children, they are usually found around the sacrococcygeal area or ovaries. Neuroblastomas are more common overall and are more commonly associated with systemic symptoms such as hypertension and fevers.

20. Answer: A. *Pediatric Surgery/Tumors/Wilms Tumor.* Wilms tumor, also known as nephroblastoma, is a type of renal tumor seen in children. It most often presents as a painless and otherwise asymptomatic abdominal mass in a child between the ages of 1 and 5 years. In 10% of patients, it presents bilaterally. Wilms tumor is often associated with other abnormalities, including aniridia, hypospadias, and hemihypertrophy. Treatment is surgical resection plus postoperative chemotherapy and possibly radiation therapy depending on the stage and grade of the tumor. Prognosis is generally good.

- **B.** Abnormalities known to be associated with Wilms tumor include aniridia, hypospadias, and hemihypertrophy. Clubbed feet are not known to be associated with Wilms tumor.
- **C.** Abnormalities known to be associated with Wilms tumor include aniridia, hypospadias, and hemihypertrophy. Cryptorchidism is not known to be associated with Wilms tumor.
- **D.** Abnormalities known to be associated with Wilms tumor include aniridia, hypospadias, and hemihypertrophy. Imperforate anus is not known to be associated with Wilms tumor.
- **E.** Abnormalities known to be associated with Wilms tumor include aniridia, hypospadias, and hemihypertrophy. Webbed digits are not known to be associated with Wilms tumor.

21. Answer: A. *Orthopedic Surgery/Pathology/Ankle Injury.* This patient has most likely injured his anterior talofibular ligament (ATFL). This ligament is the most commonly injured with ankle sprains and often occurs when the ankle is slightly plantar flexed. The anterior drawer test evaluates the ATFL and can be performed by securing the distal leg with one hand and applying an anterior pull to the heel with the ankle slightly planar flexed. Treatment depends on the degree of sprain, with physical rehabilitation almost always required. Surgical intervention is sometimes needed for severe ligament tears or serious athletes.

- **B.** Injury to the calcaneofibular ligament does not increase the amount of displacement with the anterior drawer test.
- **C.** The deep deltoid ligament functions to prevent lateral displacement and external rotation of the talus. The anterior drawer test does not test the deep deltoid ligament.
- **D.** The posterior talofibular ligament prevents posterior and rotary subluxation of the talus. It is not tested by the anterior drawer test.
- **E.** The talonavicular ligament is a wide, sheetlike band that stabilizes the talocalcaneonavicular joint. It is not tested by the anterior drawer test.

22. Answer: C. *Orthopedic Surgery/Pathology/Multiple Myeloma.* This patient is most likely suffering from multiple myeloma, a neoplastic process involving proliferating monoclonal plasma cells. Multiple myeloma is associated with chronic pain, fevers, and anemia. There may be lytic lesions identified on radiography. The proliferating plasma cells produce nonfunctional monoclonal antibodies that may include both light and heavy chains. Urinalysis will show an increased amount of paraprotein (also called Bence Jones protein), which is composed of only monoclonal light chains.

- **A.** Hypercalcemia rather than hypocalcemia is characteristic of multiple myeloma.
- **B.** Increased heavy chains are not found in the urine of patients with multiple myeloma.
- **D.** The erythrocyte sedimentation rate is typically elevated in patients with multiple myeloma.
- **E.** The serum creatinine is typically elevated in patients with multiple myeloma.

23. **Answer:** D. *Orthopedic Surgery/Pathology/Knee Dislocations.* Posterior knee dislocations should always be evaluated for vascular injury due to the high rate of popliteal artery injury. Patients with obvious signs of decreased perfusion (absent peripheral pulses, expanding hematomas, palpable thrills, audible bruits, pulsating hemorrhage) should receive surgical re-vascularization immediately. Indexes less than 0.9 indicate an abnormal result and further workup, often with duplex ultra-sonography or CT angiography, is required. Additionally, serial perfusion checks should be performed.

    A. Although anxiolytics may be administered, vascular evaluation should take precedence.

    B. Although NSAIDs may be important for pain control, this patient's vascular status should be evaluated.

    C. Patients without hard evidence of arterial compromise should receive radiographs and arterial evaluation prior to reduction.

    E. Although plain radiography is important in this patient's evaluation, the vascular status of the limb should be evaluated first.

24. **Answer:** A. *Orthopedic Surgery/Pathology/Legg-Calvé-Perthes Disease.* This patient is most likely suffering from Legg-Calvé-Perthes disease, or avascular necrosis of the femoral head. The condition is most common in boys between the ages of 3 and 12 years of age. It is not associated with obesity. Although the mechanism of action is not thoroughly understood, it is thought to be caused by temporary disruption of vascular supply. Symptoms include an insidious onset of intermit-tent knee, hip, groin, or thigh pain. Limping with a Trendelenburg gait is caused by the femoral head collapse, leading to decreased abductor muscle tension. The diagnosis is made with plain radiographs of the pelvis and "frog-leg" laterals. The prognosis is excellent in children with a bone age of less than 6 years. Treatment is aimed at keeping the femoral head con-tained within the acetabulum and maintaining good range of motion. This can usually be accomplished with observation, activity restriction, partial weight bearing, traction, and/or physical therapy. Rarely, surgery may be needed.

    B. This patient does not have a fever or history of trauma; thus, osteomyelitis of the hip is less likely.

    C. This patient's lack of morning stiffness makes rheumatoid arthritis less likely.

    D. The physical exam of this patient's knee is unremarkable, and there is no fever, making septic arthritis unlikely.

    E. Slipped capital femoral epiphysis is more common in obese and older (average age of 13) patients.

25. **Answer:** A. *Orthopedic Surgery/Pathology/Meniscal Injuries.* This patient has suffered a meniscal injury. First-line treat-ment for meniscal injuries includes NSAID use and observation. Goals of therapy are to minimize the effusion, normalize the gait, and maintain fitness. A trial of conservative treatment should be used for almost all meniscal injuries with the exception of the most severe. In this patient, his symptoms have not responded to conservative therapy; thus, surgery is needed. Arthroscopic partial meniscectomy is a procedure used for treating meniscal tears nonresponsive to more conserva-tive treatment or areas of the meniscus that are avascular.

    B. Continued NSAID use and observation would not be appropriate because he has not responded to trials of conservative treatment.

    C. Published clinical trials have failed to show a significant benefit for this treatment.

    D. Although observation is part of the treatment, it should be combined with pain relief, physical therapy, and other treat-ment modalities to maximize rehabilitation.

    E. Total knee replacement is invasive and rarely necessary for meniscal tears.

26. **Answer:** E. *Surgery/Esophagus and Stomach/Stomach/MALT.* The pathology describes a gastric MALToma (mucosa-asso-ciated lymphoid tissue), the most common extranodal lymphoma. Gastric MALTomas may transform into widespread ma-lignant disease, but their pathophysiology is strongly related to chronic gastritis as well as *H. pylori* infection. Surprisingly, eradication of *H. pylori* successfully treats most patients and exhibits low rates of recurrence. Eradication of this infectious process, therefore, is the first-line form of treatment given that the disease only involves the lamina propria.

    A. A PET scan would be effective if metastatic disease was present (i.e., exam or biopsy suggested lymphomatous spread outside of the stomach).

    B. Radiation therapy is effective for MALTomas and is an option for early-stage disease, but it is typically reserved for *H. pylori*–negative gastric MALTomas.

    C. Although MALTomas can resemble the Peyer patches of the small intestine, we can be fairly certain given this patient's history and symptoms that this biopsy was obtained from the correct area.

    D. Finally, surgical resection is rarely advised for gastric MALToma given the success of *H. pylori* treatment and radiation; furthermore, advanced disease proceeds to immuno- or chemotherapy, not surgery.

27. **Answer:** C. *Surgery/Esophagus and Stomach/Stomach/Dumping Syndrome.* Dumping syndrome describes a common condition secondary to gastric bypass surgery, particularly the Roux-en-Y bypass. Symptoms are similar to those described here. Dumping syndrome is thought to be caused by rapid dumping of food into the Roux-en-Y limb with rapid distention of the small intestine with hyperosmolar food content that rapidly bypasses the stomach. It commonly occurs during this postoperative time period (10 weeks). Foods that provoke symptoms (sugar-laden foods) can be avoided for initial conservative measures, or antimotility drugs that slow the passage of food through the stomach can be used.

   A. Anastomotic ulceration is a rare complication of Roux-en-Y gastric bypass, but patients develop the complication quickly (within days) with signs of peritonitis and/or sepsis.

   B. Conversion disorder as an answer choice entertains the idea that undergoing gastric bypass surgery is a major physiologic and psychiatric adjustment for the patient. Depression, not conversion disorder, can be a serious nonsurgical patient issue.

   D. A bowel obstruction due to iatrogenic causes (postoperative adhesions) would be expected to occur much later than dumping syndrome; additionally, the presentation would be similar to any bowel obstruction (and thus different from this patient's symptoms).

28. **Answer:** D. *Surgery/Esophagus and Stomach/Stomach/PPI Mechanism of Action.* This patient appears to have a fairly straightforward case of GERD, and we are told in the question that he is proceeding to medical management. Although many drugs are useful for GERD, proton pump inhibitors (PPIs) have become the first line drug for patients with GERD based on efficacy. This question asks, therefore, for the mechanism of action of PPIs, with distracters being his medication list and past medical history. PPIs work by binding irreversibly to the H^+-K^+ ATPase exchange and reduce gastric acid secretion. Their efficacy is largely based on the fact that they act on the terminal source of acid secretion in the stomach (as opposed to H_2 antagonists, for example, which exert their mechanism upstream of hydrogen ion pumps).

   A. Decreased production of prostaglandins via inhibition of COX-1 and COX-2 enzymes describes NSAIDs' causal link to gastritis, which is an adverse effect and not a therapeutic mechanism.

   B. Formation of a viscous gel along the gastric lining for protection against ulceration is the mechanism of action of sucralfate (a cytoprotective GERD drug).

   C. A histaminergic antagonist that decreases gastric acid secretion would describe any H_2-receptor blockers.

   E. Finally, a synthetic prostaglandin analogue that decreases acid secretion and increases bicarbonate secretion would be misoprostol (a PGE_1 analogue).

29. **Answer:** E. *Surgery/Esophagus and Stomach/Stomach/Most Common Cause of Upper GI Bleed.* The most common cause of an upper GI bleed regardless of age is peptic ulcer disease, which is causative as often as 40% of cases. This patient's previous diagnosis of GERD could simply be a misdiagnosis, which would explain the progression of his peptic ulcer disease to melena as well as anemia. His situation deserves a workup with upper endoscopy with biopsy and, likely, triple therapy.

   A. Gastric adenocarcinoma is undoubtedly included on this patient's differential, albeit at much lower rates compared to peptic ulcer disease.

   B. Although GERD is not a typical cause of an upper GI bleed, progression of GERD to Barrett esophagus may cause subtle blood loss via the GI tract.

   C. Epistaxis is not a common cause of GI bleeds as this adult patient presents; however, it can be a source of massive, acute, intractable hemorrhages in patients with severe cirrhosis.

   D. Although low-dose daily aspirin as secondary prevention for cardiovascular disease is not a common cause of GI bleeding, it does have noteworthy risk in terms of GI bleeds, particularly in repeat GI bleeds, and its risk, therefore, should be assessed per patient circumstances.

30. **Answer:** C. *Surgery/Esophagus and Stomach/Stomach/Hyperplastic Polyps.* Hyperplastic polyps are a type of benign tumor of the stomach that commonly arise secondary to chronic atrophic gastritis. They are small (<2 cm), rarely undergo malignant transformation (1% to 3%), and respond with eradication of *H. pylori*. The incorrect answers in this question refer to other pathologies involving the stomach.

   A. Rates of adenocarcinoma as high as 20% are found in adenomatous polyps.

   B. Stomach polyps commonly found in familial polyposis syndromes describe fundic gland polyps, a pathology that lacks malignant potential altogether.

   D. An artery eroding through the gastric mucosa and contributing to a potentially dangerous bleed describes a Dieulafoy lesion.

   E. And, finally, nitrate consumption (a substance found in smoked meats common to the Japanese diet) is a risk factor for the development of malignant adenocarcinoma.

31. **Answer:** D. *Surgery/Neurosurgery/Pediatrics/Medulloblastoma.* Medulloblastomas occur for the most part in the pediatric population (75%), which is typically tested. They are typically located below the tentorium cerebelli, usually around the cerebellum with or without extension into the fourth ventricle. Because of their involvement with the cerebellum, gait imbalances can occur, as with this patient. Ideal treat for medulloblastoma begins with maximal surgical resection with which staging and diagnosis can be confirmed.

    A. Despite being a mainstay in the treatment for medulloblastoma, the benefits of chemotherapy for medulloblastoma remain largely unknown. Chemotherapy typically begins after an ideal surgical resection and diagnostic confirmation.

    B. There is no reason to suggest that palliative therapy is indicated. Furthermore, proper staging and adequate resection both begin with surgical intervention, which this answer does not include.

    C. Radiation therapy is also used for medulloblastoma; however, it typically begins following surgical resection and histologic confirmation and staging.

32. **Answer:** C. *Surgery/Neurosurgery/Pediatrics/Myelomeningocele.* Myelomeningocele is a neural tube defect in which the meninges and neural tissue herniate through a vertebral defect in the lumbosacral region. The commonly tested associated anomaly is the Chiari II malformation. The defect may be open, may blend into the skin, or may be covered by a thin cutaneous membrane.

    A. Anencephaly is the most common congenital malformation and is typically detected prenatally. The calvarium is absent with a thickened and flattened skull base. Cerebral material is disorganized, leaving a flattened cerebral remnant only.

    B. The Arnold-Chiari malformation describes elongation of the cerebellar tonsils and extension into the fourth ventricle. This is a temping question for those who know the association with myelomeningocele, but this is not confirmed yet and is not the primary diagnosis in this child.

    D. Spina bifida occulta tends to be a more subtle presentation of spina bifida variations.

33. **Answer:** A. *Surgery/Neurosurgery/Pediatrics/Horner Syndrome.* Horner syndrome presents with the classic triad of ptosis, miosis, and hemi-anhidrosis. It is a very rare condition, with no epidemiologic predilection for that reason. Commonly tested scenarios for Horner syndrome include dissection status post-trauma, iatrogenic Horner syndrome (status postsurgery), and Pancoast tumor invasion. Remember that it can present congenitally in the pediatric population as idiopathic Horner syndrome, as it is here.

    B. Acoustic neuromas present with tinnitus, hearing loss, and balance disturbances. Involving the eighth cranial nerve, they would not cause the symptoms seen in this patient.

    C. Medulloblastoma occurs in the pediatric population (75%) and is typically located below the tentorium cerebelli, usually around the cerebellum with or without extension into the fourth ventricle. Gait abnormalities are common presentations.

    D. Prolactinoma describes the condition of a prolactin-secreting adenoma. Found in the pituitary fossa, the common presentation involves visual disturbances and headache, not ptosis and miosis.

    E. Right-sided facial nerve palsy describes a right-sided Bell palsy, which is a unilateral paralysis of the peripheral portion of the facial nerve. Facial droop and inability to blink are typical symptoms. It, similarly, has a wide range of etiologies.

34. **Answer:** C. *Surgery/Neurosurgery/Neurovascular/Berry Aneurysms and Autosomal Dominant Polycystic Kidney Disease.* The question is twofold; specifically, it is asking you to recall the association between autosomal dominant polycystic kidney disease (ADPKD) and the presence of berry aneurysms. Additionally, you must know that bleeding of cerebral aneurysms releases blood into the subarachnoid space. Remember that any uncontrolled hypertension predisposes to cerebral aneurysms, and there is nothing special about ADPKD's predisposition to aneurysms other than its hypertension component. Finally, patients are also prone to intracerebral hemorrhage, but note that this is not an answer choice.

    A. Epidural hematomas are commonly due to trauma and appear as convex bleeds beneath the skull as their boundaries are made by dural attachments. There is no association with ADPKD.

    B. Subdural bleeds can be due to trauma or involve chronic bleeds such as those seen in the elderly. There is no association with ADPKD.

    D. Intraventricular hemorrhage can occur not only in preterm neonates but also in patients who suffer trauma. In traumatic scenarios, it is often considered a poor prognostic indicator. The presence of blood within the ventricles is pathognomonic, typically with blood in the lateral ventricles or all ventricles.

35. **Answer:** C. *Surgery/Neurosurgery/Infection/Hematogenous Epidural Abscess.* This is a classic presentation of spinal epidural abscess, where infectious signs and meningeal-like signs coincide. Spinal epidural abscesses are caused by hematogenous seeding of infection, typically with *Staphylococcus* or *Streptococcus* bacterial species. This specific etiology of this infectious process is a commonly tested phenomenon.

   A. Although infectious complications from epidural anesthesia are fairly rare, they do occur; however, we are not provided any information from the clinical history to suggest that this should be included in the differential.

   B. Lumbar disk herniation commonly occurs at lower lumbar levels with pain, paresthesia, or dysesthesias occurring along the nerve roots that are compressed. The suggestion of infection and altered mental status of this patient seem to suggest a diagnosis other than disk herniation.

   D. A malignant process of the spinal cord would present with a more chronic progression of disease. We are told that the signs seen in this patient began acutely. Note that epidural abscesses can present chronically, in which case they can mimic malignant processes.

   E. There is no reason to believe that this is a reaction to a meningococcal vaccination because it is not mentioned in the vignette and a reaction of this type is atypical. The most serious reaction to the meningococcal vaccine is anaphylaxis. There is also a concern for Guillain-Barré syndrome with some meningococcal vaccine types.

36. **Answer:** C. *Hepatobiliary System/Internal Medicine/Emphysematous Cholecystitis.* Emphysematous cholecystitis is caused by an infection by gas-forming bacteria (*E. coli, Enterococcus, Klebsiella,* or *Clostridia* spp.). These patients are commonly diabetic and present with RUQ pain and sepsis. The treatment of emphysematous cholecystitis first is IV fluids. There are required to replenish any dehydration and, more importantly, to address the sepsis.

   A. Laparoscopic cholecystectomy is indicated to remove the source of the infection, but the sepsis needs to be addressed first with IV fluids.

   B. Percutaneous cholecystostomy is indicated for poor surgical candidates to decompress the gallbladder initially, to be followed by a cholecystectomy in 4 to 6 weeks.

   D. Broad-spectrum antibiotics are also imperative in the treatment of emphysematous cholecystitis, but IV fluids should be started first.

   E. ERCP can be used to assess for blockage of the common bile duct, but it is to follow the acute treatment of sepsis with IV fluids.

37. **Answer:** D. *Hepatobiliary System/Internal Medicine/Ascending Cholangitis.* Ascending cholangitis is a bacterial infection of the biliary ductal system, due to ductal obstruction leading to increased bacteria in the bile. Causes of cholangitis include choledocholithiasis, benign stricture, or tumors. The classic presentation of ascending cholangitis is *Charcot triad* (fever, RUQ pain, and jaundice). In severe presentations, the addition of mental status change and hypotension yields *Reynold pentad.* Initial management involves fluid resuscitation and empiric IV antibiotics. The next step is decompression of the biliary tree, which is achieved with either percutaneous transhepatic cholangiography or endoscopic retrograde cholangiopancreatography. In the case of choledocholithiasis, cholecystectomy is indicated once the patient is stabilized to prevent recurrence.

   A. Intravenous fluids and antibiotics alone will not address the built-up pressure in the biliary tree.

   B. Cholecystectomy is not indicated for the acute treatment of cholangitis; ERCP or PTHC is preferred over surgical intervention.

   C. Cholecystectomy is not indicated for the acute treatment of cholangitis; ERCP or PTHC is preferred over surgical intervention.

   E. Empiric intravenous antibiotics are indicated to treat the infection in the biliary tree, especially in this case where the patient presents with sepsis.

38. **Answer:** A. *Hepatobiliary System/Radiology/Primary Sclerosing Cholangitis.* Primary sclerosing cholangitis is a chronic progressive cholestatic disease. It is an autoimmune inflammatory process that targets the intrahepatic and extrahepatic bile ducts, leading to strictures. It is associated with inflammatory bowel disease, with 85% having ulcerative colitis and 15% having Crohn disease. Males are affected more than females, with peak incidence in the fourth decade of life. Patients present with signs/symptoms of biliary obstruction, jaundice, pruritus, weight loss, and fatigue. Diagnosis is based off of cholestasis or cirrhosis on liver biopsy. ERCP or MRCP can be performed, which shows the characteristic beaded appearance of the bile ducts due to areas of strictures and dilatation.

   B. Proximal dilation is associated with a single stricture, obstructing stone, or tumor.

   C. Double duct sign is highly suggestive of a tumor at the head of the pancreas.

   D. Dilated common duct with filling defects is associated with choledocholithiasis, with the filling defects representing the stones.

   E. Ectasia of branches of the pancreatic duct is associated with chronic pancreatitis.

39. **Answer: C.** *Hepatobiliary System/Surgery/Gallbladder Adenocarcinoma.* Gallbladder cancer is 90% adenocarcinoma and is more common in women, especially those with a history of gallstones. Other risk factors include Native American heritage, gallstones >2.5 cm, porcelain gallbladder, choledocha cysts, primary sclerosing cholangitis, and cholecystenteric fistula. At diagnosis, 25% are localized to the gallbladder, 25% have regional lymph node or organ metastasis, and 40% already have distant metastasis. Patients present with RUQ pain, often appearing similar to other biliary conditions. Other symptoms include weight loss, jaundice, and an RUQ abdominal mass (Courvoisier sign). Diagnosis can be made with RUQ ultrasound or abdominal CT. Management depends on the stage of the cancer. If the cancer is into the muscle or beyond, an additional resection with a 2-cm margin in the adjacent tissue is indicated with a regional lymphadenectomy.

   A. If the cancer is localized to the gallbladder (remains submucosal with no muscular invasion), open cholecystectomy is all that is required.

   B. There is no role for a biopsy of Calot node in the management of gallbladder cancer.

   D. In the case of the cancer spreading into the muscle of the gallbladder, a 2-cm margin is indicated, not 1 cm. In addition, a regional lymphadenectomy is also indicated.

   E. In the case of the cancer spreading into the muscle of the gallbladder, a 2-cm margin is indicated, not 1 cm.

40. **Answer: A.** The patient is presenting with a cholangiocarcinoma, which is a cancer originating in the biliary tree. It is more likely in patients with history of biliary stasis, infection, stones, and chronic inflammation, which can be due to conditions like primary sclerosing cholangitis, choledocha cysts, hepatolithiasis, and biliary enteric fistulae. Cholangiocarcinoma is classified based on location: intrahepatic, perihilar, and distal. Most patients present with jaundice, pruritus, fever, and abdominal pain. For diagnosis, abdominal CT is the initial test of choice for visualization of the dilated bile ducts, regional lymph nodes, and vascular anatomy.

   B. ERCP may be used to further evaluate the patency of the pancreatic duct and biliary tree, but a CT scan is less invasive and evaluates the organ parenchyma.

   C. MRCP may be used to evaluate the ductal patency but is not the best initial test.

   D. HIDA scan is a good initial test for cholecystitis, not cholangiocarcinoma.

   E. RUQ ultrasound is the initial test of choice for gallstones and cholecystitis.

41. **Answer: C.** *Principles of Surgical Physiology/Breast Disease/Hormone Therapy for Breast Cancer.* Hormone therapy in breast cancer works for those tumors with estrogen receptor/progesterone receptor (ER/PR)–positive cells. Patients with these tumor types have better outcomes in general, and for postmenopausal women, hormone therapy is as effective as chemotherapy in treating ER/PR-positive breast cancer. Hormone therapy works by blocking the growth that natural hormones would cause in the cancer cells either by blocking estrogen receptors (tamoxifen and raloxifene) or by inhibiting excess estrogen synthesis (aromatase inhibitors such as anastrozole).

   A. Heritable breast cancers are not necessarily good candidates for hormone therapy. Response to hormone therapy can be predicted only by the presence or absence or hormone receptors on tumor cells.

   B. Males with breast cancer are not necessarily good candidates for hormone therapy. Response to hormone therapy can be predicted only by the presence or absence or hormone receptors on tumor cells.

   D. Patients with the *BRCA-1* mutation are not necessarily good candidates for hormone therapy. Response to hormone therapy can be predicted only by the presence or absence or hormone receptors on tumor cells.

   E. Patients with the *BRCA-2* mutation are not necessarily good candidates for hormone therapy. Response to hormone therapy can be predicted only by the presence or absence or hormone receptors on tumor cells.

42. **Answer: B.** *Principles of Surgical Physiology/Breast Disease/Cancer of the Male Breast.* Men can develop breast cancer, but it is both a small percentage of all cancers in men (<1%) and a small percentage of total breast cancers (also <1%). Workup is the same as that in women, including clinical examination, mammography, and fine-needle aspiration. Features that suggest cancer rather than a benign etiology for a breast mass in a male include unilateral lesions (although gynecomastia is commonly unilateral, breast cancer is almost exclusively unilateral), painless lesions, fixed lesions (to the chest wall or to the skin), and ulceration. Gynecomastia generally produces tenderness.

   A. Fixation of the mass to the skin or to the chest wall suggests malignancy rather than gynecomastia or some other benign disease.

   C. Ulceration is often seen in cancer. Gynecomastia and other benign conditions would generally not cause ulceration.

   D. Gynecomastia may present unilaterally, but breast cancer in men is almost exclusively unilateral. Bilateral lesions would suggest gynecomastia rather than cancer.

   E. All of the responses are suggestive of cancer except pain on palpation. Pain or tenderness is more likely due to a benign lesion. Breast cancer lesions are generally painless.

43. **Answer:** E. *Principles of Surgical Physiology/Breast Disease/Gynecomastia Treatment.* Gynecomastia is common, occurring in 60% to 70% of early teenage boys (12 to 15 years old). In this age group, the condition is benign and almost always regresses spontaneously. Less commonly, it can occur in older men as well. Causes in older men include certain medications, alcohol abuse, marijuana abuse, and cirrhosis. Mastectomy can be performed if the gynecomastia is severe or distressing to the patient.

   A. Gynecomastia in a male of this age (15 years old) is common and benign and generally requires no treatment. Chemotherapy is used in the treatment of breast cancer in patients with positive lymph nodes or metastases.

   B. Gynecomastia is not caused by blocked ducts but by the abnormal development in males of normal, female-appearing breast tissue. Most cases resolve spontaneously and require no treatment.

   C. Hormone therapy is useful in patients with estrogen receptor/progesterone receptor–positive tumors. This patient most likely has gynecomastia, which requires no treatment at his age.

   D. Simple mastectomy can be performed if the gynecomastia is distressing to the patient or becomes very large.

44. **Answer:** C. *Principles of Surgical Physiology/Breast Disease/Postmastectomy Recurrence of Breast Cancer.* The standard treatment for recurrence of breast cancer that involves the chest wall after a mastectomy is radiation therapy. Prognosis is worse for patients with recurrent disease within 2 years versus those with recurrence after 5 years. The recurrence is usually in the same quadrant as the original disease. Ten percent of patients with recurrence will also have metastatic disease.

   A. Chemotherapy would be a good choice for a patient known to harbor distant metastases. This patient, with apparently localized chest wall involvement, would best be treated with radiation therapy.

   B. Hormone therapy would be a good choice for a patient who was originally treated with hormone therapy and had good response. This patient was treated with mastectomy and now has recurrence in the chest wall. She would best be treated with radiation therapy.

   D. The best treatment for recurrence involving the chest wall after mastectomy is radiation therapy.

   E. The best treatment for recurrence involving the chest wall after mastectomy is radiation therapy.

45. **Answer:** A. *Principles of Surgical Physiology/Breast Disease/Axillary Node Status in Breast Cancer.* Cancer staging is done to predict a patient's prognosis and to direct treatment methods. Clinical staging involves the physical exam and mammogram and possibly additional tests in the setting of metastasis. Pathologic staging is based on the TNM (tumor, node, metastasis) system. Parameters such as tumor size, tumor extent, axillary node status, and metastases are evaluated. Of these, axillary node status bears the highest correlation with survival and has the best prognostic value.

   B. Cellular appearance on FNA is useful in the sense that findings direct possible further interventions such as excisional biopsy for samples with cellular atypia. The FNA biopsy is not as useful as the axillary node status for predicting outcome.

   C. Mammography is useful to evaluate whether a mass found on exam has benign or malignant features. Findings on mammography do not correlate to outcome nearly as well as axillary node status.

   D. Weight changes have not been shown to accurately predict outcomes in breast cancer as axillary node status does. Axillary node status would be the best prognostic indicator in this patient.

   E. Poor prognostic features of the tumor itself include swelling around the tumor, dimpling, or fixation of the tumor to the chest wall or skin. Axillary node status, however, is still the best predictor of survival.

46. **Answer:** E. *Skin and Soft Tissue/Pathology/Keloid Scar.* This patient is most likely suffering from a keloid scar. Features that suggest a keloid scar include the initiating event (biopsy or trauma), patient's race (much more common in black patients), location (most commonly occurs on the ear lobe), and histologic features. This type of scar is composed of mainly type III or type I collagen, depending on the maturity. They are benign but can sometimes be painful or itchy.

   A. Basal cell carcinomas are the most common skin malignancy. They usually develop in sun-exposed areas in fair-skinned individuals. Although slow-growing, they may erode into adjacent structures. Histologically, they are composed of nests of basophilic cells. This patient's presentation is not consistent with this diagnosis.

   B. Chronic folliculitis is defined as inflammation of a hair follicle and will histologically be composed of increased inflammatory cells. This patient's history and histologic features are not consistent with chronic folliculitis.

   C. Dermatofibromas are hard, solitary, slow-growing papules that are benign tumors. They may be related to previous insect bites or thorn pricks. They are composed of disordered collagen and are usually found on the leg.

   D. Hypertrophic scars may often be confused with keloid scars. However, there are some key differences. The primary difference is that hypertrophic scars do not grow beyond the original boundaries of the wound. Additionally, they often appear as erythematous raised fibrotic lesions and may undergo spontaneous regression.

47. Answer: D. *Skin and Soft Tissue/Pharmacology/Electrical Soft-Tissue Burns.* This patient has suffered an electrical injury to his arm. Unfortunately, electrical burn injuries are usually much more extensive than they may superficially appear. Extensive surgical debridement of the soft tissues along the path of the electrical current is often necessary. Adequate hydration is extremely important in the initial management for these patients. If severe muscle damage is expected, an osmotic diuretic such as mannitol and/or an alkalinizing agent is indicated to prevent acute renal failure from myoglobinuria. In addition to mannitol administration, urine alkalization with sodium bicarbonate increases the rate of myoglobin clearance.

A. Aluminum chloride is a medication used to acidify the urine. It would be contraindicated in the use with electrical burn injuries because acidification of the urine would increase the chance of developing acute renal failure.

B. Dopamine is a vasopressor that increases medullary oxygen demand. Withdrawal from dopaminergic agents may cause rhabdomyolysis. However, this is not a medication that will help this patient avoid renal failure.

C. Epinephrine will not help avoid acute renal failure in this patient.

E. Oxacillin is a penicillinase-resistant beta-lactam antibiotic and will not help this patient avoid renal failure.

48. Answer: D. *Skin and Soft Tissue/Pathology/Melanoma.* This patient's presentation is concerning for melanoma. Melanoma risk factors include fair skin, ultraviolet light exposure, history of precursor lesions, history of peeling or blistering sunburns, family history of melanoma, and immunosuppression. Diagnosis is clinically made with the ABCDE rule, where A stands for asymmetry, B for border irregularity, C for color variation, D for diameter greater than 6 mm, and E for evolution. The next best step for patients with lesions greater than 1.5 cm in diameter is a full-thickness punch biopsy of the thickest part of the lesion because this will allow for adequate histologic characterization as well as depth. If the diagnosis of melanoma is established, then surgical excision is the primary treatment.

A. 5-Fluorouracil is uncommonly used for treating advanced melanoma.

B. Excisional biopsy is appropriate for lesions less than 1.5 cm in diameter.

C. Observation is not appropriate when melanoma is suspected in a young individual such as this.

E. Shave biopsies should be avoided in patients with suspected melanoma because the prognosis is highly dependent on the depth of the malignancy. Shave biopsy will make it very difficult to determine the depth in the future.

49. Answer: A. *Skin and Soft Tissue/Pathology/Basal Cell Carcinoma.* This patient's history and exam are most consistent with a diagnosis of basal cell carcinoma. Basal cell carcinomas are the most common skin malignancy. They usually develop in sun-exposed areas in fair-skinned individuals. Although slow-growing and rarely metastatic, they are locally invasive. These patients are at a much greater risk for developing new lesions, especially in areas exposed to sunlight. Histologically, basal cell carcinomas are composed of nests of malignant and basophilic cells. Treatment involves surgical resection. If the margins are tumor-free, then no additional treatment is necessary. Other treatment options include topical 5-fluorouracil or radiation.

B. Congenital melanocytic nevi are benign lesions usually discovered at birth. They are often located on the head and neck and are characterized by a well-circumscribed patch of light brown to black pigmentation with a heterogeneous consistency. Microscopically, congenital melanocytic nevi appear similar to acquired nevi, with the exception that cells are often found deeper within the dermis. Surgery is sometimes used for treatment because large lesions have an increased malignant potential.

C. Malignant melanoma is clinically characterized by asymmetry, irregular borders, variation in color, diameter greater than 6 mm, and an evolving appearance. This patient's presentation is not consistent with melanoma.

D. Sarcomas are malignant soft-tissue tumors that rarely occur on the face. Although they may erode into the skin, this patient's presentation is highly inconsistent with this diagnosis.

E. Squamous cell carcinoma is the second most common form of skin cancer. It often occurs on the lower lip or below. It typically grows faster than basal cell carcinoma and is also locally invasive.

50. Answer: A. *Skin and Soft Tissue/Pathology/Squamous Cell Carcinoma.* This patient is most likely suffering from squamous cell carcinoma on his lower lip. This occurs in greater frequency in sun-exposed areas. Smoking and alcohol are both risk factors, although more so for oral lesions. The first step in diagnosis is a punch biopsy on the edge of the lesion for histologic diagnosis. Smaller lesions may be diagnosed with excisional biopsy. Once the diagnosis is confirmed, treatment involves excision with clear and wide (greater than 1 cm) margins.

B. Although 5-fluorouracil may be an option for precancerous skin lesions, including carcinoma in situ and actinic keratosis, it is not appropriate for the initial management of invasive squamous cell carcinoma.

C. A shave biopsy may not obtain enough information for pathologic diagnosis and is not recommended as an initial biopsy method.

D. Observation when localized malignancy is suspected is not appropriate.

E. Although they may be appropriate for infectious lesions, topical antibiotics are ineffective for treating squamous cell carcinoma.

51. **Answer: E.** *Pancreas and Spleen/Pathology/Immune Thrombocytopenic Purpura.* Assuming this patient is a good surgical candidate, splenectomy is the next best step in management of this patient's ITP because it is refractory to glucocorticoid therapy. The reason for this is a higher long-term success rate with splenectomy when compared to alternative therapy options such as rituximab.

   A. Aspirin is contraindicated in patients with ITP because it further reduces platelet function.

   B. Cyclophosphamide is sometimes used in ITPs that no longer have a response to splenectomy and other medications.

   C. Because the underlying autoimmune dysfunction will also destroy donor platelets, platelet transfusions are normally not recommended in patients with ITP unless there is an emergency.

   D. Rho(D) immunoglobulin has been effective in some cases of ITP. However, the treatment is costly and only produces short-term improvement.

52. **Answer: D.** *Pancreas and Spleen/Pathology/Splenic Abscess.* This patient is presenting with signs and symptoms of splenic abscess. Splenic abscess typically occurs secondary to septic emboli from endocarditis or other sites of infection. Typical manifestations include fever and left upper quadrant pain. Occasionally, patients may present with left-sided pleural effusion and shoulder pain related to inflammation of the left hemidiaphragm. The best way to diagnose splenic abscess is with CT imaging. The gold standard for treating splenic abscess is broad-spectrum antibiotics and splenectomy. Although percutaneous drainage may be attempted with certain abscesses (uncomplicated), it would not be recommended in this patient.

   A. Although broad-spectrum antibiotics would be important to start in this patient, percutaneous drainage would most likely not be successful with multiple lesions.

   B. Although diagnostic percutaneous aspiration would be helpful in confirming the diagnosis and providing a specimen for culture, it is not necessary in this patient because he already has positive blood cultures.

   C. Although intravenous support and broad-spectrum antibiotics are appropriate for this patient, they do not provide definitive treatment for splenic abscess.

   E. Splenic artery embolization is sometimes used for splenic lacerations. It would not be an appropriate treatment for splenic abscess.

53. **Answer: D.** *Pancreas and Spleen/Pathology/Pancreatic Carcinoma.* This patient is presenting with weight loss, depression, jaundice, and migratory thrombophlebitis, all potential indicators of pancreatic cancer. Pancreatic cancer is the fourth leading cause of cancer deaths among both men and women. Because it is very difficult to diagnose during its early stages, patients more often present late in the disease.

   A. Although this patient does present with signs of clinical depression, studies have shown that depression may be an early sign of pancreatic malignancy. Additionally, depression would not explain the other symptoms the patient is experiencing.

   B. Although hypothyroidism could account for the signs of depression, the patient would be expected to experience weight gain. Additionally, jaundice and migratory thrombophlebitis are not features of hypothyroidism.

   C. This patient's symptoms are not consistent with Paget disease.

   E. Although this patient does have a history of alcoholism and depression, this patient's symptoms are better explained by pancreatic malignancy.

54. **Answer: A.** *Pancreas and Spleen/Epidemiology/Pancreatic Carcinoma.* This patient has multiple risk factors for pancreatic cancer. However, multiple studies have shown that alcohol is most likely not a risk factor for pancreatic cancer.

   B. Diabetes mellitus has been linked to pancreatic cancer. Studies also suggest that late-onset diabetes may be an early sign of pancreatic cancer.

   C. Patients with multiple endocrine neoplasia type 1 have an increased risk for certain types of pancreatic malignancies, including gastrinomas and insulinomas.

   D. Obesity has been noted to be a risk factor for pancreatic cancer in multiple studies. In particular, central obesity patterns have the highest risk.

   E. Smoking is the most common environmental risk factor for pancreatic cancer. Studies have shown that smoking may be responsible for up to 30% of cases.

55. **Answer: B.** *Pancreas and Spleen/Pathology/Acute Necrotizing Pancreatitis.* Acute necrotizing pancreatitis is a severe form of acute pancreatitis. The natural history of acute pancreatitis is often described in the literature as consisting of two phases, with an initial systemic inflammatory response resulting in release of inflammatory mediators and possible organ failure. The second phase, usually described as a sepsis picture with organ failure, usually occurs several weeks later. Several physical exam findings are associated with acute necrotizing pancreatitis, including Cullen sign and Grey-Turner sign. Cullen sign is characterized by superficial bruising and edema in the subcutaneous tissues surrounding the umbilicus. Grey-Turner

sign is characterized by retroperitoneal hemorrhage and flank bruising. Other signs may include subcutaneous nodules as a result of fat necrosis.

A. This physical exam finding is a description of dermatitis herpetiformis, a skin condition associated with celiac disease.

C. This physical exam finding is a description of Virchow node, which also may represent malignant disease (often gastric cancer) in the abdomen.

D. This description is that of a Sister Mary Joseph nodule, which classically represents metastatic cancer in the pelvis or abdomen.

E. This physical exam finding is a description of Trousseau sign of malignancy, associated with pancreatic adenocarcinoma.

56. **Answer: B.** *Principles of Surgical Physiology/Invasive Monitoring/Pulmonary Capillary Wedge Pressure.* A pulmonary artery catheter consists of a long tube with a balloon at one end, which is inserted usually through a subclavian or jugular vein into the right ventricle. The balloon allows the catheter to be floated through the heart along with normal blood flow into one of the pulmonary arteries. The balloon follows the flow until it becomes lodged in a pulmonary artery too small to let it pass. A port on the distal end of the balloon allows accurate measurement of venous pressure from the left side of the heart. The catheter's pulmonary capillary wedge pressure (PCWP) is a close approximation of left atrial and left diastolic ventricular pressures.

A. The pressure in the inferior vena cava or any other central vein would not be measured by a pulmonary artery catheter. Additionally, central venous pressure is normally between 3 and 8 mm Hg.

C. Right atrial pressure would not be measured with a pulmonary artery catheter. Right atrial pressure is normally between 3 and 8 mm Hg.

D. Right ventricular pressure during diastole would be essentially the same as central venous pressure or right atrial pressure. These pressures are not measured by pulmonary artery catheterization and are normally between 3 and 8 mm Hg.

E. Right ventricular systolic pressure is normally between 15 and 30 mm Hg. A pulmonary artery catheter would not measure this pressure because the balloon at the catheter's tip ensures that the distal port is in contact only with left cardiac venous blood.

57. **Answer: A.** *Principles of Surgical Physiology/Shock/Cardiogenic Shock.* Shock refers to any situation in which the cardiovascular system is unable to maintain adequate tissue perfusion. This can be due to inappropriate systemic vasodilation (as occurs in septic and neurogenic shock), inability of the heart to pump with sufficient contractility (cardiogenic shock), insufficient intravascular volume (hypovolemic shock), or some obstruction causing decreased cardiac output (obstructive shock). This woman's findings of cold, clammy skin suggest systemic vasoconstriction (ruling out septic and neurogenic shock). Her distended neck veins suggest congestion (ruling out hypovolemic shock). The otherwise normal pulmonary and cardiac exams make cardiogenic shock the most likely of the remaining two choices. Examples of obstructive shock include cardiac tamponade and tension pneumothorax and would likely have some abnormality on physical exam.

B. Hypovolemic shock is due to insufficient circulating volume (such as following a major bleed). The finding of distended neck veins effectively rules out this possibility.

C. Neurogenic shock is characterized by a decrease in autonomic tone of the vasculature, resulting in warm, well-perfused skin. Cold, clammy skin is characteristic of hypovolemic and cardiogenic shock.

D. Obstructive shock occurs when cardiac output is impaired by some physical obstruction such as a tension pneumothorax or cardiac tamponade.

E. Septic shock would present with a similar appearance to neurogenic shock—warm, well-perfused skin.

58. **Answer: E.** *Principles of Surgical Physiology/Shock/Septic Shock.* Shock refers to any situation in which the cardiovascular system is unable to maintain adequate tissue perfusion. This can be due to inappropriate systemic vasodilation (as occurs in septic and neurogenic shock), inability of the heart to pump with sufficient contractility (cardiogenic shock), insufficient intravascular volume (hypovolemic shock), or some obstruction causing decreased cardiac output (obstructive shock). This man's findings of warm, flushed skin suggest systemic vasodilation (ruling out cardiogenic and hypovolemic shock). His history of a dirty wound with a background of diabetes is concerning for infection and sepsis, making septic shock more likely than neurogenic shock.

A. Cardiogenic shock occurs when some injury to the heart (such as in an MI) impairs the heart's contractility, leading to poor perfusion. The skin of the extremities will be cold and clammy from the vasoconstrictive response to decreased cardiac output.

B. Hypovolemic shock is due to insufficient circulating volume (such as following a major bleed). The skin of the extremities will be cold and clammy from the vasoconstrictive response to decreased cardiac output.

C. Neurogenic shock is characterized by a decrease in autonomic tone of the vasculature, resulting in warm, well-perfused skin. The history of a dirty wound in a patient with diabetes, fever, and chills makes septic shock more likely.

D. Obstructive shock occurs when cardiac output is impaired by some physical obstruction such as a tension pneumothorax or cardiac tamponade.

59. Answer: B. *Principles of Surgical Physiology/The Intensive Care Unit/Ventilator Support.* The ventilator addresses two different issues the lungs normally handle: ventilation (ridding the body of CO_2) and oxygenation. Depending on the patient's underlying problem, the ventilator may be correcting one aspect more than the other. The variety of settings on the ventilator allow the physician to modify oxygenation and ventilation independently of each other. In this case, the patient's ABG shows a "normal" PaO_2 of 90 mm Hg; this represents an inappropriate response to her FiO_2 of 40%. The normal ratio of PaO_2 (normally about 100 mm Hg) to FiO_2 (approximately 0.2 for room air) is 500. A ratio less than 200 defines ARDS. Her ratio is $90 / 0.4 = 225$, suggesting respiratory distress and a level close to the diagnostic level for ARDS. An increase in her FiO_2 would be prudent. Her pH, $PaCO_2$, and bicarbonate levels are within normal limits, so no changes in ventilation are necessary at this time. Breathing rate affects ventilation more than oxygenation. She requires better oxygenation while her pH, $PaCO_2$, and bicarbonate levels are within normal limits, so no changes in ventilation are necessary at this time.

A. A PEEP of 6 mm Hg is appropriate for this patient. Increasing the PEEP may compensate for some degree of hypoxia, but high PEEP decreases venous return to the heart and can lead to hypotension and poor perfusion. Her relative hypoxia would best be corrected by increasing the FiO_2.

C. Appropriate tidal volume for a patient on a ventilator can be calculated by estimated between 8 and 10 mL/kg (500 mL is appropriate for this patient). Increasing the tidal volume affects ventilation more than oxygenation.

D. She requires better oxygenation while her pH, $PaCO_2$, and bicarbonate levels are within normal limits, so no changes in ventilation are necessary at this time.

E. This patient's relative hypoxia suggests oxygenation is inadequate. To increase oxygenation, PEEP can be increased (already is above 5 mm Hg for her) or FiO_2 can be increased.

60. Answer: D. *Principles of Surgical Physiology/Nutrition and the Surgical Patient/Protein.* Adequate protein intake for a normal adult is approximately 0.8 g/kg/day, but this can increase to 2 g/kg/day during times of illness and stress. A number of indicators can be used to evaluate adequate protein intake. These include measuring nitrogen output (urine plus stool) versus nitrogen intake (grams of protein/6.25) to maintain a positive balance, monitoring weight gain (although this is the least reliable), and measuring visceral protein levels (albumin, prealbumin, transferrin). Of the choices listed, measuring a prealbumin level would be the most reliable indicator in this patient.

A. Calculating the protein content of food is only part of the steps needed to determine nitrogen balance. This amount must be compared with excreted nitrogen (urinary nitrogen and estimated stool nitrogen) to determine whether the patient has a positive or negative balance.

B. Daily weights is the least accurate method of determining protein nutrition because many other unrelated factors also affect weight.

C. Hemoglobin levels do not fluctuate with changes in protein metabolism nearly as much as prealbumin. Albumin and transferrin levels may be used to evaluate protein nutritional status, but hemoglobin may not.

E. Calculating the excreted urinary nitrogen is only part of the steps needed to determine nitrogen balance. This amount of excreted nitrogen (urinary nitrogen and estimated stool nitrogen) must be compared to the dietary intake of nitrogen (protein grams / 6.25) to determine whether the patient has normal nitrogen intake.

61. Answer: D. *Small Bowel/Pathology/Celiac Disease.* Celiac disease is a chronic diarrheal disease characterized by intestinal malabsorption. It is caused by ingestion of gluten-containing foods. Common presenting complaints include diarrhea, cramps, abdominal pain, flatulence and distention, and other gastrointestinal complaints. Additionally, patients with celiac sprue are at increased risk for many complications of their disease, including lymphomas and adenocarcinomas of the small intestine, short stature and stunted growth, subfertility, anemia, osteopenia, and seizure disorders. Women of childbearing age also have a higher rate of miscarriage than the general female population. However, sarcoma of the small bowel does not occur at increased rates in patients with celiac disease.

A. Anemia is a common problem in patients with celiac sprue and may be a result of vitamin and/or mineral malabsorption or chronic inflammation.

B. Women with celiac disease who are of childbearing age are at increased risk of having miscarriages.

C. Patients with celiac disease are at increased risk of intestinal lymphomas.

E. Numerous studies have shown that both men and women with celiac disease may suffer from fertility problems.

62. Answer: C. *Small Bowel/Pathology/Crohn Disease.* This patient is most likely suffering from Crohn disease. Common symptoms of Crohn disease include nonbloody diarrhea, abdominal pain and cramping, fatigue, malaise, and low-grade fevers. The most common section of bowel affected by Crohn disease is the terminal ileum. Strictures may form and manifest as stenotic bowel on imaging.

A. Adenocarcinoma of the colon is unlikely, considering the patient's age and clinical picture.

B. Celiac disease is associated with ingestion of gluten-containing foods and may have a similar presentation to Crohn disease. However, this patient's clinical picture, including imaging and oral ulcers, is more characteristic of Crohn disease.

D. Although gastritis presents with gastrointestinal symptoms, it is more often acute in nature and would not have this patient's oral ulcer or imaging findings.

E. Ulcerative colitis shares many of the same features of Crohn disease and is also an inflammatory bowel disease. However, the ileum is not involved in inflammatory bowel with the exception of so-called backwash ileitis.

63. **Answer: B.** *Small Bowel/Pathology/Peptic Ulcer Disease.* This patient is most likely suffering from a duodenal ulcer. Duodenal ulcers are the most common location of peptic ulcers in the gastrointestinal tract. Epigastric pain is the most common complaint in patients with peptic ulcer disease and is characterized by a gnawing or burning sensation that occurs after meals. This patient's nighttime pain is a common complaint in duodenal ulcers and characteristically occurs several hours after meals. Most patients with duodenal ulcers have a combination of decreased duodenal bicarbonate secretion and increased gastric acid secretion. Upper endoscopy is the preferred diagnostic test in evaluation of patients with peptic ulcer disease. Additionally, testing for *H. pylori* is an essential part of the workup because it has been found to be a major cause of duodenal ulcers.

A. Crohn disease is a form of inflammatory bowel disease that can affect any part of the gastrointestinal tract from mouth to anus. There are numerous manifestations of Crohn disease that may include both those gastrointestinal and extraintestinal in nature. Biopsy with histologic examination is important for confirming the diagnosis. This patient's symptoms are not consistent with a diagnosis of Crohn disease.

C. Esophageal spasms are abnormal contractions of the esophageal muscle that may cause impairment in swallowing. Common symptoms include difficulty swallowing and chest pain. This patient's symptoms are not consistent with a diagnosis of esophageal spasms.

D. Gastric ulcers may appear similar to duodenal ulcers but are less common. They too are associated with infection with *H. pylori*. Signs and symptoms that suggest gastric ulcer over duodenal ulcer include pain immediately after eating and pain made worse with food. This patient's symptoms are more suggestive of a duodenal ulcer because there is delayed and nocturnal pain temporarily relieved by food intake.

E. Although epigastric pain does occur in pancreatitis, it usually radiates to the back and also occurs with food intake. This patient's symptoms are more characteristic of peptic ulcer disease than pancreatitis.

64. **Answer: C.** *Small Bowel/Pathology/Volvulus.* This patient has questionable viability of a segment of small bowel. During surgery, if ischemic bowel is present, these segments should be removed. If the viability of the bowel cannot be determined, a second operation may be necessary to reassess the viability of bowel. This surgery is typically performed 12 to 36 hours after the initial surgery.

A. Although the patient should be closely monitored for signs of peritonitis, failure to remove ischemic portions of bowel would greatly increase this patient's chance of mortality. Thus, a second operation is necessary at this point.

B. The initial management of suspected volvulus involves nasogastric suction, antibiotics, and intravenous support. Although this will continue to be important postoperatively, the bowel in this patient will need to be reexamined.

D. Removing the entire small bowel is unnecessary and would most likely result in death or long-term morbidity for the infant.

E. Removing the portion of small bowel before viability is determined could result in the infant having short bowel syndrome. Short bowel syndrome is a dreaded and unfortunate complication when significant portions of bowel are removed. A better approach would be to re-examine the small bowel with repeat surgery.

65. **Answer: A.** *Small Bowel/Pathology/Carcinoid Tumor.* Although carcinoid tumors of the intestine are often asymptomatic, they may present with symptoms such as those described in this patient. Additional signs may include facial telangiectasias, rashes (from niacin deficiency), wheezing, and edema. The initial workup for carcinoid tumors involves a 24-hour urine test for urinary levels of 5-HIAA, a metabolite of tryptophan metabolism. The levels are usually greatly increased in patients with carcinoid tumors. Additional testing may include noncontrast CT imaging of the abdomen, which is the imaging modality of choice due to the vascularity of the tumors.

B. Abdominal ultrasounds may have limited use in tumors less than 1 cm, but they are generally not useful in the diagnosis of carcinoid tumors.

C. Although CT imaging of the abdomen would be useful as an additional test to identify the location of the tumor, the head is a very unlikely location for this tumor.

D. Although niacin levels may be diminished in carcinoid tumors because it is involved in the metabolism of serotonin, low levels of niacin are very nonspecific for the diagnosis of carcinoid tumors.

E. A radionucleotide scan (OctreoScan) may be useful in the diagnosis of carcinoid tumors when other imaging modalities have failed to localize the tumor.

66. Answer: D. *Endocrine System/Internal Medicine/VIPoma.* This patient's history of chronic watery diarrhea with skin flushing indicates he has a VIPoma. Other clues of a VIPoma are hypokalemia, achlorhydria, and dehydration. VIPomas are tumors that secrete vasoactive intestinal peptide (VIP). Ninety percent of VIPomas originate in the pancreas from a nonbeta islet cell. The excess VIP secreted increases intestinal motility and secretion of water and electrolytes, which causes the diarrhea. The medical treatment of choice is octreotide, which blocks the action of VIP to decrease the intestinal motility and quell the diarrhea. Surgical excision of the tumor is the next step.

A. Carcinoid tumors are neuroendocrine tumors that secrete serotonin. Patients usually are asymptomatic until the tumor metastasizes to the liver, which causes carcinoid syndrome (patients experience flushing, diarrhea, wheezing, abdominal cramps).

B. Tropical sprue is a malabsorption syndrome seen typically in the tropical regions. It can become a chronic steatorrhea, leading to weight loss and malnutrition.

C. Bacterial gastroenteritis can present with diarrhea, but patients typically present more acutely with fever and vomiting. The 2-month duration of the diarrhea makes this diagnosis unlikely.

E. Laxatives are used to treat constipation and act through a variety of mechanisms to soften stool. Abuse of laxatives can cause watery diarrhea, but there is nothing in the history that indicates this patient is abusing laxatives.

67. Answer: A. *Endocrine System/Pathology/Glucagonoma.* This patient has a glucagonoma, which is a rare tumor of the pancreas that produces excess levels of glucagon. Glucagon is a hormone produced by pancreatic alpha cells that acts to increase blood levels of glucose via stimulation of glycolysis and gluconeogenesis in the liver, stimulation of lipolysis in peripheral adipose, and stimulation of protein breakdown in skeletal muscle. Excess glucagon levels causes hyperglycemia, anemia, and a dermatologic condition called necrolytic migratory erythema (NME). NME appears as erythematous blisters and swelling, which occurs in areas subject to greater friction and pressure, like the buttocks and perineum in this patient. The origin of this tumor is the pancreatic alpha cells in the islets of Langerhans.

B. The zona fasciculata is the middle zone of the adrenal cortex responsible for glucocorticoid production. Tumors from this region can cause Cushing syndrome.

C. Pancreatic carcinoma originates from the pancreatic acinar cells. It classically presents with painless jaundice.

D. The adrenal medulla is the main source of catecholamines into the bloodstream. Pheochromocytomas are tumors of the adrenal medulla.

E. Malignant transformation of pancreatic delta cells can form somatostatinomas, which manifest as steatorrhea and hyperglycemia.

68. Answer: C. *Endocrine System/Biochemistry/Carcinoid Syndrome.* This patient's history of episodic diarrhea, flushing, and wheezing is classic for carcinoid syndrome. Carcinoid syndrome is caused by liver metastasis of a carcinoid tumor, which is a neuroendocrine tumor of the GI tract that produces excess serotonin. In the case of a localized carcinoid tumor, this excess serotonin is removed from the bloodstream by the liver and the patient is asymptomatic. But with liver metastasis, as in our patient with a low albumin and elevated INR, the normal liver tissue is unable to remove the serotonin. It then enters the systemic circulation and patients become symptomatic. The amino acid precursor of serotonin is tryptophan, which is readily consumed by the carcinoid cells. Tryptophan is quickly depleted by this outflow of serotonin.

A. Alanine does not play a role in the synthesis of serotonin. Its most important role is in the alanine-glucose cycle, where it travels from skeletal muscle to the liver to aid in gluconeogenesis.

B. Tyrosine is the main building block of the catecholamines dopamine, norepinephrine, and epinephrine.

D. Threonine is not used in the synthesis of neurotransmitters or hormones.

E Histidine is the precursor of histamine, which is released by mast cells in type I hypersensitivity reactions.

69. Answer: B. *Endocrine System/Surgery/Carcinoid Tumor.* The surgical management of carcinoid tumor varies depending on the tumor size, site, and whether or not metastatic disease is present. This patient has a large duodenal tumor, which is treated with a Whipple procedure (also known as a pancreaticoduodenectomy). For tumors smaller than 1 cm without any metastasis, segmental intestinal resection is indicated. For tumors larger than 1 cm, multiple tumors, or lymph node involvement, the surgery indicated is a wide excision of bowel and mesentery. For tumors of the terminal ileum, a right hemicolectomy is indicated. For small duodenal tumors, local excision is indicated. And for extensive disease that cannot be locally controlled, surgical debulking is indicated for palliation.

A. Local excision is indicated for small duodenal tumors.

C. Segmental intestinal resection is indicated for localized tumors smaller than 1 cm.

D. For tumors larger than 1 cm, wide resection of bowel and mesentery is indicated.

E. This surgical procedure is not indicated for any carcinoid tumors.

70. **Answer: E.** *Endocrine System/Pharmacology/Carcinoid Syndrome.* The patient's episodes of flushing, wheezing, and diarrhea are consistent with carcinoid syndrome. Carcinoid syndrome is caused by a malignancy of neuroendocrine cells of the GI tract, which secrete excess amounts of serotonin. When this malignancy invades the liver, the excess serotonin is able to enter the systemic circulation, causing symptoms. The medical treatment of choice for carcinoid syndrome is octreotide. Octreotide is a somatostatin analog that decreases the symptoms of diarrhea and flushing caused by carcinoid syndrome. It does this by decreasing the amount of serotonin released by the carcinoid tumor cells.

A. Labetalol is a nonselective beta-blocker that has alpha-blocking effects as well. It can be used in the treatment of pheochromocytoma.

B. For the treatment of pheochromocytoma, alpha- and beta-blockers are used. Phenoxybenzamine and atenolol are examples of these, respectively.

C. Diphenhydramine is a first-generation antihistamine that may be used as an adjunct medication for symptomatic relief of carcinoid syndrome. It is not very effective alone.

D. This answer choice is a distractor; atenolol can be used for treatment of pheochromocytoma after alpha blockade is established. Diphenhydramine may be used for some symptomatic control of carcinoid syndrome.

71. **Answer: C.** *Urology/Pathology/Stress Incontinence.* This patient is presenting with pure stress incontinence, which should always be managed conservatively if possible. Conservative treatments include weight loss, diet modification (avoiding coffee, alcohol, carbonated beverages, etc.), bladder training, and pelvic floor (Kegel) exercises. If these interventions do not work, then more aggressive measures such as surgery may be considered.

A. Although diet modification may help with stress incontinence, intermittent catheterization generally does not.

B. Oxybutynin is an anticholinergic agent used to treat urge incontinence. It is generally not helpful for stress incontinence.

D. Sacral nerve stimulation involves implantation of a programmable stimulator that delivers low amplitude electrical signals to sacral nerves to treat urinary incontinence, retention, and other issues. Because it is noninvasive and effective, it is gaining popularity for treating neurogenic bladder. However, it is not useful for stress incontinence because the problem is not neural in nature.

E. Vaginal slings are an option for treating stress incontinence in select patients when more conservative therapy has failed.

72. **Answer: C.** *Urology/Pathology/Testicular Cancer.* This patient is most likely suffering from a seminoma, a type of germ cell tumor. Germ cell tumors are the most common malignancy of men age 15 to 35 years. Of these, seminomas account for approximately one-third of the diagnoses. The most common clinical presentation is a painless testicular lump. They are usually found at stage 1, and the prognosis for such patients is excellent. Seminomas appear grossly yellow and histologically as uniform populations of large cells that form sheets and nests. Serum placental alkaline phosphatase is elevated in a majority of patients.

A. Gonadoblastomas grossly appear lobulated and histologically as complex mixture of different gonadal cells. It occurs almost exclusively in patients with disorders of sex development.

B. Leydig tumors are tumors of the gonadal interstitium. Because the tumors are typically hormonally active, feminizing or virilizing symptoms are common complaints. Grossly, they appear as a solid and well-circumscribed nodule with a gold-brown cut surface. Microscopically, the tumor will appear as sheets of round/polygonal cells with eosinophilic cytoplasm. Occasionally, Reinke crystals may be present.

D. Sertoli cell tumors are a type of sex cord stromal tumor derived from Sertoli cells, which are located in the seminiferous tubules. These cells normally function to support spermatogenesis. The tumors grossly appear as well-circumscribed yellow, white, or gray masses. Histologically, they are composed of solid tubules containing Sertoli cells arranged in cords, nests, or sheets. Because these cells secrete testosterone, females may have masculinization.

E. Teratomas are germ cell tumors composed of multiple cell types from three or more germ cell layers. Testicular teratomas usually present as a painless, firm scrotal mass without accompanying symptoms. Histologically, there are multiple cell types, which may include skin, hair, sebaceous glands, sweat glands, and many other tissue types.

73. **Answer: D.** *Urology/Pathology/Testicular Torsion.* This patient's presentation could be explained by several conditions, including acute epididymitis and testicular torsion. This patient will need a testicular ultrasound to rule out testicular torsion since it is the most damaging possibility. If the testicle is found to be torsed, the patient will need immediate exploration and detorsion in the operating room.

A. Ceftriaxone might be appropriate if the patient has acute epididymitis. However, testicular torsions should be ruled out first.

B. Observation would be inappropriate because this patient is in severe pain and testicular torsion must be ruled out.

C. Scrotal biopsy is unnecessary at this point. If continued workup fails to identify the problem, biopsy may be considered.

E. Although this patient's urine should be sent for culture, testicular torsion is the most damaging possibility and should be ruled out first.

74. **Answer: A.** *Urology/Pharmacology/Orchitis.* Viral orchitis is an acute inflammatory condition of the testicles secondary to a viral infection. There are many viruses that can cause orchitis, including coxsackievirus, Ebstein-Barr virus, varicella, echovirus, paramyxovirus (mumps), and many others. The diagnosis of viral orchitis can generally be made without an extensive workup. Treatment for viral orchitis is supportive with bed rest, hot and/or cold packs, and scrotal elevation.

   B. Ceftriaxone would help treat orchitis caused by *Neisseria gonorrhea.*

   C. Doxycycline would help treat orchitis caused by *Neisseria gonorrhea.*

   D. Although acyclovir may help with some viral infections such as herpes, most cases of orchitis are self-limited and are not helped by antiviral drugs.

   E. Ganciclovir is an antiviral commonly used to treat cytomegalovirus infections. It is not useful for viral orchitis.

75. **Answer: A.** Both epispadius and bladder exstrophy are most likely caused by the same congenital defect of cloacal membrane instability. Failure of mesenchyme to migrate between the ectodermal and endodermal layers of the lower abdominal wall results in this instability and potential cloacal rupture.

   B. Cryptorchidism is caused by a blunted testosterone embryologic response and other hormone disturbances. It is not caused by the same defect in the cloaca as epispadius.

   C. Ectopic scrotal tissue is uncommon congenital abnormality where there is an abnormally positioned hemiscrotum. It usually occurs near the inguinal ring. It is not generally associated with bladder exstrophy.

   D. Hypospadias is caused by incomplete fusion of the urethral groove, which results in a urethra on the ventral surface of the penis. It is not caused by the same embryologic defect as epispadius.

   E. Penile agenesis is a rare disorder caused by developmental failure of the genital tubercle. It is associated with cryptorchidism but is rarely associated with bladder exstrophy.

76. **Answer: C.** *Hernias/Anatomy/Femoral Hernias.* Femoral hernias occur within the femoral canal, below the inguinal ligament. From laterally to medially, the femoral triangle contains the femoral nerve, artery, vein, a space, and the lymphatics. Femoral hernias occur in the space between the vein and lymphatics.

   A. The femoral artery and vein lie next to each other and do not provide enough space for the hernia to occur here.

   B. The femoral nerve is outside the femoral canal and is not involved in a femoral hernia. The femoral artery is found lateral to the femoral vein and is not a border of the femoral hernia.

   D. The rectovesical pouch is the space between the rectum and bladder. It is not involved in a femoral hernia.

   E. The retropubic space is an extraperitoneal space between the pubic symphysis and bladder. It is not involved in a femoral hernia.

77. **Answer: E.** *Hernias/Pathology/Parastomal Hernia.* Parastomal hernias may occur after stomal construction because an artificial point of weakness is made in the abdominal wall. If the weakness is great enough, the abdominal contents may protrude through the defect and often into the subcutaneous tissue. Some studies show that the rate of parastomal hernia may be as high as 30% following stomal construction. Factors that increase the risk of parastomal herniation include (1) placement of the stoma lateral to the rectus sheath, (2) poor abdominal muscle tone (pregnancy, aging, etc.), (3) creation of an oversized stomal incision, (4) factors that increase intra-abdominal pressure such as chronic cough or ascites, (5) location of the stoma in a midline incision, and (6) wound infection. Small bowel has the lowest rate of parastomal herniation. Multiple methods are described for parastomal hernia repair, including meshes, localized fascia repair, and moving the stoma to a different site in the abdomen.

   A. Larger stomal incisions are associated with an increased risk of parastomal herniation

   B. Placement of the stoma lateral to the rectal sheath is associated with an increased risk of parastomal herniation.

   C. Tension suturing is associated with an increased risk of parastomal herniation. Tension-free techniques are most often used when constructing stomas.

   D. Use of large bowel for stoma formation is associated with an increased risk of parastomal herniation.

78. **Answer: D.** *Hernias/Pathology/Umbilical Hernia.* This patient most likely has an umbilical hernia that is exacerbated by his ascites. Because there is skin breakdown and necrosis of the hernia, repair is a necessary and urgent part of this patient's management. However, repair of the hernia should be accompanied by treatment of his ascites because failure to do so would most likely make the repair unsuccessful. Of the previous choices, only using a peritovenous shunt along with hernia repair would address both problems. In stable patients, treatment of ascites should precede hernia repair.

   A. Although intravenous hydration and broad-spectrum antibiotics may be part of this patient's management, avoiding correction and observing the patient could be disastrous.

   B. This patient would not be a candidate for liver transplant due to his current alcoholism.

   C. Primary umbilical hernia repair without addressing the ascites would result in a very high rate of repair failure.

   E. Reassurance is not appropriate because this patient's condition is quite serious.

79. **Answer: B.** *Hernias/Pathology/Spigelian Hernia.* Spigelian hernias are an uncommon form of ventral hernia that protrudes between the attachment of the internal oblique and transversus abdominis muscle to the rectus sheath (semilunar line). Patients often present with swelling and/or pain in the mid to lower abdomen. Because they occur submuscularly, they may not be palpable on exam and are thus difficult to clinically diagnose. Imaging with abdominal ultrasound (preferred) or CT may be helpful. Peak incidence is at age 50 years. Repair is performed using an open, tension-free approach similar to repair of incisional hernias.

    A. Although Spigelian hernias do occur between the internal oblique and transversus abdominis muscle, they are posterior (not anterior) to the external oblique aponeurosis.

    C. Indirect inguinal hernias originate lateral to the inferior epigastric vessels and protrude through the inguinal ring.

    D. Direct inguinal hernias originate medial to the inferior epigastric vessels (in Hesselbach triangle) through a weak point in the fascia of the abdominal wall.

    E. Obturator hernias occur through the obturator canal.

80. **Answer: B.** *Hernias/Anatomy/Inguinal Hernias.* Direct and indirect inguinal hernias are often defined anatomically by their relation to the inferior epigastric vessels. Direct inguinal hernias occur medially to the vessels (from a weak spot in the fascia of the abdominal wall), and indirect inguinal hernias occur laterally (via a patent processus vaginalis).

    A. Cooper ligament (also called the pectineal ligament) is an extension of the lacunar ligament and rungs along the pectineal line of the pubic bone. It is often used in hernia repair because it is strong and holds sutures well.

    C. The inguinal ligament does not separate indirect and direct inguinal hernias because both defects occur at or above the inguinal ligament.

    D. The rectus abdominis muscle is a large paired muscle that runs vertically on each side of the anterior abdominal wall. It does not separate indirect and direct inguinal hernias.

    E. The superficial epigastric artery distributes blood to the superficial fascia and skin of the lower abdominal wall. It originates below the inguinal ligament and passes through the femoral sheath. It is found between Camper and Scarpa fascia. The inferior, not superficial, epigastric artery is a major separating landmark between direct and indirect inguinal hernias.

81. **Answer: A.** *Trauma and Burns/Trauma/Airway Injury.* This patient has a penetrating wound to the upper left chest and symptoms of a hemothorax. However, the patient remains stable, and the amount of blood draining from the chest tube is decreasing and below the value requiring surgical exploration. In general, surgical exploration should be considered if there is evacuation of more than 1,000 mL of blood immediately after tube thoracotomy, continued bleeding from the chest tube at a rate of greater than 150 to 200 mL over 2 to 4 hours, and/or repeated blood transfusion requirements to maintain hemodynamic stability of the patient.

    B. Although CT scanning can be helpful for quantification of blood amount or diagnosis when an X-ray is unequivocal, it is generally not needed when the diagnosis has already been made, the patient is stable, and the amount of blood draining from the chest tube is minimal and decreasing.

    C. Emergent bedside thoracotomy is generally indicated in thoracic injuries when survival rate without immediate intervention is low. It is not needed in this patient who is hemodynamically stable with mild blood loss.

    D. Exploratory thoracotomy would be indicated if this patient was hemodynamically unstable, had greater than 1,000 mL of blood loss immediately after chest tube placement, or had increasing and/or significant continued bleeding from the chest tube.

    E. Ventilation perfusion scans are sometimes helpful in the diagnosis of pulmonary embolism. It would not be indicated in this case.

82. **Answer: B.** *Trauma and Burns/Trauma/Acute Subdural Hematoma.* This patient is most likely suffering from an acute subdural hematoma. After securing an airway and stabilizing circulation, the most important next step in head trauma is emergent noncontrast CT scanning of the head. This will establish the diagnosis of an acute subdural hematoma and will often show a hyperdense, crescent-shaped mass between the skull and the surface of the cerebral hemisphere. The hematoma may push on the brain and cause herniation or other mass effects, as evidenced by this patient's fixed and dilated pupil. Treatment will involve a neurosurgical consultation with surgical decompression.

    A. Prior to emergent decompression, medical therapy may be initiated to reduce intracranial pressure. One approach is using osmotic diuretics such as mannitol. It is not indicated for long-term use.

    C. Hyperventilation, not hypoventilation, may be used to decrease intracranial pressure. It works by decreasing cerebral blood flow.

    D. MRI is less useful than CT imaging in acute subdural hematoma due to the time it takes to obtain the study and the lack of equipment in the suites for emergent resuscitation.

    E. Although a neurosurgical consult followed by emergent craniotomy is the correct treatment of an acute subdural hematoma, the diagnosis should be first established with CT imaging.

83. Answer: E. *Trauma and Burns/Trauma/Neck Injury.* This patient has a penetrating injury to zone 2 of his neck, which contains many vital structures. Patients who are exsanguinating from a zone 2 neck wound, have a stroke, or have evidence of an expanding hematoma should have immediate exploration of the neck to control the bleeding. Neck wounds with an expanding hematoma in zones 1 or 3 of the neck can sometimes be initially imaged with emergent angiography or CT angiography, although they may also require immediate surgical exploration.

A. Admission and observation in critical care area may be needed after surgery but is not the next best step in management of this patient.

B. Angiography is the gold standard for evaluating stable patients with penetrating wounds to zones 1 and 3 of the neck.

C. Direct laryngoscopy might be indicated in this case because the patient may have an airway injury. However, this patient's airway has now been secured with intubation, and the possible major vessel injury in the neck should be addressed now.

D. Removal of objects protruding from the neck should not be done in the emergency department. It is possible that the knife is currently preventing significant blood exsanguination. The knife may be carefully removed in the operating room during surgical exploration.

84. Answer: E. *Trauma and Burns/Trauma/Spinal Injuries.* Most trauma patients are suspected of having cervical spinal injury until proven otherwise. Cervical trauma often occurs from hyperflexion, hyperextension, vertical compression, or lateral rotation of the neck during an injury. It is possible that this patient injured his neck, and he should be checked for signs of spinal injury. Examination involves assessing midline tenderness, sensation, motor function reflexes, and performing a rectal exam. Exam findings that suggest spinal injury include pain with movement, tenderness, gaps or steps in the spine, edema or bruising over the spine, or spasm of associated muscles. Patients without these symptoms can be cleared, assuming other risk factors (such as increased age, mechanism of injury, falls greater than 1 m, axial loads on the spine, high speed, or dramatic injuries) are not present.

A. Mild bruising over the left temple does not necessarily indicate neck or back trauma.

B. Patients who are intoxicated should have imaging to assess the cervical spine. A history of alcohol abuse does not necessarily mean the patient is intoxicated.

C. This patient sustained a knee injury; thus, impaired function of his right knee might be expected. This is not a contraindication to clearing the cervical spine without additional imaging.

D. Normal sensation and reflexes would imply an intact spinal cord.

85. Answer: D. *Trauma and Burns/Trauma/Abdominal Injury.* This patient has an obvious penetrating injury to the abdomen with evisceration. She is stable, but the abdomen needs to be surgically explored and any injuries, if found, repaired. Other imaging modalities will most likely not be helpful in this case and may only serve to delay care.

A. Abdominal ultrasound imaging is not necessary in this case because the injury is apparent and it would only serve to further delay care.

B. CT imaging of the abdomen is not necessary for the same reason as in A.

C. Diagnostic peritoneal lavage is most useful in the case of questionable abdominal bleeding in an unstable patient. It would not be helpful in this case.

E. Some trauma centers have advocated immediate reduction with closure of the defect with evisceration because many laparotomies are found to be negative for additional injury. However, recent studies have shown prompt operative intervention to be the best management. An exception might be applied to a select few patients with only omentum evisceration and benign abdominal findings.

86. Answer: A. *Hematologic Diseases and Neoplasms/Pathology/Anemia of Chronic Disease.* This patient is most likely suffering from anemia of chronic disease secondary to her Crohn disease. Anemia of chronic disease is most often a normocytic normochromic anemia and may result from any chronic inflammatory condition as a response to inflammatory cytokines. In more severe cases, the anemia of chronic disease may be microcytic. Iron studies will show a low serum iron and a low total iron-binding capacity. Ferritin may be elevated because it is an acute phase reactant. Treatment for anemia of chronic disease is to treat the underlying condition. In some more severe cases, transfusions or erythropoietin can be helpful.

B. Decreased total iron-binding capacity and increased serum iron could be seen in iron overload conditions such as hemochromatosis.

C. Howell-Jolly bodies are basophilic nuclear remnants found in erythrocytes. These inclusions are normally removed by the spleen and can be seen in patients with asplenia or a hypofunctioning spleen.

D. Increased total iron-binding capacity and decreased serum iron is found in iron deficiency anemia.

E. Large red blood cells on a peripheral smear indicate a macrocytic anemia, of which folate and vitamin B12 deficiency should come to mind. This patient's MCV is within normal limits, and the presentation is not consistent with a macrocytic anemia.

87. **Answer: C.** *Hematologic Diseases and Neoplasms/Pathology/Iron Deficiency Anemia.* The most likely cause of this patient's fatigue, malaise, and conjunctival pallor is anemia. Women with heavy and irregular periods who are not taking iron supplements are predisposed to becoming deficient in iron. Iron deficiency anemia is characterized by an increase in total iron-binding capacity, decreased ferritin, and decreased serum iron. Treatment for this patient would include iron supplements.

   A. Anemia of chronic disease is often caused by a chronic inflammatory condition. This patient is young and has no history of other medical problems. A history of heavy menstrual bleeding is more consistent with iron deficiency anemia.

   B. Folate deficiency will cause a macrocytic anemia and is caused by a lack of folate in the diet. Folate can be found in fruits and vegetables. A history of heavy menstrual bleeding is more likely to be the cause of this patient's anemia.

   D. Symptoms of vitamin B_6 deficiency may include dermatitis, atrophic glossitis, angular cheilitis, somnolence, and neuropathy. Anemia is generally not a feature.

   E. Vitamin B_{12} deficiency results in a macrocytic anemia. Symptoms may include anemia along with neurologic problems. This patient's presentation is more consistent with iron deficiency.

88. **Answer: C.** *Hematologic Diseases and Neoplasms/Immunology/Pernicious Anemia.* This patient has a macrocytic anemia. The differential for macrocytic anemias includes vitamin B12 or folate deficiency, alcoholism, rapid red cell turnover, and myelodysplastic syndrome. Of these, the most consistent with this patient's presentation is vitamin B12 or folate deficiency. Her associated symptoms of vitiligo suggest an autoimmune etiology; thus, pernicious anemia is the most likely diagnosis. Pernicious anemia is caused by autoimmune atrophic gastritis in which antibodies against gastric parietal cells or intrinsic factor are produced. Serum B_{12} and anti-intrinsic or parietal cell antibody studies can confirm the diagnosis.

   A. Adenocarcinoma of the colon could potentially cause a macrocytic anemia if the terminal ileum was involved but usually is characterized by an iron deficiency anemia from chronic blood loss. This patient's vitiligo suggests an autoimmune etiology.

   B. Excessive alcohol consumption can cause a megaloblastic anemia, but elevated liver enzymes or a history of greater alcohol use would be present.

   D. Lack of dietary folate is a common cause of macrocytic anemia. Folate is found abundantly in foods such as green leafy vegetables. Stores can be depleted after several months. This patient's vitiligo and well-balanced diet point away from this etiology.

   E. Lack of dietary vitamin B_{12} is most likely not the cause of this patient's anemia because her diet is well balanced. This patient's presentation is more consistent with a lack of vitamin B_{12} absorption due to an autoimmune process.

89. **Answer: E.** *Hematologic Diseases and Neoplasms/Pathology/Paroxysmal Nocturnal Hemoglobinuria.* This patient is presenting with a normocytic anemia from chronic hemolysis, pancytopenia, episodes of hemoglobinuria, and abdominal pain. This is highly suggestive of paroxysmal nocturnal hemoglobinuria. In this disease, there is a deficiency of anchor proteins that link complement-inactivating proteins to red blood cell membranes. This in turn causes increased complement-mediated lysis of red blood cells, white blood cells, and platelets. Patients with paroxysmal nocturnal hemoglobinuria have an increased tendency for venous thrombosis, such as Budd-Chiari syndrome and renal vein thrombosis. Unfortunately, paroxysmal nocturnal hemoglobinuria may evolve into aplastic anemia, myelodysplasia, myelofibrosis, or leukemia.

   A. Autoimmune hemolytic anemia is also characterized by hemolysis, but pancytopenia is generally not a feature.

   B. Hemolysis is generally not a feature of chronic myelogenous leukemia.

   C. Glucose-6-phosphate dehydrogenase deficiency may present with hemolysis, but pancytopenia is not a feature.

   D. Immune thrombocytopenic purpura usually presents with easy bruising and bleeding. It would show a decreased platelet count, but the other findings in this patient would not be present.

90. **Answer: A.** *Hematologic Diseases and Neoplasms/Pathology/Disseminated Intravascular Coagulation.* This patient is most likely in disseminated intravascular coagulation. Disseminated intravascular coagulation is caused by an abnormal activation of the complement cascade that results in consumption of platelets, fibrin, and other coagulation factors and resulting microthrombi throughout circulation. Simultaneously, hemorrhage occurs as a result of fibrinolytic activation. Laboratory studies will show increased prothrombin time, partial thromboplastin time, and bleeding time. Fibrin split products will also be increased. Infection is a major cause of disseminated intravascular coagulation, especially sepsis from gram-negative organisms.

   B. Hemolytic uremic syndrome is a thrombotic microangiopathy that most often occurs in children. It is characterized by hemolytic anemia, acute kidney failure, and a low platelet count. It is usually preceded by an infectious diarrhea, most commonly *E. coli* O157:H7.

   C. Immune thrombocytopenic purpura usually presents with easy bruising and bleeding. It would show a decreased platelet count. Increased fibrin split products would not be present.

   D. Rebleeding at the operative site would generally not present with oozing from intravenous sites. An abdominal drain would most likely show bloody drainage.

   E. Thrombotic thrombocytopenic purpura (TTP) presents with neurologic changes, acute renal failure, thrombocytopenia, hemolytic anemia, and fever. This patient's presentation is more consistent with disseminated intravascular coagulation.

91. **Answer: A.** *Reproductive System/Pathology/Uterine Prolapse.* A common result of normal aging is the increased laxity of the broad round ovarian and cardinal ligaments, usually combined with loss of tone in myofascial structures such as the urogenital diaphragm. This results in uterine prolapse into the vagina, most commonly presenting as dysuria. A tear in the diaphragm can also cause uterine prolapse but is less common and is usually accompanied by symptoms of incontinence.

  B. Endometrial hyperplasia occurs due to unopposed estrogen effects on the endometrium lining the uterus. This increases the patients' risks for endometrial cancer.

  C. Fecal impaction of the sigmoid colon would not lead to uterine prolapse.

  D. Nulliparity has been associated with an increased risk of breast cancer.

  E. A tear in the urogenital diaphragm could cause bladder prolapse.

92. **Answer: A.** *Reproductive System/Pathology/Endodermal Sinus Tumor.* This child has an endodermal sinus (yolk sac) tumor. This is a malignant germ cell tumor that has its peak incidence in infancy and early childhood; it is the most common testicular tumor in this age group. It is analogous to endodermal sinus tumor of the ovary and causes an increase in serum alpha-fetoprotein, which is also associated with hepatocellular carcinoma.

  B. High levels of FSH are seen with gonadotrophic pituitary adenomas.

  C. High levels of hCG is associated with seminomas.

  D. High levels of LH are seen with gonadotrophic pituitary adenomas.

  E. Thyrotrophic pituitary adenomas will secrete high levels of TSH.

93. **Answer: C.** *Reproductive System/Anatomy/Lymphatics.* Lymph from the lower 25% of the vagina (below the hymen) drains downward to the perineum, where it is received by the superficial inguinal lymph nodes. The upper three-quarters of the vagina, on the other hand, drains upward to the internal iliac nodes. Since the fornix lies adjacent to the cervix, it is classified as lying within the upper three-quarters of the vagina.

  A. This deep inguinal nodes receive lymphatics after the superficial nodes.

  B. The external iliac nodes receive lymphatics after the superficial and deep nodes.

  D. This answer is incorrect.

  E. This answer is incorrect.

94. **Answer: B.** *Reproductive System/Interdisciplinary Topics/Immature Teratoma.* Immature teratoma is usually a malignant tumor in females, as opposed to mature teratoma, which is usually benign. This is, however, reversed for males, in whom mature teratomas are more likely to be malignant.

  A. Adenomyosis is a benign extension of endometrial glands and stroma into the myometrium, most often causing uterine enlargement.

  C. Human papillomavirus (HPV) type II is a benign strain of HPV.

  D. Leiomyomas, or fibroids, are extremely common benign tumors of the uterus. They may very rarely transform into leiomyosarcomas.

  E. Mature teratomas in females are commonly benign

95. **Answer: B.** *Reproductive System/Interdisciplinary Topics/Breast Cancer.* The presence of bilateral cancerous lesions, especially in such a young woman, is highly suggestive of a germline mutation. Of those listed, a derangement of the p53 allele is most highly correlated with the development of breast cancer. Genes implicated in the development of breast cancer include BRCA-1, BRCA-2, and p53.

  A. The c-erb allele is a growth factor receptor gene and is upregulated in some breast cancers.

  C. The mutated Rb allele is associated with retinoblastoma.

  D. The CCG trinucleotide repeat has not been implicated in the pathogenesis of breast cancers.

  E. The loss of an enzyme in the excision repair system has not been implicated in the pathogenesis of breast cancers.

96. **Answer: D.** *Reproductive System/Pathology/Leiomyomas.* Leiomyomas, otherwise known as fibroids, are the most common benign tumors of the uterus. They are also commonly estrogen responsive, causing them to enlarge in a cyclic pattern. When they are severe, they may cause mass effects in the abdomen, such as bloating.

  A. Adenomyosis also commonly causes uterine enlargement, but this is usually bilateral and non-nodular.

  B. The same is true for endometrial hyperplasia, which also rarely reaches the size of leiomyomas or adenomyosis.

  C. Endometriosis can result in chocolate cysts, but these rarely reach the size needed to cause mass effects.

  E. A molar pregnancy could also result in an asymmetric abdominal mass, but in this case, the pregnancy test would have been positive.

97. Answer: B. *Reproductive System/Pathology/Adrenogenital Syndrome.* This question is a little tricky because the mother has the misconception that her child is male. The presence of ovaries in the absence of testicles, however, is definitive of the female gender. The child is therefore referred to as a female pseudohermaphrodite. The most common cause of this is the adrenogenital syndrome. It results from the body's inability to hydroxylate 17-hydroxyprogesterone adequately, leading to decreased or absent levels of 11-deoxycortisol.

   A. There is consequent congenital adrenal hyperplasia, decreased levels of cortisol, increased levels of ACTH, and increased production of androgens. Therefore, these females are 46XX and have ovaries, but their external genitalia are masculinized.

   C. The lack of receptors for dihydrotestosterone is seen in androgen insensitivity syndrome.

   D. The XO karyotype is defined as Turner syndrome and the gender is female, although the ovaries are fibrous streaks.

   E. Point mutations in the SRY gene and adrenal hypofunction are both variable according to the severity of the lesion; however, neither represent the most common cause of female pseudohermaphroditism.

98. Answer: A. *Infectious Diseases/Microbiology/Mechanism of Bacterial Overgrowth.* Antibiotic therapy can reduce normal flora in the bowel, allowing pathogenic organisms normally present in low numbers to overgrow. Patients with antibiotic-induced diarrhea usually are on antibiotics for a chronic period of time. Symptoms can include diarrhea and lower quadrant abdominal pain. Stool cultures can be positive for clostridium difficile.

   B. Botulinum toxin food poisoning will not cause overgrowth of *Clostridium difficile*.

   C. Compromised immune system will not cause overgrowth of *Clostridium difficile*.

   D. Gastric ulcer will not cause overgrowth of *Clostridium difficile*.

   E. Mechanical obstruction of the left colon will not cause overgrowth of *Clostridium difficile*.

99. Answer: A. *Infectious Diseases/Microbiology/Mechanism of Bacterial Invasion.* Invasive bacteria are those that can enter host cells or penetrate mucosal surfaces, spreading from the initial site of infection. *Streptococcus pyogenes* produce several toxins, including C5a peptidase, which inactivates complement component C5a. Streptolysin O and S are also produced, which damage mammalian cells, resulting in cell lysis and release of lysosomal enzymes.

   B. Hyaluronidase is an enzyme that can degrade components of the extracellular matrix to allow bacteria easier access to host cells.

   C. Elastase breaks down elastin. It has a limited role in *facilitating* bacterial entry into cells.

   D. Telomerase breaks down ends of chromosomes, which may facilitate cell death.

   E. Urokinase facilitates breakdown of blood and blood products.

100. Answer: D. For patients with recurrent cancer, using a different chemotherapeutic agent than was used initially is often favored. This is due to the fact that cancer cells can become resistant to chemotherapy drugs to which they are exposed. In this patient's case, paclitaxel (a microtubule inhibitor) was used during her initial treatment. The physician chose to use irinotecan, an agent that inhibits topoisomerase, this time in hopes to avoid any resistance the cancer cells may have to microtubule inhibitors.

   A. Cisplatin is a DNA-binding agent that forms cross-links in DNA strands. It does not interfere with topoisomerase.

   B. Docetaxel and paclitaxel are taxanes, which inhibit microtubule depolymerization. They do not interfere with topoisomerase.

   C. Erlotinib inhibits cell proliferation by blocking the epidermal growth factor receptor. It does not interfere with topoisomerase.

   E. Vincristine destabilizes microtubules, inhibiting normal cell cycle progression. It does not interfere with topoisomerase.

Page numbers followed by *f*, *t*, and *b* indicate figures, tables, and boxed material, respectively.